THE COMPLETE MEDICINE BOOK

By Thomas A. Gossel, R.Ph., Ph.D.
and Donald W. Stansloski, R.Ph., Ph.D
with John A. Kramer, M.D. as medical consultant
And By The Editors of CONSUMER GUIDE®

Manufactured in the United States of America
1 2 3 4 5 6 7 8 9 10

Library of Congress Catalog Card Number: 80-81315
ISBN: 0-671-25501-0

Cover Design: Frank E. Peiler

*Note: Neither the authors nor the publisher take responsibility for any possible conse-
quences from any treatment, action, or application of medication or preparation by any
person reading or following the information in this book. The publication of this book
does not constitute the practice of medicine, and this book does not attempt to
replace your physician or your pharmacist. The authors and publisher advise the
reader to check with a physician before administering or consuming any medication or
using any health care device.*

Contents

PART III: DRUG PROFILES 293

More than 1,000 of the most commonly used prescription
and nonprescription medications are profiled.
Arranged alphabetically for easy reference, these profiles
tell you about possible adverse reactions and drug
interactions, how to take the drug to achieve maximum
benefit, and what to do should you experience certain
side effects.

PART IV: HEALTH CARE ACCESSORIES 630

In this overview of what's available in the typical well-
stocked pharmacy, you'll learn about the latest in heating
pads, fever thermometers, and blood pressure kits, as

well as how to choose the essentials for your medicine cabinet.

Introduction

More and more people want to participate in their own health care; they want to be able to make decisions that affect their treatment. *The Complete Medicine Book* is intended to help you make those decisions. It combines information on over 1,200 drug products—both prescription and over-the-counter—with descriptions of over 300 common medical problems and their treatment. Furthermore, it includes a buying guide of the health care accessories (fever thermometers, heating pads, foot care products, blood pressure kits) available in every pharmacy.

The Complete Medicine Book encourages the consumer to take an active role in health care. Part I tells you how and why you should be keeping health records, what you should do in case of drug overdose, and what to keep in the home medicine cabinet. For your own safety, you should learn how to read prescriptions, and *The Complete Medicine Book* includes an easy-to-use chart explaining the abbreviations and symbols most commonly used on prescriptions. Using medications properly means that you get the full benefit of the drug and full value for your money. This book tells how to use most dosage forms properly, giving special instructions for individual drug products.

Part II describes hundreds of common symptoms, diseases, and conditions, and their treatment. In it you will learn about the significance of certain symptoms, the characteristic course of each disease, how long the period of contagion is for the common infectious illnesses of childhood, and how to tell when your condition merits medical attention. Each disease description is cross-referenced to the drugs and health care accessories you're likely to use in its treatment. And these cross references include recommended choices among OTC drugs. These recommendations pinpoint the basic items that are effective in relieving many ailments. You'll also learn which OTC items are a waste of money.

Part III of *The Complete Medicine Book* includes information on hundreds of the most commonly used brand-name prescription and nonprescription drugs in the form of profiles. The profiles are listed alphabetically by the name most frequently used; that is, if a prescription product is prescribed most often by its generic name, it is listed by generic name. Equivalent products are cross-referenced so that you will be able to turn immediately to the appropriate profile if your drug is not the most commonly prescribed form. These profiles concisely state what you should know before you ever swallow a pill or pour a spoonful of cough syrup. Each profile identifies the components of the product, its available dosage forms, its use, and the possible side effects and adverse reactions.

People with certain conditions should not take certain drugs—for these people the drug is contraindicated. People with other conditions should use some drugs cautiously. Each drug profile identifies the conditions in which it may be harmful or dangerous to use the drug. Possible adverse effects are also described for every drug profiled in the book, and each drug description indicates the precautions that should be taken to monitor for those adverse effects, whether those precautions include laboratory testing or simply watching for certain symptoms. Certain drugs should not be taken with other drugs; one may diminish or increase the action of the other, or in combination they may produce a toxic reaction. *The Complete Medicine Book* cautions the reader about possible drug interactions, including those that involve substances as common as aspirin and alcohol. For both prescription and over-the-counter products, it lists possible side effects and special administration instructions.

Part IV surveys the health care accessories available in the typical well-stocked pharmacy. Among the items included are some that we use every day (toothbrushes, for example) and others (such as crutches) that we may use only once or twice in a lifetime. Information on these devices is slanted for the consumer—telling what's available, what features to look for, whether a device serves its intended purpose. *The Complete Medicine Book* fills the gap, providing information on the necessities found in most home medicine cabinets and also the extras—such as foot massagers, electronic pulse-meters, digital blood pressure kits, and oral irrigating devices—that you may want to add to your collection of personal health care items. Specific items that stand out among others in their class are pinpointed and recommended.

The Complete Medicine Book also includes a comprehensive index that will guide you to information about a particular drug and the diseases for which it might be used, as well as to the specifics about health care and accessories contained in the book.

Your informed responsibility in matters of health care is essential. *The Complete Medicine Book* is not a substitute for consulting your doctor. It is a guide to your health care. Your doctor and your pharmacist are your primary health reference sources, and this book will aid you in working with these health care professionals so that you can achieve the greatest benefit from your partnership.

Part I
Your Health Care

Drugs and How They Work

A drug is any substance used to diagnose, treat, cure, or prevent a disease. Over the centuries, man has used thousands of substances as drugs. In ancient Egypt, prescribed medication included the testicles of the black ass and the eggs of the babzu bird. The dried leaf of the common foxglove has been used for hundreds of years to treat cardiovascular problems and is still in use as the drug digitalis today. In the sixteenth and seventeenth centuries, science turned to chemicals as a drug source and often employed substances now known to be toxic (lead, mercury, arsenic, copper). One can only surmise that patients who improved after receiving these chemicals had been given very small doses.

Modern drug therapy began in 1935, with the introduction of the first sulfa drug, prontosil. Before prontosil, there were no drugs to counter infections. The slightest cut or bruise might cause quick death. A chest cold that today is treated for several days with modern medicines frequently led to pneumonia and death before prontosil. As prontosil's benefits became known, interest in developing new medications spurted, and other drugs soon followed. Penicillin was developed in the early 1940s. It was soon followed by the antibiotics streptomycin, tetracycline, and chloramphenicol, as well as dozens more.

Severe disorders of the heart and blood pressure were brought under control in the 1950s with the development of hydralazine and rauwolfia. Further research on rauwolfia isolated reserpine, which, along with another new drug of the 1950s, Thorazine, almost emptied the nation's mental wards. Later that same decade, drugs that could be taken by mouth became available to treat diabetes.

The achievements in health-related discoveries and developments continued in the 1960s and 1970s. Arthritis and similar crippling diseases largely were controlled by using drugs like cortisone, Butazolidin, and, later, Indocin. Polio was conquered with the Salk vaccine. Dozens of drugs to stall the spread of cancer appeared, and, while cancer remains a major health problem, patients at least have hope for longer, more comfortable lives. Drugs to treat diseases of the heart, lungs, kidneys, and brain were introduced. Vaccines to immunize people against severe infections appeared, and as a result, one of the most dreaded diseases known to the world—smallpox—has been practically eradicated, and others have been brought under control.

The Drug Market Today

Today we have literally hundreds of thousands of drug products to choose from. There may be half a million drug products available to Americans over-the-counter, that is, without a prescription. All these products are made from fewer than 300 significantly active ingredients. The 200 most frequently used prescription drugs are available as at least 1500 different brand-name products, and most of these products are available in multiple dosage forms and strengths. To thread their way through this maze, all consumers should know certain basics about the medicines they use to treat their ailments.

Over-the-counter drugs. OTC drugs can be purchased without a doctor's prescription. They are also called proprietary medicines, nonprescription drugs, patent medicines, family medicines, or home remedies. OTC drugs are intended to be used by consumers without assistance.

Various studies have shown that fewer than 25 percent of all people who are ill are seen by doctors. This means that most of us prescribe our own treatment. And many times, we decide to treat our ailments with OTC products.

OTC products offer the consumer a wide range of medication, much of it as strong as what a doctor would prescribe if one were consulted. For example, aspirin is still the drug of choice for treating rheumatoid arthritis as well as a dozen or so other inflammatory diseases, and the antacids are the most useful of all drugs for treating pain from peptic ulcers.

Prescription (R_x) drugs. In general, prescription drugs are more potent and potentially more harmful than nonprescription medication, although drugs are designated prescription-only for a variety of reasons. Some prescription drugs are too dangerous to use without the supervision of a doctor. Others may mask certain symptoms of serious illness. Others may cause addiction or other problems if they are taken over a long period of time or by the wrong individual. Examples of such drugs include the narcotics, amphetamines (such as those in diet preparations), and a few of the sleeping medications.

Other drugs require a prescription because of the way in which they must be taken. For example, certain drugs must be injected into the body. A prescription tells the pharmacist that the doctor knows that the individual can inject the drug properly, or can have it done by someone qualified.

Generic drugs. "Generic" means not protected by trademark registration. The generic name of a drug is like a shortened form of its chemical name. For example, the chemical name of a common antibiotic is "4-dimethylamino-1,4,4a,5,5a,6,11,12a-octahydro-3,6,10,12,12a-pentahydroxy-6-methyl-l,11-dioxo-2-naphthacenecarboxamide." Tetracycline is the drug's generic name. Anyone may use this name when describing the drug or when marketing and selling it, but usually a manufacturer uses a trade name as well as a generic name for a drug. A trade name is a copyrighted name that no one else may use when marketing the product. Only Lederle Laboratories may market Achromycin brand tetracycline, and only The Upjohn Company may market Panmycin brand tetracycline.

Many consumers already know about the savings to be gained by "shopping generic." Generic products are generally priced lower than similar trademarked products, largely because they are not widely advertised. And the same type of savings can often be gained by purchasing drugs generically.

When a company develops a new drug and applies for a patent on it, it has 17 years to market the drug and regain the investment. The manufacturer can use the generic name but usually uses a trade name. As long as the patent is in effect, no other companies can legally sell the same drug regardless of whether they use the generic name or apply their own trade name.

But once a patent runs out (after 17 years) any drug manufacturer can manufacture the drug. Another company may choose to call it by its generic name or apply its own trade name. And, usually, when a drug begins to be manufactured by several companies after the original patent has run out, competition drives the price down.

Not every drug is available generically, and not every generic is significantly less expensive than its trademarked equivalent. For certain drugs, it's inadvisable to "shop around" for a generic equivalent. Although the Food and Drug Administration has stated that there is no evidence to suspect serious differences between trade-name and generic drugs, differences have been shown between brands of certain drugs, for example, the heart drug digoxin.

However, for other drugs, consumers may be able to save as much as 75 percent. One hundred capsules of Darvon Compound-65 analgesic may cost $10 to $12. One hundred capsules of the generic equivalent product may cost as little as $3, a savings of $7 to $9. Pavabid may cost $12 to $15 per 100 capsules, but if bought generically, the drug may cost as little as $5 per 100 capsules—again, a savings of $7 to $10 per prescription. And these savings do not affect only prescription drugs—Bayer aspirin, for example, costs two to three times more than the less well-known St. Joseph brand, and the generic brand carried by your pharmacy may cost even less.

In most states, consumers can now request that their pharmacist fill their prescriptions with the cheapest generic brand. If such substitution is not yet legal in your state (contact your state pharmacy association to find out), ask your doctor to prescribe drugs by generic name, thus allowing your pharmacist to dispense the least expensive generic drug.

How Drugs Work

Anyone taking a drug should know how it basically works. The more a patient knows about a drug, the more likely that she or he will comply with the doctor's directions in taking it and will recognize side effects should they occur. Following are brief definitions of many of the most widely used drug types.

adrenergic—a substance which mimics the effects of adrenalin; stimulates the part of the nervous system that controls involuntary actions such as blood vessel contraction, sweating, etc.; used in the treatment of low blood pressure, asthma, shock, and respiratory congestion
Examples: Actifed; Ornade

amphetamine—a substance that acts as a central nervous system stimulant; increases blood pressure, reduces appetite, and reduces nasal congestion; used as an anorectic and to treat hyperkinesis

analgesic—having pain-relieving properties; a pain-relieving substance; may be narcotic
Examples: aspirin; Darvon; Demerol

anesthetic—causing loss of feeling and sensation; a substance that causes loss of feeling and sensation

anorectic—a substance that decreases the appetite; usually a sympathomimetic amine
Examples: Fastin; Ionamin

antacid—a drug that neutralizes excess acidity, usually of the stomach; most frequently used to relieve gastrointestinal distress and to treat peptic ulcers
Examples: Gelusil; Maalox

anthelmintic—an anti-infective used to kill worms infecting the body
Example: Povan

antianginal—a substance used to relieve or prevent the chest pain known as angina; causes a sudden drop in blood pressure

12

Examples: Isordil; nitroglycerin

antiarrhythmic—a drug that improves abnormal heart rhythms
Example: quinidine sulfate

antibacterial—a drug that destroys or prevents the growth of certain bacteria
Example: Gantrisin

antibiotic—a drug that destroys or prevents the growth of certain bacteria
Examples: ampicillin; penicillin; tetracycline

anticholinergic—a drug that blocks the passage of certain nerve impulses; frequently used to treat peptic ulcer and diarrhea, and as an antiemetic
Examples: atropine; Pro-Banthine

anticoagulant—"blood-thinner"; a substance that slows the clotting of blood
Example: Coumadin

anticonvulsant—a substance used to treat or prevent seizures or convulsions
Example: Dilantin

antidepressant—a substance used to treat symptoms of depression; drugs currently used as antidepressants are generally tricyclic antidepressants, monoamine oxidase inhibitors, and amphetamines
Examples: Elavil; Tofranil

antidiabetic—a drug used to treat diabetes mellitus
Examples: insulin; Orinase

antidiarrheal—a drug used to treat diarrhea; may act by absorbing fluid in the bowel or by slowing the action of the bowel
Example: Lomotil

antidote—a substance that counteracts the effects of an ingested poison

antiemetic—a drug used for symptomatic control of vomiting
Example: Compazine

antiflatulent—a drug that reduces gas in the gastrointestinal tract
Example: Mylicon

antifungal—a drug that destroys and prevents the growth and reproduction of fungi
Example: Mycostatin

antihistamine—a drug used to relieve the symptoms of an allergy; works by blocking the effects of histamine
Examples: brompheniramine maleate; chlorpheniramine maleate; Dimetapp

antihypertensive—a drug that counteracts or reduces high blood pressure
Examples: Apresoline; reserpine

anti-infective—a drug used to treat an infection; included among the anti-infectives are antibiotics, sulfonamides, and antifungals

anti-inflammatory—a substance that counteracts or suppresses inflammation

Examples: aspirin; Butazolidin

antinauseant—a drug used to relieve nausea; most work by blocking the transmission of nerve impulses that stimulate vomiting
Examples: Bendectin; Compazine

antispasmodic—a drug that relieves spasms (violent, involuntary muscular contractions or sudden constrictions of a passage or canal); antispasmodics are typically used to treat dysfunctions of the gastrointestinal tract, the gallbladder, or the urinary system
Examples: atropine sulfate; Bentyl

antitussive—a drug used to relieve coughing; may be narcotic
Examples: codeine (narcotic); dextromethorphan (non-narcotic)

barbiturates—a class of drugs used as sedatives or hypnotics; can be addictive
Example: phenobarbital

beta blocker—an adrenergic used to slow the heart rate and reduce blood pressure
Example: Inderal

bronchodilator—a drug used to help breathing; works by relaxing bronchial muscles which expands the air passages of the lungs
Example: aminophylline

cathartic—a substance that causes evacuation of the bowel; for all purposes, the same as a laxative

central nervous system depressant—a drug that acts on the brain to decrease alertness and concentration
Examples: barbiturates; codeine; morphine; all hypnotics and sedatives

contraceptive—an agent used to prevent conception or diminish its likelihood

cough suppressant—a drug that suppresses the impulse to cough

decongestant—a drug that relieves congestion in the upper respiratory system; a decongestant product may be composed of a sympathomimetic amine, or it may combine a sympathomimetic amine with an antihistamine
Examples: ephedrine; phenylephrine; phenylpropanolamine

digitalis drug—a drug used to improve heart rhythm or increase the output of the heart in heart failure; slows the heart rate and increases the force of contraction
Example: Lanoxin

diuretic—a drug that affects the kidneys to cause an increase in urine flow; also called water pills
Example: Aldactone; Diuril; Lasix

emetic—a substance that causes vomiting
Example: ipecac syrup

expectorant—a drug used to increase the secretion of mucus in the

respiratory system, thus making it easier to "bring up" phlegm from the lungs; in a cough remedy, an expectorant promotes a productive cough
Example: guaifenesin

hormone—a chemical substance produced by glands in the body; regulates the action of certain organs
Examples: insulin; thyroid

hypnotic—a drug that is used to induce sleep
Examples: Nembutal; phenobarbital; Quaalude

keratolytic—an agent that softens the skin and causes the cells of the outer layer of the skin to slough off

laxative—a substance that causes evacuation of the bowel; for all purposes, the same as a cathartic

monoamine oxidase (MAO) inhibitor—a drug used to treat severe depression; acts by inhibiting the enzyme monoamine oxidase

narcotic—an addictive drug derived from the opium poppy; used to relieve pain and/or coughing
Examples: codeine; morphine

pediculocide—a preparation used to treat a person infested with lice
Example: Kwell

phenothiazine—a drug used to relieve anxiety and as an antinauseant
Examples: Compazine; Thorazine

salicylates—a class of drugs prepared from the salts of salicylic acid; the most commonly used pain relievers in the U.S.
Example: aspirin

scabicide—a preparation used to treat a person infested with scabies
Example: Kwell

sedative—a drug given to reduce nervousness and promote calm, thereby inducing sleep
Examples: Librium; phenobarbital

smooth muscle relaxant—a drug that causes the relaxation of smooth muscle tissue (i.e., muscle tissue such as that in the lungs, stomach, and bladder that performs functions not under voluntary control)
Examples: papaverine hydrochloride; theophylline

steroid—any one of a group of compounds secreted primarily by the adrenal glands; often used to treat allergic reactions and skin irritations
Examples: Aristocort; prednisone

sulfa drug—an antibacterial drug belonging to the chemical group of sulfonamides
Example: Gantrisin

sympathomimetic amine—a drug that raises blood pressure, acts as a decongestant, improves air passage into the lungs, and decreases the appetite

Examples: amphetamines; ephedrine; epinephrine

thyroid preparation—drug used to correct thyroid hormone deficiency; may be natural or synthetic; affects the biochemical activity of all body tissues and increases the rate of cellular metabolism
Examples: Synthroid; thyroid hormone

tranquilizer—a drug that calms part of the brain without affecting clarity of mind or consciousness when taken in normal doses
Examples: Librium; Valium

tricyclic antidepressant—a drug used to suppress symptoms of depression; differing slightly in chemical structure from the phenothiazines
Example: Tofranil

uricosuric—a drug that promotes the excretion of uric acid in the urine; used to prevent gout attacks
Example: Benemid

vaccine—a medication containing weakened or killed germs; stimulates the body to develop an immunity to those germs

vasoconstrictor—a drug that constricts blood vessels, thereby increasing blood pressure and decreasing blood flow

vasodilator—a drug that expands blood vessels to increase blood flow
Examples: Cyclospasmol, Vasodilan

vitamin—a chemical present in foods that is vital to normal body functions

Side Effects and Adverse Reactions

Drugs have certain desirable effects—that's why they are taken. The desirable effects of a drug are known as the drug's activity or therapeutic effect. Most drugs, however, have undesirable effects as well. Undesirable effects are called side effects, adverse reactions, or, in some cases, lethal effects. A side effect is any undesirable effect of a drug—even a minor one that is not dangerous. An adverse reaction is serious and may outweigh the desirable effects of the drug. A toxic or lethal effect is one capable of causing death. Often, the terms "side effect" and "adverse reaction" are used interchangeably. They have different meanings, however. Although all adverse reactions are side effects, not all side effects are adverse reactions.

Some side effects are expected and unavoidable, but others may surprise the doctor as well as the patient. Unexpected reactions may be due to a person's individual response to the drug.

Side effects may fall into one of two major groups—those that are obvious and those that are subtle and cannot be detected without laboratory testing. The discussion of a drug should not be restricted to its easily recognized side effects; other, less obvious, side effects may also be harmful.

If you know a particular side effect is expected from a particular drug, you can relax a little. Most expected side effects are temporary and need not cause alarm. You'll merely experience discomfort or inconvenience for a short time. For example, you may be drowsy after taking an antihistamine or have a stuffy nose after taking reserpine or certain other drugs that lower blood pressure. Of course, if you find minor side effects especially bothersome, you should discuss them with your doctor who may be able to prescribe another drug, or at least assure you that the benefits of the drug far outweigh its side effects. Sometimes side effects can be minimized or eliminated by changing your dosage schedule or taking the drug with meals. Consult your doctor or pharmacist before making such a change.

Many side effects, however, signal a serious—perhaps dangerous—problem. And when these side effects appear, you should consult your doctor immediately. The following discussion should help you determine whether your side effects require attention from your physician.

Obvious Side Effects

Certain organs and body systems are commonly associated with symptoms of an adverse reaction. And if you are alert, you may discover the first indications of an adverse reaction.

Ear. Although a few drugs may cause loss of hearing if taken in large quantities, hearing loss is uncommon. Drugs that are used to treat problems of the ear may cause dizziness, and many drugs produce tinnitus, a sensation of ringing, buzzing, thumping, or hollowness in the ear. Discuss with your doctor any problem with your hearing or your ears if it persists for more than three days.

Eye. Blurred vision is a common side effect. Drugs such as digitalis may cause the patient to see a "halo" around a lighted object (a television screen or a traffic light), and other drugs may cause night blindness. Indocin anti-inflammatory (used in the treatment of arthritis) may cause blindness. Atropine and Librax sedative may make it difficult to accurately judge distance while driving and may make the eyes sensitive to sunlight. While the effects on the eye caused by digitalis and Indocin are dangerous signs of toxicity, the effects caused by atropine and Librax are to be expected. In any case, if you have difficulty seeing while taking drugs, contact your doctor.

Gastrointestinal system. A side effect affecting the gastrointestinal system can be expected from almost any drug. Many drugs produce dry mouth, mouth sores, difficulty in swallowing, heartburn, nausea, vomiting, diarrhea, constipation, loss of appetite, or abnormal cramping. Other drugs cause bloating and gas, and some cause rectal itching.

Diarrhea can be expected after taking many drugs, and in most cases, the diarrhea is temporary and self-limiting. But diarrhea may signal a problem. For example, Cleocin antibiotic may cause severe diarrhea, leading to intestinal ulceration and bleeding. If you develop severe diarrhea while taking Cleocin, or any other drug, or if diarrhea lasts more than three days, call your doctor. During the three days, do not take any antidiarrheal medication. Be sure to drink liquids to replace the fluid you are losing.

As a side effect of drug use, constipation is less serious than diarrhea and is more frequent. It occurs when a drug slows down the activity of the bowel. Drugs such as atropine and Pro-Banthine anticholinergic slow down bowel activity, and the constipation they produce lasts a few days to a week. Other drugs absorb moisture in the bowel, causing constipation. And constipation may occur if a drug—for example, Aldomet antihypertensive—acts on the nervous system and decreases nerve impulses to the intestine. Constipation produced by a drug may last several days, and you can help relieve it by drinking at least eight glasses of water a day. If constipation continues, call your doctor.

Heart and circulatory system. Drugs may speed up or slow down the heartbeat. If a drug slows the heartbeat, you may feel drowsy and tired or even dizzy. If a drug accelerates the heartbeat, you probably will experience palpitations (thumping in the chest). You may feel as though your heart is skipping a beat occasionally, and you may have a headache. For most people, none of these symptoms indicates a serious problem. If, however, they bother you, consult your doctor who may adjust the dosage of the drug or prescribe other medication.

Some drugs cause edema (fluid retention). When edema occurs, fluid from the blood collects outside the blood vessels. Ordinarily, edema is not serious. But if you are steadily gaining weight or have gained more than two or three pounds in a week, talk to your doctor.

Drugs may increase or decrease blood pressure. When blood pressure decreases, you may feel drowsy and tired. Or, you may become dizzy and even faint, especially when you rise from a reclining position. When blood pressure increases, you may feel dizzy, have a headache or blurred vision, or hear ringing or buzzing in your ears. If you develop any of these symptoms, call your doctor.

Nervous system. Drugs that act on the nervous system may cause drowsiness or stimulation. If the drug causes drowsiness, you may become dizzy, or your coordination may be impaired. If a drug causes stimulation, you may become nervous or have insomnia or tremors. Neither drowsiness nor stimulation is cause for concern for most people. When you are drowsy, however, you should be careful around machinery and avoid driving. Some drugs cause throbbing headaches, and others produce tingling in the fingers or toes. These symptoms are expected and should disappear in a few days or a week.

Respiratory system. Side effects common to the respiratory system include stuffy nose, dry throat, shortness of breath, and slowed breathing. A stuffy nose and dry throat usually disappear within days, and you may use nose drops or throat lozenges or gargle with warm salt water to relieve them. Shortness of breath is a characteristic side effect of some drugs (for example, Inderal antiarrhythmic). Shortness of breath may persist, but it is not usually serious. Barbiturates or drugs that promote sleep retard respiration. Slowed breathing is expected, and you should not be concerned as long as your doctor knows about it.

Skin. Skin reactions include rash, swelling, itching, and sweating. Itching, swelling, and rash frequently indicate a drug allergy, and you should not continue to take a drug if you have developed an allergy to it. Some drugs increase sweating; others decrease it. Drugs that decrease sweating may cause problems in hot weather when the body must sweat to reduce body temperature.

Another type of skin reaction that requires consultation with your doctor is photosensitivity (or phototoxicity or sun toxicity)—that is, unusual sensitivity to the sun. Tetracyclines, such as Declomycin antibiotic, can cause photosensitivity. If, after taking such a drug, you remain exposed to the sun for a brief period of time, say 10 or 15 minutes, you may receive a severe sunburn. You do not have to stay indoors while taking these drugs, but you should be fully clothed while outside, and you should not remain in the sun too long. Since these drugs may be present in the bloodstream after you stop taking them, you should continue to take these precautions for two days.

If you have a minor skin reaction that does not indicate an allergy or photosensitivity, ask your pharmacist for a soothing cream. He may also suggest that you take frequent baths and dust the area with a suitable powder.

Subtle Side Effects

Some side effects are difficult to detect. You may not notice any symptoms at all or you may only notice slight ones. And laboratory testing may be necessary to confirm the existence of a side effect or adverse drug reaction.

Blood. A great many drugs affect the blood and the circulatory system but do not produce symptoms for some time. If a drug lowers the level of sugar in the blood, for example, you probably will not have any symptoms for several minutes to an hour. If symptoms develop, they may include tiredness, muscular weakness, and perhaps palpitations or tinnitus. Low blood levels of potassium produce similar symptoms.

Some drugs decrease the number of red blood cells, which carry oxygen and nutrients throughout the body. If you have too few red blood cells, you have anemia, and you may be pale and feel tired, weak and perhaps hungry.

Some drugs decrease the number of white blood cells, which combat bacteria. Having too few white blood cells increases susceptibility to infection and may prolong illness. If a sore throat or a fever begins after you begin taking a drug and continues for a few days, you may have an infection and too few white blood cells to fight it.

Kidney. If a drug reduces the kidney's ability to remove chemicals and other substances from the blood, they begin to collect. Over a period of time, this buildup may cause vague symptoms such as edema, nausea, headache, or weakness. Obvious symptoms, especially pain, are rare.

Liver. Drug-induced liver damage may result in fat accumulation. Often, liver damage occurs because the drug increases or decreases the liver's ability to metabolize other drugs and substances.   Liver damage may be quite advanced before it produces any symptoms.

COMMON MINOR SIDE EFFECTS

Side effect	Management
Blurred vision	Avoid operating machinery
Decreased sweating	Avoid work or exercise in the sun
Diarrhea	Drink lots of water; if diarrhea lasts longer than 3 days, call your doctor
Dizziness	Avoid operating machinery
Drowsiness	Avoid operating machinery
Dry mouth	Suck on candy or ice chips, or chew gum
Dry nose and throat	Use a humidifier or vaporizer
Fluid retention	Avoid adding salt to foods
Headache	Remain quiet; take aspirin or acetaminophen
Insomnia	Take last dose of the drug earlier in the day; drink a glass of warm milk at bedtime; ask your doctor about an exercise program
Itching	Take frequent baths or showers
Nasal congestion	If necessary, use nose drops
Palpitations (mild)	Rest often; avoid tension; do not drink coffee, tea, or cola; stop smoking
Potassium loss	Eat a banana or dried fruit such as apricots or figs, or drink a glass of orange juice every day
Upset stomach	Take the drug with milk or food

Psychological changes. Drugs not intended to affect the nervous system often cause psychological changes. For example, women taking oral contraceptives often become depressed, yet oral contraceptives do not act on the brain.

Other Types of Drug Reactions

Superinfection. Superinfection occurs when a drug such as an antibiotic or sulfa drug kills or inhibits the growth of some bacteria needed by the body while others flourish.

The body needs bacteria to digest food, to synthesize vitamins, and to carry out other vital functions. Infecting bacteria are also present in the body, but usually they are held in check by other bacteria and by the body's defense system. As long as the infecting bacteria must compete with the other bacteria, the body maintains a system of checks and balances.

When you take an antibiotic or a sulfa drug, it begins to attack some kinds of infecting bacteria. After several doses, the drug may also attack the bacteria the body needs. Other infecting organisms may multiply (even in the presence of the drug) and cause symptoms. The most common symptoms of superinfection in the gastrointestinal tract are diarrhea, sores in the mouth, and rectal itching. If the superinfection is located in the lungs, you may develop a cough. If it is located in the kidneys or urinary tract, you may urinate more frequently and notice itching and pain.

Superinfection usually poses no problem as long as it is recognized early. If you are taking an antibiotic or a sulfa drug and detect any of these symptoms, call your doctor immediately. Most likely, you will be told to stop taking the drug and that the symptoms will disappear in a few days.

Allergy. An allergic reaction can happen with almost any drug, prescription or over-the-counter, and to almost any person. If you have ever been allergic to any drug you are more likely than most people to be allergic to another one. If you are allergic to a food item, to animal fur, or if you have had hay fever or asthma attacks, you may be more allergic than most people to a drug. And, if you have ever been allergic to a drug, you should be allergic to that drug from then on.

You cannot have an allergic reaction the first time you are exposed to a drug. An allergic reaction requires prior exposure in order for sensitization to occur. However, we are often exposed to drugs that we don't know about. For example, estrogens (female hormones) were fed to animals to help them grow faster. When we ate the meat of those animals we were exposed to small doses of estrogens. Or, certain foods or drugs may be contaminated. When a manufacturer makes penicillin and other drugs, the other drugs may accidentally be contaminated with penicillin dust. So anyone taking the contaminated drug unknowingly also takes penicillin.

In either situation a drug was taken unintentionally, and the user perhaps became allergic to it. When that person later received a prescription for the drug, or began to take an over-the-counter product, an allergic reaction occurred.

Most of the time allergy does not cause an upset stomach, diarrhea, or drowsiness. Allergy causes rashes, or hives, or difficulty in breathing, or even death. See your doctor if a rash or hives appear and intensify or fail to go away after two days. If you have difficulty breathing or feel that you have fluid in your lungs, you should see your doctor immediately.

Birth defects. Would-be parents often wonder whether the drugs they take can cause birth defects. Expectant mothers worry about taking drugs during pregnancy. Indeed, the current rate of birth defects from all causes is about 2 percent of all live births. Some of these birth defects may be caused by drug use.

Drug manufacturers must prove that their products, both old and new, do not cause birth defects and can be used safely by pregnant women. But until 1962, testing a drug to determine if it caused birth defects was just another routine step in the process of getting the drug on the market. Manufacturers injected the drug or chemical into a pregnant mouse or rat or into a fertilized chicken egg and looked for abnormalities in the offspring.

What happened in 1962? Thalidomide. Thalidomide was commonly used as a sleeping aid in Europe, particularly in Germany and Great Britain, and the drug was thought to be so safe that it was sold without a prescription. However, the drug caused severe birth defects. By 1962, more than 8,000 malformed infants had been delivered to mothers who had taken thalidomide early in their pregnancies.

The severity of the birth defects due to thalidomide use prompted a widespread effort in this country to determine whether other drugs could cause birth defects. The findings of this research indicate that expectant mothers should not take medication — even coffee, tobacco, alcohol, and marijuana. Sometimes, of course, they must, but they should avoid the use of drugs if they can.

A fetus is most susceptible to birth defects from drugs during the first trimester, or first three months, of pregnancy. Generally, after the fourth month, the chances of causing damage to the unborn child are reduced. However, tetracycline taken during the last three months of pregnancy may cause

Drugs That May Be Dangerous If Taken During Some Period Of Pregnancy*

anabolic hormones (Dianabol, Maxibolin, etc.)
androgen hormones (testosterone, etc.)
anticoagulants (Coumadin, etc.)
busulfan (Myleran)
chlorambucil (Leukeran)
chlorpropamide (Diabinese)
corticosteroids (hydrocortisone, Decadron, prednisone, etc.)
cyclizine (Marezine)
cyclophosphamide (Cytoxan)
dextroamphetamine (Dexedrine, etc.)
dienestrol
diethylstilbestrol
ergot alkaloids
ethionamide (Trecator-SC)
iodides
lithium carbonate (Eskalith, Lithane, etc.)
meclizine (Antivert, etc.)
methotrexate
opiates (codeine, morphine, etc.)
penicillamine (Cuprimine)
phenmetrazine (Preludin)
phenothiazines (Thorazine, Stelazine, etc.)
phenytoin (Dilantin, etc.)
phytonadione (vitamin K)
progestins (oral contraceptives)
propylthiouracil (PTU)
reserpine (Serpasil, etc.)
streptomycin
sulfonamides (Gantrisin, etc.)
tetracyclines (Achromycin, Sumycin, Panmycin, etc.)
thyroid hormone
vaccines for measles, mumps, smallpox
vitamin A
vitamin D

*Only the more common drugs are listed. Not included are items, such as thalidomide, that are not available in the United States, and the general anesthetics, which people don't administer to themselves.

discoloration of the child's teeth. A thyroid hormone taken during the last trimester may cause a thyroid disorder in the infant. A child's teeth discolored by tetracycline will not whiten completely, but a thyroid disorder caused by thyroid hormone can be corrected by proper treatment. Other drugs may also affect the infant when taken during the last trimester.

By the time a woman discovers she is pregnant, the damage may have already been done. Usually, a fetus is not affected until the 20th day after conception. If a woman misses a period, she may continue taking drugs after the 20th day following conception and unwittingly endanger the fetus. If for any reason a woman believes she may be pregnant, she should see her doctor at once. The doctor probably will advise her to stop taking medication. A drug manufacturer's instructions for use of a drug usually warn against taking the drug during pregnancy. The key is to use extreme caution with any drug. Never take any drug without your doctor's knowledge if there is even the remotest chance that you may be pregnant or may become pregnant.

Cancer. Think of your body's resistance to cancer as a bridge. Now start driving automobiles onto that bridge. One car won't break it and neither will two. But if you put enough weight on it, the bridge topples.

Those weights that you are adding might be cancer risks such as smoking tobacco, or eating foods containing chemicals that may cause cancer, inhaling polluted air, or taking a drug which may cause cancer. None of these things alone will break the bridge. But if you do enough of them, or enough of any one of them, the bridge may break and your resistance to cancer will be gone.

Not everyone has the same resistance to cancer, and even in the same individual, that resistance declines with age. Therefore, not everyone who smokes cigarettes gets lung cancer. Some smokers have more resistance or fewer other risk factors. The reason that we are so aware of the cancer risks associated with smoking is that many Americans smoke. Far fewer people take any one prescription drug, so the damage from tobacco became apparent first. Some very careful measurements of cancer rates have begun to show that some drugs might also be connected with cancer. Among those involved are some of the very drugs used to treat the disease. They appear to be "double-edged" swords. Reserpine, isoniazid, diethylstilbestrol, methapyrilene and the oral contraceptives are under strict investigation.

Does this mean that you will get cancer if you take one of these drugs? No, but your risk of getting cancer may be increased. What you must do is weigh the risk of cancer against the benefit of taking the drug in question.

Drug Interactions

Two drugs taken at the same time may produce dangerous side effects. Perhaps the best example is the alcohol and sleeping pill combination. Many "suicides" are probably due to accidentally taking alcohol and sleeping pills together. Both are depressants, and together they can cause unconsciousness and death.

When two drugs are taken at the same time, one may interfere with the action of the other. The antibiotic Lincocin causes diarrhea in a great many people, but taking Kaopectate antidiarrheal remedy will prevent the absorption of Lincocin. Similarly, iron tablets inhibit the absorption of tetracycline.

Not all drug interactions are adverse. Bactrim antibacterial contains two antibacterial drugs, and each intensifies the action of the other. The two together are more effective than either alone.

But because drug interactions may be adverse, your doctor and your pharmacist should have a complete record of the medication you take (including over-the-counter drugs such as aspirin or a laxative) as well as tobacco, marijuana, and alcohol.

Examples of Potentially Serious Drug Interactions*

If you take	And then start taking	The result may be
Aldactone or Dyrenium	potassium products such as potassium chloride, K-Lyte	overdose of potassium
Antabuse	alcohol	flushing, fall in blood pressure, vomiting
antidiabetic drugs	alcohol	loss of control of blood sugar
antidiabetic drugs	Butazolidin; Dicumarol; Parnate or other monoamine oxidase inhibitors	fall in blood sugar
antidiabetic drugs	Inderal	rise in blood pressure, loss of control of blood sugar
antihypertensive drugs	amphetamine, anorectics, oral decongestants	rise in blood pressure
Anturane or Benemid	aspirin	worsening of gout
Coumadin	a barbiturate or Doriden	hemorrhage if latter medication is stopped
Coumadin	Dianabol	hemorrhage
Dilantin	Antabuse or isoniazid	clumsiness
Inderal	decongestants	lessened effect of both
Ismelin	tricyclic antidepressants	rise in blood pressure
levodopa	pyridoxine (vitamin B₆)	worsening of Parkinson's disease
Lincocin	Kaopectate	lessened effectiveness of Lincocin
Mandelamine	Diamox	lessened effectiveness of Mandelamine; worsening of infection

If you take	And then start taking	The result may be
methotrexate	aspirin	increase in toxicity of methotrexate
methotrexate	vaccinations	infection develops
Parnate or other monoamine oxidase inhibitors	tricyclic antidepressants	high temperature, excitement
Parnate or other monoamine oxidase inhibitors	amphetamines or anorectics, ephedrine, Neo-Synephrine, Propadrine, Sudafed, some foods (including cheese, broad-pod beans, chicken livers, herring, wines)	rise in blood pressure, stroke, possible death
sedatives	any other sedative	increased sedation (especially when alcohol is used with any other sedative)
tetracycline antibiotics	antacids or dairy products	lessened effectiveness of tetracycline; worsening of infection
Zyloprim	Azathioprine or mercaptopurine	increase in toxicity of Azathioprine or mercaptopurine

Your doctor may decide that you need both drugs despite these possible interactions. He will regulate the dosages you take or tell you to take the drugs several hours apart to reduce the chance of interactions. Follow these instructions very carefully.

Weighing the Risks Against the Benefits

No drug is 100 percent safe and 100 percent effective for 100 percent of the people who take it. Whenever a drug is taken, its risks must be weighed against its benefits for that particular patient. We cannot predict exactly how anyone will react to a specific drug. However, we can prepare ourselves by learning about how drugs work and about the reactions other people have had. To minimize the likelihood of adverse reactions, the patient should take responsibility for following the doctor's instructions carefully and for giving the doctor a full health history.

The Patient's Responsibility

To receive the best medical care for yourself and your family you must take responsibility for communicating fully with your doctor and pharmacist and for conscientiously following through on their instructions. You can assure the safety and effectiveness of any drug products that you use by administering them properly in the correct dosage. You should be able to read and understand your prescription, and you should make the effort to have anything you don't understand explained to you. Your active participation throughout the process is good insurance on your health.

Communicating with Your Doctor and Pharmacist

One important attribute of health care professionals is their willingness to answer your questions. Equally important is your willingness to answer theirs—or your eagerness to volunteer information. You should know what to tell your doctor and your pharmacist as well as what to ask.

Talking to your doctor. What should you tell your physician about the drugs you are taking? Mention all the over-the-counter drugs you take—even an occasional aspirin tablet. Aspirin may cause significant problems, such as stomachache, itching, or difficulty in breathing. It may interact with a drug your doctor wishes to prescribe, and it could cause serious bleeding. Discuss with your doctor any laxatives, "stay awake" tablets, or vitamins you use. A laxative such as mineral oil may be responsible for a tired, run-down feeling; and, if you take a laxative at the wrong time, it may interfere with the action of an antibiotic you may also be taking. Your physician should also know whether you take birth control pills, and if you have seen another doctor or dentist recently or plan to soon.

Do not ask your doctor how much a prescription will cost. Doctors usually don't know. The question is important to you, but it is one you should save for your pharmacist.

Talking to your pharmacist. Give the same information to your pharmacist that you gave to your doctor. Doctors and pharmacists should complement one another. If one misses an important possible drug interaction or toxicity or has made an error in drug dosage, the other should catch it. In checking for possible drug interactions, your pharmacist must know about drugs you get from another drugstore and those the doctor dispenses directly to you.

What information should you get in return? You should be told about how long you will have to take the drug. Of course, people's treatments vary tremendously, but you should know whether you will have to take medication for five to ten days (for example, to resolve a mild respiratory infection) or for a few months (for example, to resolve a kidney infection).

Your pharmacist should advise you of possible side effects, describe their symptoms in understandable terms, and tell you which side effects require prompt attention from your physician. For example, one of the major side effects of Butazolidin, an anti-inflammatory, is a blood disorder. One of its first symptoms is a sore throat. Your pharmacist should tell you to consult your physician if you develop a sore throat.

Your pharmacist should also explain how to take your medicine. "One tablet four times a day" is not enough. You must know whether to take the drug before or after a meal or along with it. When you take a drug can make a big difference, and the effectiveness of each drug depends on following the directions for its use. Your pharmacist should describe what "as needed," "as directed," and "take with fluid" mean. You may take water but not milk with some drugs. With other drugs, you should take milk. Your pharmacist should tell you how many refills you may have and whether you may need them. You should know all this information before putting a tablet, capsule, or spoonful of liquid medication in your mouth.

Your pharmacist should not be asked certain questions. "Why am I taking this drug?" is a question to ask your doctor. Most drugs have several uses. Your pharmacist may tell you about only one of them; if it is not the one for which your doctor prescribed the drug, you may become needlessly worried. Second, your pharmacist may not be able to answer such questions as, "Will this drug work for me," or "Will it cure me?" No one can guarantee a patient's response to a drug. Remember, your doctor prescribed it because he or she believed it would work for you.

Reading Your Prescription

You should understand what your doctor has written on the prescription to be sure the label on the drug container you receive from your pharmacist repeats the information from the prescription. And, by understanding what has been written on a prescription, you can be sure you are following your doctor's directions exactly.

Prescriptions are not mysterious, and they do not contain secret messages. Many of the symbols and phrases doctors use on prescriptions are abbreviated Latin or Greek words. These are holdovers from the days when doctors actually wrote in Latin. For example, "gtts" comes from the Latin word *guttae*, which means drops, and "bid" is a shortened version of *bis in die*, Latin for twice a day.

The accompanying chart lists the symbols and abbreviations most commonly used on prescriptions.

Common Abbreviations and Symbols Used in Writing Prescriptions

Abbreviation	Meaning	Derivation and Notes
A₂	both ears	*auris* (Latin)
aa	of each	*ana* (Greek)
ac	before meals	*ante cibum* (Latin)
AD	right ear	*auris dextra* (Latin)
AL	left ear	*auris laeva* (Latin)
AM	morning	*ante meridiem* (Latin)
AS	left ear	*auris sinistra* (Latin)
bid	twice a day	*bis in die* (Latin)
c̄	with	*cum* (Latin)
cap	capsule	—
cc or cm³	cubic centimeter	30 cc equals one ounce
disp	dispense	—

Common Abbreviations and Symbols
Used in Writing Prescriptions

Abbreviation	Meaning	Derivation and Notes
dtd#	give this number	*dentur tales doses* (Latin)
ea	each	—
ext	for external use	—
gtts	drops	*guttae* (Latin)
gutta	drop	*gutta* (Latin)
h	hour	*hora* (Latin)
H₂O	water	two molecules of hydrogen, one of oxygen
HOH	water	hydrogen-oxygen-hydrogen
HS	bedtime	*hora somni* (Latin)
M ft	make	*misce fiat* (Latin)
mitt #	give this number	*mitte* (Latin)
ml	milliliter	30 ml equals one ounce
O	pint	*octarius* (Latin)
O₂	both eyes	*oculus* (Latin)
OD	right eye	*oculus dexter* (Latin)
OJ	orange juice	—
OL	left eye	*oculus laevus* (Latin)
OS	left eye	*oculus sinister* (Latin)
OU	each eye	*oculus uterque* (Latin)
pc	after meals	*post cibum* (Latin)
PM	evening	*post meridiem* (Latin)
po	by mouth	*per os* (Latin)
prn	as needed	*pro re nata* (Latin)
q̄	every	*quaqua* (Latin)
qd	once a day	*quaqua die* (Latin)
qid	four times a day	*quater in die* (Latin)
qod	every other day	—
s̄	without	*sine* (Latin)
Sig	label as follows	*signetur* (Latin)
sl	under the tongue	*sub lingua* (Latin)
SOB	shortness of breath	—
sol	solution	—
ss	half-unit	*semis* (Latin)
stat	at once, first dose	*statim* (Latin)
susp	suspension	—
tab	tablet	—
tid	three times a day	*ter in die* (Latin)
top	apply topically	—
ung or ungt	ointment	*unguentum* (Latin)
UT	under the tongue	—
ut dict	as directed	*ut dictum* (Latin)
x	times	—

Practice reading prescriptions with the sample prescriptions provided. The first is for Darvon Compound-65 (Darvon Cpd-65), a painkiller. The prescription tells the pharmacist to give you 24 capsules (#24), and it tells you to take one capsule (cap i) every four hours (q̄4h) as needed (prn) for pain. The prescription indicates that you may receive five refills (5x) and that the label on the drug container should state the name of the drug (yes).

Let's try another one. Look at the prescription for a 3-percent solution of Isopto-Carpine eyedrops. It states you will receive 15 ml (disp: 15 ml). Because Isopto-Carpine is packaged in 15-ml containers, the pharmacist will give you one bottle. The bottle's label will direct you to place two drops (gtts ii) in your left eye (OL) every (q̄) morning (AM) and evening (PM) as directed (ut dict). No refills are indicated; so you or your pharmacist must contact your doctor before you can have the prescription refilled. And the prescription states that the name of the drug should be on the bottle's label (✓).

Let's do one more. Look at the last prescription. It shows you will receive 100 (dtd C) tablets of Lanoxin, 0.125 mg. You will take three tablets at once (iii stat), then two (ii) tomorrow morning (AM), and one (i) every (q) morning (AM) thereafter with (c̄) orange juice (OJ). You may receive refills as needed (prn), and the name of the drug will be on the package (✓). '

Do remember to check the label on the drug container. If the label is not the same as the prescription, question your pharmacist. Make doubly sure that you are receiving the right medication and the correct instructions for taking it.

John D. Jones MD
Anytown, U.S.A.

DEA#123456789   PHONE #123-4567

NAME _Your name_   AGE _25_
ADDRESS _Anytown, U.S.A_   DATE _10-15-80_

℞ Darvon cpd - 65
    #24
    Sig: cap i q̄4h prn pain

REFILLS _5X_   _John D. Jones, MD_
LABEL _yes_   **MD**

John D. Jones MD
Anytown, U.S.A.

DEA #123456789   PHONE #123-4567

NAME _Your Name_   AGE _25_
ADDRESS _Anytown, USA_   DATE _10-15-80_

℞   I sop to - Carpine 3%
    disp: 15 ml
    Sig: gtt ii OL q̄ AM & PM ut dict

REFILLS_____   _John D Jones, MD_
LABEL __✓____   MD

John D. Jones MD
Anytown, U.S.A.

DEA #123456789   PHONE #123-4567

NAME _Your name_   AGE _25_
ADDRESS _Anytown, USA_   DATE _10-15-80_

℞   Lanoxin 0.125
    dtd C
    Sig: iii stat, ii tomorrow AM ⊤ then
    i q̄ AM c̄ OJ

REFILLS _prn_   _John D Jones, MD._
LABEL __✓____   MD

Purchasing Drug Products

In a prescription, your doctor specifies exactly how many tablets or capsules or how much liquid medication you will receive. If you must take a drug for a long period of time, you might consider asking about the possibility of purchasing a larger amount. You may be able to save money in the long run.

The amount of medication to buy depends on several factors. The most obvious is how much money you have, or, for those who have a comprehensive insurance program, how much the insurance company will pay for each purchase. But you must also consider the kind of medication you will be taking. For example, you should buy enough antibiotics to last at least ten days unless your doctor has specifically directed otherwise. Antibiotics often cure an infection within ten days and liquid antibiotic preparations may lose potency after ten days. If you have more than a ten-day supply, you may waste money on medication you do not need or should not take.

But medication to treat heart disease, high blood pressure, diabetes, or a thyroid condition may be purchased in large quantities. Patients with such chronic conditions take medication for prolonged periods of time, and chances are they will pay less per tablet or capsule by purchasing large quantities of drugs. Generally, the price per dose decreases with the amount of the drug purchased. In other words, a drug that usually costs six cents per tablet may cost four or five cents per tablet if you buy a supply of 100 at a time. Many doctors prescribe a month's supply of drugs that will be taken for a long period of time. If you wish to buy more, check with your pharmacist.

When buying OTC medications, you decide how much you need or can afford to buy and base your judgement on this decision, but you should also consider the kind of product you will be taking. For example, you should buy enough of a cold remedy to last for five to seven days. Antacids are taken for ulcer pain for two to three months or more, and if you can save money by buying a larger quantity, you should do so. A headache, on the other hand, usually lasts only a few hours or less, and if you don't have frequent headaches, a smaller quantity of medication would be best for you.

When buying drugs, also consider how far away from the pharmacy you live and how many trips you will have to make to restock your supply. If you have small children around, you may wish to buy smaller containers to reduce the amount of drugs you have in the house. Above all, buy enough medication to be economical but not so much that you may have to throw some away.

If you have been plagued with annoying side effects or have had allergic reactions to some drugs, ask your pharmacist to dispense just enough medication on initial prescriptions for a few days or a week. Then you can determine whether it agrees with you before you buy a large quantity of the drug. Pharmacists cannot take back prescription drugs once they have left the pharmacy. You may have to pay more by asking the pharmacist to give you a small amount of the drug, but at least you will not be paying for a supply of medication you cannot take. But be sure you can get the remainder of the prescribed amount of the drug. After you have received part of the intended amount of some drugs, such as narcotics, you cannot receive more without obtaining another prescription.

Dosage

One of the least understood aspects of drug therapy is dosage. Most people believe that dosage simply represents the amount of the drug to be taken. But dosage also involves when the drug should be taken.

Obviously, it is important to take the correct amount of a drug. People can become seriously ill by taking an overdose, and taking just a little too much can often cause problems. Many cases of aspirin poisoning in children are caused by parents or guardians who give just "a little too much" aspirin just "a little too soon." On the other hand, diabetics may go into shock if they wait too long between injections of insulin or miss an injection altogether.

A prescription that states "one tablet four times daily" seems plain enough. But exactly what does "four times daily" mean?

For some antibiotics prescribed for serious infections, it may mean one dose every six hours around the clock. For some medications used for nervous conditions, it may mean one in the morning, one at noon, one in the early evening, and one at bedtime. And for medication to treat intestinal worms, it may mean one every hour for the first four hours after you get up in the morning.

Let's go back to the prescription for Darvon Compound-65. It tells you to take one capsule every four hours as needed. How many capsules can you take each day—four, six, or more? The phrase "as needed" is not clear, and unless you completely understand your prescription, you may leave the pharmacy with unanswered questions.

The phrases "as needed," "as directed," "with meals," and "on an empty stomach" seem specific. Your doctor and pharmacist understand these phrases and sometimes assume that you do too. But these expressions are not always as clear as they seem. To get the most benefit from your medication and to minimize harmful side effects, you must take drugs as directed. Do not be afraid to ask your pharmacist for an explanation.

Overdosage

It has been reported that several million Americans are poisoned every year, and another study has shown that only one out of every 50 cases of poisoning is reported—the actual number of Americans poisoned each year is unknown. What is known is that half of all poisonings are caused by drugs.

Over 50 percent of all reported cases of poisoning involve children under the age of five. Children are naturally curious. Their curiosity takes them up onto tabletops and sinks and even into medicine cabinets. They see their parents consume drugs, and since youngsters are imitative, they wish to follow suit. Parents unwittingly encourage them when they call a flavored tablet "candy" or liquid medication "sweet syrup."

Sometimes poisoning in children is caused by well-meaning but careless adults. Some parents may give their children aspirin at the first wheeze or sniffle. The first aspirin is quickly followed by a second, and a third, and before long, the child has been poisoned. Of course, aspirin is not the only drug given to children, but it is the most common agent of drug poisoning of children.

Barbiturates and sleeping aids are the leading agents in adult drug poisoning. Other drugs commonly involved in poisonings are listed in the accompanying table. Always remember that any drug product may be toxic if taken in sufficient quantity.

Most drug overdoses can be reversed by observing a few simple rules. Luckily, these rules can be used in the emergency treatment of overdoses from many drugs, and you need not follow a specific treatment for an overdose of a particular drug.

Act fast. After an adult or child has taken an overdose of a drug, your primary objective is to lessen the toxicity of the drug or to get rid of it as quickly as possible. Act fast! As soon as an overdose has been discovered, dilute the drug.

Dilute the poison. Diluting the drug helps prevent it from damaging the lining of the stomach. Also, adding fluid to the stomach aids vomiting.

One cup of water may be given to a child, and two to three cups are suitable for an adult. Carbonated beverages (soda pop) should not be given. Carbonated beverages produce gas, which can distend the stomach wall and increase the chance of a stomach rupture. Besides water, fruit juice or milk is commonly used to dilute a drug. However, only water should be given until a doctor or pharmacist has been consulted regarding the use of milk or fruit juices.

Make a Call. Then immediately call a doctor, pharmacist, or your Poison Control Center. Tell him or her what was swallowed and ask for instructions.

Drugs That Most Often Cause Poisoning

Drug Name	Symptoms
aspirin or aspirin products	Nausea, vomiting (may have blood in vomitus), fever, rapid breathing, weakness, confusion; may have white spots in the mouth
sedatives (barbiturates, meprobamate, Valium, Librium, Quaalude, etc.)	Drowsiness, dizziness, weakness, slow breathing, pinpoint pupils; may breathe with a "gurgling" sound
cold medicines containing antihistamines	Drowsiness, dizziness, weakness, nervousness, dry mouth, fever, pounding in chest; children may experience excitement, increased pulse and breathing
narcotics (codeine, meperidine, morphine, etc.)	Drowsiness, dizziness, weakness, pinpoint pupils, slow breathing; may breathe with a "gurgling" sound
acetaminophen or acetaminophen products	Nausea, vomiting, loss of color, weakness, difficult breathing; symptoms may disappear in four to eight hours, but it still is extremely important to call your doctor for help
tricyclic antidepressants (Tofranil, Elavil, etc.) or items containing anticholinergics	Excitation, dry mouth, pounding in chest, nervousness; respiration increases for first several hours, then decreases
vitamins and iron	Nausea, vomiting
	vitamin A—above, plus loss of appetite, headache
	vitamin D—above, plus twitching of muscles, nervousness
	iron—above, plus diarrhea (may contain blood, or dark spots), drowsiness

In most cases you should then get ready to induce vomiting or administer activated charcoal to keep the drug from entering the bloodstream.

Induce vomiting—sometimes. Vomiting (emesis) can be used to rid the body of any poison except an acid, (usually) a petroleum derivative, a corrosive such as lye, or a convulsive such as strychnine. These poisons can burn the throat as they are being vomited. Containers of these poisons have clearly marked labels that warn against inducing vomiting. Always check the label on the container of the poison that has been ingested before attempting to induce vomiting.

Drugs generally do not contain any such poisons. And inducing vomiting in a child or adult who has taken a drug overdose usually is safe as long as the victim is conscious. If the victim of a drug overdose is unconscious, do not try to induce vomiting because you may cause the victim to choke.

To induce vomiting, you may follow one of several methods. You should know the benefits and risks of each.

Ipecac syrup—Undoubtedly, ipecac syrup is the emetic of choice for home emergency treatment of drug poisoning. One teaspoon of ipecac syrup usually is given to a child, and one tablespoonful to an adult. Make the victim drink water after the ipecac syrup is administered, if he or she has not drunk any before. Vomiting should occur in about 15 minutes. If it does not, the dose can be repeated once, 15 to 30 minutes after the first dose. Ipecac syrup is available in one-ounce bottles in first-aid kits and it can be purchased from most pharmacies.

Mechanical stimulus— To induce vomiting by mechanical stimulus, place the victim in a spanking position and gently stroke the back of his tongue with your finger or a blunt object, such as a spoon. Be careful if you stroke the back of the tongue with your finger. The victim may bite down on it as he gags.

Mechanical stimulus is a common way to induce vomiting, but it usually is not effective. In a study of 30 children who had ingested a poison, only two vomited after this procedure was followed, and the volume actually vomited was small, even though the children had been given a cup of water. The time wasted trying to induce vomiting by mechanical stimulus could be better spent by administering an effective agent, such as ipecac syrup.

Mustard—Mustard powder (one or two teaspoonsful in a cup of water) has not been shown to effectively induce vomiting, even though its use has been advocated for years. Mustard powder is not available in most households, and the mustard used on hotdogs does not substitute for it.

Table salt—Table salt has long been thought to be a safe and effective agent for inducing vomiting but it is not. It should *never* be used to induce vomiting because the salt itself can be toxic and may be lethal. Unfortunately, many first-aid charts and package labels still recommend that it be used. Such recommendations should be disregarded. If you have any further questions, ask your doctor or pharmacist.

Go to the hospital. Remember that even after the victim has vomited, you must still get him or her to the hospital or to a doctor. Vomiting seldom removes all traces of a poison, and the victim may need further treatment.

Recommended Antidotes For Drug Poisoning

Ipecac Syrup:
For children: 1 teaspoonful accompanied by 1 or 2 glasses of water.
For adults: 1 tablespoonful accompanied by 2 or 3 glasses of water.
(Dose may be repeated once, 15 to 30 minutes later.)

Activated Charcoal:
For children and adults: 2 heaping tablespoonsful (about 2 ounces) mixed with 1 cup of water to form a slurry.
(Dose may be repeated 30 to 60 minutes later, and again as frequently as necessary.)

Administer an antidote. In practically all cases of drug poisoning, activated charcoal can be used as an antidote. An ounce or two should be mixed as a slurry in a cup of water and drunk as soon as possible after poisoning. This dose is not absolute, and because activated charcoal is nontoxic, the victim of drug poisoning need not worry about consuming too much. To ensure complete removal of the drug, the dose of activated charcoal can be repeated once or twice at 30- to 60-minute intervals.

Activated charcoal prevents absorption of a drug into the bloodstream. Even though the benefits of activated charcoal in the treatment of drug overdoses have been known for years, many doctors and pharmacists largely have ignored it.

One reason for its rather poor acceptance is that charcoal has some disagreeable characteristics. It is black and stains the gums and mouth. It has a bitter taste and it creates a gritty sensation in the mouth.

When using activated charcoal to treat a drug overdose, you may want to remember a few "tricks of the trade." Mix a little cocoa powder with the charcoal solution or place a small amount of cocoa or powdered sugar directly on the victim's tongue before he drinks it. Mix the activated charcoal with water in an amber-colored container so that the victim cannot see the color of the mixture while drinking. Or have the victim drink it through a straw.

Prompt use of activated charcoal is effective for home emergency treatment of an overdose from a number of drugs. It is inexpensive, can be purchased without a prescription, and is not irritating to the stomach.

One other thing to remember is that you should not administer both ipecac syrup and activated charcoal at the same time. Your doctor or pharmacist will help you decide which is better to use and whether to administer activated charcoal after the victim has vomited.

To be ready to take prompt action in the case of a drug overdose, get some ipecac syrup and activated charcoal *now*. Do not wait until you need them. Get them today and keep them handy. You may never need them, but do not take that chance.

What comes next? Home emergency treatment of a drug overdose is not enough. You must also seek professional care. If you live near a Poison Control Center, call for instructions. Look up the Center's phone number and keep it handy in case of an emergency.

If you are not near a phone or a Poison Control Center, start for the hospital as soon as the antidote has been administered. Be sure to take the poison container and all remaining tablets, capsules, or liquid with you so an estimate of the amount of drug ingested can be made.

Take a sample of the vomit with you in a dish, or at least take an empty dish or pan to collect any material vomited on the way to the hospital. Your doctor may want to analyze it if the identity of the drug is not known.

By all means, stay calm. Note symptoms, and keep track of time. Your doctor will want to know how much time elapsed between swallowing the drug and the first symptoms.

Most cases of drug poisoning are not fatal. But survival depends on the drug, how much was taken, how soon the overdose was discovered, the age of the victim, and the emergency measures taken.

Prevention of overdoses. Obviously, preventing drug poisoning is better than having to treat it. These tips may help you avoid a potential tragedy.

1. Store drugs out of the reach of children. Place drugs in a cabinet, closet, or trunk that can be locked.
2. Store medication intended for external use separate from drugs intended to be swallowed.
3. Use child-resistant drug containers if children live with you or visit often. Refasten the lid securely after use.

4. Read the label carefully, paying particular attention to warnings and precautions.
5. Do not take or give drugs in the dark—one bottle easily can be mistaken for another. Always turn on a light and check the label.
6. Do not keep unlabeled drugs in the house.
7. Do not take drugs when your children are nearby. They are apt to mimic you.
8. Do not refer to any drug (including vitamins) as "candy."
9. Do not leave medication within the reach of children. Take it with you or return it to its locked storage area if you are called to the telephone or the door.
10. Do not use drugs prescribed for someone else. They may be dangerous to you.
11. Keep handy the telephone numbers of your doctor, your pharmacist, and the local Poison Control Center.
12. Teach your children never to place anything strange in their mouths. Instruct them on what may happen if they accidentally swallow anything poisonous, and make sure they understand that in such situations they should get help as quickly as possible.
13. Take no chances. If your child may have swallowed a drug (if you see him handling an open container or if there are particles of the drug in his mouth, for example), do not wait for symptoms of an overdose. Follow the procedures for emergency measures. Some drugs, such as aspirin, may not produce symptoms until several hours after poisoning.
14. Dispose of old drugs. Once a drug has served its purpose, discard it. Flush it down the toilet or pour it down the sink. Rinse the container and discard it.
15. Purchase some ipecac syrup and activated charcoal now. The best antidote in the world is no good if you don't have it when you need it.

Your Medicine Cabinet

Almost everyone keeps OTC medicines and prescription drugs in the bathroom medicine cabinet, one of the worst places to keep such items. Small children can easily climb onto the sink and reach items stored above it. The temperature and humidity in the bathroom vary greatly over the course of the day, and the changes in humidity and temperature may adversely affect the stability of many drug products.

What are ideal storage conditions? Most drug products need to be protected from heat and moisture; otherwise, they may lose potency. You can safely store most drug products at room temperature and out of direct sunlight. If you have small children, you'll want to keep drugs locked up. You can get an inexpensive lock for a cabinet or closet at your local hardware store, but you must remember to use it. If you do not lock up drugs, have them packaged in child-resistant containers. Child-resistant caps and containers, despite the frustration you may feel when trying to open them, have reduced the number of accidental poisonings. If you have trouble opening child-resistant containers, ask your pharmacist to place your medication in a regular container. And please remember to store these containers out of the reach of your children.

Many drug containers are more difficult to open than they once were because the container tops and lids fit more tightly to keep out moisture. Containers with tightly fitting lids can help assure the safety and effectiveness of the drugs they house.

To find out how to store a particular drug item, check the label on the package. If the label states that the product should be stored at a certain temperature, use the accompanying table as a guide.

If a label says to store the item in a "cool" place, a refrigerator is appropriate. If it indicates the item should be stored at room temperature, ask your pharmacist if it is alright to keep it in the refrigerator. If you bought the item from a store shelf, don't worry about keeping it in the refrigerator. If you had to ask your pharmacist to get the item for you, then be sure to ask if it needs to be stored in the refrigerator. The label should describe optimal storage conditions, but you still want to be sure.

Some items do require storage in the refrigerator. But the statement "keep in the refrigerator" does not mean that you can keep the product in the freezer. If frozen and thawed, some liquid medications will separate into layers that cannot be remixed. This is especially true for thick medicines such as Pepto Bismol diarrhea remedy and Maalox antacid.

Other liquid drugs cannot be stored in the refrigerator, because as they become cold they will thicken and will not pour from the bottle.

Some people keep nitroglycerin tablets in the refrigerator because they believe the drug will be more stable. Nitroglycerin, however, should not be stored in the refrigerator.

Definitions Of Ideal Storage Temperatures

Cold	Any temperature under 46° F (8° C)
Refrigerator	Any cold place where the temperature is between 36°-46° F (2°-8° C)
Cool	Any temperature between 46°-59° F (8°-15° C)
Room Temperature	Temperature usually between 59°-86° F (15°-30° C)
Excessive heat	Any temperature above 104° F (40° C)

Be careful about purchasing tablets of aspirin or other pain relievers in small tin or plastic flat boxes. These containers do not close tightly and allow moisture to seep in. The slightest amount of moisture may destroy your tablets. If you ever smell vinegar when you open a drug container, do not take the tablets as they will be at least partially destroyed. They may not relieve your pain, and worse yet, they may cause harsh stomach pain.

Your medicine cabinet should not contain any prescription drugs you no longer need or any drugs whose expiration date has passed. Expiration dates are established by drug manufacturers. An expiration date indicates the time beyond which the drug may no longer be totally effective. An expiration date usually is set for five years after the drug was made, and it is based on the time at which 5 percent of the drug will have been destroyed or converted.

The expiration date on certain antibiotics, such as the tetracyclines, is especially important because it indicates when the antibiotic may become toxic. After the expiration date, tetracycline, for example, converts into another chemical that may fatally damage the kidneys. Other antibiotics, such as penicillin, do not become toxic after their expiration dates, but they do lose potency.

The Home Medicine Cabinet

Medication	Purpose
Emetrol antinauseant	nausea; vomiting
antihistamine	colds and allergy
decongestant	colds and allergy
cough syrup	coughs of colds
aspirin, acetaminophen	pain and fever
activated charcoal	poisoning
ipecac syrup	poisoning
rubbing alcohol	mild antiseptic
anti-infective cream	minor cuts
anesthetic cream	burns, insect bites, etc.
hydrogen peroxide	mild antiseptic
petroleum jelly	soothe irritated skin
epsom salts	swollen tissues (sprained ankle, etc.)
antidiarrheal	diarrhea

Supplies

adhesive tape (½ " wide)
sterile bandages (2" x 2", 3" x 3", and 4" x 4")
cotton-tipped swabs
gauze bandage rolls (1" wide and 4" wide)
adhesive bandages (assorted sizes)
elastic bandage (3" wide)
triangle bandage
scissors
tweezers
thermometer (oral and rectal)
wooden tongue depressors
flashlight
stethoscope
sphygmomanometer
first-aid manual
insect sting kit (if someone in family is allergic to insect stings)
ice bag
heating pad

While a drug may be effective beyond its expiration date, you cannot be sure and should not take chances. So, never use a drug after the expiration date on the label.

Flush any outdated or leftover medication down the toilet or pour it down the sink, and wash and destroy the empty container. Regularly clean out your medicine cabinet and discard all drugs you are no longer using. These drugs can be dangerous to your children, and you might be tempted to take them in the future if you develop similar symptoms. Though similar, the symptoms may not be due to the same disease, and you may complicate your condition by taking medication prescribed to treat a different ailment. So be cautious—always dispose of leftover prescription drugs.

Ideally, your home medicine cabinet should contain the drugs you use frequently plus those items you might need suddenly. Right now, your medicine cabinet probably has over-the-counter and current prescription drugs, assorted first aid "odds and ends," cosmetics, toiletries, disinfectants, and the like. It probably has some items that don't belong there—unused prescription medications, outdated OTC drugs, and empty bottles.

Now is a good time to take stock of your medicine cabinet, to remove anything that is not intended to treat sickness—perfumes, aftershave lotions, and household cleaning products—and to separate drugs for external use from those for internal use.

The ideal home medicine cabinet deliberately leaves out drugs that should be picked up when you need them rather than stocked in advance. Many health problems progress slowly enough for you to purchase an OTC drug or see a doctor and get a prescription before the symptoms get too bad: for example, constipation, diarrhea, athlete's foot, diaper rash, poison ivy, nasal congestion, and fever blisters. The ideal home medicine cabinet also contains a sphygmomanometer (used to measure blood pressure) and a stethoscope.

Your medicine cabinet should have an emergency first aid section. It should contain a supply of adhesive bandage strips, an elastic bandage, a triangle bandage, gauze rolls and gauze pads, cotton swabs, a bottle of rubbing alcohol, a tube of anti-infective cream, a tube of anesthetic cream, activated charcoal, and ipecac syrup. Additionally, you should have a small pair of scissors, a pair of tweezers, and wooden tongue depressors which you may buy from most drug stores. We also recommend that you buy and study a first-aid manual. This will help you in time of emergency, and should answer most of your questions about common first-aid measures.

Administering Medicine Correctly

If you use drug products correctly, you will get full benefit from them. If you do not follow the directions explicitly, you may not receive the desired effect and you will be wasting your money as well.

Liquids. Liquids may be used externally on the skin; they may be placed into the eye, ear, or nose; or they may be taken internally.

Before taking or using any liquid medication, look at the label to see if there are any specific directions, such as shaking the container before measuring the dose.

If a liquid product contains particles that settle to the bottom of the container, it must be shaken before you use it. If you don't shake it well each time, you may not get the correct amount of the active ingredient. As the amount of liquid remaining in the bottle becomes smaller, the drug will become more concentrated. You will be getting more of the active ingredient with each dose. The concentration may even reach toxic levels.

When opening the bottle, point it away from you. Some liquid medications may build up pressure inside the bottle; the liquid could spurt out quickly and stain your clothing.

If the medication is intended for application on the skin, pour a small quantity onto a cotton pad or a piece of gauze. Do not use a large piece of cotton or gauze as it will absorb the liquid and much will be wasted. You can spread medication over a small area with your finger. If you must apply the liquid to a large area (such as a whole arm or leg), you should not pour it into your cupped hand because you may spill some of it. And never dip cotton-tipped applicators or pieces of cotton or gauze into the bottle of liquid as this might contaminate the rest of the medication.

Liquid medications that are to be swallowed must be measured accurately. When your doctor prescribes one teaspoonful of medication, he is thinking of a 5 cc medical teaspoon. The teaspoons you have at home may contain anywhere from 2 cc to 10 cc. Thus, if you use a regular teaspoon to measure your liquid medication, you may get too little or too much with each dose. Consequently, you should ask your pharmacist for a medical teaspoon or for one of the other plastic devices for accurately measuring liquid medications. Most of these cost only a few cents, and they are well worth their cost to assure accurate dosages. These plastic measuring devices have another advantage. While many children balk at medication taken from a teaspoon, they often seem to enjoy taking it from the special measuring devices.

Capsules and tablets. Many people find it hard to swallow a tablet or capsule. If you're one of them, rinse your mouth with water, or at least wet your mouth, before taking a tablet or capsule. Place the tablet or capsule on the back of your tongue, take a drink of water, and swallow.

If you cannot swallow a tablet or capsule because it is too large or because it "sticks" in your throat, empty the capsule or crush the tablet into a spoon and mix it with applesauce, soup, or even chocolate syrup. But be sure to check with your pharmacist first. Some tablets and capsules must be swallowed whole, and your pharmacist can tell you which ones they are.

If you have trouble swallowing a tablet or capsule and do not wish to mix the medication with food each time you take it, ask your doctor to prescribe a liquid drug preparation or a chewable tablet instead.

Sublingual tablets. Some drugs, such as nitroglycerin, are prepared as tablets that must be placed under the tongue. To take a sublingual tablet properly, place the tablet under your tongue, close your mouth, and hold the saliva in your mouth and under your tongue as long as you can before swallowing. If you have a bitter taste in your mouth after five minutes, the drug has not been completely absorbed. Wait five more minutes before drinking water. Drinking water too soon may wash the medication into the stomach before it has been absorbed thoroughly.

Eyedrops and eye ointments. Before administering eyedrops or ointments, wash your hands. Then, lie down, or sit down and tilt your head back. Gently and carefully pull your lower eyelid down to form a pouch. To insert eyedrops, hold the dropper close to the eyelid without touching it. Place the prescribed number of drops into the pouch. Do not place the drops directly on the eyeball; you may blink and lose the medication. Close your eye and keep it shut for a few moments. Do not wash or wipe the dropper before replacing it in the bottle. Tightly close the bottle to keep out moisture.

To administer an ointment to the eye, squeeze a one-quarter to one-half inch line of ointment into the pouch and close your eye. Roll your eye a few times to spread the ointment. As long as you do not squeeze the ointment directly onto the eyeball, you should feel no stinging or pain.

Be sure the drops or ointments you use are intended for the eye. Also, make sure your pharmacist has indicated the expiration date of the drug on the label. Do not use a drug product after that date.

Eardrops. Eardrops must be administered so that they fill the ear canal. To administer eardrops properly, tilt your head to one side, turning the affected ear upward. Grasp the earlobe and pull it upward and back to straighten the ear canal. When administering eardrops to a child, gently pull the child's earlobe downward and back. Fill the dropper and place the prescribed number of drops (usually a dropperful) in the ear, but be careful to avoid touching the ear canal. The dropper can be easily contaminated by contact with the ear canal.

Keep your ear tilted upward for five to ten seconds, then gently insert a small piece of cotton into the ear to be sure the drops do not escape. Do not wash or wipe the dropper after use; replace it in the bottle and tightly close the bottle to keep out moisture.

You may warm the bottle of eardrops before administering the medication. The best way to warm eardrops is to roll the bottle back and forth between your hands to bring the solution to body temperature. Do not place the bottle in boiling water. The eardrops may become so hot that they will cause pain when placed in the ear, and boiling water can loosen or peel the label off the bottle.

Nose drops and sprays. Before using nose drops and sprays, gently blow your nose if you can. To administer nose drops, fill the dropper, tilt your head back, and place the prescribed number of drops in your nose. Do not touch the dropper to the nasal membranes. This will prevent contamination of the medicine when the dropper is returned to the container. Keep your head tilted for five to ten seconds and sniff gently two or three times.

Do not tilt your head back when using a nasal spray. Insert the sprayer into the nose, but try to avoid touching the inner nasal membranes. Sniff and squeeze the sprayer at the same time. Do not release your grip on the sprayer until you have withdrawn it from your nose to prevent nasal mucus and bacteria from entering the plastic bottle and contaminating its contents. After you have sprayed the prescribed number of times in one or both nostrils, sniff two or three times.

Unless your doctor has told you otherwise, nose drops and sprays should not be used for more than two or three days at a time. If they have been prescribed for a longer period, do not administer nose drops or sprays from the same container for more than one week. Bacteria from your nose can easily enter the container and contaminate the solution. If you must take medication for more than a week, purchase a new container. Never allow anyone else to use your nose drops or spray.

Rectal suppositories. A rectal suppository may be used as a laxative or to relieve the itching, swelling, and pain of hemorrhoids. Regardless of the reason for their use, all suppositories are inserted in the same way.

In extremely hot weather, a suppository may become too soft to handle properly. If it does, place it inside the refrigerator or in a glass of cool water until firm. Before inserting a suppository, remove any aluminum wrappings. Rubber finger coverings or disposable rubber gloves may be worn when inserting a suppository, but they are not necessary unless your fingernails are extremely long and sharp.

To insert a suppository, lie on your left side (if you are right-handed) and push the suppository, pointed end first, into the rectum as far as is comfortable. If you feel like defecating, lie still until the urge has passed. If you cannot insert a suppository, or if the process is painful, coat the suppository with a thin layer of Vaseline petroleum jelly or mineral oil before trying to insert it.

Manufacturers of many suppositories that are used in the treatment of hemorrhoids suggest that the suppositories be stored in the refrigerator. Be sure to ask your pharmacist if the suppositories you have purchased should be stored in the refrigerator.

Vaginal ointments and creams. Most vaginal products contain complete instructions for use. If a woman is not sure how to administer vaginal medication, she should ask her pharmacist.

Before using any vaginal ointment or cream, read the directions. They probably tell you to screw the applicator to the top of the tube and squeeze the tube from the bottom until the applicator is completely filled. Then lie on your back with your knees drawn up. Hold the applicator horizontally or pointed slightly downward and insert it into the vagina as far as it will go comfortably. Press the plunger down to empty the cream or ointment into the vagina. Withdraw the plunger and wash it in warm, soapy water. Rinse it thoroughly and allow it to dry completely. Once it is dry, return the plunger to its package.

Vaginal tablets and suppositories. Most vaginal tablets or suppositories have complete directions for their use. But you may wish to review some general instructions.

Remove any foil wrapping. Place the tablet or suppository in the applicator that is provided. Lie on your back with your knees drawn up. Hold the applicator horizontally or tilted slightly downward and insert it into the vagina as far as it will go comfortably. Depress the plunger slowly to release the tablet or suppository into the vagina. Withdraw the applicator and wash it in warm, soapy water. Rinse it and let it dry completely. Once it is dry, return the applicator to its package.

Unless your doctor has told you otherwise, do not douche two to three weeks before or after you use vaginal tablets or suppositories. Be sure to ask your doctor for specific recommendations on douching.

Throat lozenges or discs. Lozenges are crystal sugar-coated; discs are not. Both contain medication that is released in the mouth to soothe a sore throat, reduce coughing, or to treat laryngitis. Neither should be chewed, but should be allowed to dissolve in the mouth. After the lozenge or disc has dissolved, try not to swallow or drink any fluids for awhile.

Throat sprays. To administer a throat spray, open your mouth wide and spray the medication as far back as possible. Try not to swallow but hold the spray in your mouth as long as you can, and try not to drink any fluids for several minutes.

External ointments and creams. Ointments and creams are topical medications that have local effects—that is, they affect only the area on which they are applied. Most creams and ointments are expensive (especially products containing steroids, such as hydrocortisone, Aristocort A, Cordran, Kenalog, Lidex, Synalar, Valisone, Vioform-Hydrocortisone, Mycolog) and should be applied to the skin as thinly as possible. A thin layer is as effective as a thick layer, and some steroid-containing creams and ointments can cause toxic side effects if applied too heavily.

Before applying the medication, moisten the skin by immersing it in water or by dabbing the area with a clean, wet cloth. Blot the skin dry and apply as directed. Gently massage it into the skin until it has disappeared. You should feel no greasiness or wetness on the skin after applying a cream. After applying an ointment, the skin will feel slightly greasy.

If your doctor has not indicated whether you should receive a cream or an ointment, ask your pharmacist for a cream. Creams are greaseless and will not stain your clothing. Creams are best for use on the scalp or other hairy areas of the body.

If, however, your skin is dry, ask your pharmacist for an ointment. Ointments help keep the skin soft for a longer period of time.

If your doctor tells you to place a wrap on top of the skin after the cream or ointment has been applied, you may use a wrap of transparent plastic film. A wrap will hold the medication close to the skin and help keep the skin moist so that the drug can be absorbed. To use a wrap correctly, apply the cream or ointment as directed, then wrap the area with a layer of transparent plastic film. Be careful to follow your doctor's directions. If he tells you to leave the wrap in place for a certain length of time, do not leave it in place longer. If you keep a wrap on the skin too long, too much of the drug may be absorbed, which may cause side effects.

Powders. Powders may be applied to any part of the body. They should be sprinkled evenly over dry skin. Powders are used when the area is tender and should be kept dry, such as in fungal and bacterial infections. They can be applied without touching the area, and because they absorb moisture, they help keep the area dry. Whenever you use a powder on your feet—in the treatment of athlete's foot or other infections—sprinkle some of the powder in your socks and shoes. Also, regardless of the type of powder, avoid inhaling it. Even a small amount of powder used for a skin infection may cause a respiratory problem if inhaled.

Aerosol sprays. Many topical items that are used on the skin are packaged as pressurized aerosol sprays. Generally, we do not recommend these sprays because they cost more than the cream or ointment form of the same product. On the other hand, they are useful on very tender or hairy areas of the body where it is difficult to apply a cream or ointment.

Before using an aerosol, shake the can. Hold it upright four to six inches from the skin. Press the nozzle for a few seconds, then release.

Never use an aerosol around the face or eyes. If your doctor tells you to use the spray on a part of your face, apply it to your hand and then rub it onto the area. If you get it in your eyes or on a mucous membrane, it will be very painful and it may damage the eyes.

Aerosol sprays also feel cold when they are applied. If this sensation bothers you, ask your pharmacist or doctor whether another form of the same product is available.

Keeping Health Records

When you go to the doctor with a medical problem, your history is probably the single most important component in the diagnosis. You should be prepared to describe your symptoms exactly. Note their time of onset and the nature of your activity (eating supper, raking the lawn, shoveling snow) at that time. Be prepared to describe the rapidity with which your symptoms appear. In some cases, the symptoms themselves provide fewer clues than does the manner in which they occur. For example, you may tell your doctor that you have a headache and a stiff neck and feel dizzy. All of these symptoms could apply to a wide variety of disorders. But when you tell your doctor that these symptoms all appeared within three to four minutes of each other and that they have persisted and grown worse since then, your doctor can zero in on the probable cause of your disorder. In this instance, a hemorrhage of the blood vessels in your brain may be suggested and immediate treatment is required.

Your daily habits and lifestyle may have some bearing on your diagnosis, and you should be prepared to tell the doctor about your diet (composition and quantity), any drugs that you may be taking (including over-the-counter preparations such as aspirin and antacids), whether you live or work under a great deal of stress, if you smoke or drink alcohol, and how much exercise you get. Other factors that may be important in your diagnosis include recent travel—people sometimes pick up "bugs" away from the home environment—and the health of your family and friends.

All this information will be helpful to the doctor in pinpointing the cause of your complaint. You can be even more helpful by beginning now, before you feel unwell, to note the state of your health on a regular basis and to keep track of bodily changes in a personal health record. A personal health record need not be elaborate—its utility depends most upon the regularity and accuracy with which you record the information. A simple spiral-bound notebook is sufficient. Write the date on a page and record the necessary information diary fashion. You may want to design a chart that has spaces for you to fill in pertinent information—body weight, respiration rate, blood pressure, etc.—and have it duplicated. Some people keep a health record on graph paper, plotting body weight and other functions so that any variation is obvious. Or, you might find a desk-type calendar with writing space appropriate.

By checking yourself regularly, you may detect certain diseases that can be successfully treated if caught early but that may cause problems if treatment is delayed, or your health record may alert you to a potentially serious drug reaction. Keeping a personal health record serves as a reminder that you are gaining or losing weight, that your insomnia is persisting, or that your stomach pain is getting worse. It's a constant record that discretely nudges you to eat properly, get more exercise, have your eyes checked, visit your doctor about that mole that seems to be getting bigger, and in general to take better care of yourself.

How often should you examine yourself? Frequency is less important

than regularity. Some measurements should be taken weekly. Certain variations, in your bowel habits for example, may occur occasionally and they
should be noted when they occur. Women should note when they do their
monthly breast examination. Make note of headaches, allergic reactions,
stomach pains—a pattern may begin to appear and that pattern may be
characteristic of some disease. Once you have devised a schedule that is appropriate for you, keep to it, whether you decide to make daily or weekly
notes about your health. Following is a list of what you should look for when
you do your health examination.

Body Appearance

To start your health record, look at the overall appearance of your body. Does
there appear to be an accumulation of fat someplace? Try the pinch test at
your waistline. Is that roll getting thicker? Do you have a different pattern of
hair growth or do you see stretch marks appearing on your skin? Are you losing your hair or gaining more? When you stand upright, does one leg bow to
the side? Do your knees appear to be the same size? Are your shoulders more
rounded or padded than they were a while back? Does your face seem to be
puffy?

And don't neglect what other people are telling you. Have you been told
that you appear heavier or thinner than before, even though your scale does
not show a weight change? Are you told that you look unusually tired or pale,
or that you are walking with a slight limp? Are people commenting that you
seem to be sweating more than usual, even though you personally haven't
thought much about it? If you are hearing such comments regularly, maybe
something is wrong, even though you feel fine. Remember that we tend to
become used to our own appearance. We accept changes as the natural
result of aging, but sometimes the changes are not those natural ones we
expect.

Weight

You don't have to weigh yourself daily, but you should weigh yourself on a
regular schedule. Once or twice a week is enough, and each time, your body
weight should be carefully charted. Unexplained weight losses or increases
of two or more pounds per week should lead you to suspect that something
may be wrong, and if this loss or increase continues over several weeks, you
should seek medical assistance.

Weighing yourself properly is more complicated than haphazardly step-
ping on a scale and recording the figure. You should always weigh yourself
on the same scale under the same circumstances. For example, many people
prefer to weigh themselves in the morning after emptying their bladder, but
before breakfast. If you always weigh yourself at this time, your weight
should be nearly constant. However, if you weigh yourself in the morning
before breakfast one day, and at night after supper the next, you can't really
tell if you've gained or lost weight. Any change might simply reflect a normal
daily fluctuation.

And you should always weigh yourself on the same scale. Because many
bathroom scales are not accurate, weighing yourself one day on one scale
and another day on another scale may not show any real changes. Likewise,
do not be surprised if your scale at home shows one weight and the scale at
your doctor's office shows a different weight. The important thing is to use
the same scale each time and to look for changes from your previous weight.

The height-weight tables that are available from most insurance companies or from any doctor's office should be used only as a general guideline
for determining your ideal weight. The figures are based on averages for

many thousands of people, and they may not necessarily represent your ideal weight. For example, the tables may say that your ideal weight is 165 pounds, but you might feel much more comfortable at 150 pounds. If this is the case, you should strive for 150 pounds. But if you feel more comfortable at a weight that exceeds the recommended weight, be careful. You may need to talk this over with your doctor.

Blood Pressure

Your blood pressure is a very important indication of overall health. Everyone should learn how to take blood pressure correctly, especially if there is a family history of high blood pressure, or if some family member has a disease of the heart or blood vessels. And, everyone should take this measurement regularly—at least once a week. At least one out of every ten Americans has high blood pressure, and only half of these people are aware of their condition. And, of course, if the blood pressure is higher than it should be, it must be lowered immediately.

Many people go to their doctor regularly and have their blood pressure taken. Many pharmacists have the equipment to measure blood pressure and are willing to provide this service if asked. Likewise, many employers have the required apparatus in their infirmary, and in most cases a company nurse would be happy to comply with an employee's request for a blood pressure reading.

However, perhaps the best way for you to keep track of your blood pressure would be to purchase a stethoscope and sphygmomanometer and learn how to use them. Of course, it is most important that people who have high blood pressure or a tendency toward high blood pressure have and use a sphygmomanometer, but everyone should at least consider the purchase.

Before you take your blood pressure, sit down and relax for a few minutes. Do not drink coffee, tea, or cola beverages, nor should you smoke. Do not take your pressure immediately after exercise, work, or climbing steps. Here are instructions for using the typical mercury type blood pressure kit.

Place the blood pressure cuff on either arm, and inflate it to about 160 to 170 as shown on the scale. The scale measures how high in millimeters a column of mercury (mm Hg) will move under applied pressure. Place the stethoscope on the inside of the arm in front of the elbow, and slowly release the pressure on the cuff. When you first hear your heart beating, note the reading on the gauge. This will be your systolic pressure. As the pressure continues to drop, listen for the point at which you can no longer hear your pulse beating. This reading is called your diastolic pressure. These two figures are commonly written one on top of the other: 120/80 for example, which shows the systolic over diastolic blood pressures.

You should take your blood pressure at least twice in a row to make sure that the readings are consistent. If you get readings that vary by five or ten points, take a third reading and then average the two closest readings and call that your blood pressure reading.

Normal blood pressure varies with age, physical build and athletic prowess, sex, and genetics. Generally, a blood pressure of 120/80 is considered normal for most adults. But blood pressure readings tend to go up with age. If you are 65, your blood pressure may normally be 160/80, 150/85, 163/90, or some other value. There is a normal blood pressure range calculated by age. Ask your doctor for information on your normal range.

It is true, within certain limits, that the lower your blood pressure, the better off you are. Most doctors agree that people with lower blood pressure live longer. On the other hand, if your blood pressure is too low, you might feel so badly throughout the day that your doctor will work to elevate it to a normal value.

46

Pulse Rate

Learn to check your pulse rate. The pulse rate is the number of times your heart beats each minute, and a normal pulse rate range is 65 to 90 beats per minute.

If your pulse rate is more rapid than it should be—100 or 120 beats per minute—it may indicate that you are under stress or tension, that you have a hyperthyroid condition or an infection, that you are anemic, or that you have heart disease, or one of several other diseases. If your pulse rate is lower than normal—say 40 to 50 beats per minute—you may be taking too much of some medication that lowers your heart rate. Or you may have some condition of the nervous system that is keeping your heart from beating more rapidly. Athletes may have slower resting heart rates than normal.

Because some drugs may affect your heartbeat, as may coffee, tea, cola beverages, smoking, and alcohol, try not to consume any of these substances prior to checking your pulse. And do not expect your pulse to be normal immediately after exercise.

To take your pulse, turn your palm upward and find the artery that runs from the arm to your hand. This will be in line with your middle finger. Lay two or three fingers over this artery and, with the second hand on a clock or watch, count the number of beats during a 15-second interval. Multiply this number by four to get the number of beats per minute (for example, 20 beats per 15 seconds $\times$ 4 = 80 beats per minute).

While you are determining your heart rate, pay close attention to whether the beats are regular. Your heart should be beating rhythmically. If your heart seems to speed up or slow down, or if it seems to skip beats sporadically, you should report this to your doctor.

Respiration

Most people never stop to count the number of breaths they take per minute. However, respiration that is faster or slower than normal can be an important symptom of disease.

To take your respiration rate, count the number of breaths that you take for 15 seconds and then multiply that number by four, as you did for your pulse rate. If you have not exercised or worked before taking this count, or consumed any coffee, tea, or carbonated beverages, or smoked, your normal respiration rate should be around 16 to 18 breaths per minute. If you find that it is abnormally high (say over 20 to 25 respirations per minute), then you should contact your doctor. You may have some disease that would cause you to breathe more rapidly. If you are breathing at a rate lower than normal (say 12 to 13 per minute), you should also see your doctor, especially if you have other symptoms such as tiredness or weakness. Because many drugs will elevate the respiration rate while others decrease it, make sure that your doctor is aware of all the drugs that you take.

Skin

Examination of your skin may furnish the first clues to identification of internal diseases as well as to diseases of the skin itself. Include an examination of your skin in your personal checkup.

Observe your skin for moisture. If it seems dry, and especially if it has been dry over the past several days, you may be dehydrated and need more fluid in your diet. Or, you may suffer from a lack of vitamin A, or have certain types of kidney trouble, or thyroid disease. On the other hand, if your skin feels more moist than usual, this may reflect overactive sweat glands, extreme stress or tension, or an overactive thyroid gland.

If your skin feels firm when it is pinched slightly between two fingers, then you may have a localized edema (collection of water) under the skin. This may be a symptom of congestive heart failure or of certain types of kidney disease. If, on the other hand, your skin feels loose when it is pinched, you may be losing weight.

Look at your skin color. If it appears paler than it should, you may have an anemia. If it looks yellowish, this may mean that you have a liver disease. It could also mean that you are taking certain drugs or are eating certain foods (carrots, etc.) that cause your skin to become yellow. A yellowish color may also denote a pernicious anemia or a hypothyroid condition.

If you have black and blue marks, and if you do not remember hitting the affected area, you may bruise too easily. Blood that has come out of the blood vessels will appear to be bluish or blackish in color after it has been out of the vessel for several hours.

If your skin appears dark red and you have not been in the sunshine or under a sunlamp, you may be photosensitive from disease or drugs.

Pay careful attention to rashes. If a rash appears and leaves in a day or so and doesn't return, you should not be particularly concerned. If, on the other hand, a rash reappears regularly, then you may be allergic to something in your diet or environment, and you will want to see your doctor. There may be nothing you can do to treat these rashes other than alleviating minor itching or irritation. On the other hand, if it is an allergic reaction you will want to identify it and then try to avoid future contact with the substance that is causing the allergy. If you don't identify it, you may someday subject yourself to the causative agent and have a more severe allergic reaction that may leave you very sick.

Always look for changes in the appearance of moles, warts, or birthmarks. Pay attention to their size, shape, and color. If any of them change, phone your doctor right away. One of the seven warning symptoms of cancer is any change in a wart or mole. Skin cancer is an extremely dangerous condition if not treated early.

Observe the hairy areas of your body (scalp, eyebrows, and underarm) for changes in quantity or texture of hair. If your hair becomes more brittle or even more silky than normal, you may have a thyroid disease or some other glandular disorder. If your hair is simply falling out, this may reflect no more than inherited baldness. On the other hand, if such a pattern does not run in your family or if hair on the eyebrows, underarms, or on areas of your body other than the scalp is falling out, you should call your doctor. Again, you may have a thyroid disease, cancer, or one of several other diseases of the endocrine system. Or, you may be taking some drug that causes hair loss as a side effect.

Because we see our skin each day, slight changes may be difficult to detect. Thus, it is important to take the advice of those who see you less frequently. You should consider their comments carefully.

Eyes

The appearance of your eyes or the skin around them can tell a lot about your condition. If the white part of your eyes appears to be yellowish, you may have a liver disease. If your eyes are bloodshot, this may reflect simple fatigue and eyestrain. It may also suggest an eye infection or high blood pressure. If the area around your eyes appears puffy and swollen, you may have kidney or heart disease. If your eyes are bulging outward, you may have hyperthyroid disease, or you may even have a tumor behind your eye that is pushing one or both of them outward.

If your eyelids appear to be droopy, you may be tired and need more sleep, but you also may have one of several diseases of the nervous system, such as myasthenia gravis. Or you may have a tumor that is pressing on certain nerve fibers and interfering with nerve impulses to your eyelids. A virus infection may cause the eyelids to look droopy. In any case, you should see your doctor as soon as possible.

Glaucoma is the major cause of blindness in the United States. In most cases, blindness can be prevented if people simply recognize that eye pain is one of glaucoma's first symptoms.

Look at your pupils (the clear spot inside the colored portion of your eye). If they appear to be larger than normal, you may have a fever, or you may have a tumor or other type of brain damage. And certain drugs cause the pupils to become larger, while other drugs cause the pupils to become smaller.

If one pupil appears to be larger than the other, you may have a disease of the nervous system. You should see your doctor right away. Each time you are looking at your pupils, make sure that you have the same amount of light shining in each eye. Light itself will cause your pupils to become smaller. Thus, if you look at your pupils in a mirror with a bright light they will appear to be smaller than when you look at them in a mirror with less light.

Tongue

People have, for centuries, examined their tongues in front of a mirror each morning. In fact, early advertisements for nearly all proprietary medications advised people that if their tongue was nice and red, they were healthy. If their tongue was paler than normal, or if it was rough or painful, these people were advised that they had certain diseases. While it is nearly impossible to tell the state of your health from the appearance of your tongue, you can get some idea of whether certain diseases are present.

For example, if your tongue seems unusually large for your mouth or if it is bulky, if you find it difficult to form your words properly or to move your tongue when you chew, you may have hypothyroid disease. On the other hand, a swollen tongue may also be a sign of increased activity of the pituitary gland. In either case, you must get medical help.

If your tongue is coated or fuzzy, it may signal the consumption of certain foods or excessive alcohol the day before. If the unnatural appearance persists, it may mean you have certain nutritional deficiencies and you should see your doctor. If you see small white spots on your tongue and on the inside of your cheeks, and you know they are not fever blisters or cold sores, you should see your doctor. Such spots are frequently noticed by pipe smokers, and they are irritated areas that some doctors consider to be precancerous.

Fingernails

If your nails are pale, you may be anemic. If they are blue or purplish, you may have a disease of the lungs or of the heart. If they are yellowish, especially if they also look thicker, you may have a fungus infection.

Look at the shape of your nails. If they seem to have valleys in the middle (a convex appearance), this may be a symptom of iron-deficiency anemia. If your nails are rounded in their center (hills), you may have tuberculosis, certain heart diseases, or a lung condition. If any of these symptoms appear, you should contact your doctor.

Special Notes for Women

Every woman over 20 should examine her breasts once a month. The American Cancer Society recommends a three-step examination. First, while in the shower or bath, feel the entire breast with flat fingers, checking for any lump or thickening. After the shower, stand in front of a mirror with your hands on your waist and look for any changes in the contours of your breasts and any swellings or dimples in the skin. Then, raise your arms overhead and check again. Finally, lie down, put your right hand behind your head. With the left hand gently feel your right breast with fingers flat. Press gently in small circular motions over the entire breast. Squeeze the nipple to check for discharge. Then reverse the position, and examine the other breast. Any lump, thickening, dimple, or discharge should be reported to a doctor.

Most women also find it helpful to make note of the beginning of the menstrual cycle, as well as any premonitory symptoms such as bloating or cramps.

Urine

You should look at your urine as it is voided to see if it has blood in it. The presence of a reddish, orangish, or brownish tint may denote bleeding within the kidneys. This is a medical emergency and you should call your doctor right away. A tea-colored urine may indicate the presence of bile, which could be the result of certain types of liver disease.

Certain foods may also make your urine reddish. Beets are a common cause. Several laxatives also make the urine appear red. Other medicines may also change the urine's color, including phenacetin which may make it gray, brown, or blackish. Thorazine and Compazine phenothiazines may turn the urine brown or red; and Elavil antidepressant may turn the urine bluish. Vitamin B complex may impart an orange to extreme yellow color. Other medicines may color urine blue or purple.

Do not be concerned if your urine appears milky or cloudy one day and clear the next. This change is normal and is dependent on many factors including the time of day, the amount and types of foods that you eat, and the amount of fluid you are drinking each day.

A wide variety of OTC urine-testing supplies is available from your pharmacy. You may want to talk to your pharmacist or doctor about using one or more of these products on a routine basis, especially if you are prone to certain diseases. For example, if you have a family history of diabetes, you may want to check your urine every month or so for the presence of sugar. If you have a family history of certain types of kidney disease, you may want to check your urine for the presence of other substances such as protein.

Your body requires a minimal amount of regular maintenance to keep it in good condition. A regular self-examination may detect the early signals of serious disorders, which, if caught early, can be treated easily, inexpensively, and successfully. The few minutes your personal health record may cost could save you the expense and pain of protracted illness.

Family Health Records

Your personal health record should be supplemented by records that list illnesses suffered in the family, allergies and allergic reactions, immunizations, hospitalizations, and the dates of medical, dental, and eye examinations. Women should record when they have Pap tests and gynecological exams. People who have a family history of certain disorders thought to be hereditary—glaucoma, diabetes mellitus, and hypertension for example—should obtain from their doctors a suggested schedule of examinations and tests and should use the family health record to make sure that they comply with the schedule.

Part II
Symptoms, Diseases, and Conditions

Pain and Fever

Pain and fever are the two symptoms that most frequently prompt people to get medical relief, and they are two primary diagnostic tools. The severity, location, duration, and type of pain give important clues to its causes, and certain diseases are characterized by the course of the fever they produce. Your doctor and pharmacist, therefore, will want a full and accurate description of these symptoms before suggesting any treatment.

Pain

People react to pain differently. If two people were pinched with the same degree of pressure, their account of the pain, how they reported it, would no doubt vary a great deal, although each would actually feel the same degree of pain. One might find it trivial and not worth mentioning; the other might find it severe enough to demand some treatment. Because of this difference, health care professionals often try to gauge the personality of the patients they treat by asking questions. The response should give some idea of whether the patient reacts strongly to pain or tends to downplay its severity.

Just as it is sometimes difficult to judge the severity of a person's suffering by how they tell about it, it is sometimes difficult to gauge the severity of a disease by the amount of pain it causes. Even a minor ache or pain can be a symptom of a serious disorder. On the other hand, severe pain may be caused by a minor illness.

In order to help your doctor diagnose the cause of your pain, you should be able to report exactly where your pain is, and also whether any of the surrounding areas are at all painful or tender. Usually, the site of the pain is the site of the disorder. Sometimes, however, pain occurs in areas of the body that are not affected by the disease. Such pain is called referred pain, and it occurs because of the way the nerve fibers run throughout the body. For example, heart disease is more likely to cause pain in the left arm or perhaps along one side of the body than around the heart. Pain caused by an ulcer is generally felt above or below the stomach rather than right over the ulcer. And, pain coming from an infection or inflammation of the sinuses may be felt above or below the eyes or even in the back of the head. Thus, a doctor or pharmacist may treat a headache with medication ordinarily used for a sore back, or a painful shoulder with medication usually employed to treat an ulcer.

Your doctor will also want you to describe the type of pain that you feel. Is the pain intermittent or constant—does it come and go or is it present all of the time? Is it dull, or sharp, or colicky? A pain associated with a bone disease is often said to be aching or boring, whereas pain associated with muscle disease is said to be sore and achy. Pain from heart disease or a heart attack is said to be crushing. The pain from an ulcer may be described as burning or gnawing.

You should record and report whether the pain comes on spontaneously or if it is precipitated by exercise, or certain foods, or certain weather conditions. Does the pain occur at the same time every day, or only at certain times of the year? Some pain is precipitated by certain movements (such as coughing, sneezing, or shaking the head). All such information is helpful in a diagnosis.

Also note what usually relieves the pain. For example, does aspirin or acetaminophen relieve the pain or do you require stronger medication? If a medication does relieve the pain, about how long does it take for relief to occur? Do antacids or tranquilizers relieve the pain? Do certain types of foods, such as milk or dairy products, relieve the pain?

Treatment

For relief of mild headache, toothache, and other minor pains, over-the-counter pain remedies are usually sufficient. Most OTC pain remedies are primarily aspirin or acetaminophen; some have added ingredients—caffeine, phenacetin, antihistamines, or antacids for example. No test has shown that a combination of ingredients is more effective than an equivalent dose of plain aspirin or acetaminophen. Aspirin effectively reduces pain, fever, and inflammation; acetaminophen does not provide anti-inflammatory effects. It is, therefore, less useful than aspirin for treating arthritic pain. However, acetaminophen is less likely to upset the stomach and interfere with blood clotting than is aspirin.

If pain persists for longer than several days, or if nonprescription pain relievers give only temporary relief, medical attention is warranted. Do not continue to take any pain medication if you do not know what is causing the pain. The pain may be caused by a severe disease that, if left untreated (remember pain relievers treat the symptom, not the disease), may progress to cause serious and severe complications.

Fever

Your body temperature is normally regulated at a set point by certain mechanisms in the brain. A "normal" body temperature is considered to be 98.6° F, although many people normally have body temperatures ranging from 97° F to 99.6° F. The normal body temperature varies among people of different ages and when taken at different body locations. It also varies at different times during the day. In the late afternoon or early evening, it may be a half degree or more higher than it is during the night and early morning.

You have a fever whenever your body temperature is about 100.5° F when measured orally, above 101.5° F when measured rectally, or above 99.5° F if you take your temperature under your arm.

The presence of a fever is frequently one of the first signs that something is wrong with your body. A fever indicates that the body's defense mechanism is working. When the body temperature is higher than usual, infecting viruses or bacteria cannot survive. Increased body temperature also triggers the production of interferon, a protein that protects the body cells from serious damage caused by viral infections.

Many people do not feel a low fever per se, but rather feel other symptoms that are caused by the fever—muscular aches and pains or the "blahs." The most common cause of fever is infection due to bacteria or virus. The cause may be obvious, such as a sore on your arm or leg, or it may not be so obvious, as when you have a head or chest cold and perhaps the only other symptom you initially feel is a slight cough and runny nose.

Treatment

Fever itself is not a disease, and "treating" the fever by attempting to bring the body temperature down to normal should not be confused with treating the illness that caused the fever. The primary aim in treating the fever should be to diagnose and treat its cause. However, prolonged fever may cause weakness and dehydration, and lowering the fever somewhat usually makes a patient more comfortable. Aspirin or acetaminophen will effectively lower a fever, and administration of these drugs and increasing the intake of fluids is recommended treatment.

In addition, when you have a fever, you should make a chart listing when you took your temperature and the thermometer readings. Always take your temperature in the same fashion. Do not take it orally in the morning and rectally at night. And, if your fever persists for several days, compare the temperature readings taken at similar times. Do not tell your doctor that your fever was 101° F one day, and then 99° F the next day unless you tell him that one reading was taken in the morning and the other at night.

When should you seek medical help to relieve your fever? First of all, if your fever is high (103° to 104° F) for 12 to 24 hours or more, you should get medical help. Second, if you have a moderate fever (101° to 102° F) that has lasted for two to three days or more, do not let it go any longer without getting medical attention. Third, if your body temperature swings from points of high fever (103° F or so) to lower points (maybe 100° to 101° F) over the day and then the same pattern repeats the following day, get medical attention. Fourth, if you had a fever and after treatment your body temperature returned to normal and stayed there for several days to a week or two but then your fever returned, seek medical attention. The return of a fever is usually a sign that you have developed a secondary infection—an infection other than the one that originally caused your fever.

If any of these criteria apply, even if you have no other symptoms such as runny nose, or a cough, or a sore on your body, get medical help. Possible serious causes of fever include poisoning from various foods or drugs, certain types of cancer, heat stroke, trauma (damage) to the body, or diseases of the thyroid gland, gastrointestinal system, heart, or blood vessels.

Drugs Used In Treatment

Recommended treatment with OTC drugs—*The most economical, safe, and effective drugs to be used in treating pain and fever are plain aspirin and acetaminophen. Choose a moderately priced product; bargain-priced drug items may not be absorbed at the same rate, and they may be less effective than other brands. Buffered products contain aspirin and antacids; no substantial difference in effectiveness between buffered and nonbuffered products has been shown. Buffered products may produce less gastric upset in some people. Enteric-coated products are formulated with a special coating so that they dissolve in the intestines rather than the stomach, thus preventing stomach upset. Among the enteric-coated aspirin products, we recommend Ecotrin, although we suggest you try acetaminophen or a buffered product first if aspirin upsets your stomach.*

OTC analgesics—*Alka-Seltzer; Anacin; Anacin-3; Arthritis Pain Formula; Arthritis Strength Bufferin; Ascriptin; Ascriptin A/D; Aspergum; Bayer; Bayer Children's Aspirin; Bayer Non-Aspirin; Bayer Timed-Release Aspirin; Bromo-Seltzer; Bufferin; Congespirin; Ecotrin; Empirin Compound; Excedrin; Excedrin P.M.; Liquiprin; Measurin; PAC; Percogesic; Sine-Aid; Tempra; Tylenol; Tylenol Extra Strength; Vanquish*

Health Care Accessory—*fever thermometer*

Skin

The skin is a waterproof barrier that protects the body from invasion of bacteria, dirt, and other elements that may be injurious to health. It helps to regulate the body's temperature and also acts as a sensory organ. The skin is richly supplied with sensitive nerve endings. It is the body's largest organ and weighs approximately seven pounds.

The skin is composed of two major layers. The outer layer (the epidermis) and the underlayer (the dermis) cover a layer of fatty tissue. The dermis is sometimes called the true skin because it contains blood vessels, nerve endings, hair follicles, sweat glands, and lymph vessels. The epidermis layer is continuously sloughing off and being rebuilt. Burns or injury to the epidermis usually result in very little trauma to the body because this layer repairs itself quickly. However, damage to the dermis can mean severe damage to the body. Breaks in the dermal layer may allow the entry of bacteria and other infective organisms to the blood or lymph vessels. Through these vessels, the organisms can reach all parts of the body.

Acne

Common acne is an inflammatory disease of the skin characterized by overactivity of the oil-secreting glands. The excess oil (or sebum) tends to clog the pores. While the exact cause is unknown, acne is thought to be genetically related. Acne is more common in males, although it does occur in females. Usually it first appears at the time of the increase in sex hormones during puberty. Acne may continue through the fourth or fifth decade of life although it usually ends by the late teens or early twenties.

Several factors seem to be associated with the course of the disease:

Diet or drugs. Certain foods seem to aggravate acne in some patients. These include nuts, cola, chocolate, seafood, and sometimes milk. If a food is suspected of aggravating the condition, it should be discontinued for at least three weeks to see if the acne improves. Certain birth control pills may make acne worse.

Trauma. Trying to remove blackheads or pinching pimples may contribute to the spread of acne and cause permanent pitting and scarring. Resting the chin on the hands or reading in a reclining position may also aggravate the condition.

Climate. Acne often improves during the summer and gets worse during the winter. However, excessive heat and humidity may cause an exacerbation.

Menses. Acne often seems to get worse around the time of the menses.

Emotion. Stress seems to affect the activity of the oil-secreting glands and may aggravate the condition.

Symptoms

Acne involves the formation of pimples and open and closed comedones (blackheads and whiteheads).

In addition to lesions on the face, neck, back, chest, and shoulders, acne sometimes causes pain, itching, or mild soreness. Someone with acne may feel self-conscious or embarrassed and therefore be inhibited in social relations.

Treatment

If acne is not treated, cyst formation with severe pitting and scarring may occur.

Home treatment includes washing the affected area two or three times a day with soap and lots of water. More frequent washing usually does not eliminate excess oil and, in fact, may cause drying of the skin. A soft complexion brush or a soap that is slightly abrasive may help but should be avoided if lesions are inflamed. Picking at or pinching lesions may cause deep-pitted permanent scar formation.

Someone with acne should avoid greasy cleansing creams and cosmetics, should shampoo once or twice a week, and should remove any blackheads with a comedo extractor. If the comedones are severe, Retin-A in lotion, cream, or gel form is recommended. Fostex, Sulforcin, Oxy-5, Oxy-10, and Vanoxide acne preparations are also useful.

The use of an abrasion cream or product may be beneficial if it is not used to excess. It should be gently applied as directed. Those with especially dark skin should talk to a doctor before using one of these abrasive products. A doctor should also be consulted about the use of a sunlamp or ultraviolet lamp.

A variety of drugs are also used to treat acne. Tetracycline, a widely used antibiotic, may be taken orally on a daily basis to control flare-ups. Some antibiotics are also used topically. These include tetracycline, erythromycin, and clindamycin. These usually require special solutions mixed by a pharmacist from a doctor's prescription.

Females with certain types of acne may be treated successfully with certain birth control medications.

Drugs Used in Treatment

Recommended treatment with OTC drugs—*The contents of OTC products used for acne are changing rapidly. We suggest that you check the labels of the products you buy and look for a product containing either 5 or 10 percent benzoyl peroxide in a pleasantly colored base. Examples of such products among our profiled drugs include Oxy-5, Oxy-10, and Vanoxide.*
OTC acne preparations—*Acne-Aid; Acnomel; Brasivol; Clearasil; Epi-Clear; Fostex; Fostril; Ionax; Komed; Liquimat; Microsyn; Oxy-5; Oxy-10; Porox 7; Rezamid; Stri-Dex; Sulforcin; Topex; Vanoxide*
℞ acne preparation—*Retin-A*
℞ antibiotics—*erythromycin; tetracycline hydrochloride*
℞ oral contraceptives

Bedsores

Bedsores may occur whenever there is prolonged pressure on one part of the body. The pressure cuts off the blood supply to the underlying tissue, which then suffers from the loss of nutrients and dies. Bedsores are seen most frequently among patients who are bedridden or paralyzed.

Symptoms

A bedsore begins as a shiny red area in which loss of sensation is experienced. Because the patient no longer feels pressure on the area, there is little motivation to shift position and relieve that pressure. Gradually the skin sloughs off, and the sore becomes a large ulceration. Bedsores occur most often on bony parts of the body that are not well protected by layers of fat and muscle: hips, ears, elbows, heels, and ankles. They also occur frequently on the buttocks. Bedsores may become infected if not treated.

Prevention and Treatment

Treatment is slow and difficult, and it is far easier to prevent bedsores than it is to treat them. Prevention is as simple as taking care to move the patient once every hour to prevent prolonged pressure on any single area. Inflated rubber cushions or sheepskin pads should be placed under the area if redness or tenderness becomes apparent. Every effort should be made to keep the area clean and dry.

If bedsores do occur, they often can be treated with products such as Vioform-Hydrocortisone cream, a steroid hormone and anti-infective, or with an anti-infective powder. An effective older method of treatment is the application of an aqueous merthiolate solution followed by an application of milk of magnesia. Surgery is sometimes required to excise dead tissue.

Drugs Used in Treatment

Recommended treatment with OTC drugs—*To treat bedsores choose the generic brands of milk of magnesia and merthiolate carried by your pharmacy.*
OTC miscellaneous—*merthiolate; milk of magnesia*
OTC external anti-infective—*B.F.I.*
R_x **steroid hormone**—*Vioform-Hydrocortisone*

Health Care Accessories—*invalid cushions; sheepskin pads*

Boils and Carbuncles

A boil is an infection, usually due to staphylococcus bacteria, that affects a hair follicle and the surrounding tissue. Boils commonly develop on the neck, face, armpit, and back. Occasionally boils develop where petroleum jelly products have been used, presumably because of the constant blockage of the hair follicles.

A carbuncle results when several boils have formed at the same spot and have merged together into a single large unit.

Symptoms

Boils appear as abscesses that range from pea-size to the size of a ping pong ball. They may appear to be rounded or slightly conical with a seeping head. As the boil fills with pus, it presses on the underlying nerves and causes severe pain. The area around the boil will be swollen, tender, and red. Someone with boils may have a fever and feel tired and weak.

Carbuncles are larger than boils and will have more than one seeping head. The pain and tenderness caused by a carbuncle will be more severe than that caused by a boil.

Treatment

Boils are very communicable. Thus, the towels and washcloths used by a person with boils should be kept separate from those used by the rest of the household.

It may take several days or several weeks for the boil to fill with pus. Throughout this period, the boil will be painful. To hasten the boil's development, the area should be soaked in warm water several times a day to increase blood supply to the area and speed up the inflammatory process. Frequently, the soaking causes the boil to burst open by itself. If the boil bursts, the pus that drains out should be caught on a piece of gauze, and the area around the boil should be carefully washed with soap and water and then wiped with rubbing alcohol and blotted dry with gauze. An antibiotic cream or ointment should be applied, and the area should then be covered with a sterile gauze pad. Once the boil bursts and drainage is complete, the boil usually heals rapidly. If it does not seem to be healing after two or three days, it should be seen by a doctor.

Boils should never be pinched as this may force the pus deeper into the skin and possibly into the bloodstream, causing serious systemic infection. All boils on the face, any that do not seem to be healing, and all carbuncles should be treated by a doctor. The doctor may lance and drain the boil and then prescribe oral antibiotics such as penicillin or erythromycin.

Drugs Used in Treatment

Recommended treatment with OTC drugs—*Your pharmacy's generic brand of rubbing alcohol is recommended to clean around a boil that has burst. Recommended antibiotic ointments include Mycitracin, Neo-Polycin, Neosporin, or Polysporin.*
OTC external anti-infective—*Baciguent; Mycitracin; Neo-Polycin; Neosporin; Polysporin*
Rx antibiotics—*erythromycin; penicillin; tetracycline hydrochloride*

Health Care Accessories—*dressings; gauze and gauze bandages*

Bunion

A bunion is a thickening and swelling at the base of the big toe. The deformity pushes the big toe toward the other toes, causing pain that is made worse by walking. Bunions occur more commonly in women, and they usually appear on both feet. There may be a familial tendency to develop bunions, and wearing ill-fitting shoes may be a contributing factor. Prolonged pressure on the area causes inflammation, and infection may also occur.

Treatment

Placing strips of cotton, pads of cloth, or bunion pads between the big toe and the second toe usually does not alleviate the problem.

It is helpful to cut out the section of shoe that rubs against the enlarged area and to purchase special shoes designed not to press against the bunion. The only truly beneficial treatment is surgical removal of the bunion and correction of the bony deformity.

Drugs Used in Treatment

OTC analgesics—*see the list under Pain and Fever*

Health Care Accessories—*foot care products*

Canker Sores and Fever Blisters

Canker sores. Canker sores occur on the mucous lining of the lips, cheeks, tongue, or gums, usually around areas already irritated. For example, they may arise where lips or cheeks have been bitten repeatedly or where improperly fitted dentures have been rubbing against the gums. They also may appear after eating certain foods, including chocolate, tomatoes, walnuts, melons, vinegar, spices, or citrus fruits. Their cause is not always clear; some causes appear to be psychosomatic.

Canker sores produce a burning or tingling sensation that may be extremely painful. Sometimes pain precedes the appearance of the canker sore by as much as a day. Usually only a few canker sores appear at one time, although there may be as many as 60 present, and they last for about 10 to 14 days. They tend to recur. They usually heal without scarring.

Fever blisters. Fever blisters, or cold sores, occur on the lips, on and around the nostrils, and in the mouth, and they are caused by the herpes simplex virus. They can be painful and irritating, and usually accompany a fever. Bad breath, loss of appetite, increased flow of saliva, and pain or a tingling sensation are frequent forerunners of fever blisters. These symptoms may occur as early as two days before the sore appears. Fever blisters rarely last more than ten days.

Treatment

OTC drugs for canker sores and fever blisters have the same objective: to relieve pain.

Lactinex diarrhea remedy has been suggested as a remedy for canker sores. However, Lactinex has not yet proved to be effective, and the extra cost of this product over the cost of other, more medically sound drugs is not warranted.

Many OTC drugs used to relieve the pain of a fever blister come in solutions of 70 percent or more alcohol. While these products may provide temporary relief, they do not remain where they have been applied, but run off. Instead of using one of these solutions, choose an ointment or a gel.

Herpes simplex may be treated by using an anti-infective powder or camphor spirits on the lesion twice daily. A moistened styptic pencil can be applied to the lesion several times daily. If these agents do not bring about relief in a couple of days, see a doctor. The drying action of these agents may cause the lesion to crack open, leading to secondary infection. Never use one of the topical corticosteroid creams unless the doctor specifically recommends it. Many doctors prefer that their patients keep the lesion moist by applying petroleum jelly and allow the disorder to run its course.

Cold sores accompanied by other symptoms—an extremely sore throat, fever, joint pain, or palpitations—can indicate more serious diseases and require diagnosis by a doctor.

Drugs Used in Treatment

Recommended treatment with OTC drugs—*OTC products for canker sores that contain carbamide peroxide (Gly-Oxide) are more effective than those containing other ingredients. Carbamide peroxide releases oxygen in the mouth, and the oxygen acts as an antiseptic to clean and promote healing. B.F.I. powder or camphor spirits (the generic brand your pharmacy carries) will effectively help to dry fever blisters.*
OTC canker sore and fever blister remedies—*Blistex; Gly-Oxide*
OTC external anti-infective—*B.F.I.*

Chafing

Chafing is irritation of the skin caused by moisture, warmth, and friction when two surfaces of skin rub against one another. Infection by bacteria or fungi is a common complication.

The use of dusting powder on a regular basis and weight reduction by obese individuals will help prevent chafing. In hot weather, wearing cool clothing and avoiding exertion will reduce the likelihood of irritation.

Cool compresses usually relieve the initial manifestations of redness, itching, and burning. On occasion, steroid preparations used locally may help the itching and inflammation.

Drugs Used in Treatment

Recommended treatment with OTC drugs—*Johnson's Baby Powder is pure talc; it will soothe irritated skin.*
OTC rash remedies—*A and D; Ammens Medicated; Baby Magic (lotion, oil, and powder); Borofax; Desitin (ointment and powder); Diaparene; Diaparene Peri-Anal; Johnson's Baby Cream; Johnson's Baby Powder; Johnson & Johnson Medicated Powder; Mexsana Medicated Powder*
R steroid hormones—*Aristocort; Medrol; Mycolog; prednisone; Synalar; Valisone; Vioform-Hydrocortisone*

Chigger Bites

Chiggers are tiny red mites. When the young chigger bites human skin, it secretes saliva that destroys surrounding cells. The chigger itself does not burrow into the skin, but the skin hardens into a tube around the chigger. Within the tube the chigger feeds on the host until it becomes engorged with blood. Then the mite drops to the ground.

While harboring the chigger, the host experiences irritation and intense itching. Scratching the area may lead to infection, inflammation, and blistering.

Symptoms

Chigger bites occur most frequently around the waist, under garters, on the feet (especially the soles), between the toes, and around the ankles. The first apparent symptom is small flat red spots. The mite will be visible as a pinpoint in the center of each spot. Within a day, the spots develop into itchy bumps, sometimes with clear blistery tops.

Treatment

Treatment involves asphyxiating the mite and relieving the irritation. An application of mineral oil can safely accomplish this. A pharmacist can supply a flexible collodion containing camphor or phenol which will serve the same purpose. A collodion is a liquid applied to the skin that dries to a transparent film. An application of clear fingernail polish can be tried, but it may cause further irritation in some individuals.

If the area becomes extremely red or irritated, it should be carefully washed with soap and water, and then a cream or ointment containing an antibiotic should be applied several times a day.

Drugs Used in Treatment

Recommended treatment with OTC drugs—*Mineral oil and flexible collodion (consult your pharmacist) will asphyxiate the mite. If the bite becomes inflamed, it is likely to be infected and an antibiotic ointment (Mycitracin, Neo-Polycin, Neosporin, or Polysporin) should be applied.*
OTC external anti-infectives—*Baciguent; Mycitracin; Neo-Polycin; Neosporin; Polysporin*

Contact Dermatitis

Contact dermatitis is an inflammation of the skin resulting from contact with some irritant, or allergen. The lesions appear on parts of the skin exposed to the irritant. Often, contact dermatitis is due to soaps or detergents or other solvents in household cleaners. Other cases are caused by certain drugs (such as antibiotics or antihistamines) and by other chemicals in foods, preservatives, and cosmetics. A reaction to poison ivy or poison oak is also contact dermatitis.

Symptoms

The primary symptoms of contact dermatitis include burning, itching, and stinging. The itching may be severe. The affected area may become swollen and may develop blisters that ooze a clear fluid. Fluid which becomes cloudy, yellow or straw-colored may indicate bacterial infection.

Treatment

The first order of treatment is to identify and remove the irritant or allergen. The location of the rash is often the first clue to the identity of the irritant. If the inflammation is on the face, then makeup, soaps, or shaving materials may be the cause. A rash on the neck can be caused by cosmetics or even a soap or detergent residue left on the necks of shirts or sweaters. If the dermatitis is on the scalp, then hair tints, sprays, or shampoos may be the cause. An allergist can run tests to narrow down the list of suspected culprits.

Once the irritant has been identified, every attempt should be made to eliminate it from the patient's environment to prevent recurrence of the dermatitis. If the irritant is a soap or detergent, the patient should try switching brands, wearing rubber gloves while washing dishes, and if possible avoiding tasks which require the use of soaps or detergents. If cosmetics are at fault, a switch to unscented or hypoallergenic brands may be helpful. If the reaction is caused by the metals in jewelry, metal jewelry should not be worn.

The itching of contact dermatitis can be relieved by orally administered steroids such as prednisone or triamcinolone (found in Aristocort steroid hormone). Topical steroids may also be used, but they do not provide the same relief. Antihistamines are sometimes prescribed but they are not usually as effective as the steroids.

Drugs Used in Treatment

Recommended treatment with OTC drugs—*Johnson's Baby Powder is pure talc; it will soothe minor irritation. If irritation is severe, prescribed medication may be necessary.*
OTC rash remedies—*A and D; Ammens Medicated; Baby Magic (lotion, oil, and powder); Borofax; Desitin (ointment and powder); Diaparene; Diaparene Peri-Anal; Johnson's Baby Cream; Johnson's Baby Powder; Johnson & Johnson Medicated Powder; Mexsana Medicated Powder*
OTC topical steroids—*Cortaid; Dermolate*
Rx steroid hormones—*Aristocort; Medrol; Mycolog; prednisone; Synalar; Valisone; Vioform-Hydrocortisone*
Rx antihistamines—*Benadryl; Periactin; Polaramine*

Related Topics—*Hives; Itching; Poison Ivy/Poison Oak*

Corns and Calluses

A corn is a mass of tightly packed, dead skin cells that occurs at a point of constant pressure on the toes or between them. Corns on the toes may be white, gray, yellow, or dark red; corns between the toes (soft corns) absorb moisture and are white, gray, or yellow spongy sores.

Corns. Corns are usually caused by pressure due to poorly fitting shoes, irregularities in shoes or stockings, or walking on hard surfaces. The pressure enlarges the small blood vessels and reddens the skin. Then, as dead skin cells accumulate, the skin in one small area thickens and becomes swollen. At first, the thickened area may cause no pain, but as a corn grows larger, pain increases due to the compression of underlying nerves.

Calluses. Like a corn, a callus is a mass of dead skin cells. Unlike a corn, a callus appears on the ball of the foot or around the heel, and it is due to prolonged friction, irritation, or constant pressure.

Treatment

Severe corns and calluses should be seen by a podiatrist (foot doctor), but a mild case can be treated with OTC pads or cushions or medication.

Pads or cushions insulate the corn or callus and help alleviate the pain. Medication helps loosen the corn or callus so it can be removed. Most OTC products for corns and calluses contain keratolytics, which soften the skin and cause the cells of the outer layer of the skin to slough off.

Corns and calluses may take a week or more to remove, and the medication must be applied as directed each day. When using a product to remove a corn or a callus, be sure to keep it away from the skin that surrounds the affected area. Place tape around the corn or callus, and then apply medication in the center. Or cover the surrounding tissue with petroleum jelly or some other protective ointment before applying the medication.

Corn and callus removers generally are contraindicated only for those people who are allergic to them. However, people who have diabetes should never take care of corns and calluses themselves.

Corn and callus removers should not be applied to broken skin and should be discontinued if a rash develops. Products of this type are intended for use on a temporary basis until the cause of the problem has been corrected.

To help prevent corns and calluses, use an ointment such as petroleum jelly that will lubricate the area and keep it soft. The best way to avoid corns and calluses is to get shoes and socks that fit well and have no irregularities that continually rub against the toes.

Drugs Used in Treatment

Recommended treatment with OTC drugs—*All of the following products contain salicylic acid, a mild keratolytic, and all are effective corn and callus removers.*
OTC corn and callus removers—*Dr. Scholl's corn and callus remedy; Dr. Scholl's "2" corn and callus remedy; Freezone*
OTC miscellaneous—*Vaseline petroleum jelly*

Health Care Accessories—*foot care products*

Cradle Cap

Cradle cap is a type of dermatitis commonly found among infants under six months of age.

Symptoms

It is characterized by yellowish, scaling, crusty areas on the scalp. Other areas of the body, including the face and crotch area, may also be affected. It may cause temporary loss of hair. Cradle cap causes an increased susceptibility to infection by bacteria and fungi.

Treatment

Mild cases of cradle cap can be treated by carefully washing the skin with a soft cloth and soap. A product like pHisoHex cleanser is very effective,but its directions for use must be followed explicitly. The scales can be rubbed away gently with a washcloth; then, the area should be carefully rinsed and dried.

Drug Used in Treatment

℞ cleanser—*pHisoHex*

Related Topic—*Seborrheic Dermatitis*

Diaper Rash

Almost every baby gets diaper rash. Babies' skin is very sensitive and easily irritated. Diaper rash is basically an irritation caused by moisture and the interaction of urine and the skin.

Symptoms

A slightly rough, red rash confined to the diaper area is likely to be diaper rash, particularly if an ammonia odor is noticed when the diaper is changed. The baby may also be reacting to the soap used to wash the diapers. A simple diaper rash can be complicated by a bacterial or fungal infection, and if the rash is blistery or bumpy, very severe, or extends beyond the diaper area, a doctor's diagnosis should be sought.

Treatment

A simple diaper rash may be relieved by the use of a soothing powder. A protective ointment applied to the skin may help prevent the rash. Make sure that diapers are thoroughly rinsed when they are washed, and if the rash was preceded by a switch in brands of soap, it may be necessary to change brands again.

Keeping the baby as dry as possible—changing diapers promptly—is helpful, as is allowing the baby to go without diapers when possible.

Drugs Used in Treatment

Recommended treatment with OTC drugs—*Johnson's Baby Powder should be soothing. To help prevent the rash, use zinc oxide ointment or Vaseline petroleum jelly.*
OTC rash remedies—*Baby Magic (lotion, oil, and powder); Diaparene; Diaparene Peri-Anal; Johnson's Baby Cream; Johnson's Baby Powder*
OTC miscellaneous—*Vaseline; zinc oxide ointment*

Drug Eruptions

Almost any drug can cause a skin reaction. Reaction to a drug applied locally is called contact dermatitis; reaction to a drug which has been swallowed, inhaled, injected, or otherwise administered is called a drug eruption or dermatitis medicamentosa. A sensitive individual may experience identical reactions to a variety of drugs, or different reactions to the same drug when it is administered at different times.

Symptoms

Symptoms usually include severe itching, redness, joint pain, headache, fever, nausea, vomiting, and loss of appetite. If reaction to a drug is severe, swelling and spasm of the respiratory system may occur, causing breathing difficulty. In some cases drug reactions damage the liver and kidneys, the central nervous system, and the eyes and ears.

Treatment

People who know they react adversely to certain drugs should always avoid those drugs. If a drug is absolutely necessary to the health of someone sensitive to it, it is sometimes possible to desensitize that individual. However, this procedure rarely solves the problem and sensitivity usually returns.

Severe drug eruptions are treated with bronchodilators—intravenously or intramuscularly—to relieve the respiratory distress. Antihistamines and corticosteroids are used to treat other symptoms of the reaction.

Drug Used in Treatment

R_x antihistamine—*Benadryl*

Related Topics—*Allergy; Contact Dermatitis; Photodermatitis*

Eczema

Eczema (atopic dermatitis) is an inflammatory disorder of the skin that has a genetic predisposition. Frequently, people who have eczema display the eczema "triad" of hay fever-asthma-eczema, and eczema is considered by some an allergic disorder. Generally the disorder appears in infancy and then disappears by the age of three years. It may recur in early youth and after that tends to come and go.

Symptoms

Severe itching is a primary symptom. A red rash usually appears over the area including the face, neck, and upper trunk. The bends of the elbows and knees are other common sites. In infants, the rash is usually seen on the cheeks and appears dry and leathery. In adults, the rash is also dry and leathery but may occur on any area of the body.

Treatment

Eczema is best treated with one of the glucocorticoid steroid medications either taken orally or applied topically. Additionally, the area may be cleansed with Cetaphil lotion. Oral antihistamines are also occasionally used to control the itching and to minimize rash.

Someone with eczema should avoid any food or chemical that is known to cause the rash and should consider becoming desensitized to these agents. Also, severe temperature changes and stress should be avoided to help control the eczema rash.

Ointments containing coal tar may be used. Iodochlorhydroxyquin ointment or cream (Vioform-Hydrocortisone) may be used for persons allergic to coal tar preparations.

Drugs Used in Treatment

Recommended treatment with OTC drugs—*Cetaphil skin cleansing lotion should be used in place of soap by someone with eczema. Although sometimes mentioned as an aid in eczema, vitamin A—either topical or oral—is of no proven benefit if there is no vitamin A deficiency.*
OTC miscellaneous—*Cetaphil skin cleansing lotion*
OTC nutritional supplement—*vitamin A*
OTC topical steroids—*Cortaid; Dermolate*
OTC rash remedies—*A and D; Ammens Medicated; Baby Magic (lotion, oil, and powder); Borofax; Desitin (ointment and powder); Diaparene; Diaparene Peri-Anal; Johnson's Baby Cream; Johnson's Baby Powder; Johnson's Medicated Powder; Mexsana Medicated Powder*
OTC antipsoriasis cream—*Tegrin*
℞ steroid hormones—*Cordran; Kenalog; Lidex; Mycolog; Synalar; Valisone; Vioform-Hydrocortisone*
℞ antihistamines—*Benadryl; Periactin; Polaramine*

Hair Loss

Hair loss is a common symptom of several diseases, including various ringworm (fungus) infections and syphilis. It may indicate general ill health. It may also result from localized injury to the head caused by overuse of curlers, continual scalp-rubbing in neurotic children, or hair-pulling in some psychotic patients.

Hair loss may be characteristic of hypothyroid disease, in which case, the eyebrows and the hair under the arms will fall out also. In some cases, the presence of a high fever (104° F or higher) for a long period of time may cause the hair to come out in patches. Additionally, some drugs, chemotherapy, and nervous disorders can be associated with hair loss.

Familial baldness and hair loss due to disease should not be confused. Nothing can be done about familial baldness. However, sudden hair loss in an individual without a family history of baldness demands a doctor's attention.

Related Topic—*Ringworm Infections*

Heat Rash

Heat rash (also known as prickly heat or miliaria) is a mild form of dermatitis that usually occurs on the upper areas of the body and on any area of the body that is easily chapped. The usual cause is a hot, moist environment, and obese people are most often affected. In severe heat rash, the sweat ducts become clogged and eventually rupture, producing an irritating or stinging sensation.

Symptoms

Severe itching and burning are the usual symptoms. If a heat rash is severe enough, heat prostration or fever may occur. Death may result in the most severe forms, but this is not usual. Heat rash usually occurs on areas of the skin that are covered.

Treatment

The most obvious treatment is to move to an air-conditioned room or other cool environment where the airflow over the skin's surface is increased. Once the stimulus to sweat is gone, the heat rash usually disappears within hours or days. The individual should remain in a cool environment, wear light clothing, and abstain from drinking alcoholic beverages. Bathing in a colloidal-oatmeal bath is soothing.

Heat rash may be treated by applying an antipyretic cooling lotion. The doctor can prescribe a lotion containing menthol, phenol, and glycerin in alcohol. OTC rash preparations and bland dusting powders are also beneficial.

Drugs Used in Treatment

Recommended treatment with OTC drugs—*Aveeno Colloidal Oatmeal bath is recommended for soothing the rash. Johnson's Baby Powder is the OTC rash remedy of choice because it is pure talc.*
OTC miscellaneous—*Aveeno*
OTC rash remedies—*A and D; Ammens Medicated; Baby Magic (lotion, oil, and powder); Borofax; Desitin (ointment and powder); Diaparene; Diaparene Peri-Anal; Johnson's Baby Cream, Johnson's Baby Powder; Johnson's Medicated Powder; Mexsana Medicated Powder*

Hirsutism

Hirsutism is a term meaning excessive hair growth on areas of the body that are not normally hairy. There may be a genetic predisposition to hirsutism, or it may be a symptom of disease (for example, cancer) or a drug reaction. Drugs that may cause hirsutism include the corticosteroids and phenytoin. Women who receive testosterone may develop the condition, and hirsutism also sometimes develops at menopause.

If hirsutism is caused by a medical problem, the cause must be identified and treated. Electrolysis is the only permanent, safe method to remove excess hair, but plucking, shaving, chemical depilatories, or bleaches may be used to remove the hair growth temporarily or to make it less obvious.

Hives

Hives (urticaria) is an inflammatory condition of the skin caused by an allergen and characterized by rapidly changing welts. Most cases of hives are caused by food allergies; common offenders include shellfish, pork, strawberries, eggs, milk, tomatoes, or chocolate. Certain drugs, food dyes, molds, bacteria, and emotional disturbances can also cause hives, as can contact with animals. A hidden infection in the body may be the cause and should always be looked for in any acute hives attack.

Symptoms

Red welts may appear all over the body or only in certain areas. The welts vary widely in size and come and go rapidly, sometimes lasting only a few minutes, sometimes a day or two. Usually the rash lasts for a week or two. It causes intense itching. Tiredness, fever, and nausea may also be present. Someone with hives may have difficulty breathing.

Treatment

Hives can be prevented by avoiding the causative agent once it is known. If the allergy is to a certain food and that food is accidentally ingested, an attack of hives may be avoided by taking a dose of castor oil to remove the irritant from the system. Antihistamines taken immediately after exposure help to control swelling. Oral glucocorticoid steroids (prednisone) are used for severe cases which affect the breathing. If someone is prone to developing hives, a source of oxygen for emergency use should be kept available.

Drugs Used in Treatment

Recommended treatment with OTC drugs—*Your pharmacy's generic brand of castor oil is suitable. Chlor-Trimeton antihistamine will help control swelling.*
OTC miscellaneous—*castor oil*
OTC cold and allergy remedy—*Chlor-Trimeton*
OTC topical steroids—*Cortaid; Dermolate*
R̖ antihistamines—*Benadryl; Polaramine*
R̖ steroid hormones—*Aristocort; Medrol; prednisone*
R̖ sedative—*Atarax*

Related Topics—*Allergy; Drug Eruptions; Itching*

Hyperhidrosis

Hyperhidrosis is the term used to describe excessive perspiration caused by overactive sweat glands. It may be local (often confined to the soles, palms, underarms, and groin), or it may be general, as in fever.

Generalized hyperhidrosis can be caused by obesity and certain glandular disorders. Often, the cause of localized hyperhidrosis is unknown. It may be related to anxiety and tension, and it is sometimes treated with mild tranquilizers. Other possible causes include alcoholism and diabetes mellitus.

Symptoms

The skin in the affected area may appear red and swollen or bluish white. In severe cases, hyperhidrosis may cause scaling and fissuring. Bacterial or fungal infections may complicate the condition and cause intense itching and irritation. Hyperhidrosis is frequent during adolescence.

Treatment

Anticholinergic agents are sometimes used to treat the condition, and aluminum chloride solutions or potassium permanganate compresses (both prepared by a pharmacist) can also be helpful.

Drugs Used in Treatment

R̖ anticholinergics—*Librax; Pro-Banthine*
R̖ sedatives—*Atarax; Ativan; Librium; meprobamate; Nembutal; phenobarbital; Serax; Tranxene; Valium*

Impetigo

Impetigo is a highly contagious disease caused by staphylococci and/or streptococci bacteria. It usually affects infants or children but it can affect adults as well. The disease is spread by direct contact with an infected person or with personal objects of an infected individual. Impetigo can be very dangerous to an infant, possibly leading to systemic infection.

Symptoms

The primary symptom of impetigo is itching. The lesions or sores begin as red patches and quickly change to oozing blisters. The scalp and face—especially around the lips and mouth—are common sites for infection. The yellowish or straw-colored fluid that oozes from the vesicles of impetigo may dry on the skin to cause an uncomfortable sensation.

Treatment

Impetigo should be treated by gently removing the crusts from the lesions and blotting dry any fluid that is present underneath. First, hold a piece of gauze or cotton moistened with warm soapy water against the crust for a few minutes to soften it. The area should then be thoroughly washed with soap and water. An antibiotic ointment should be applied. The lesions must not be covered unless they are oozing a lot of fluid, and then the covering must be loose to allow air to get in.

Be sure to dispose of cotton or tissue used to absorb the oozing liquid. Also, keep towels or washcloths used by a person with impetigo separate from those used by other people. After treating the lesions, wash the sink and counter area well and then swab with rubbing alcohol. Also, be sure to scrub the hands carefully, especially under the fingernails.

The impetigo should clear within several days to a week. However, in more severe cases, oral antibiotics such as erythromycin or penicillin may be necessary.

Drugs Used in Treatment

Recommended treatment with OTC drugs—*Impetigo is an infection; therefore an antibiotic ointment (Mycitracin, Neo-Polycin, Neosporin, or Polysporin) is indicated. Rubbing alcohol (your pharmacy's generic brand is recommended) will be needed to clean the sink area after treating the lesions.*
OTC external anti-infectives—*Baciguent; Mycitracin; Neo-Polycin; Neosporin; Polysporin*
R antibiotics—*amoxicillin; ampicillin; erythromycin; Keflex; Minocin; penicillin G; penicillin potassium phenoxymethyl; Terramycin; tetracycline hydrochloride; Vibramycin*

Health Care Accessory—*gauze*

Ingrown Toenails

Ingrown toenails are a common foot problem initiated by tightly-fitting shoes, injury to the toes, or improper cutting of the toenails.

Symptoms

The pain and tenderness of an ingrown toenail result when the corner or edge of the toenail breaks the skin surrounding the nail. The break in the skin may encourage infection that causes swelling of the tissues surrounding the nail. There may be a discharge of thin, watery pus. The toe becomes extremely sensitive to pressure.

Treatment

An ingrown toenail can be treated by soaking the toe in hot water to soften the skin. Then the nail can be gently lifted up, and a small piece of gauze or cotton can be inserted underneath the edge of the nail. Moistening the gauze first with castor oil will make it easier to insert and will also help further soften the skin. The nail will grow out, eventually extending over the flap of the skin. Wearing sandals while the nail grows out will reduce pressure and pain. If the skin or nail begin to change color or pus appears, a podiatrist should be consulted.

An OTC product, Outgro ingrown toenail remedy, can be used to toughen the skin around ingrown toenails, allowing the nail to be cut.

Once the nail has grown out, future problems can be prevented by trimming the toenails straight across. The corners of the cut nail should not be curved. In addition, care should be taken that shoes fit properly.

Drugs Used in Treatment

Recommended treatment with OTC drugs—*Outgro ingrown nail remedy is effective. If you use castor oil, choose your pharmacy's generic brand.*
OTC miscellaneous—*castor oil; Outgro*

Insect Bites and Stings

In most cases, a bite or sting from an insect is no more than an inconvenience. It may hurt briefly or itch for a few days. It may cause a slight rash. However, people who have developed hypersensitivity to insect stings can be very seriously affected by a bite or sting. The injection of the insect's venom may initiate a potentially fatal allergic reaction.

Symptoms of Allergic Reaction

Someone who reacted adversely to the bite or sting of an insect in the past is likely to be sensitive. The pattern of the reaction varies with the individual. One person may not experience any discomfort for several hours after the sting; another may react immediately. Possible reactions include: swelling, shortness of breath, palpitations (sudden, rapid heartbeat), coughing, wheezing, and light-headedness. The area around the bite may swell to immense size and become quite tender, or it may become completely numb.

Treatment

Anyone allergic to insect stings should rush to a doctor after being stung. Immediate medical treatment includes an adrenalin injection. The adrenalin will help the body to fight off the reaction.

If an ice pack is available, it should be used over the stung area as soon as possible. A tourniquet is useful for a bite on an extremity as long as it is not so tight that it completely stops the blood flow. Both measures will slow the spread of venom through the body.

Many allergic people keep insect bite kits with them. These kits contain adrenalin for injection, as well as other first aid measures that may be needed. The kits are prescribed by a doctor. Some doctors are able to conduct tests to determine whether someone is sensitive to insect bites and stings.

Symptoms of Nonallergic Reaction

Most people are not allergic to insect stings and bites, but no one is immune to the mild skin reaction caused by them. Normally, both stings and bites cause local irritation, swelling, and itching that provoke intense rubbing and scratching. Secondary infections may occur and may result in impetigo or other dangerous skin diseases.

Treatment

To treat an insect sting or bite, apply an ice pack over the affected area to help reduce swelling. Treat other symptoms of itching and irritation with OTC remedies.

Drugs Used in Treatment

Recommended treatment with OTC drugs—*To treat the itching caused by an insect sting or bite, use Bactine antiseptic, which contains alcohol and other ingredients that counteract itching. Or the area can be doused with a half-and-half solution of water and rubbing alcohol (your pharmacy's generic brand).*
OTC insect sting and bite remedies—*Americaine; Bactine; Foille; Medi-Quik; Noxzema; Nupercainal; Solarcaine*

Health Care Accessory—*ice bag*

Related Topics—*Chigger Bites; Impetigo; Itching; Poison Ivy/Poison Oak*

Itching

Itching is any disagreeable sensation that causes the desire to scratch. It may be experienced as a stinging, crawling, or burning sensation. It is the single most common symptom of skin disorders, and some people feel that they can tolerate pain better than they can tolerate itching.

Itching is commonly caused by an allergen, a fungus infection (athlete's foot), or by contact with some irritant like poison ivy or poison oak. Excessive dryness of the skin due to overbathing or wind or sun exposure can aggravate itching. Emotional upsets make some people itchy. This type of itching usually lasts for only a few days and can be relieved by soaking the affected area in hot water, by using medications containing mild local anesthetics, or by using lotions and oils formulated for dry skin.

However, if the itching persists for more than a week, or if there are seeping lesions on the skin's surface, the condition demands a doctor's attention. This type of itching may be due to an infection or to a serious disease such as cancer, syphilis, certain types of liver disease, gout, and uremia. Certain drugs can also cause generalized itching.

Treatment

The best treatment for a minor itch due to an irritant, allergen, or emotional upset is to remove the causative agent. If a feeling of itchiness always follows the use of certain soaps or detergents, a switch to a different brand may solve the problem. If the itching is a reaction to a certain fiber, that fiber should be avoided.

If the itching is aggravated by dryness of the skin, bathing in lukewarm water for 15 minutes two or three times a day may be helpful. If the entire body is dry and itchy, bath oil should be used in the bathwater. If only a few specific areas are affected, the skin should be blotted dry after getting out of the water, and Vaseline petroleum jelly should then be rubbed into the dry areas. A colloidal-oatmeal preparation added to the water can also be soothing, but bubble baths may aggravate itchiness. Elderly people with excessively dry skin should not take a tub bath more than once a day. A doctor may even recommend that baths be limited to once a week.

If such measures fail to bring relief, or if signs of infection are present, a doctor's examination is recommended.

The glucocorticoid creams such as Aristocort cream may be applied to the itchy spot if the itch is caused by an allergen, by dermatitis, or by certain infections. Glucocorticoid tablets may be taken if itching occurs over large parts of the body. Antihistamine medications, such as chlorpheniramine or cyproheptadine, may be taken orally. Antihistamine creams applied to the skin have not been shown to be truly efficacious. Local anesthetic creams and ointments have limited value and may further aggravate the condition because of the sensitivity they induce. Sedatives may relax the body enough to relieve the itching. If only a small area is itchy, the application of an ice bag often helps.

Drugs Used in Treatment

Recommended treatment with OTC drugs—*Vaseline petroleum jelly and Aveeno Colloidal Oatmeal preparation are recommended OTC products to relieve itching.*

OTC miscellaneous—*Aveeno; Vaseline*

OTC rash remedies—*A and D; Ammens Medicated; Baby Magic (lotion, oil, and powder); Borofax; Desitin; Diaparene; Diaparene Peri-Anal; Johnson's Baby Cream; Johnson's Baby Powder; Johnson & Johnson Medicated Powder; Mexsana*

OTC burn remedies—*Americaine; Bactine; Foille; Medi-Quik; Noxzema; Nupercainal; Solarcaine*

OTC topical steroids—*Cortaid; Dermolate*

R steroid hormones—*Aristocort; Cordran; Medrol; Mycolog; prednisone; Synalar; Valisone; Vioform-Hydrocortisone*

R antihistamines—*Benadryl; Periactin; Polaramine*

R sedatives—*Atarax; Ativan; Librium; meprobamate; Nembutal; phenobarbital; Serax; Tranxene; Valium*

Health Care Accessory—*ice bag*

Related Topics—*Chigger Bites; Contact Dermatitis; Drug Eruptions; Eczema; Heat Rash; Hives; Impetigo; Insect Bites and Stings; Lice Infestation; Poison Ivy/Poison Oak; Pruritus Ani/Pruritus Vulvae; Psoriasis; Ringworm Infections; Scabies; Seborrheic Dermatitis; Shingles*

Lice Infestation

Pediculosis is the medical term for an infestation of body lice. The infestation may involve the head, the entire body, or the pubic area (in which case, the lice are known as crabs). The head louse and the pubic louse live directly on the host; body lice usually live in the seams of undergarments. Lice are carriers of typhus, and if an infestation is left untreated, severe disease may result.

Lice depend on blood for their food. When they infest a body, their mouth parts penetrate the skin and seek out small blood vessels from which they can suck blood. When they have found a source of food, the lice quickly reproduce. The female may lay from three to ten eggs per day. The eggs are white or yellow in color. The eggs of head lice and crabs are firmly attached to hair shafts or the skin. The eggs of the body louse may be found in the underclothing.

Head Lice. Head lice are transmitted by personal contact or by sharing personal items such as a towel or comb. Infestation with head lice is now common among schoolchildren. Head lice can be identified by their visible eggs (called nits), about the size of a flake of dandruff, clinging to hair shafts.

Body Lice. Infestation with body lice is uncommon in the United States. Transmitted by contact with an infested person, the lice live in the seams of undergarments and leave only when they must feed.

Pubic Lice. Crab infestation is the most frequent type of pediculosis in the United States. Usually transmitted during sexual intercourse, crabs can also be picked up from infested clothing, bed linens, or toilet seats. The lice may be found in the scalp or beard as well as in the pubic area.

Symptoms

Pediculosis causes intense itching. Scratching should be avoided because it may lead to infection or it may transmit the lice or their eggs to other parts of the body. Inspection for eggs or lice is the most reliable method of diagnosis.

Treatment

OTC products can rid the body of parasitic head, body, or crab lice. The chemicals in these products act only on the insects. After applying the product as directed, use a fine-toothed comb to remove dead insects and eggs from the hair. Or apply a solution of vinegar and water (half-and-half) and then shower. The entire family should be inspected for lice.

These products should not be used more frequently than indicated on the label, and care should be taken that none of the solution gets into the eyes. These products may cause irritation and should not be used on children except with a doctor's direction. If the condition does not respond quickly with one of these products, medical attention is necessary. A product containing gamma benzene hexachloride (Kwell or Gamene pediculocides) will probably be prescribed.

Linens, personal objects, clothing, hats, and furniture should be cleaned or dry-cleaned to kill lice and their eggs. An OTC product (Li-Ban lice control spray) is designed to be used on objects that would be difficult to clean otherwise (mattresses, for example).

Drugs Used in Treatment

Recommended treatment with OTC drugs—*Either of the antilouse preparations (A-200 Pyrinate, Rid) listed will effectively kill the insects and their eggs. Li-Ban lice control spray is also effective for the purpose listed above.*
OTC antilouse preparations—*A-200 Pyrinate; Rid*
OTC lice control spray—*Li-Ban*
R̵ pediculocide—*Kwell*

Photodermatitis

Photodermatitis, or contact photodermatitis, is an inflammation of the skin due to overexposure or hypersensitivity to sunlight. Increased sensitivity to sunlight may be a side effect of certain drugs, or it may be caused by certain genetic disorders or by allergy to certain chemicals in cosmetics, antiseptics, and other products.

Symptoms

Photodermatitis is characterized by inflammation in areas of the skin that have been exposed to sunlight. Accompanying symptoms may include pain, nausea, vomiting, fever, and malaise. Sometimes unconsciousness occurs. There may be oozing lesions and swelling.

Treatment

If the condition is caused by a drug reaction or allergen, either the offending substance should be avoided or exposure to sunlight should be avoided while taking or using that substance. If exposure is unavoidable, the skin should be covered and protected as much as possible. Para-aminobenzoic acid, contained in protective sunscreening agents, may help, but it may interact with other drugs. Check with your pharmacist. Two or three tablets of aspirin taken every three to four hours before going out and while in the sun may help, due to aspirin's anti-inflammatory properties. If the inflammation is already present, corticosteroids may be beneficial.

Cool, soothing wet dressings and soothing skin lotions may also help reduce irritation. Severe irritation should be treated by a doctor.

Generally the condition is self-limiting if it is due to allergy or drug reaction. The hypersensitivity ceases as soon as the drug is stopped or the irritant is avoided. However, in some cases, hypersensitivity persists after discontinuation of the drug. In this case a doctor should be consulted.

Drugs Used in Treatment

OTC analgesics—*see the list under Pain and Fever*
OTC topical steroids—*Cortaid; Dermolate*
R̟ steroid hormones—*Aristocort; Medrol; prednisone*

Related Topics—*Burns and Sunburn; Contact Dermatitis; Drug Eruptions*

Poison Ivy/Poison Oak

The plant family called Rhus has caused an enormous amount of summertime misery, for it is this family that includes poison ivy and poison oak. These plants contain the chemical urushiol. If someone who is sensitive to this chemical comes in contact with it, it causes severe itching, blistering, and watering. Sensitivity to poison ivy or poison oak usually produces a reaction only on the skin, but if fumes from burning the plants are inhaled, the respiratory tract may be affected. About 70 percent of the American population is susceptible. Dark-skinned people are less susceptible than others. Children under age three are seldom susceptible.

Prevention

Everyone should be guided by the old saying, "leaves three, let them be," because the triple-leaf growth habit of these plants is their most distinguishing feature. However, many people aren't able to recognize the plants in all seasons and locales. Depending on the habitat, poison ivy, for example, can be a trailing vine or a free-standing bush ten feet tall. The leaves may be thick and glossy or broad and dull, and they change color during the year. They're purplish in the spring, green in the summer, and yellow, red, or orange in the fall.

If the plant is recognized only after contact has been made, a shower should be taken immediately to abate the reaction. Someone who has been exposed should take care to wash completely with soap and shampoo, to scrub under the nails, and to dry thoroughly after the shower.

Any clothing, sports equipment, or garden tools that could have been contaminated must be washed. If the family dog was romping through a patch of poison ivy or poison oak, it should be bathed and the bather should be sure to wash the hands and arms afterward.

Symptoms

Itching usually develops within two to twenty-four hours of contact. Pin-sized clear blisters then develop. They may appear in straight lines, but the rash may also be spread generally over the skin and may look similar to other rashes.

Treatment

Most rashes due to poison ivy or poison oak go away without treatment in one or two weeks. The following treatment will reduce discomfort somewhat: Wash the hands and the affected area in hot, soapy water. Rinse well, and dry. Using a clean, wooden tongue depressor, or other blunt object—such as a butter knife—gently scrape across the skin until the tops of the blisters are loose. Allow the fluid to escape from the blisters so it will not interfere with medication, and pat the area dry. Then, apply an OTC product that contains calamine or zinc oxide. Repeat the process each evening or as often as needed.

Calamine and zinc oxide protect underlying tissue and dry the affected area. However, they are messy and will leave a crust on the skin after they have dried. Therefore, many people do not want to use them during the day. An alternative to calamine or zinc oxide is a solution of rubbing alcohol and water (half-and-half). It will sting for a minute, but it will relieve the itching. Witch hazel, aftershave lotion, or even hot water can be used in place of rubbing alcohol. If itching is still intense, soak in a tub of hot water for 15 to 20 minutes. Avoid scratching. Scratching can cause skin damage and infection.

Topical OTC products for poison ivy or poison oak that contain either an anesthetic or an antihistamine are not recommended. Anesthetics in OTC products include benzocaine, diperodon hydrochloride, dibucaine, tetracaine hydrochloride, cyclomethycaine, and pramoxine hydrochloride. Of these, benzocaine is the best for the relief of itching. However, at least a 5 percent concentration of benzocaine is needed, and a 20 percent concentration is even better.

Antihistamines are included in these products to help relieve itching, but only one antihistamine—diphenhydramine hydrochloride—actually offers any significant relief. And anesthetics and antihistamines may cause the skin to blister and itch more than it already does.

A topical steroid is now available over-the-counter. It may be tried to relieve inflammation, but it has not been proven effective for this purpose.

Avoid any product that contains zirconium oxide (or zirconia). After one or two weeks of use, it has been shown to cause severe skin irritation in some people.

For severe cases of poison ivy or poison oak or any case that seems to affect the breathing, see a doctor. A prescription for a strong glucocorticoid steroid product may be used. These medications are taken orally and are applied directly to the area in the form of creams, ointments, and sprays.

Drugs Used in Treatment

Recommended treatment with OTC drugs—*Your pharmacy's generic brands*

of calamine lotion and rubbing alcohol are recommended for relief of itching.
OTC miscellaneous—*calamine lotion; zinc oxide ointment*
OTC topical steroids—*Cortaid; Dermolate*
OTC poison ivy remedies—*Caladryl; Ivy Dry; Neoxyn; Rhulicream; Rhulihist; Ziradryl*
℞ steroid hormones—*Aristocort; Cordran; Kenalog; Lidex; Medrol; Mycolog; prednisone; Synalar; Valisone*

Poison Sumac

See treatment for Poison Ivy/Poison Oak.

Pruritus Ani/Pruritus Vulvae

The terms "pruritus ani" and "pruritus vulvae" refer to severe itching of the anal or genital area. These parts of the body are particularly susceptible to the development of itching because the area is always moist and it is exposed to fecal material retained in the anal-rectal folds.

Causes of the itching may be rough toilet tissue, hemorrhoids, hard stools, diarrhea, certain vitamin deficiencies (A and the Bs), and poor sanitary habits. Additionally, certain infections (yeast and fungal), as well as intestinal worms may be the cause. The itching may be due to irritation from soaps, douches, cosmetics, or contraceptives. Certain drugs, including antibiotics, may cause pruritus ani. Occasionally, psoriasis or seborrheic dermatitis is also present.

Symptoms

The major symptom is itching, which is aggravated by scratching. If the itching occurs primarily at night, the condition may be due to pinworms, and if accompanied by other symptoms—bleeding from the area and weight loss—medical assistance is required. The sensation may also be described as burning, tingling, or mild pain, and it may cause restlessness or sleeplessness.

Treatment

In general, these disorders should be treated by identifying and treating the cause. Someone with pruritus ani and pruritus vulvae should avoid hot, spicy foods which can irritate the anal or genital area.

If the itching is due to diarrhea, a mild soap solution should be used after each bowel movement to cleanse the area thoroughly. Then the area should be wiped with a soft tissue moistened with witch hazel or diluted rubbing alcohol. Tucks or Gentz wipes will serve the same purpose. Then the area should be dusted with a medicated powder to absorb moisture. Taking a sitz bath twice a day or simply sitting in a tub of lukewarm water may help to alleviate the condition.

Local anesthetic ointments should not be used to relieve pruritus ani and pruritus vulvae; they may numb the area enough so that proper treatment is neglected.

If these measures fail and itching persists for more than a couple of days, medical assistance should be sought. Glucocorticoid steroid creams or ointments may be prescribed. Vioform-Hydrocortisone cream can be useful.

Drugs Used in Treatment

Recommended treatment with OTC drugs—*Use your pharmacy's generic brand of rubbing alcohol or witch hazel to moisten the tissue used to wipe the anal-genital area. Then dust the area with medicated powder.*

OTC hemorrhoid products—*Gentz; Tucks*

OTC laxatives—*see the list under Constipation*

OTC diarrhea remedies—*see the list under Diarrhea*

OTC rash remedies—*A and D; Ammens Medicated; Baby Magic (lotion, oil, and powder); Borofax; Desitin (ointment and powder); Diaparene; Diaparene Peri-Anal; Johnson's Baby Cream; Johnson's Baby Powder; Johnson & Johnson Medicated Powder; Mexsana Medicated Powder*

OTC topical steroids—*Cortaid; Dermolate*

R̲ steroid hormones—*Aristocort; Medrol; Mycolog; prednisone; Synalar; Valisone; Vioform-Hydrocortisone*

Related Topics—*Chafing; Hemorrhoids; Itching; Lice Infestation; Pinworms; Psoriasis; Seborrheic Dermatitis*

Psoriasis

Psoriasis is a common noncontagious skin disease of unknown cause. It may be hereditary. Most patients are between the ages of 20 and 50. Psoriasis usually occurs in an eruptive fashion—especially during periods of stress.

Symptoms

Other than the skin lesions, there are no discomforting symptoms, although the appearance of the dry, scaly, red skin may make someone self-conscious.

The disease is usually chronic; the lesions tend to appear in the winter and abate in the summer. The lesions are bright red and sharply outlined. Frequently they are covered with silvery scales. They may be itchy. The lesions most commonly occur on the knees, scalp, and elbows. If the fingernails are involved, they may look finely stippled as though a severe fungal infection were present; they may also look discolored or pitted. The nails may separate from the nail bed.

Treatment

There is no treatment to cure psoriasis, but several procedures will cause temporary remission of the symptoms. The remission may last for months or years.

The most effective treatment is a warm climate and regular, controlled exposure to the sun. Using a sun lamp is also beneficial. If any drugs or chemicals seem to aggravate the condition, they must be avoided. A daily warm bath is important, and the lesions should be thoroughly scrubbed with a surgical brush, soap, and water. A bland ointment containing 5 percent coal tar can be applied over the lesions, followed by a mild keratolytic agent to stimulate removal of the plaque. Glucocorticoid steroid creams or lotions are applied over the psoriatic lesions. These drugs may be taken internally, but topically-applied medications are probably just as effective. Methotrexate can be taken for severe psoriasis, but because of its toxicity, it should be tried only after all other methods of treatment have failed.

When using a glucocorticoid steroid cream or lotion, the doctor may direct that the skin be covered with an occlusive dressing. A special plastic exercise suit is available to wear when the medication is applied. It can be ordered through a pharmacist.

Drugs Used in Treatment

OTC antipsoriasis cream—*Tegrin*
OTC topical steroids—*Cortaid; Dermolate*
R steroid hormones—*Aristocort; Medrol; Mycolog; prednisone; Synalar; Valisone; Vioform-Hydrocortisone*
R antimetabolite—*methotrexate*

Ringworm Infections

All ringworm infections are caused by fungi; the designation ringworm is a misnomer. Superficial ringworm infections can be divided by the parts of the body they affect. All are contagious.

Ringworm of the scalp. This is an especially contagious infection that occurs almost exclusively among children. It usually disappears by puberty.

The infection begins with small, itching, scaly lesions. These quickly spread over the skin to form patches. Any hair located in the path of the spread may lose its luster and break off. The appearance of the infection is an irregular, grayish area of hair stumps surrounded by sores.

Ringworm of the scalp is best treated with griseofulvin taken orally. Miconazole cream or clotrimazole cream or lotion may also be rubbed into the area.

Ringworm of the body. This is also called ringworm of the smooth skin. The lesions may vary from simple scaling to deep roughening of the tissue. The infection usually occurs on the trunk and upper extremities. The lesions are round. The centers may appear to be scaly, and they tend to heal as the wound spreads outwards. This is what gives rise to the name "ringworm." However, several lesions may coalesce to form a single, larger infected area—each lesion having a healed central area. Lesions itch intensely, especially in warm weather.

Specific treatment consists of griseofulvin taken orally. Additionally, an ointment containing salicylic acid and sulfur may be rubbed into the lesions. Undecylenic acid ointment or a tolnaftate product may be applied to the area. Haloprogin, miconazole and clotrimazole are also useful when rubbed onto the area.

Ringworm of the groin. This is also called "jock itch." It's common among males. The lesions extend from the crural fold (the area at the crease between the inner thigh and the pelvis), up over the adjacent area, inner thigh, and possibly into the area of the anus. It may affect the vulva in females. Symptoms include intense itching. The affected area will look like it's covered with an intense red rash. There may be small vesicles in the area. See athlete's foot (below) for treatment.

Athlete's foot. Athlete's foot is the most common fungal infection in the United States. Up to 70 percent of the population will have athlete's foot at some time in their lives. It easily spreads in gyms and locker rooms, and it may produce severe itching and pain.

Some OTC drugs used to treat athlete's foot or jock itch contain keratolytics (agents that soften and peel off the outer layer of the skin) like salicylic acid. Keratolytics must be used long enough to allow the skin on the affected area to become softened. Softening of the skin may take weeks or months. In the meantime, the skin may become irritated from the keratolytic.

Products containing tolnaftate are the first line of therapy for athlete's foot or jock itch. Tolnaftate is safe; toxic reactions are rare and mild. And it is available as a cream, solution, powder, and aerosol powder. Where the skin is thick, a keratolytic agent may be applied first to soften the skin so tolnaftate can penetrate more easily.

When using an OTC drug to treat athlete's foot or jock itch, choose an ointment or cream. With ointments and creams, the active ingredient in the drug remains close to the skin longer than it does with a liquid. If using a liquid, allow it to air dry completely. Aerosol sprays are expensive to use and are not recommended.

Between applications of a cream, ointment, or liquid, use a powder. Sprinkle the powder into socks and shoes to counteract athlete's foot or into underwear to treat jock itch. If there is no improvement within three to four weeks, see a doctor. The infection may be caused by something other than a fungus.

To avoid spreading a fungal infection, do not use anyone else's bathmat, and do not walk barefooted through the house.

Ringworm of the Nails. This is called onychomycosis. It is the most difficult ringworm infection to treat.

The infected nails—usually the toenails—become thickened and distorted, taking on a yellowish-brown color. Debris accumulates underneath; their plates become separated from underlying tissue. The nail is often destroyed. Women are affected more often than men, and the most common age is between 40 and 50.

Ringworm of the nails is usually treated with oral griseofulvin. It may take many months to a year of continuous therapy for the infection to heal. None of the topically applied antifungal agents will effectively treat ringworm of the nails.

Drugs Used in Treatment

Recommended treatment with OTC drugs—*Traditionally sulfur and salicylic acid ointments were used for topical fungal infections. If you choose this mode of treatment, use your pharmacy's generic brand. Undecylenic acid is an extremely effective medication which has generally replaced sulfur and salicylic acid combinations. Desenex brand products are preferred among the products containing undecylenic acid. Tolnaftate is the newest and most effective treatment. Recommended brands of tolnaftate include Aftate and Tinactin.*

OTC athlete's foot remedies—*Aftate; Blis-To-Sol; Campho-Phenique; Cruex; Desenex (aerosol powder, liquid, ointment, powder, and soap); Enzactin; NP 27 (aerosol powder, cream, liquid, and powder); Sopronol; Tinactin (aerosol powder, cream, powder, solution)*

℞ antifungal agents—*Fulvicin-U/F; Lotrimin*

Scabies

Scabies, also known as "the itch," is an extremely contagious type of skin infection caused by mite infestation. The mites themselves are barely discernible to the naked eye, but under close inspection they may be seen as tiny white dots on the skin. The infection begins when the impregnated female burrows into the skin where she deposits her eggs. The larvae hatch in a few days. When they mature, they mate, and the cycle begins again.

Symptoms

Scabies causes intense itching that is so severe at night it causes loss of sleep. The burrows appear as tiny streaky lesions ⅛ to ¼ inch in length. These lesions are called "runs" or "galleries," and they usually appear on the sides of the fingers, heels, palms, genitalia, buttocks, elbows, and under the arms. The face is rarely affected. The runs may be obscured by the patient's scratching. If the infection has persisted for two weeks or longer, the runs may be covered by a rash or dermatitis.

Treatment

Treatment consists of a prolonged hot bath and vigorous scrubbing of the affected areas with a brush. Scrubbing removes the tops of the runs, allowing medication to penetrate and kill the mites. Gamma benzene hexachloride or lindane (as found in Kwell or Gamene pediculocides) should be applied after the bath. These must be obtained through a doctor. At one time, sulfur ointments were used, but these are less effective than lindane. To control the itching, calamine lotion with 1 percent menthol and 1 percent camphor may be beneficial. Consult your pharmacist.

All the infested person's underclothing must be laundered thoroughly in hot water. Scabies is readily transmitted by personal contact, and an infested person should be isolated until completely healed. Other members of the family should also be checked for infestation.

Drugs Used in Treatment

Recommended treatment with OTC drugs—*Your pharmacy's generic brand of calamine lotion will help control the itching.*
OTC miscellaneous—*calamine lotion*
OTC scabicides—*A-200 Pyrinate; Rid*
OTC lice control spray—*Li-Ban*
R̠ scabicide—*Kwell*

Sebaceous Cyst

A sebaceous cyst is a benign skin tumor formed when the sebaceous (oil-secreting) glands become blocked or clogged. Sebaceous cysts are most commonly found on the ears, face, back, scalp, and scrotum.

Symptoms

A sebaceous cyst feels like a firm, round, movable hard object. It may be marble size or larger. If a sebaceous cyst is opened, a rancid-smelling material may exude.

Treatment

Sebaceous cysts may lead to secondary bacterial infection with or without abcess formation. One method of treatment is to apply hot packs three or four times a day to dilate the duct to allow expulsion of the contents. A corticosteroid product may be applied to relieve inflammation, but this treatment is not as reliable as the hot compresses.

Only a doctor should attempt to lance or drain a sebaceous cyst. The area must be thoroughly sterilized to avoid secondary infection. After drainage, an antibiotic ointment may be applied. Persistent or cosmetically objectionable sebaccous cysts may be surgically excised in some instances.

Drugs Used in Treatment

Recommended treatment with OTC drugs—*Ointments containing polymyxin, neomycin, or bacitracin, or a combination of any two of these antibiotics (Mycitracin, Neo-Polycin, Neosporin, Polysporin), are effective treatment after the cyst has been drained.*
OTC external anti-infectives—*Baciguent; B.F.I.; Mercurochrome; Mycitracin;*

Neo-Polycin; Neosporin; Polysporin
OTC topical steroid—*Cortaid*
℞ steroid hormones—*Aristocort; Medrol; Mycolog; prednisone; Synalar; Valisone; Vioform-Hydrocortisone*

Seborrheic Dermatitis

Seborrheic dermatitis is an inflammatory disease in which the skin flakes off. It affects the scalp, face, and occasionally other parts of the body. The most common form is dandruff. The cause is unknown, but the condition does seem to be associated with a sebaceous (oil-secreting) dysfunction. It does have a genetic component and is probably precipitated by stress, various nutritional disorders, infection, hormonal imbalances, and dry skin.

Symptoms

The symptoms sometimes include itching. Dry scales or oily, yellowish flakes are also common. The face, scalp, back, chest, and body folds may be either oily or dry. The affected areas may appear to be red.

Treatment

Seborrheic dermatitis of areas of the body other than the scalp is best treated with an ointment or cream containing hydrocortisone. Additionally, other corticosteroid creams or topical preparations may be used.

For the scalp, Selsun shampoo should be used once a week after a regular shampoo. If the seborrhea is especially oily, Fostex Cream is efficacious. The use of one of the glucocorticoid steroid sprays is also useful.

For areas where scales are flaking off abundantly, an ointment containing 3 to 5 percent sulfur with 1 percent salicylic acid will aid in the removal of these scales.

Dandruff will not be controlled by using a shampoo for oily hair. An oily scalp has nothing to do with the formation of dandruff.

Drugs Used in Treatment

Recommended treatment with OTC drugs—*Sulfur and salicylic acid ointments are usually marketed as generic products, and the product carried by your pharmacy is recommended to hasten the removal of flakes. For dandruff, Selsun Blue shampoo is recommended because it contains selenium sulfide, which acts directly on scalp cells to reduce their rate of growth, thus slowing dandruff formation.*

OTC dandruff remedies—*Head and Shoulders; pHisoDan; Selsun Blue; Tegrin*
OTC topical steroids—*Cortaid; Dermolate*
℞ seborrheic shampoo—*Selsun*
℞ steroid hormones—*Aristocort; Medrol; prednisone; Synalar; Valisone; Vioform-Hydrocortisone*

Shingles

Shingles (herpes zoster) is an eruption of the skin caused by a virus that is similar to, if not identical with, the virus that causes chicken pox. Blisters and a rash form on the skin; they usually follow the paths of certain nerves. Shingles usually occurs in adults, although it can occur at any age. The person may or may not have a history of chicken pox during childhood. Usually, an attack of shingles provides immunity against further attacks.

A shingles attack that includes the eye area can be very painful and dangerous. The condition, called ophthalmic herpes zoster, can destroy vision if the cornea is badly scarred.

Symptoms

Symptoms include intense pain and a flu-like response up to 48 hours before the first lesion appears. The lesions are usually grouped, small-seeded vesicles which occur on the face or trunk. The blisters usually last for two to three weeks.

Shingles may cause severe pain; among the elderly the pain may persist for many years, making strong pain relievers necessary. Scarring usually does not occur, although in severe cases, it may.

Treatment

Calamine lotion applied over shingles helps relieve the itching. Mild sedatives may be used to relieve tension. Analgesics such as aspirin or an aspirin-codeine combination are used. Prednisone or another glucocorticoid is taken internally and may help to ease the inflammation and swelling. Although vitamin B_{12} deficiency may cause nerve damage, this is not a valid reason for vitamin B_{12} supplements in shingles.

Drugs Used in Treatment

Recommended treatment with OTC drugs—*Use the generic brand of calamine lotion that your pharmacy carries to relieve itching. One of the OTC analgesics may be used to help relieve pain.*
OTC analgesics—*see the list under Pain and Fever*
OTC miscellaneous—*calamine lotion*
OTC topical steroids—*Cortaid; Dermolate*
℞ sedatives—*Atarax; Ativan; Librium; meprobamate; Nembutal; phenobarbital; Serax; Tranxene; Valium*
℞ analgesics—*Darvocet-N; Darvon; Darvon Compound-65; Demerol; Empirin Compound with Codeine; Fiorinal; Fiorinal with Codeine; Motrin; Percodan; Synalgos-DC; Talwin; Tylenol with Codeine*
℞ steroid hormones—*Aristocort; Medrol; prednisone*

Staph Infections

See Boils and Carbuncles; Impetigo.

Warts

A wart is a skin tumor caused by a virus. Warts may appear abruptly and disappear just as abruptly days, months, or years later. They may appear at any age and on any part of the body. They vary widely in size. They are most common in children and young adults, and are uncommon among the aged. There are several types of warts.

Common warts. Common warts are light-grey or greyish-black areas. They are round or irregular, firm, and rough. They usually appear on parts of the body that are subject to pressure or trauma—fingers, elbows, knees or scalp—but they may be located anywhere. Moisture helps their spread to other locations.

Filiform warts. Also called "thread" warts, these are found in the anal-genital region. They may join together to form larger plaques.

Plantar warts. Plantar warts are common warts that develop on the soles of the feet. They are usually flattened by pressure and are surrounded by extremely hard skin. They are usually extremely tender.

Flat warts. Flat warts are smooth, yellow-brown, flat lesions. They are usually seen on children and young adults on the face and along scratch marks through self inoculation.

Symptoms

Warts may cause mild tenderness, soreness, or pressure. Some may itch. Occasionally, they may cause an obstruction if located in the nose or ear.

Treatment

There is no completely satisfactory treatment for warts. They can be surgically removed, but the virus frequently remains in the skin and the warts recur either at the same site or later on at different sites. Unless the wart causes discomfort or obstruction, it is usually best to leave it alone.

Some OTC agents are available to help in the removal of warts. These must be applied to the top of the wart and not to the surrounding skin. No warts should ever be cut, filed, or pulled away by anyone other than a doctor. The use of a 40 percent salicylic acid plaster will help to soften the wart for its easy removal, but again this should be attempted only by a doctor.

Drugs Used in Treatment

Recommended treatment with OTC drugs—*If a wart is especially unsightly or bothersome, Compound W wart remedy can be used to remove it.*
OTC wart removers—*Compound W; Vergo; Wart-Off*

Eye Disorders

The eye is a sphere about one inch in diameter, filled with fluid, resting in a bony socket, cushioned by a layer of fat, and moved by its own muscles. The conjunctival membrane, a thin layer of mucous membrane, lines the inner surface of each eyelid and covers the exposed surface of the eyeball. Lacrimal glands continuously secrete lacrimal fluid (tears) to keep the eyeball moist and clean.

The cornea is the transparent outermost layer of the eyeball. It has been called the window of the eye, and it helps to focus light. Behind the cornea is the iris, the colored part of the eye. In the center of the iris is an opening, the pupil, whose size determines the amount of light admitted to the eye. Behind the iris is the lens. The lens is held in place by muscles that change its shape to accommodate different depths of vision. This fine-focuses the images we see. Fluid located between the lens and the cornea is called the aqueous humor. The fluid filling the eyeball behind the lens is called the vitreous humor.

The inner lining of the eyeball is the retina, which is rich in nerve endings. The optic nerve and blood vessels enter the eyeball at the rear. Light waves focused by the lens stimulate the nerve endings, whose impulses are transmitted to the brain via the optic nerve.

Like the rest of the body, our eyes are subject to injury and infection. Although they are less delicate than may be commonly thought, they are so important to the quality of life that they deserve expert care.

Black Eye

A black eye is caused by an injury to the eye and the surrounding area. The "black" color is caused by bleeding into the eye. While many black eyes represent minor injuries which will heal after several days, any condition that persists or causes severe pain should be brought to the attention of a doctor—preferably an eye specialist—as soon as possible. If severe bleeding occurs within the eye, glaucoma may develop, possibly leading to permanent visual loss. Such an injury may also damage the optic muscles and nerves, and cause cataract formation and retinal damage.

Treatment

Severe eye damage may necessitate bed rest for a week with both eyes bandaged to reduce the chances of secondary hemorrhaging.

A minor black eye can be treated with ice packs the first day to reduce swelling. On the second day, warm compresses should be used to aid in the absorption of blood.

In emergency situations, a doctor will dilate the pupil with atropine drops and then apply an antibiotic drop to the eye to prevent infection. Corticosteroid drops may also be used if inflammation is present. If an excessive amount of blood has leaked into the eye, a doctor may refer the patient to an ophthalmologist who may administer an enzyme drug to help dissolve the blood.

Drugs Used in Treatment

R antibiotic ophthalmic solution—*Neosporin*
R ophthalmic suspension—*Cortisporin*

Health Care Accessories—*eye pad; heating pad; ice bag*

Blepharitis

Blepharitis is an inflammation of the margins of the eyelids. Most cases are due to bacterial infections, usually staphylococcal, although some may be allergic in origin or associated with seborrheic dermatitis. The condition is contagious; people with blepharitis should keep their towels and washcloths separate from those of the rest of the household.

Symptoms

Blepharitis causes pain, burning, swelling, and severe itching of the eyelids. The eyes water. Bacterial blepharitis is ulcerative, characterized by the formation of crusts and eventual shallow ulcers. During sleep, the eyelids may become glued together by dried secretions which can be gently washed off with warm water.

Seborrheic blepharitis causes the formation of greasy scales on the lid margins.

Treatment

Blepharitis tends to be chronic and difficult to treat. Attacks may recur, possibly leading to loss of eyelashes, scarring of the eyelids, and vision impairment.

Treatment involves the application of an eye ointment containing an antibiotic or sulfonamide. Antibiotic-glucocorticoid combination eyedrops may help prevent further infection.

Drugs Used in Treatment

R antibiotic ophthalmic solution—*Neosporin*
R ophthalmic suspension—*Cortisporin*

Related Topic—*Seborrheic Dermatitis*

Cataract

The purpose of the lens is to focus rays of light as they enter the eye. A healthy lens is clear. A cataract is an opacity of the lens. The formation of cataracts is a normal part of aging; however, cataracts may also be caused by certain diseases (diabetes, for example) and some drugs and chemicals.

Symptoms

The opacity of the lens allows less light to enter the eye, and the major symptom of a cataract is a gradual, usually painless loss of vision. Almost complete blindness may result from severe cataracts.

Treatment

Surgically removing the affected lens and wearing special contact lenses or eyeglasses thereafter helps restore vision.

Conjunctivitis

Conjunctivitis (pinkeye) is an inflammation of the conjunctiva, the delicate membrane that lines the eyelids and covers part of the eyeball. It is usually due to bacterial infection, although it may also be due to a virus, allergy, or irritation from pollutants (such as smoke, dust, sand) or from intense light. Diseases such as the common cold and measles may aggravate conjunctivitis.

Symptoms

Symptoms of conjunctivitis include a discharge from the eye. The discharge is first watery, but later becomes thickened with pus. The eyelids burn and itch and may swell. Someone with conjunctivitis may find it painful to look at light. The discharge may seal the eyes shut overnight, but the dried discharge can be gently washed away with warm water. The conjunctiva becomes bright red (thus, the name pinkeye.) Symptoms of mild conjunctivitis may last for a few days; a severe case may last two weeks or more.

Vernal (spring) conjunctivitis occurs in the spring and may last through the summer. It is usually seen in males ages 5 to 20, and the symptoms are nearly identical, although the inflammation usually lasts longer.

Treatment

Conjunctivitis is extremely contagious. Someone with conjunctivitis should not use towels and washcloths used by the rest of the family and should avoid contact with other people.

The eyes should be washed periodically with warm water and blotted dry with sterile gauze or cotton. An antibiotic or sulfonamide-containing eyedrop should be applied as directed. Over-the-counter items advertised for removing the "redness" should not be used unless a doctor has been consulted and has approved.

Vernal conjunctivitis is controlled by frequent applications of corticosteroid-containing eyedrops. The use of oral antihistamines may help to prevent symptoms in milder cases.

Conjunctivitis usually does not cause permanent eye damage.

Drugs Used in Treatment

Recommended treatment with OTC drugs—*Chlor-Trimeton antihistamine is appropriate for vernal conjunctivitis.*
OTC decongestant cold and allergy remedy—*Chlor-Trimeton*
℞ antibiotic ophthalmic solution—*Neosporin*
℞ ophthalmic suspension—*Cortisporin*
℞ eyewash—*Collyrium*
℞ antihistamines—*Benadryl; Periactin; Polaramine*

Corneal Ulcer

The cornea is a transparent membrane over the lens of the eye. A corneal ulcer results from irritation to this membrane, often due to infection (bacterial or viral) following trauma to the eye. It could also be caused by infection elsewhere in the body that has been transported to the eye, or it could result from diseases such as gonorrhea, conjunctivitis, blepharitis, and from certain nutritional disorders.

Symptoms

Symptoms of corneal ulcer include excessive tearing, pain, and photophobia. The lesion may appear a dullish gray. The sore area may spread to involve the entire width of the cornea. The lesion may penetrate into the eye, although it usually does not.

Treatment

Corneal ulcers are treated with antibiotics placed directly into the eye. Sulfacetamide eye solution and ointment are also used. There is no home treatment; a corneal ulcer must be treated by a doctor. If the condition is severe, an eye patch should be worn to protect the eye from air and light. Corticosteroid drops may be used if antibiotic therapy is insufficient. Warm compresses may be used when the eye patch is not worn.

Drugs Used in Treatment

℞ **antibiotic ophthalmic solution**—*Neosporin*
℞ **ophthalmic suspension**—*Cortisporin*
℞ **ophthalmic drops**—*Sodium Sulamyd*

Health Care Accessories—*eye pad; heating pad*

Related Topics—*Blepharitis; Conjunctivitis*

Dacryocystitis

Dacryocystitis is an infection of the lacrimal sac that usually results from obstruction of the tear duct. The condition may be acute or chronic. It occurs most commonly in infants and adults over age 40.

Symptoms

Symptoms include pain and swelling in the area underneath the eye. A discharge of pus and extreme tearing are present.

Treatment

Hot, moist compresses may be used to alleviate the condition. Antibiotics placed in the eye may be helpful, but they are usually not necessary. An examination should be made for upper respiratory tract infections, and if any are present, they should be treated.

Drugs Used in Treatment

℞ **antibiotic ophthalmic solution**—*Neosporin*

Health Care Accessories— *eye pad; heating pad*

Eye Bleeding

Bleeding or hemorrhages in the eye may occur as a result of sneezing, coughing, straining, or other minor trauma. Although the bright red appearance of a hemorrhage on the eyeball may be alarming, such an injury is usually not considered serious. As a rule, it will disappear spontaneously within about two weeks. The only treatment recommended is cold compresses two or three times a day for the first two to three days to stop the bleeding. After the first few days, warm packs may be used to aid in the reabsorption of the blood.

If such hemorrhages occur frequently, or if this symptom is accompanied by pain or disturbances of vision, a doctor should be contacted. Some types of bleeding into the eye are serious and demand immediate treatment. They may be associated with potential damage to the retina or they may be a symptom of underlying disease such as diabetes mellitus, hypertension, kidney disease, or blood disorders.

Eye Floaters

Eye floaters, or "spots before the eyes," may be annoying and worrisome, but they are usually without clinical significance. They are caused by opacities floating in the vitreous humor within the eye. They are more common in adults than in children, and they are accentuated by bright light.

However, if eye floaters are seen frequently, or if this symptom is accompanied by disturbances of vision, or if the floaters seem to get worse over time, a visit to the doctor is in order. The floaters may be caused by a foreign body in the eye, or they may be a sign of infection or other damage to the eye, or they may be a precursor to retinal detachment.

Eye, Foreign Body in

Contamination of the eye by foreign bodies is among the most common of eye injuries. A foreign body in the eye can lead to severe infection or to loss of the eye. Physical abrasion of the object against delicate tissues can damage the eyeball.

Treatment

Removal of a foreign body from the eye is a very delicate procedure. Rubbing the eye in an attempt to move the body into view can cause further damage to the eye, as can other home methods of treatment. If the object does not wash out with the tears, or if pain persists after the object has been removed, the best treatment is to go to the doctor. The doctor's probable treatment will be to anesthetize the eye with drops and then locate and remove the foreign body with a special instrument or with a sterile cotton-tipped applicator. Antibiotic eye ointment or drops may be used to curtail the possibility of infection.

If the eye is dry, moisturizing eyedrops can be used for several days to lubricate the eye and aid in the healing of any scratched or irritated areas.

If the cornea is scratched or the eye is severely irritated, a sterile gauze eye pad can be worn to help retard eye movement, thus easing pain and promoting healing.

Drugs Used in Treatment

Recommended treatment with OTC drugs—*Isopto artificial tears is meant to be used to lubricate the eyes; it is not medicated. It is the treatment of choice for mild irritation.*
OTC artificial tears—*Isopto*
Rx antibiotic ophthalmic solution—*Neosporin*

Health Care Accessory— *eye pads*

Glaucoma

Glaucoma is a disorder of the eye characterized by an elevated internal pressure. This pressure pushes against the sensitive optic nerve endings in the eye and can cause irreparable damage. Glaucoma accounts for about 15 percent of all blindness in the United States. It is estimated that over two million Americans have glaucoma. There are two major types of glaucoma.

Acute glaucoma. Acute glaucoma is also referred to as angle closure glaucoma, narrow angle glaucoma, or acute congestive glaucoma. This is the more dangerous but less common type of glaucoma; 5 to 10 percent of glaucoma patients have acute glaucoma. Most people experience their first attacks during the nighttime or while in a theatre or a dimly lit room. In the darkness, the pupils of the eyes dilate and the pressure within the eyeballs builds up to serious levels, causing intense, almost blinding pain. The attacks are sudden and obvious.

Chronic glaucoma. Chronic glaucoma is also known as wide angle glaucoma, open angle glaucoma, or chronic simple glaucoma. Over 90 percent of all patients who have glaucoma have chronic glaucoma. It usually has its onset around age 40 and continues for the rest of a person's life.

The major difference between chronic and acute glaucoma is in the severity and symptoms. Chronic glaucoma may produce no symptoms or only occasional pain around the eyes, but generally the pain is not severe. Other early warning signals are seeing halos or rainbows around lights and poor night vision.

Treatment

Either type of glaucoma, if left untreated, can cause blindness. Blindness may occur within two to five days after symptoms of acute glaucoma first appear. With chronic glaucoma, blindness may not occur for 10 or 20 years.

Glaucoma is best prevented by having the eyes checked at least once a year. A doctor uses a device called a tonometer to check the pressure inside the eyes. The examination is painless and is usually completed before the person realizes what is going on.

Since a person may have a tendency toward glaucoma and still have a normal intra-ocular pressure, other tests may also be run, especially if the patient complains of the classical symptoms of glaucoma.

The treatment for acute glaucoma is surgery on the eye. Treatment for chronic glaucoma includes using the drug Diamox, which keeps the pressure within the eye low. Drops that are put directly into the eye to achieve the same purpose include pilocarpine, epinephrine, and others.

Drugs Used in Treatment

℞ diuretic—*Diamox*
℞ ophthalmic solution—*Isopto Carpine*

Iritis

Iritis is an inflammation of the iris, the colored portion of the eye. It is usually caused by infection due to bacteria or fungi. If left untreated, iritis can result in glaucoma.

Symptoms

Iritis causes pain in the area of the eye; the pain may extend to the temples. The eye will appear red, and vision will be blurred. There may be tearing and photophobia. Eventually the entire iris will look swollen and the pupils contracted.

Treatment

Iritis is treated by using atropine or similar drops in the eye. Atropine enlarges the pupil and helps to hold down inflammation. A glucocorticoid will also help prevent inflammation.

Drugs Used in Treatment

℞ ophthalmic suspension—*Cortisporin*

Related Topic—*Glaucoma*

Keratitis

Keratitis is an inflammation of the cornea, the transparent outermost covering of the eyeball. The inflammation is usually caused by a viral or bacterial infection. If left untreated, keratitis can cause blindness.

Symptoms

Primary symptoms include pain in the area of the eye, tearing, and redness. The eye is sensitive to light, and vision is blurred. There may be a sensation of an object in the eye.

Treatment

Keratitis demands immediate treatment. If due to bacterial infection, it is treated with antibiotics; if viral, with idoxuridine. Glucocorticoid therapy is indicated to prevent excessive inflammation, but it must be supervised by a doctor.

Drugs Used in Treatment

℞ ophthalmic suspension—*Cortisporin*
℞ antibiotic ophthalmic solution—*Neosporin*

Night Blindness

Night blindness (nyctalopia) is less than normal vision in faint or dim light. Someone with night blindness can see at night but is unable to make out images clearly.

The primary cause of night blindness is a deficiency of vitamin A. Treatment is supplemental vitamin A. If left untreated, night blindness can lead to permanent vision impairment.

Drugs Used in Treatment

Recommended treatment with OTC drugs—*If your physician has determined that your night blindness is due to a vitamin A deficiency, your pharmacy's generic brand of supplemental vitamin A is suggested. If you prefer to take a multivitamin, Unicap is recommended.*
OTC nutritional supplements—*see the list under Nutritional Disorders*

Retinitis

The retina is the light-sensitive tissue that covers the back of the inside of the eyeball. It is the part of the eye on which the lens focuses images and that transmits the images to the brain.

Retinitis is an inflammation of the retina. It may be caused by infection, trauma to the eye, or ruptured blood vessels. Retinitis causes visual impairment, and if it is not treated quickly, it can cause permanent impairment, or even loss of vision.

Symptoms

A person with retinitis will have pain in the area of the eye and blurred vision. In addition, someone with retinitis may not be able to discriminate shapes well and may have an altered field of vision.

Treatment

The pain is usually not severe and can be relieved with aspirin or acetaminophen. However, such relief may delay necessary medical treatment. If pain and vision impairment persist after the initial dose of analgesics has worn off (three to four hours) an eye doctor should be contacted. Glucocorticoid therapy in the eye usually heals the condition.

Drugs Used in Treatment

OTC analgesics—*see the list under Nutritional Disorders*
℞ ophthalmic suspension—*Cortisporin*

Sty

A sty (hordeolum) is an infection of an ocular gland usually caused by staphylococcus bacteria. Sties may be external or internal. The external sty is well localized and appears on the base of the eyelash. The internal sty may be seen through the conjunctiva.

Symptoms

A sty usually begins with a feeling of having a foreign body in the eye. Other initial symptoms include pain, tearing, redness, and the appearance of small, round, tender areas. The eye is sensitive to touch and light. Slight swelling may be present. Eventually, small yellowish boils appear. These boils are filled with pus. When they burst, the pus escapes and the pain subsides.

Treatment

A sty is best treated through the use of antibiotic eye solutions or ointments. The application of warm, moist heat three to four times a day for ten minutes at a time may help bring the sty to a head. A sty should never be opened by anyone but a doctor.

Drugs Used in Treatment

Recommended treatment with OTC drugs—*Yellow mercuric oxide eye ointment, an old time remedy, can be tried for mild cases.*
OTC eye ointment—*yellow mercuric oxide*
℞ antibiotic ophthalmic solution—*Neosporin*
℞ eyewash—*Collyrium*

Ear, Nose, and Throat

In medicine, the ears, nose, and throat are often grouped together, as they are connected. The eustachian tubes extend from the ears to the nasopharynx, the upper part of the throat, which opens into the nose. And because they are connected, infection in one structure often spreads into one of the others.

Ear. The ear is composed of three portions—the external ear, the middle ear, and the inner ear. The external ear is largely ornamental, although it does collect sound waves and transmits them through the eardrum to the middle ear. The middle ear transmits these sound waves through a series of tiny bones to the opening of the inner ear. The middle ear buffers the inner ear from harsh vibrations and exceedingly loud noises. The inner ear changes the vibrations to nerve impulses that are sent to the brain. Within the inner ear are tiny sensory hairs that detect motion as the head is moved. These sensory hairs tell the brain about the position of the head and body.

The eustachian tubes, which extend from the middle ear to the nasopharynx, allow the air pressure in the middle ear to equalize with that outside the body, thus protecting the eardrum from rupturing. However, these same tubes also pose a threat, for they serve as a passageway for infecting microorganisms into the middle ear. It is not uncommon for a respiratory system infection to enter the middle ear from the nose and throat through the eustachian tubes. This results in middle ear infections.

Nose. Air can enter the respiratory system through the nose or mouth, but only the nose warms and adds moisture to the air and filters out large particles such as dust and insects. The nose is also the site of our sense of smell. It contains specialized nerve receptors that detect odorous molecules in the air and transmit signals to the brain. Our sense of smell is far more delicate and specialized than our sense of taste, and many of the "tastes" that we relish are actually discerned by our olfactory sense. Thus, when we have a cold or a stuffy nose, foods often seem bland and tasteless.

Throat. The throat, or pharynx, is a tube approximately five inches long extending from the base of the skull to the esophagus. It is divided into three parts: the nasopharynx, which opens into the nose; the oropharynx, which opens into the mouth; and the laryngopharynx, which includes the larynx, or voice box. Air and food pass through the throat; it is part of both the respiratory and the digestive systems.

Common Cold

A cold is not a simple, clear-cut disease. It is a set of symptoms brought on by an infecting organism. At one time, bacteria were considered to be the sole cause of colds, but they really account for only 5 percent of colds. Viruses are responsible for all the rest. There are over 200 viruses that can cause a cold. And the only way to avoid exposure to any of them is to stay away from people who have colds. A single cough or sneeze can spread viral germs more than 20 feet. And those germs can start the cold process in any recipient.

Symptoms

A cold begins abruptly—usually with a dry, itching throat and nose. Dryness in the throat may or may not produce a cough, but the itchy feeling in the nose aggravates certain cells that line the inside of the nose. These cells release histamine, a substance that causes blood vessels in the nose to dilate and swell. This leads to sneezing, teary eyes, and congestion.

As the cold continues, its symptoms worsen. Secretions accumulate in the nose, throat, and lungs, producing a stuffy nose, sore throat, and cough. The secretions sometimes partially block the eustachian tubes and cause earaches.

Eventually, the secretions are released, and the nose runs. The watery discharge from the nose, called coryza, and the secretions in the throat then thicken and pass into the lungs. Coughing removes them from the lungs, but the throat becomes irritated from the coughing. At this point, a rash may appear, especially in children who have a fever.

Usually, most symptoms ease within four to five days and are completely gone in seven to ten days. A cough may persist for another week or so, depending on the degree of irritation to the throat.

Colds are classified by their symptoms. A head cold affects the nose and upper throat and causes sneezing, a runny nose, and a slight cough but not a fever. A chest cold affects the lungs as well as the nose and throat, and a fever is common—especially in children.

Treatment

No drug can treat the cause of the common (viral) cold. Therefore, treatment is directed toward alleviating symptoms of nasal congestion, headache, muscle ache, sneezing, cough, watery eyes, and, sometimes, fever. These symptoms are kept in check until the body's natural defense mechanisms can restore the patient to normal health.

Unfortunately, no single therapeutic agent can effectively modify all the symptoms of the common cold. As a result, most OTC cold products have multiple ingredients. Among the ingredients included in some of these "shotgun" products are: analgesics (aspirin or acetaminophen), decongestants (pseudoephedrine hydrochloride, for example), anticholinergics (such as belladonna alkaloids), antihistamines (chlorpheniramine maleate, for example), and stimulants (often caffeine). There are some problems with such products. Not surprisingly, a multiplicity of different drug actions is likely to produce a multiplicity of adverse effects. In addition, there is a danger of double dosing with these products. For example, if someone were taking Comtrex cold remedy for a stuffy nose and also decided to take acetaminophen for achiness, the person would be receiving a double dose of acetaminophen.

The use of certain ingredients in cold products is controversial. For example, antihistamines are generally ineffective in treating most cold symptoms, although they may alleviate a stuffy nose, tearing, and sneezing. Anticholinergics are used in cold treatment because of their drying effects. They decrease the amount of secretions produced by the nose and throat, and thereby may make those secretions thicker. The problem is that the thickened secretions may remain in the lungs, obstruct air flow, and increase the possibility of lung infection. In addition, anticholinergics should not be used by anyone with glaucoma. Stimulants included in cold remedies have no proven benefit in treating a cold. The same effect can be obtained by drinking a cup of coffee.

We feel that the additional expense of these "shotgun" cold preparations is unjustified. When treating a cold with OTC remedies, choose single-ingredient products aimed at treating the specific symptoms you have.

Vitamin C has also been touted as a preventative or treatment for the common cold. The FDA Advisory Review Panel on cold remedies reports that current data does not confirm any benefit from the use of vitamin C to prevent or treat a cold.

Many people go to their doctors and request antibiotics when they have colds. In cold therapy, antibiotics are indicated only for those people who are prone to other respiratory illnesses or for those who have a cold caused by bacteria. Antibiotics have no effect on the vast majority of colds that are viral in nature. Furthermore, antibiotics can become toxic. Taking antibiotics unnecessarily is both dangerous and a waste of money.

It has frequently been said that if you treat a cold it will go away in a week, whereas if you allow it to run its course, it usually takes seven days. Generally, the intent of treatment is to make those seven days more comfortable.

Most of the discomfort associated with a cold involves the nose, and an estimated 20 percent of all illnesses involving the nose are the result of insufficient moisture in the air. Thus, adding moisture to the air with a humidifier or vaporizer can bring much relief.

Someone with a cold need stay in bed only if the cold is especially severe and a high fever is present. Otherwise, taking it easy and avoiding overexertion usually suffices. In addition, a light liquid diet should be followed, and at least eight to ten glasses of water a day should be drunk.

Dozens of other diseases affect the head and chest and have symptoms similar to a cold. They include hay fever, tonsillitis, sinusitis, laryngitis, tracheitis, and pharyngitis. Cold symptoms also may be brought on by allergic reaction, or they may stem from a severe infection such as pneumonia. Consequently, if OTC remedies don't bring relief of symptoms in two or three days, or, if your pharmacist suggests it, see your doctor. You may have a disorder much more serious than a cold. Also, call your doctor whenever any of your symptoms become more severe than normal: if, for example, your throat is so sore that mild lozenges do not ease the pain, if a fever lasts more than 24 to 36 hours, or if a rash doesn't disappear when the fever breaks. Otherwise, you can do the doctoring yourself.

Drugs Used in Treatment

Recommended treatment with OTC drugs—*Treat only the symptoms you have. If you feel feverish and achy, take an analgesic, aspirin or acetaminophen. Either will reduce the fever enough to make you more comfortable. Decongestants reverse congestion by constricting the minute blood vessels located within the nasal mucosa. This results in decreased vessel permeability with a reduction in fluid production and, subsequently, larger breathing passages, improving both nasal and sinus drainage. In addition, these decongestants are thought to open the passage from the ear to the upper respiratory tract and thereby allow air pressure to equalize between the outside environment and the inner ear, thus relieving earache somewhat. Sudafed cold remedy is recommended as an oral decongestant. Decongestants in the form of a nasal spray or drops can be used for two to three days effectively, but longer use is likely to produce "rebound congestion," leaving the patient more congested than before. Recommended brands include Afrin and Neo-Synephrine Intranasal. For a cough, choose Cheracol, Cheracol D, or one of the Robitussin cough remedies. Relieving the cough should help a sore throat. In addition, gargling with warm salt water and sucking on hard, sour candy may relieve the discomfort somewhat. Anesthetic throat lozenges (Chloraseptic) help relieve the minor pain associated with a sore throat.*
OTC analgesics: *see the list under Pain and Fever*

OTC cold and allergy remedies–*Alka-Seltzer Plus; Allerest; A.R.M.; Bayer (children's and decongestant formulas); Chlor-Trimeton; Comtrex; Congespirin; Contac; Contac Jr.; Coricidin; Coricidin "D"; Coricidin Demilets; Coryban-D; Co Tylenol (regular and for children); Covangesic; Dristan (tablet and time capsule); 4-Way; Neo-Synephrine Compound; Ornade 2 for Children; Ornex; Sinarest; Sine-Off; Sinutab; Sinutab II; Sudafed; Sudafed Plus; Triaminicin; Viro-Med (liquid and tablet)*

OTC nasal decongestants—*Afrin; Allerest; Benzedrex; Coricidin; Dristan (inhaler and spray); Neo-Synephrine Intranasal; NTZ; Privine; Sine-Off Once-A-Day; Sinex; Sinex-L.A.; Sinutab; Triaminicin; Vicks*

OTC cough remedies—*Benylin DM; Breacol; Cheracol; Cheracol D; Chlor-Trimeton Expectorant; Chlor-Trimeton Expectorant with Codeine; Coricidin; Coryban-D; Dimacol; Formula 44; Formula 44D; Hold (lozenge and liquid); Novahistine DH; Novahistine DMX; Novahistine Expectorant; Nyquil; Ornacol; Pediaquil; Pertussin 8-Hour; Robitussin; Robitussin A-C; Robitussin-CF; Robitussin-DM; Robitussin-DM Cough Calmers; Robitussin-PE; Romilar CF; Silence is Golden; Triaminicol; Triaminic Expectorant; Triaminic Expectorant with Codeine; Trind; Trind-DM; 2/G; 2/G-DM; Vicks*

OTC throat lozenges—*Cēpacol (anesthetic and regular); Chloraseptic; Listerine; Sucrets; Synthaloids; Throat Discs*

℞ cough and cold remedy—*Tuss-Ornade*

℞ expectorants—*Actifed C; Phenergan VC*

Health Care Accessories—*dosage cup; fever thermometer; heating pad; hot water bottle; humidifier; vaporizer*

Related Topics—*Cough; Nasal Congestion; Pain and Fever; Sore Throat*

Earache

A pain in the ear can be caused by infection, water in the ear, physical trauma (a blow to the ear), cold air, or impacted earwax. An earache that is not easily relieved by one or two doses of aspirin or acetaminophen, or one that recurs after the instillation of a mild earache solution, should be appraised by a doctor. Anyone with a severe earache should be seen by a doctor right away to avoid possible rupture of the eardrum in case an infection is present.

A discharge coming from the ear may mean an infection is present. The infection may not be in the ear, but in the nose, sinus, or throat. Never neglect a discharge from an ear. Seek medical assistance at once.

Treatment

Aspirin or acetaminophen may be beneficial in relieving an earache. If you suspect the earache is due to impacted earwax, try taking a hot shower in a shower stall or an unventilated bathroom to help soften the wax and thus ease the pain. A vaporizer or humidifier may also be beneficial in that added moisture in the air may also soften the wax.

Other than adding one of the OTC drops for removing impacted earwax, you should never attempt to remove the wax yourself. Do not insert cotton-tipped swabs, hairpins, toothpicks, or other objects into the ear. You are likely to cause serious and perhaps irreversible damage to the eardrum. Do not use an ear syringe unless advised to do so by your doctor, and even then, make sure you know how to use it properly.

If you have a bottle of eardrops containing benzocaine around the house, discard it. Benzocaine is a local anesthetic that effectively relieves an earache. It is so effective, in fact, that many people use it instead of seeing their doctors for recurring earaches. Treatment of the pain without treatment of the cause of an earache can cause permanent damage to the ear. Because of this danger, benzocaine is no longer used in OTC ear products.

People with nose or throat infections or congestion often feel pain in the ear upon descent during an airplane flight. If this occurs, it indicates that the eustachian tube is blocked, and pressure within the ear cannot equalize. Chewing, swallowing, or yawning often relieves the pain. Anyone with a severe upper respiratory infection should postpone flying until the infection heals. People who are congested may get relief by using an oral decongestant before departing, and a topical decongestant before the plane descends.

Do not use any OTC drops for severe or persistent earaches. These conditions may signal a more serious disorder and the need for a doctor's help. Most severe earaches are due to bacterial infection in the middle ear. If such infections are neglected for a few days, they may proceed into other parts of the body to cause severe disease. Infections of the middle ear require antibiotic therapy and possibly the insertion of a tube to drain the ear of fluid. See your doctor for any severe earache.

Drugs Used in Treatment

Recommended treatment with OTC drugs — *Try aspirin or acetaminophen to relieve the pain. If the earache is due to congestion, Sudafed oral decongestant or Afrin or Neo-Synephrine Intranasal topical decongestants will relieve the pressure.*
OTC analgesics — *see the list under Pain and Fever*
OTC nasal decongestants — *Afrin; Allerest; Benzedrex; Coricidin; Dristan (inhaler and spray); Neo-Synephrine Intranasal; NTZ; Privine; Sine-Off Once-A-Day; Sinex; Sinex-L.A.; Sinutab; Triaminicin; Vicks*
OTC eardrops — *Auro; Debrox*
R̥ otic solution — *Auralgan*

Health Care Accessory — *ear syringe*

Related Topics — *Impacted Earwax; Middle Ear Infection; Swimmer's Ear*

Hay Fever

Hay fever is an allergic reaction of the nasal membranes to inhaled substances. Acute seasonal attacks of hay fever are generally reactions to pollen. Typically, spring attacks are reactions to tree pollen; summer attacks are due to grass pollen; and autumn attacks are due to weed pollen. Year-round hay fever may be a reaction to pet dander, certain fibers, feathers, housedust, or molds.

Symptoms

Hay fever symptoms are identical, regardless of the type of allergen involved. The nose, roof of the mouth, and eyes itch severely. A thin, constant, watery discharge from the nose is characteristic, and the eyes may water as well. Sneezing and headache are common. Someone with hay fever is often irritable, feels exhausted, and sometimes suffers from insomnia and loss of appetite. As the season progresses, the hay fever sufferer may begin to cough and wheeze.

Treatment

A severe allergy may best be treated by a change in environment. Someone living in a rural area and allergic to weed pollen may find relief by moving to an urban area. An air conditioning system with filters will help to keep pollen levels low. Relief of year-round hay fever may require giving away the family pet; eliminating carpets, drapery, and feather pillows; or daily dusting and damp moppings.

Oral antihistamines will bring satisfactory relief in a majority of patients. Severe cases may respond to corticosteroids taken orally or sprayed into the nose or lungs. Decongestant eyedrops will relieve itching and redness in the eyes.

In severe cases, hyposensitization may be advisable, especially for those who cannot take corticosteroids or for whom corticosteroids are not effective.

Drugs Used in Treatment

Recommended treatment with OTC drugs—*Sudafed or Chlor-Trimeton antihistamine cold and allergy remedies are recommended for relief of allergy symptoms. Decongestant eyedrops, such as Visine, shrink blood vessels and therefore tend to reduce the redness in the eyes characteristic of hay fever.*
OTC cold and allergy remedies—*Allerest; A.R.M.; Chlor-Trimeton; Contac; Contac Jr.; Neo-Synephrine Compound; Ornade 2 for Children; Sudafed*
OTC decongestant eyedrops—*Allerest; Isopto-Frin; Murine; Ocusol; Visine*
OTC nasal decongestants—*Afrin; Allerest; Benzedrex; Coricidin; Dristan (inhaler and spray); Neo-Synephrine Intranasal; NTZ; Privine; Sine-Off Once-A-Day; Sinex; Sinex-L.A.; Sinutab; Triaminicin; Vicks*
R~x~ **antihistamines**—*Actifed; Dimetapp; Naldecon; Periactin*
R~x~ **allergy and congestion remedy**—*Drixoral*
R~x~ **steroid hormones**—*Aristocort; Medrol; prednisone*

Impacted Earwax

Earwax, or cerumen, is a normal secretion from cells lining the ear. It serves to lubricate, protect, and clean the ear. Some individuals accumulate more earwax than others. The accumulated wax may become dry, hard, and impacted within the ear canal and cause scaling of the skin or obstruction of the ear canal. There are usually no symptoms of impacted earwax until the ear canal is almost completely closed. Then, the individual may feel pain or a dullness in the ear, or may hear thumping or ringing. Hearing may be impaired. Some people may feel dizzy.

Treatment

OTC products containing carbamide peroxide, aluminum acetate, or acetic acid are used to soften earwax. In addition to dissolving earwax, these substances will remove dirt and other debris from the ear. They will not produce any major side effects as long as they are used as directed. No one should attempt to clear the ear of wax by inserting cotton-tipped swabs, hairpins, toothpicks, or similar objects. Such objects can puncture the eardrum. Use an ear syringe only on the advice of your doctor, and make sure you know how to use it properly.

Taking a hot shower in a shower stall or an unventilated bathroom may help soften the wax. A vaporizer or humidifier may be beneficial in that added moisture in the air may also soften the wax. If pain persists, see the doctor.

The doctor will remove the earwax with a cotton applicator or he may, after determining that no infection is present, irrigate the ear with warm water to remove the wax. If an infection is present, irrigation could spread it. Eardrops, glycerin, or hydrogen peroxide may also be used to loosen the earwax.

Drugs Used in Treatment

Recommended treatment with OTC drugs—*Debrox eardrops contain carbamide peroxide and will help remove earwax when used as directed.*
OTC eardrops—*Auro; Debrox*
OTC miscellaneous—*hydrogen peroxide*
℞ otic solution—*Auralgan*

Health Care Accessories—*ear syringe; humidifier; vaporizer*

Related Topics—*Earache; Middle Ear Infection*

Laryngitis

Laryngitis is an inflammation of the voice box (larynx). Laryngitis is usually associated with a respiratory tract infection such as a cold, bronchitis, pneumonia, or whooping cough; or with sinusitis, tonsillitis, or measles. If hoarseness persists for months or longer, it may be due to the inhalation of irritants in the air, smoking, alcoholic overindulgence, or polyps on the vocal cords.

Laryngitis that recurs frequently is called chronic laryngitis. It is caused by inhalation of irritants, abuse of the vocal cords, chronic infections of the throat or sinus, or allergy.

Symptoms

Hoarseness or loss of voice is the most obvious symptom. The throat will be raw, red, and swollen, and the patient will have a constant urge to clear the throat. If the laryngitis is due to an infection, a fever may be present. People with chronic laryngitis often feel a dryness in the throat before hoarseness develops. They also cough and bring up thick fluids.

Treatment

Laryngitis associated with another illness will clear up as the other disease is cured. Additional treatment involves resting the voice, sipping warm liquids, and avoiding irritants to the throat. Do not smoke, and stay out of heavily polluted air. Use a vaporizer or humidifier; the added moisture in the air should bring some relief, as will the application of either hot or cold packs to the neck. Start by applying moist heat for 30 to 60 minutes. If this does not bring relief in several hours, try applying a cold pack.

Cough suppressants and expectorants are of no benefit.

If laryngitis is prolonged for more than seven to ten days, the doctor should be contacted to determine and treat the cause. Persistent laryngitis may cause the vocal cords to be covered with hardened masses, making the voice continually hoarse. Persistent laryngitis may also be a symptom of a more serious disorder such as cancer. For bacterial laryngitis, antibiotics will be prescribed.

Drugs Used in Treatment

℞ antibiotics—*amoxicillin; ampicillin; erythromycin; Keflex; Minocin; penicillin G; penicillin potassium phenoxymethyl; Terramycin; tetracycline hydrochloride; Vibramycin*

Health Care Accessories—*humidifier; vaporizer*

Related Topic—*Sore Throat*

Ménière's Syndrome

Ménière's syndrome is a disorder of the membranous labyrinth of the inner ear characterized by repeated episodes of severe vertigo. The cause of the disease is not known, although the symptoms are associated with extremely high amounts of fluid in the inner ear. The disease may be due to a tumor, an allergy, or to a drug response.

Symptoms

The most obvious symptom is severe vertigo which may cause loss of balance and a momentary loss of consciousness. Objects surrounding the individual may appear to be spinning. Nausea, vomiting, headache, and intense perspiration are frequently associated with the attacks of vertigo. The attacks come on abruptly and may last for a period ranging from several minutes to several hours.

The disease is also associated with loss of hearing and ringing in the ears (tinnitus). Hearing loss usually affects only one ear, but in 10 to 15 percent of the cases, both ears are affected.

Ménière's syndrome is a recurrent disease, and once it appears, the person will probably suffer from it for several years.

Treatment

Ménière's syndrome is treated with diuretics such as Diamox and Diuril. Diuretics help to reduce the fluid present in the inner ear. Certain antihistamines and atropine sulfate may help relieve the vertigo.

Additional recommendations include not smoking, avoiding salt in the diet, and the use of salt substitutes.

Drugs Used in Treatment

OTC salt substitute—*Co-Salt*
OTC vitamin supplement—*nicotinic acid*
R͟x diuretics—*Aldactazide; Aldactone; Diamox; Diuril; Dyazide; Enduron; hydrochlorothiazide; Hygroton*
R͟x antihistamine—*Benadryl*

Middle Ear Infection

The middle ear is a small bony box between the eardrum and the inner ear. The eustachian tube is a passageway running from the throat to the middle ear. Frequently, after an infection of the upper respiratory tract, such as a cold or influenza, microorganisms ascend from the throat to the middle ear via the eustachian tube. The result is often a middle ear infection (otitis media). The lining of the middle ear becomes infected and inflamed. Swelling develops, causing pressure against the eardrum, and possibly breaking or perforating it.

Middle ear infections are extremely dangerous. A perforated eardrum may not heal completely, leaving the middle ear constantly accessible to infecting microorganisms. Serious complications can develop, including mastoiditis (when the infection spreads into bony air spaces behind the ear, causing bone damage). Mastoiditis can lead to meningitis, an infection of the tissues covering the brain.

Symptoms

The major symptoms of middle ear infection include severe ear pain, deafness, chills, fever, and a feeling of pressure or fullness in the ear. A recent upper respiratory infection is another clue to possible middle ear infection. Children who have recurrent upper respiratory tract infections should be watched carefully to make sure that the infection does not spread to the middle ear.

Treatment

A middle ear infection must be treated by a physician. Analgesics help to control the pain, and penicillin or another oral antibiotic will control the infection if it is bacterial. The antibiotic must be continued for a minimum of seven days, and preferably for ten days. Even if pain or other symptoms have completely disappeared, the medication must be continued for as long as the doctor directs.

Antibiotic eardrops may also be prescribed, but these are not effective unless used with orally administered antibiotics. OTC nasal sprays and drops (Afrin or Neo-Synephrine Intranasal) are sometimes used to aid in removal of fluid from the upper respiratory tract to prevent it from ascending into the ear. This use has not been shown to be beneficial. Using an ear syringe to remove mucus or irrigate the ear is contraindicated while the ear is infected because it may spread the infection.

If middle ear infections recur frequently, the doctor may suggest removal of the tonsils and/or adenoids or the insertion of a tube in the ear. The tube allows fluid to drain out of the ear easily. The tube is implanted and left in the ear until it is automatically rejected, up to a year later.

To avoid recurrent middle ear infections, children should be taught to blow their noses properly—to gently blow through both nostrils at the same time without blocking either one and thereby forcing some nasal mucus up the eustachian tube into the middle ear.

Using a vaporizer or humidifier to add moisture to inhaled air may also help to keep the incidence of infection low.

Drugs Used in Treatment

OTC analgesics—*see the list under Pain and Fever*
OTC nasal decongestants—*Afrin; Allerest; Benzedrex; Coricidin; Dristan (inhaler and spray); Neo-Synephrine Intranasal; NTZ; Privine; Sine-Off Once-A-Day; Sinex; Sinex-L.A.; Sinutab; Triaminicin; Vicks*
℞ antibiotics—*amoxicillin; ampicillin; erythromycin; Keflex; Minocin; penicillin G; penicillin potassium phenoxymethyl; Terramycin; tetracycline hydrochloride; Vibramycin*
℞ analgesics—*Darvocet-N; Darvon; Darvon Compound-65; Demerol; Empirin Compound with Codeine; Equagesic; Fiorinal; Fiorinal with Codeine; Motrin; Percodan; Synalgos-DC; Talwin; Tylenol with Codeine*
℞ otic solution/suspension—*Cortisporin*
℞ allergy and congestion remedy—*Drixoral*
℞ antibacterial—*Bactrim*
℞ adrenergic and antihistamine—*Actifed*

Health Care Accessories—*humidifier; vaporizer*

Nasal Congestion

A stuffy nose is a symptom of the common cold, influenza, allergy, bronchitis, and a number of other disorders. The nose becomes congested when blood vessels enlarge and begin to secrete fluid. The enlarged blood vessels reduce the size of the nasal cavities, allowing less air to enter with each breath. The fluid leaking out of the blood vessels collects within the tissues of the nose and makes breathing even more difficult.

Constant nasal congestion may occur if anatomical abnormalities interfere with flow of air into the nose. Certain drugs, such as those that reduce blood pressure, may produce nasal congestion. Any persistent nasal congestion demands a doctor's attention.

Treatment

Decongestants (sympathomimetic amines) shrink the swollen blood vessels and stop them from excreting fluid. But they also shrink the blood vessels in other parts of the body and thereby raise blood pressure. They may also cause nervousness or insomnia. Decongestants should not be used by people with high blood pressure, and should be used prudently by those with heart disease, diabetes, or thyroid malfunction.

Nasal sprays cost more than drops, but they deliver medicine in a fine mist that penetrates far back into the nose, and they are easy to administer. Drops are preferred for children under age six, because they are easier to administer to the smaller nostrils.

Inhalers (like those offered as Benzedrex, Dristan, and Vicks nasal decongestants) work only if there is some airflow in the nose. Consequently they are effective only for mild congestion. Inhalers may irritate the nose and damage the cilia (tiny, hair-like projections lining the nose and respiratory passages).

Nasal sprays, drops, and inhalers should be used only for a brief period—three days is the period usually advised—to avoid "rebound congestion." These products work by constricting the blood vessels. Their repeated use fatigues the muscles that cause the blood vessels to constrict. The fatigued muscles relax completely, making the nose more congested than it was before the product was used, thus the name "rebound congestion."

Occasionally the doctor will prescribe specific medication to be placed in the nose. A variety of vaporizers and nebulizers is available to get maximum benefit out of these agents.

A nasal aspirator will help remove mucus which obstructs the breathing of a small child. A vaporizer or humidifier will help breathing by adding more moisture to the room.

Drugs Used in Treatment

Recommended treatmant with OTC drugs—*For an oral decongestant, use Sudafed. For a topical product, we recommend either Afrin or Neo-Synephrine Intranasal decongestants.*
OTC nasal decongestants—*Afrin; Allerest; Benzedrex; Coricidin; Dristan (inhaler and spray); Neo-Synephrine Intranasal; NTZ; Privine; Sine-Off Once-A-Day; Sinex; Sinex-L.A.; Sinutab; Triaminicin; Vicks*
OTC cold remedy—*Sudafed*

Health Care Accessories—*humidifier; vaporizer*

Related Topics—*Common Cold; Hay Fever; Influenza*

Nosebleeds

Nosebleeds may be caused by trauma to the nose (as when it is hit), by breathing dry air for an extended period of time, or even by repeated blowing of the nose. Constant nose picking may cause irritation that will eventually lead to bleeding. More serious causes of nosebleeds include tumors in the nose, high blood pressure, blood diseases, measles, and rheumatic fever. Usually, however, bleeding from the nose is not a symptom of serious illness, and most cases can be easily managed.

Treatment

Occasional nosebleeds are not a matter for concern. Recommendations for treatment vary widely. We recommend this procedure: Have the patient sit up and lean forward to prevent swallowing of the blood. Pinch the soft portion of the nose together for about five minutes, and then gently release. If this has not stopped the blood flow, moisten a piece of gauze with hydrogen peroxide or a nasal decongestant (such as Afrin or Neo-Synephrine Intranasal), and insert this into the nose. Leave in place for 15 to 20 minutes and remove. If this fails to stop the bleeding, try applying cold packs to the bridge of the nose and sitting still for 15 or 20 minutes. If bleeding persists, see a doctor. The nosebleed may be occurring far back in the nose and may need to be cauterized to stop the flow.

A person who suffers from frequent nosebleeds when the air is dry would benefit from having a humidifier in the home to add moisture to the air. Anyone with frequent nosebleeds should also take care not to blow the nose harshly and to blow through both nostrils simultaneously, that is, without closing one while blowing through the other.

A nasal decongestant may be helpful if the nosebleed seems to occur during a cold or other respiratory infection when the nose is tender. A dry or rough nose may benefit from a normal saline solution used as a nasal rinse.

Very frequent nosebleeds require medical attention. Once serious disease has been ruled out, the doctor may decide to cauterize small blood vessels in the nose to keep them from bleeding.

Drugs Used in Treatment

Recommended treatment with OTC drugs—*Your pharmacy's generic brand of hydrogen peroxide can be used as a simple antiseptic. The nasal decongestants (we recommend Afrin or Neo-Synephrine Intranasal) work by constricting the blood vessels. This constriction often slows or stops the flow of blood from a broken vessel.*
OTC nasal decongestants—*Afrin; Allerest; Benzedrex; Coricidin; Dristan (inhaler and spray); Neo-Synephrine Intranasal; NTZ; Privine; Sine-Off Once-A-Day; Sinex; Sinex-L.A.; Sinutab; Triaminicin; Vicks*
OTC miscellaneous—*hydrogen peroxide*

Health Care Accessories—*gauze; humidifier; ice bag; vaporizer*

Perforated Eardrum

The eardrum is closer to the outside of the ear than most people realize, and it may be perforated easily by the insertion of bobby pins, cotton swabs, or other objects into the ear. A blow to the side of the head or a sharp slap on the ear may also perforate the eardrum. A middle ear infection may cause enough pressure within the ear to perforate the eardrum, and this is why a doctor may implant a small tube into the ear of a child with a middle ear infection. The tube allows pus to drain out, relieving pressure and protecting the eardrum from perforation.

A perforated eardrum makes the middle ear more accessible to infective microorganisms. If the damage is severe, the eardrum may not heal properly and hearing will be hindered.

Symptoms

Perforation of an eardrum causes intense pain and a decrease or loss of hearing. The patient often reports a hollow sound or a feeling that the head is in a vacuum. There may be nausea, vomiting, or dizziness. Blood may ooze from the ear.

Treatment

If perforation of the eardrum is suspected, insert a small piece of cotton into the ear and go to a doctor at once. Aspirin, acetaminophen, or other analgesics may be taken to relieve the pain, but no eardrops should be used until the doctor has had a chance to examine the ear.

Most cases of small perforations will heal spontaneously, but many complications are possible and a physician's care is advisable.

Drugs Used in Treatment

OTC analgesics—*see the list under Pain and Fever*

Related Topic—*Middle Ear Infection*

Ringing in the Ears

"Tinnitus" is the medical name for the perception of noise without an external stimulus. The noise may be perceived as ringing, roaring, hissing, clicking, or thumping. Although the mechanism has not been defined with certainty, the sensation is thought to be due to irritation of nerve endings within the ear.

Tinnitus can be a symptom of a number of diseases, notably Ménière's syndrome and almost all ear disorders. It can also be caused by an overdose of certain drugs, including aspirin and quinine, and by abuse of alcohol and tobacco.

The cause of the disorder is often impossible to identify; nonetheless, it should always be sought. Tinnitus can be a symptom of a disease that can lead to permanent ear damage.

Treatment

There is no specific treatment for tinnitus. Sometimes the symptom disappears spontaneously or after the removal of impacted earwax. If tinnitus is caused by an overdose of drugs, correcting the dosage will correct the condition. Some people with tinnitus take sedatives—low doses of phenobarbital or butabarbital—but these are usually not necessary.

If tinnitus disturbs an individual's sleep, an "under pillow" speaker for the radio or stereo may be helpful. External noise often drowns out the internal sounds.

Related Topics—*Earache; Impacted Earwax; Ménière's Syndrome; Middle Ear Infection; Swimmer's Ear*

Sinus Infection

The sinuses are air-filled cavities in the face that connect with the nasal passages. Because of the connection with nasal passages, the sinuses are likely to be affected by any upper respiratory tract infection or allergy. Sometimes a bacterial infection of the nose invades the sinuses, resulting in a sinus infection, or sinusitis.

Attacks of sinusitis may be preceded by a cold or allergy attack. Swimming or dental extraction sometimes precipitates an attack. Sinusitis may also be caused by a deviated septum (an abnormality in the wall dividing the nasal cavities) or polyps that may arise after repeated attacks of sinus infection. Deviations in the septum and polyps can obstruct a sinus outlet, causing a buildup of secretions within the sinus and resulting in pressure and possible inflammation.

Acute sinusitis can cause much discomfort. In addition, there is a danger that the infection may spread, leading to complications such as meningitis, pneumonia, and middle ear infection.

Symptoms

The symptoms of an acute sinus infection are similar to those of a simple runny nose, but they are more severe. There will be tenderness and swelling around the cheekbones and eyes, a headache, and a thick, yellowish discharge from the nose. There may be a sore throat, fever, and cough. The headache is usually worse during the day, and eye movement may increase the pain.

A mild sinus infection that persists for a long time (weeks to months) is called chronic sinusitis. Chronic sinusitis may be symptom-free, or there may be a slight cough and a minor runny nose.

Treatment

Free drainage of secretions from the sinus is the first aim of treatment. A topical decongestant can be used to promote drainage of the sinus area and to open the stuffy nose. Application of warm, moist heat from an electric heating pad or hot water bottle will reduce the pain and help the infection to heal. Antibiotics will prevent spread of the infection. A vaporizer or humidifier will add moisture to the air to help promote drainage.

A nasal aspirator can be used to remove mucus from the nose of patients who are unable to blow their noses. The nose should be blown gently with the mouth kept open.

Drugs Used in Treatment

Recommended treatment with OTC drugs—*Topical decongestants (Afrin or Neo-Synephrine Intranasal) have been documented to be effective for opening nasal passages and promoting drainage.*
OTC nasal decongestants—*Afrin; Allerest; Benzedrex; Coricidin; Dristan (inhaler and spray); Neo-Synephrine Intranasal; NTZ; Privine; Sine-Off Once-A-Day; Sinex; Sinex-L.A.; Sinutab; Triaminicin; Vicks*
OTC cold and allergy remedies—*Alka-Seltzer Plus; Allerest; A.R.M.; Bayer (children's and decongestant formulas); Chlor-Trimeton; Comtrex; Congespirin; Contac; Contac Jr.; Coricidin; Coricidin "D"; Coricidin Demilets; Coryban-D; Co Tylenol (regular and for children); Covangesic; Dristan (tablet and time capsule); 4-Way; Neo-Synephrine Compound; Ornade 2 for Children; Ornex; Sinarest; Sine-Off; Sinutab; Sinutab II; Sudafed; Sudafed Plus; Triaminicin; Viro-Med (liquid and tablet)*
℞ **antibiotics**—*amoxicillin; ampicillin; erythromycin; Keflex; Minocin; penicillin G; penicillin potassium phenoxymethyl; Terramycin; tetracycline hydrochloride; Vibramycin*
℞ **adrenergic and antihistamine**—*Naldecon*
℞ **cough and cold remedy**—*Tuss-Ornade*

Health Care Accessories—*heating pad; humidifier; vaporizer; water bottle*

103

Sore Throat

A sore throat may be caused by a specific infectious agent present in the throat, middle ear, nose, or sinus area. During a cold, the throat may be sore because the nose is congested, forcing the patient to breathe through the mouth and causing the mucous membranes to dry out and become irritated. It may be sore from coughing, or the secretions of postnasal drip may be draining into the throat through ducts in the back of the nose, chafing the lining of the throat.

The inhalation of irritants such as smoke, pollen, polluted air, or dust can cause the throat to become sore. Additionally, the irritation may stimulate sinus drainage into the throat, causing more irritation. If a sore throat occurs primarily when the patient lies down, sinus drainage is the most likely cause.

Swallowing hot or stinging fluids or foods can also irritate the throat.

Treatment of a Severe or Persistent Sore Throat

If a sore throat is accompanied by fever, achiness, and fatigue, or if the throat and mouth are extremely red or have yellow or white spots, it is probably caused by a bacterial infection, and should be seen by a doctor right away. A sore throat caused by bacteria (such as streptococci) may lead to a systemic disorder such as rheumatic heart disease. A cough and stuffy nose are not characteristic of strep throat, but the patient may have a strep throat along with another illness. If strep throat is present, penicillin is given to prevent rheumatic fever, and aspirin or acetaminophen is given to reduce pain and fever.

If the sore throat persists for more than a week, if it occurs without a cold or congested nose, and if it cannot be attributed to some irritant, it needs to be evaluated by a doctor. The sore throat may be the symptom of a much more serious illness, a blood disorder, or a severe infection.

Treatment of a Minor Sore Throat

The sore throat that accompanies a cold is treated by relieving the other cold symptoms. If the sore throat results from breathing dry air, a nasal decongestant can be used to assist breathing. A humidifier or vaporizer will bring some relief by adding moisture to the air. Sucking on a piece of hard, sour candy will stimulate the flow of saliva to the throat. While the throat is sore, the patient should refrain from talking and smoking.

If the throat is irritated from coughing, a cough suppressant can be beneficial. A sore throat may also be somewhat relieved by gargling every hour with a solution of one-half-teaspoonful of table salt in a cup of warm water. Gargling with a solution containing aspirin has absolutely no value but for a slight analgesic effect that can be obtained with a warm salt water gargle or a commercially available gargle or lozenge.

OTC gargles and throat sprays offer little, if any, relief of sore throat pain. They are intended to temporarily cleanse the mouth. They do not kill germs, and their regular use may cause problems.

Lozenges that contain a pain reliever such as benzocaine or phenol bring quick and long-lasting relief, and they work best if the person lies down while the medication dissolves. But lozenges that contain nothing but an antimicrobial (for example, Cēpacol or Listerine lozenges) are no better than a piece of hard candy.

Drugs Used in Treatment

Recommended treatment with OTC drugs—_OTC analgesics will help relieve the pain of a sore throat. If your sore throat is due to nasal congestion,_ decongestants such as Sudafed (oral), Afrin, or Neo-Synephrine Intranasal (both topical) should make you more comfortable. For a cough, we recommend Cheracol D cough suppressant because it contains dextromethorphan. Chloraseptic throat lozenges will also help relieve minor pain.

OTC analgesics—*see the list under Pain and Fever*

OTC cold and allergy remedies—*Alka-Seltzer Plus; Allerest; A.R.M.; Bayer (children's and decongestant formulas); Chlor-Trimeton; Comtrex; Congespirin; Contac; Contac Jr.; Coricidin; Coricidin "D"; Coricidin Demilets; Coryban-D; Co Tylenol (regular and for children); Covangesic; Dristan (tablet and time capsule); 4-Way; Neo-Synephrine Compound; Ornade 2 for Children; Ornex; Sinarest; Sine-Off; Sinutab; Sinutab II; Sudafed; Sudafed Plus; Triaminicin; Viro-Med (liquid and tablet)*

OTC nasal decongestants—*Afrin; Allerest; Benzedrex; Coricidin; Dristan (inhaler and spray); Neo-Synephrine Intranasal; NTZ; Privine; Sine-Off Once-A-Day; Sinex; Sinex-L.A.; Sinutab; Triaminicin; Vicks*

OTC cough remedies—*Benylin DM; Breacol; Cheracol; Cheracol D; Chlor-Trimeton Expectorant; Chlor-Trimeton Expectorant with Codeine; Coricidin; Coryban-D; Dimacol; Formula 44; Formula 44D; Hold (lozenge and liquid); Novahistine DH; Novahistine DMX; Novahistine Expectorant; Nyquil; Ornacol; Pediaquil; Pertussin 8-Hour; Robitussin; Robitussin A-C; Robitussin-CF; Robitussin-DM; Robitussin-DM Cough Calmers; Robitussin-PE; Romilar CF; Silence is Golden; Triaminicol; Triaminic Expectorant; Triaminic Expectorant with Codeine; Trind; Trind-DM; 2/G; 2/G-DM; Vicks*

OTC throat lozenges—*Cēpacol (anesthetic and regular); Chloraseptic; Listerine; Sucrets; Synthaloids; Throat Discs*

Rx antibiotics—*amoxicillin; ampicillin; erythromycin; Keflex; Minocin; penicillin G; penicillin potassium phenoxymethyl; Terramycin; tetracycline hydrochloride; Vibramycin*

Strep Throat

See Sore Throat.

Swimmer's Ear

Swimmer's ear, or external otitis, is an infection of the ear canal. It may be caused by bacteria or other infective organisms. Rarely is it caused by a fungus. The infection occurs most often during the summer months when the frequent presence of fluid (from swimming) in the ear sets up ideal conditions for an infection. In addition, picking at or trying to clean the ear with a sharp object can irritate and scratch the skin, inviting infection. Allergic individuals seem to be more prone to developing swimmer's ear.

Symptoms

Major symptoms include itching and pain. The ear canal will appear dry, scaling, and crusty. There may be a watery, foul-smelling discharge from the ear.

Treatment

Aspirin or acetaminophen will help control the pain, and OTC products, such as Debrox eardrops, will help remove dirt and loosen the crusty scales. People who are prone to swimmer's ear should be careful to keep their ears as dry as possible while swimming by using a bathing cap or earplugs. To dry out the ear after swimming, instill a few drops of a product that contains at least 30 percent glycerin. If pain persists for a few days, see your doctor.

The doctor will prescribe antibiotic eardrop medications to treat a bacterial infection. Corticosteroid drops or corticosteroid-antibiotic combination drops will help to decrease the inflammation and irritation.

Drugs Used in Treatment

Recommended treatment with OTC drugs—*Debrox eardrops contain enough glycerin to be effective in removing water from the ear. A good brand of pure glycerin will work just as well. Consult your pharmacist.*
OTC analgesics—*see the list under Pain and Fever*
OTC eardrops—*Debrox*
R͓ otic solutions—*Auralgan; Cortisporin*

Tonsillitis

The tonsils are two lumps of lymphoid tissue located at the back of the throat. The tonsils trap germs as they enter the body through the respiratory tract, and they start the process that destroys the disease-causing microorganisms. Occasionally the tonsils become infected and inflamed. This inflammation is called tonsillitis. It is usually due to a bacterial infection, but it may also be caused by a viral infection. Tonsillitis is very contagious; someone with tonsillitis should be isolated and should not share personal items with other members of the household.

Tonsillitis may lead to infections in the middle ear, the sinuses, or the lymph nodes. Occasionally rheumatic fever or pneumonia may develop after tonsillitis.

Symptoms

Symptoms of tonsillitis arise suddenly: sore throat, pain that may extend to the ears, headache, fever (105° to 106° F), chills, loss of appetite, and fatigue. The tonsils will appear swollen and red. A yellowish pus may be present on the tonsils or in the area around them. Occasionally the neck and jaw become sore and stiff. The breath may smell bad and a severe cough may be present.

Treatment

Treatment consists of bed rest, fluids, and analgesics such as aspirin or acetaminophen. If the infection is bacterial, antibiotics will be given. A light diet should be maintained. Gargling with warm salt water will relieve sore throat pain, as will eating ice cream or sucking ice chips. Tonsillitis generally takes about a week to heal, and someone with tonsillitis should remain in bed and be kept quiet and inactive for the entire time.

If tonsillitis recurs frequently, it may be advisable to have the tonsils surgically removed, especially if it is associated with a middle ear infection.

Drugs Used in Treatment

OTC analgesics—*see the list under Pain and Fever*
OTC cold and allergy remedies—*Alka-Seltzer Plus; Allerest; A.R.M.; Bayer (children's and decongestant formulas); Chlor-Trimeton; Comtrex; Congespirin; Contac; Contac Jr.; Coricidin; Coricidin "D"; Coricidin Demilets; Coryban-D; Co Tylenol (regular and for children); Covangesic; Dristan (tablet and time capsule); 4-Way; Neo-Synephrine Compound; Ornade 2 for Children; Ornex; Sinarest; Sine-Off; Sinutab; Sinutab II; Sudafed; Sudafed Plus; Triaminicin; Viro-Med (liquid and tablet)*
R͓ antibiotics—*amoxicillin; ampicillin; erythromycin; Keflex; Minocin; penicillin G; penicillin potassium phenoxymethyl; Terramycin; tetracycline hydrochloride; Vibramycin*

Respiratory Tract

Respiration is the process by which cells are supplied with necessary oxygen and relieved of waste carbon dioxide. In simple animals, the exchange of carbon dioxide for oxygen may take place through a membrane, through air ducts, or through gills. But in man, the process is complex, involving the organs of two body systems, the respiratory and the cardiovascular.

The respiratory system includes the nose, the pharynx, the larynx, the trachea, the bronchi, and the lungs. Breathing is the process by which air is brought through these structures to the lungs (inhalation) and by which waste gases leave the body (exhalation).

The nose warms, moistens, and filters air entering the respiratory system. Both air and food pass through the pharynx, but the epiglottis prevents food from passing into the larynx (or voice box), a tubular passage joined at the lower end with the trachea, or windpipe. The trachea divides into the two bronchi, one leading into each lung. The bronchi divide and subdivide like the roots of a tree; hence, the term bronchial tree. The very smallest bronchial tubes end in cup-shaped air sacs, called alveoli. It is in the alveoli that the exchange of vital gases takes place. Each alveolus is richly supplied with blood vessels. Oxygen passes through the alveolar wall into the capillary, while carbon dioxide passes through the capillary wall into the alveolus. The blood then carries the oxygen to the body's cells, while the carbon dioxide is released upon exhalation.

Each lung is covered by a thin, moist membrane called the pleura, and the chest cavity is lined with a similar membrane. The two surfaces slide and glide against each other as the lungs expand and contract.

Although the lungs do expand and contract, they have no muscle tissue. They are flexible, passive organs, expanded and contracted by the movement of the ribs and diaphragm—the large muscle that divides the cavity of the chest and the cavity of the abdomen. During inhalation, this muscle contracts, chest capacity expands, and air rushes in. During exhalation, the diaphragm is relaxed, chest capacity is reduced, and air is pushed out of the body, taking with it the waste gases.

Allergy

Fifteen percent of all Americans require medical treatment for an allergy. Many more are mildly allergic. An allergy is the body's abnormal reaction to substances such as pollen, dust, smoke, ragweed, grass, grain, drugs, or certain foods. Although the substances that cause allergies, called allergens, may differ, all allergies produce symptoms by the same mechanism. Common allergic diseases include hay fever, poison ivy-oak reactions, asthma, and contact dermatitis.

Allergic people have a special type of antibody in their blood which specifically interacts with allergen, and this combination releases histamine. Here is an example.

If you have hay fever, your body makes antibody against pollen. When you come into contact with pollen, the pollen combines with the antibody. Together, the pollen and its antibody stimulate the release of histamine into the blood. The histamine then produces the symptoms of an allergy—itching, rash, runny nose, and red eyes.

Symptoms

Allergic symptoms vary widely, but they are generally caused by the release of histamine. The release of histamine leads to the dilation of small blood vessels and the contraction of smooth muscle. Thus, if the irritant is inhaled, swelling of the blood vessels in the nose leads to a runny nose and swelling in the throat may lead to difficult breathing—wheezing and coughing. An intestinal allergy may produce symptoms such as colic and diarrhea due to histamine's effects on the intestines. Contact dermatitis, caused by skin contact with an irritant, causes itching and a rash.

Treatment

Because the symptoms of an allergy are caused by histamine, the most effective drugs to relieve them contain an antihistamine. For best results, an antihistamine must be taken when the first symptom appears. Antihistamines are not very effective once all the symptoms of an allergy have become prominent; that is, when histamine has already been released.

Because an allergy often causes nasal congestion or runny noses, decongestants may be helpful. But OTC drugs that contain both an antihistamine and a decongestant should not be used unless relief of your symptoms requires both ingredients. If your allergy causes both itching and a runny nose, you can take a product with both an antihistamine and a decongestant. But if your allergy causes only itching you should use a product that contains only an antihistamine. For severe allergic reactions, a glucocorticoid steroid may be prescribed. However, these drugs must be taken exactly as prescribed and never over a long period unless the doctor specifically directs it.

Drugs Used in Treatment

Recommended treatment with OTC drugs—*OTC antihistamines are as effective as prescription products, and we recommend the least expensive generic form of the antihistamine chlorpheniramine maleate that your pharmacy carries. Chlorpheniramine-containing products are the most likely to be effective without causing excessive drowsiness. Decongestants may also be useful. If you need an oral decongestant, we recommend Sudafed. For a topical decongestant, choose either Afrin or Neo-Synephrine Intranasal.*
OTC cold and allergy remedies—*Chlor-Trimeton; Contac; Contac Jr.; Neo-Synephrine Compound; Ornade 2 for Children; Sudafed; Sudafed Plus*
OTC nasal decongestants—*Afrin; Allerest; Benzedrex; Coricidin; Dristan (inhaler and spray); Neo-Synephrine Intranasal; NTZ; Privine; Sine-Off Once-A-Day; Sinex; Sinex-L.A.; Sinutab; Triaminicin; Vicks*
℞ antihistamines—*Benadryl; Periactin; Polaramine*
℞ steroid hormones—*Aristocort; Medrol; prednisone*

Related Topics—*Contact Dermatitis; Eczema; Hay Fever; Hives; Insect Bites; Itching; Poison Ivy/Poison Oak*

Asthma

Between 2 and 4 percent of all American children under the age of 12 have asthma. Most outgrow it. Some people do not develop asthma until they are adults. Either way, the asthmatic suffers recurrent attacks of coughing, wheezing, and difficult breathing.

Asthma may be due to allergy to a certain item, possibly a food, animal dander, a plant, or grass. It may be part of a nervous disorder, in that during an attack certain nerves that lead from the brain to the lungs seem to become overactive. In many cases there is a personal or family history of allergy.

Symptoms

The word "asthma" comes from a Greek word meaning "panting," and panting is one of the primary symptoms of an asthma attack. Often the first thing noted before an attack is a feeling of tightness in the chest. The asthmatic experiences difficulty in breathing, and wheezes and coughs, possibly bringing up a thick mucus. The veins on the neck stand out; the face becomes flushed or pale. The attacks may come at any time, including during sleep. They may last less than an hour or a week or more. Despite the severity of an asthmatic attack, few are fatal.

During an asthma attack, the muscles around the tiny air-carrying tubes in the lungs become tightened and smaller, making the passage of air difficult. Mucus collects. The asthmatic finds it difficult to breathe. Some asthmatics develop enlarged "barrel" chests from the strain of attempting to breathe.

Treatment

If the asthma attacks seem to be triggered by certain substances, the first order of treatment is to avoid the offending substance. Many asthmatics find relief by moving to a relatively pollen-free environment, such as Arizona or somewhere else in the Southwest. Other asthmatics react not to pollen, but to dust, cold air, stress, or fatigue. Certain drugs, notably aspirin, may cause an asthma attack. Exposure to widely fluctuating temperatures also may precipitate asthma attacks in some people, and for these people, a cold weather mask may be helpful. These masks make the air warmer before it is taken into the lungs.

An acute asthma attack must be reversed as quickly as possible, and for this purpose, a drug containing epinephrine is the treatment of choice. Severe attacks may require an injection of epinephrine by a doctor. For milder attacks, one of the OTC inhalation devices containing epinephrine may suffice. Aminophylline (by suppository for a mild attack, and by injection for a severe attack) has also been used successfully.

Many nebulizer products are available that employ epinephrine, isoproterenol, or other substances. These products are inhaled to alleviate mild asthmatic attacks. Some can be purchased without a prescription. For more severe attacks, generally only the corticosteroid steroid drugs will be effective by inhalation. All of these products must be used cautiously and never more often than directed by the doctor. Portable vaporizers and nebulizers can be purchased to administer asthma drugs by inhalation. These allow the medication to be inhaled far into the lungs where it is needed.

Asthmatics should drink at least eight to ten glasses of water each day and should consider purchasing a vaporizer or humidifier for the home to keep sufficient moisture in the air.

The use of a portable oxygen tank may prove beneficial during an asthmatic attack. But, these should only be used at a doctor's direction.

For preventing asthmatic attacks, corticosteroids may be given by mouth on a very closely regimented schedule. Additionally, drugs containing aminophylline, theophylline, or similar bronchodilators are taken daily. Occasionally, products are taken that contain phenobarbital or other sedatives. While these drugs help relax the asthmatic and prevent the onset of asthmatic attacks, they should never be taken during an acute asthmatic attack as the sedative may cause further depression of the breathing center.

Some people advocate the use of antihistamines to prevent attacks. However, antihistamines have a drying action on the respiratory passages, and this action may induce further asthmatic attacks.

If asthmatic attacks occur too frequently or are severe when they do occur, desensitization should be considered. Although this procedure never completely stops the suffering from asthma, it does help somewhat and is worth the cost to those who have frequent, severe asthma attacks.

Drugs Used in Treatment

Recommended treatment with OTC drugs—*For mild asthma attacks, use Bronkaid mist asthma remedy, which contains epinephrine. Epinephrine is rapidly effective and useful for acute attacks of asthma. Used as an inhaler, it causes minimal side effects. However, we do not recommend that asthma be treated without a doctor's assistance.*

OTC asthma remedies—*Bronitin; Bronkaid; Bronkaid mist; Primatene M; Primatene P; Tedral*

℞ bronchodilators—*aminophylline; Brethine; Choledyl; Elixophyllin*

℞ antiasthmatic—*Tedral*

℞ expectorant and smooth muscle relaxant—*Quibron*

℞ adrenergic, sedative, and smooth muscle relaxant—*Marax*

℞ expectorant—*Actifed-C*

℞ steroid hormones—*Aristocort; Medrol; prednisone*

Health Care Accessories—*cold weather masks; filter masks; humidifier; vaporizer*

Related Topics—*Allergy; Coughing*

Bronchiectasis

Bronchiectasis is a chronic disease of the lungs in which the medium-sized bronchi become extensively dilated. The disease may be caused by infections due to diseases such as tuberculosis or pneumonia, or it may be caused by obstruction of the bronchi due to the presence of a foreign body (a peanut, for example). Many people with bronchiectasis have a long history of respiratory disease, and a relationship to sinusitis is apparent. Bronchiectasis should be suspected whenever pneumonia fails to heal within a normal period.

Symptoms

The symptoms of bronchiectasis are due to loss of the normal elasticity of the bronchi. Fluid accumulates in the lungs, and coughing, wheezing, expectoration, and other bronchitis-like symptoms are seen. Recurrent acute attacks of pneumonia are common. Thick mucus is frequently brought up, especially when the patient suddenly changes posture—for example, standing suddenly after lying in bed. Bleeding from the lungs may occur, but it is usually not severe. Possible additional symptoms include weight loss, night sweats, and fever. As the disease progresses, emaciation and clubbing of the fingers are seen.

Treatment

The danger of bronchiectasis is that a severe pulmonary infection may develop in the accumulated fluid in the lungs. Treatment therefore involves draining the lungs by having the patient lie with hips elevated for ten minutes, two to four times a day. The use of a vaporizer or humidifier will help to keep the mucus thin. Antibiotics may be given if there is a danger of infection.

Drugs Used in Treatment

℞ **antibiotics**—*amoxicillin; ampicillin; erythromycin; Keflex; Minocin; penicillin G; penicillin potassium phenoxymethyl; Terramycin; tetracycline hydrochloride; Vibramycin*

Health Care Accessories—*humidifier; vaporizer*

Related Topics—*Bronchitis; Pneumonia*

Bronchitis

Bronchitis is an inflammation of the bronchial tubes, the air passages that lead into the lungs. Bronchitis is caused by an irritation or (usually) an infection. Bronchitis frequently occurs with bacterial diseases of the lungs such as tuberculosis, or it may follow a common cold.

Bronchitis may cause emphysema and possibly other diseases of the lungs. Pneumonia and heart failure frequently follow periods of severe, chronic bronchitis. Chronic bronchitis may cause coughing severe enough to fracture a rib or cause hemorrhaging.

Symptoms

The symptoms of bronchitis include fever, coughing, wheezing, muscular aches and pains, and sometimes shortness of breath. The symptoms resemble those of a cold. The coughing begins as a tickle in the throat, then becomes hacking and unproductive, and eventually becomes productive. The fluid brought up is usually yellow and sticky. Coughing is worse at night.

Bronchitis that occurs repeatedly or that is present for a prolonged period of time (one month or so) is referred to as chronic bronchitis. Chronic bronchitis causes prolonged coughing. The chest may hurt because of the coughing and the person may be short of breath.

Treatment

A person who has bronchitis should avoid breathing irritating substances and should stop smoking. Bed rest is the preferred treatment for acute bronchitis, and at least eight to ten glasses of water should be drunk each day. Using a steam or mist vaporizer or humidifier is helpful in supplying moisture to the respiratory system and thus relieving the cough.

Antihistamines are sometimes used in cough preparations although they may further dry the respiratory passages. Severe coughing may be controlled by a cough suppressant. Expectorants may also be used.

If the bronchitis is severe, antibiotics may be given to cure the infection and to prevent complications. If asthma is also present, bronchodilators will be prescribed.

A basin should be kept at the bedside to collect sputum that is coughed up during the night. A fever thermometer will also be useful.

Whenever possible, sufferers of chronic bronchitis should avoid cold, damp climates and smoggy areas. The use of air conditioning may help.

Drugs Used in Treatment

Recommended treatment with OTC drugs—*OTC cough suppressants such as codeine (Cheracol) or dextromethorphan (Cheracol D) are effective. The risk of side effects or addiction is small when these products are taken as directed. If you need an expectorant, choose one of the Robitussin cough remedies.*

OTC cough remedies—*Benylin DM; Breacol; Cheracol; Cheracol D; Chlor-Trimeton Expectorant; Chlor-Trimeton Expectorant with Codeine; Coricidin; Coryban-D; Dimacol; Formula 44; Formula 44D; Hold (lozenge and liquid); Novahistine DH; Novahistine DMX; Novahistine Expectorant; Nyquil; Ornacol; Pediaquil; Pertussin 8-Hour; Robitussin; Robitussin A-C; Robitussin-CF; Robitussin-DM; Robitussin-DM Cough Calmers; Robitussin-PE; Romilar CF; Silence is Golden; terpin hydrate and codeine elixir; Triaminicol; Triaminic Expectorant; Triaminic Expectorant with Codeine; Trind; Trind-DM; 2/G; 2/G-DM; Vicks*

R̥ expectorants—*Actifed-C; Ambenyl; Dimetane Expectorant-DC; Phenergan; Phenergan with Codeine; Phenergan VC; Phenergan VC with Codeine*

R̥ bronchodilators—*Brethine; Choledyl; Elixophyllin*

R̥ cough suppressant—*Tussionex*

R̥ antihistamine—*Benadryl*

R̥ steroid hormones—*Aristocort; Medrol; prednisone*

R̥ antibiotics—*amoxicillin; ampicillin; erythromycin; Keflex; Minocin; penicillin G; penicillin potassium phenoxymethyl; Terramycin; tetracycline hydrochloride*

R̥ adrenergic, sedative, and smooth muscle relaxant—*Marax*

Health Care Accessories—*fever thermometer; humidifier; vaporizer; vomit basin*

Related Topics—*Common Cold; Coughing; Emphysema; Pneumonia*

Coughing

Coughing is a reflex that can be brought on by many factors. It is a symptom of some respiratory disorders; it may be associated with such diseases as influenza, tuberculosis, or pneumonia. It is a normal reflex used by the body to get rid of dust, dirt, or other irritants (including bacterial and viral germs) and secretions in the respiratory system. The very act of coughing may elicit more coughing: air rapidly moving across tissues in the throat can irritate the throat, provoking more coughing. Persistent coughs (those that last more than two or three weeks) or those present without other respiratory symptoms may suggest other diseases, including diseases of the heart or brain.

Treatment

Because coughing serves to expel foreign substances, it should never be totally suppressed. However, it may be beneficial to control a cough so that it does not disrupt sleep or spread germs. People who are over age 65, those with heart disease or excessively high blood pressure, and those who are in otherwise poor health should control coughing as much as possible. Harsh, persistent coughing can further weaken diseased heart muscle and can reduce the body's ability to ward off illness.

The type of cough present partially determines its treatment. Coughing can be either productive or nonproductive. Productive coughing originates from the lungs and usually can be traced to a bacterial infection. When infecting bacteria attack the lungs, lung tissue produces large amounts of secretions in defense. As more and more secretions accumulate, the lungs must try to remove them, and the result is coughing that brings up fluid. A yellowish or reddish fluid in particular indicates infection and requires a doctor's attention.

Nonproductive coughing does not bring up fluid. It occurs when sinuses drain into the throat or when smoke, dust, pollen, or other irritants enter the respiratory system. It may be touched off by drinking fluids that are too hot, or by eating foods that are highly spiced, and it usually can be controlled by a cough suppressant or antitussive.

Types of Cough Remedies

Coughs are treated with drugs known as cough suppressants or antitussives. Codeine and dextromethorphan are the only OTC cough suppressants that have been shown to be both safe and effective, although other ingredients may provide some relief.

Codeine is the most widely used antitussive, and it is used in both OTC and prescription cough medicines. Codeine works directly on that part of the brain that controls coughing. Codeine has a mild sedative effect on the nervous system although it may initially cause temporary stimulation. In proper dosage, this effect is so mild, in fact, that most people do not notice it. Codeine also has a drying effect that may be beneficial in relief of a runny nose but which may complicate an illness such as asthma. People who have a cold and want to suppress a nonproductive cough can use OTC medications containing codeine. But those who have a lung disease should not use these products unless directed to by their doctors.

Codeine, at doses present in OTC cough medicines, does not lead to narcotic addiction unless it is taken in large amounts for a long time. When taken as directed, codeine-containing cough medicine causes few problems.

Dextromethorphan hydrobromide is an alternative to codeine. Dextromethorphan works in the same way and is just as effective as codeine, but it is not a narcotic. It neither causes sedation nor affects breathing as codeine does. Nausea and vomiting are its only side effects.

Expectorants stimulate the production of fluid in the lungs so secretions can be coughed up more easily. The way they work is somewhat similar to the way the mouth salivates. During salivation, the glands at the back of the mouth and under the tongue produce more fluid than usual. Expectorants are used to stimulate the lungs to produce more fluid. The most commonly recommended OTC expectorant in the United States is guaifenesin. However, there is no definite proof that it always works, especially in the doses usually recommended. Some studies show that people who use guaifenesin are able to cough up secretions more easily than those who do not, but other studies report contrary results.

Still, a product containing guaifenesin is preferred if an expectorant is needed. Guaifenesin is safe. It causes no side effects other than occasional nausea or vomiting. And future studies may show it to be effective.

Nondrug Relief

Coughing can result from insufficient moisture in the air. The respiratory passages become dry and irritated, and coughing develops. This occurs especially in the winter months when the humidity is lowest. The use of a humidifier or vaporizer to add moisture to the air may provide greater relief than any drug, but do not use one of the volatile oils or products in the vaporizer. They do nothing other than impart a pleasant odor to the room.

Drugs Used in Treatment

Recommended treatment with OTC drugs—*For a codeine-containing cough syrup, we recommend Cheracol. For one that contains dextromethorphan, choose Cheracol D. Robitussin cough remedies are preferred for a brand of guaifenesin.*

OTC cough remedies—*Benylin DM; Breacol; Cheracol; Cheracol D; Chlor-Trimeton Expectorant; Chlor-Trimeton Expectorant with Codeine; Coricidin; Coryban-D; Dimacol; Formula 44; Formula 44D; Hold (lozenge and liquid); Novahistine DH; Novahistine DMX; Novahistine Expectorant; Nyquil; Ornacol; Pediaquil; Pertussin 8-Hour; Robitussin; Robitussin A-C; Robitussin-CF; Robitussin-DM; Robitussin-DM Cough Calmers; Robitussin-PE; Romilar CF; Silence is Golden; terpin hydrate and codeine elixir; Triaminicol; Triaminic Expectorant; Triaminic Expectorant with Codeine; Trind; Trind-DM; 2/G; 2/G-DM; Vicks*

R͓ **expectorants**—*Actifed-C; Ambenyl; Dimetane Expectorant-DC; Phenergan; Phenergan with Codeine; Phenergan VC; Phenergan VC with Codeine*
R͓ **cough suppressant**—*Tussionex*
R͓ **antihistamine**—*Benadryl*

Health Care Accessories—*humidifier; vaporizer*

Related Topics—*Bronchitis; Common Cold; Emphysema; Influenza; Pleurisy*

Croup

Croup is more a symptom than a disease. Acute infectious croup is the most common form, and it can be caused by any of the viruses that normally cause upper respiratory tract infections in children. The infection may not be confined to the upper respiratory tract but may extend into the lower portion, including the lungs. The severity and potential danger of croup is related to how much the upper respiratory infection has affected the lungs.

Typically, the patient is a child less than two years of age who has had an upper respiratory infection for two to three days. The weather is often cold and frosty. As evening approaches, a dry persistent cough worsens and the voice becomes hoarse. It becomes evident that the child is having trouble breathing.

Croup can be a dangerous condition. Swelling and spasm of the larynx, as well as the production of a thick, sticky mucus, may block the air passage, making it very difficult for the child to breathe. The child may get panicky because of the need to fight for air. Fever may also be present.

Treatment

Relief from uncomplicated croup often can be obtained with the use of a vaporizer or humidifier. The unit should be run continuously, and the room should be kept at a temperature no higher than 75° F. Occasionally a mild sedative such as phenobarbital may be given to allay fear. Antibiotics are occasionally given to treat secondary infection. More serious forms of croup require hospitalization and possibly surgery or intubation. Cough syrups generally have little value in croup.

Drugs Used in Treatment

R͓ **sedative and hypnotic**—*phenobarbital*
R͓ **phenothiazines**—*Compazine; Stelazine; Triavil*
R͓ **analgesics**—*Fiorinal; Fiorinal with Codeine*
R͓ **expectorant**—*Actifed-C*
R͓ **antibiotics**—*amoxicillin; ampicillin; erythromycin; Keflex; Minocin; penicillin G; penicillin potassium phenoxymethyl; Terramycin; tetracycline hydrochloride; Vibramycin*

Cystic Fibrosis

Cystic fibrosis is an inherited disease affecting the exocrine glands, those whose secretions leave the body rather than flow into the bloodstream. For example, the pancreas and the sweat glands are exocrine glands. If both parents are carriers, there is a one in four chance that each child will have the disease. The disease occurs most frequently among Caucasians. Its causes are unknown.

Cystic fibrosis causes glandular secretions to increase and become sticky. These secretions obstruct the ducts of the body. Obstruction in the lungs may lead to chronic pulmonary infections. The secretions also become more salty.

Symptoms

Symptoms affect primarily the respiratory system. The onset of symptoms occurs soon after birth. The baby seems to have a good appetite, yet gains weight slowly. Large, frequent, and foul-smelling stools are characteristic. There may be a chronic cough and a rapid respiratory rate. Respiratory symptoms resemble those of an allergy. Paroxysms of coughing may be severe enough to induce vomiting. The child may find it difficult to sleep. Children with cystic fibrosis appear very thin and have protuberant abdomens. The chest often becomes barrel-like.

Cystic fibrosis causes susceptibility to severe respiratory infections; it is the primary cause of chronic lung disease in children and long-term lung damage is the major danger in the disease. Digestive disorders—weight loss, malnutrition, diarrhea—and retarded growth and development also occur. People with cystic fibrosis characteristically have very salty sweat, and there is also real danger of dehydration, heat prostration, and death in hot climates.

Treatment

There is no preventive measure for cystic fibrosis. Anyone with a familial history of the disease should be aware of the possibility of offspring having the disease so that proper treatment can be instituted early to prevent permanent lung damage.

Treatment must be directed by a doctor. A calorie-rich diet with vitamin and mineral supplements is given. Supplementary salt is needed. Medications are used to liquify respiratory mucus and minimize its formation to prevent obstruction of the bronchioles and to control infection. During severe stages, patients should sleep in mist tents. Special breathing exercises are usually recommended. Additional medications include pancreatic enzymes, aerosol bronchodilators, and antibiotics (to prevent or treat infections).

Drugs Used in Treatment

OTC nutritional supplements—*see the list under Nutritional Disorders*
R̟ bronchodilator—*Choledyl*
R̟ adrenergic, sedative, and smooth muscle relaxant—*Marax*
R̟ expectorant—*Actifed-C*
R̟ antibiotics—*amoxicillin; ampicillin; erythromycin; Keflex; Minocin; penicillin G; penicillin potassium phenoxymethyl; Terramycin; tetracycline hydrochloride; Vibramycin*

Emphysema

Emphysema is a serious disorder of the respiratory system commonly associated with smoking. The patient with emphysema is able to breathe air into the lungs, but cannot efficiently or easily breathe out. The alveolar sacs, tiny bag-like projections in the lungs where oxygen exchange takes place, lose their elasticity and become overinflated. Eventually, the sacs may burst.

Symptoms

Emphysema can be disabling. The patient with emphysema is continually short of breath, constantly fatigued, and may cough continuously. Because the lungs can fill with air but cannot easily expel it, they are constantly overinflated, and the individual may develop a "barrel chest." In severe cases, the patient's skin may appear white or blue.

Treatment

Once the alveolar sacs are destroyed, nothing can reverse the situation. However, someone with emphysema can be made more comfortable.

A humidifier or vaporizer should be used constantly to add more moisture to the environment. A home air conditioner should be used during appropriate times to filter dust, pollen, and other irritants out of the air. Additionally, someone with emphysema should stop smoking, avoid breathing polluted air, and should follow a strict rest-exercise-diet program prescribed by a doctor. People with emphysema should also avoid excessive use of cough syrups or medications that sedate the nervous system. Coughing is essential to bring up phlegm, and it should be suppressed only when it becomes dangerous to the individual's health or disrupts sleep. Likewise, the use of sedatives may further suppress respiration, aggravating the emphysemic symptoms.

Oxygen is useful for periods of shortness of breath or for periods immediately following exertion, but the use of unmoistened oxygen, as with a Lif-O-Gen tank, can further aggravate the lungs. Thus, unhumidified oxygen should only be used in extreme emergencies.

Bronchodilator drugs used in atomizers or nebulizers are effective for many patients. Potassium iodide solution or ammonium chloride solution will help to loosen phlegm and allow it to be coughed up. If an infection is present, the use of an appropriate antibiotic will aid the condition.

Drugs Used in Treatment

℞ bronchodilators—*aminophylline; Brethine; Choledyl; Elixophyllin*
℞ expectorant—*Actifed-C*
℞ antibiotics—*amoxicillin; ampicillin; erythromycin; Keflex; Minocin; penicillin G; penicillin potassium phenoxymethyl; Terramycin; tetracycline hydrochloride; Vibramycin*

Health Care Accessories—*humidifier; vaporizer*

Related Topics—*Bronchitis; Coughing*

Influenza

Influenza (grippe, grip, or the "flu") is a highly contagious disease of the respiratory tract caused by various viruses. There is no influenza virus that attacks or significantly affects the gastrointestinal tract; the term "intestinal flu" is a misnomer.

Symptoms

Onset is usually sudden. The individual develops chills or a chilly sensation and fever. Aches and pains with headache, weakness, and loss of appetite develop. The respiratory tract itself displays few symptoms, except that a cough, sore throat, and runny nose may be present. A fever may reach 102° F and may last for two to three days in milder forms of influenza. In more severe forms, a fever of 104° F is common, and it may last for four to five days. Most symptoms begin to disappear when the fever breaks. However, weakness, sweating, and fatigue may continue for several more days to weeks.

Whenever symptoms, including fever and cough, last longer than five days, a bacterial pneumonia may be present. In this case, fluid can be detected in the lungs. Coughing will become more severe, producing a thick sputum. Unless this is treated, death can occur in as little as two days.

Treatment

In uncomplicated influenza, recovery will occur even without medical treatment. In fact, there is no real treatment per se except to alleviate symptoms. To treat pain, fever, and cough, analgesics, antipyretics, and cough suppressants may be helpful. Bed rest will reduce the intensity and severity of symptoms. Amantadine taken prophylactically will modify the symptoms of some types of influenza and lessen the severity of any infections that may occur.

Antibiotics do not affect the course of an influenza infection nor do they prevent complications. They have no effect whatsoever on virus infections. While secondary bacterial infections are possible and may even result in life-threatening pneumonia, it is considered best to closely monitor high-risk patients and to give the appropriate antibiotic if and when signs of secondary infection occur rather than to blanket everyone with protective antibiotic therapy.

People at special risk from influenza (those with heart or lung problems, or the elderly, for example) may want to consider being vaccinated before flu season starts. Consult your doctor.

Drugs Used in Treatment

Recommended treatment with OTC drugs—*For a codeine-containing cough syrup, we recommend Cheracol. For one that contains dextromethorphan, choose Cheracol D. Robitussin cough remedies are preferred for a brand of guaifenesin.*
OTC analgesics—*see the list under Pain and Fever*
OTC cough remedies—*Benylin DM; Breacol; Cheracol; Cheracol D; Chlor-Trimeton Expectorant; Chlor-Trimeton Expectorant with Codeine; Coricidin; Coryban-D; Dimacol; Formula 44; Formula 44D; Hold (lozenge and liquid); Novahistine DH; Novahistine DMX; Novahistine Expectorant; Nyquil; Ornacol; Pediaquil; Pertussin 8-Hour; Robitussin; Robitussin A-C; Robitussin-CF; Robitussin-DM; Robitussin-DM Cough Calmers; Robitussin-PE; Romilar CF; Silence is Golden; terpin hydrate and codeine elixir; Triaminicol; Triaminic Expectorant; Triaminic Expectorant with Codeine; Trind; Trind-DM; 2/G; 2/G-DM; Vicks*
R_x analgesics—*Darvocet-N; Darvon; Darvon Compound-65; Demerol; Empirin Compound with Codeine; Equagesic; Fiorinal; Fiorinal with Codeine; Motrin; Percodan; Synalgos-DC; Talwin; Tylenol with Codeine*
R_x cough suppressant—*Tussionex*

Nocardiosis

Although thought for years to be fungal, nocardiosis is a bacterial disease that primarily affects the lungs. It usually is contracted by people who have a serious underlying disease such as leukemia or other cancers.

Symptoms

Symptoms begin with loss of weight, malaise, night sweats, and fever. Coughing is common and a thick purulent sputum is brought up. Spread of the bacteria through the bloodstream to other systems in the body including the central nervous system, is common. Lesions occur most frequently in the brain or meninges.

Treatment

Nocardiosis is treated with an antibacterial. Treatment may require many months of drug therapy to make sure that all clinical manifestations of the disease have disappeared. Aspirin or acetaminophen is given to control the fever and reduce the incidence of night sweats. Water (eight to ten glasses each day) should be forced to help the passage of the thick sputum. A vitamin-mineral supplement may be given when the appetite is decreased to help maintain proper nutrition.

Drugs Used in Treatment

OTC analgesics—*see the list under Pain and Fever*
OTC nutritional supplements—*see the list under Nutritional Disorders*
R̥ antibacterial—*Bactrim*

Occupational Lung Diseases

Pneumoconiosis is the term applied to a group of lung disorders that are directly related to the inhalation of fine dust particles in the working environment. These disorders are also called dusty lung diseases. Among the occupations most likely to be involved are mining, foundry work, and asbestos manufacturing. Irritant substances include asbestos, silica, coal dust (black lung disease), and beryllium.

Symptoms

Initially, the only symptom may be an increased susceptibility to upper respiratory tract infections. Occasionally a severe cough, with or without phlegm, and wheezing develop. Dyspnea (difficult respiration) on exertion is the most commonly reported symptom. These symptoms may persist for many years until the patient becomes chronically short of breath and the coughing becomes extremely irritating and eventually productive. Occasionally blood is coughed up in the sputum. All of these respiratory symptoms may lead to an increased tendency toward pneumonia, lung cancer, and tuberculosis. In the later stages of black lung disease, the lung tissue darkens and finally becomes black because of the accumulation of coal dust in the lungs' cells. The patient frequently develops emphysema.

Treatment

Treatment is symptomatic. Coughing and wheezing are treated with cough syrups or bronchodilators. A vaporizer or humidifier will aid in breathing and lessen throat irritation. All symptoms are made worse by smoking, and all patients should stop smoking. Young people who develop the symptoms of dusty lungs should change occupations. If the condition is especially severe, it may be advisable to move to a less polluted area.

If tuberculosis develops, isoniazid (INH) is given to keep it from getting worse. Those who work in industries like those listed above should wear protective filter masks.

118

Drugs Used in Treatment

Recommended treatment with OTC drugs—*OTC cough suppressants such as codeine (Cheracol) or dextromethorphan (Cheracol D) are effective. The risk of side effects or addiction is small when these products are taken as directed.*

OTC cough remedies—*Benylin DM; Breacol; Cheracol; Cheracol D; Chlor-Trimeton Expectorant; Chlor-Trimeton Expectorant with Codeine; Coricidin; Coryban-D; Dimacol; Formula 44; Formula 44D; Hold (lozenge and liquid); Novahistine DH; Novahistine DMX; Novahistine Expectorant; Nyquil; Ornacol; Pediaquil; Pertussin 8-Hour; Robitussin; Robitussin A-C; Robitussin-CF; Robitussin-DM; Robitussin-DM Cough Calmers; Robitussin-PE; Romilar CF; Silence is Golden; terpin hydrate and codeine elixir; Triaminicol; Triaminic Expectorant; Triaminic Expectorant with Codeine; Trind; Trind-DM; 2/G; 2/G-DM; Vicks*

℞ expectorants—*Actifed-C; Ambenyl; Dimetane Expectorant-DC; Phenergan; Phenergan with Codeine; Phenergan VC; Phenergan VC with Codeine*
℞ bronchodilators—*Brethine; Choledyl; Elixophyllin*
℞ cough suppressant—*Tussionex*

Health Care Accessories—*filter mask; humidifier; vaporizer*

Related Topics—*Emphysema; Pneumonia; Tuberculosis*

Pleurisy

The pleura is a serous, normally moist membrane that covers the outside of the lungs and lines the chest cavity. Any disease causing inflammation of the lungs may also cause inflammation of the pleura. Such an inflammation is called pleurisy. Pleurisy commonly develops as a complication of tuberculosis, pneumonia, and certain other serious infections of the respiratory system. It can also occur following rheumatic fever, bronchitis, and even during severe kidney disease.

There are basically two broad types of pleurisy: wet and dry. Dry pleurisy is the simple inflammation of the pleura. If too much fluid emanates from the pleura, the condition is called wet pleurisy.   The excess fluid compresses the lungs.

Symptoms

The major symptoms of pleurisy include a sharp, knife-like pain made worse by deep breathing or by coughing. The pain is usually felt in the chest, but it may also be felt around the shoulders and neck and as low as the abdomen. Respiration is usually rapid and shallow. A fever may or may not be present. Wet pleurisy causes chills, fever, coughing, and breathing difficulty.

Treatment

The first order of treatment is to search out and treat the underlying cause.
Treatment of pleurisy itself includes analgesics such as aspirin or acetaminophen. If these are insufficient, a narcotic analgesic will be necessary. Bed rest is essential. A humidifier or vaporizer should be used to add moisture to the air. An elastic bandage may be wrapped around the chest and rib cage to reduce the pain on breathing. Treatment of wet pleurisy includes drainage of excess fluid from the pleural cavity.

Drugs Used in Treatment

OTC analgesics—*see the list under Pain and Fever*
R̟ analgesics—*Darvocet-N; Darvon; Darvon Compound-65; Demerol; Empirin Compound with Codeine; Equagesic; Fiorinal; Fiorinal with Codeine; Motrin; Percodan; Synalgos-DC; Talwin; Tylenol with Codeine*

Health Care Accessories—*elastic bandage; humidifier; vaporizer*

Related Topics—*Bronchitis; Pneumonia; Rheumatic Fever; Tuberculosis*

Pneumonia

Pneumonia is an inflammation of the lungs, generally caused by bacterial infection. The inhalation of irritating substances such as fumes or certain types of chemicals can cause pneumonia as can the presence of a small object, such as a coin, in the lungs.

The presence of bacteria or the irritant causes fluid to accumulate in the lungs. Because of the fluid, the normal exchange of oxygen and carbon dioxide in the lungs cannot take place. Left untreated, pneumonia may result in death in 40 percent of the cases. Death most often occurs when the patient is less than two or more than 45 years old.

Pneumonia is contagious, but not everyone will develop the infection if contaminated. It is only when the person's defense mechanisms are lowered, as they may be during periods of other infections or stress, that the disease normally appears. Bacterial pneumonia is usually preceded by a cold, influenza, or other upper respiratory tract infections. Any impairment in the cough reflex or anything causing problems in the movement of mucus can predispose a person to pneumonia.

Symptoms

Onset of symptoms is usually rapid, beginning with severe shaking, chills, and stabbing chest pain made worse by breathing. Sometimes the pain is noted in the abdomen or shoulder. Fever may go over 104° F. Severe coughs may produce a dark yellow or rusty sputum. Recent upper respiratory illness corroborates the diagnosis. The individual will feel ill, respiration may be rapid (30 to 40 breaths per minute) with severe wheezing and pain on respiration. The pulse rate may be as high as 125 beats per minute.

Treatment

Pneumonias are sometimes classified by the extent of the infection. If one or more of the lungs' five lobes are involved, it is lobar pneumonia. If both lungs are involved, it is double pneumonia. If the infection is localized near the bronchial tubes, the condition is called bronchopneumonia.

If the infection is mild, it occasionally can be treated with injections of antibiotics and bed rest at home. In such cases the use of oxygen is usually not required, although one of the portable products such as Lif-O-Gen may be used occasionally.

Treatment of extensive pneumonia usually requires immediate hospitalization. Antibiotics such as penicillin or tetracycline are given by injection. Sedatives such as phenobarbital, or Compazine are given to relax the patient and encourage sleep. Fluids are given either intravenously or by mouth to replace those lost through sweating. The patient may experience loss of appetite, and a liquid diet is usually prescribed to supply sufficient protein, calories, vitamins, and minerals. OTC cough suppressants may be effective, but stronger medication is usually required. The pain will be relieved with a codeine-containing analgesic or some other strong analgesic. Oxygen is necessary, but it must be humidified before it is inhaled.

Drugs Used in Treatment

Recommended treatment with OTC drugs—*For a codeine-containing cough syrup, we recommend Cheracol. For one that contains dextromethorphan, choose Cheracol D. Robitussin cough remedies are preferred for a brand of guaifenesin.*
OTC analgesics—*see the list under Pain and Fever*
OTC nutritional supplements—*see the list under Nutritional Disorders*
OTC cough remedies—*Benylin DM; Breacol; Cheracol; Cheracol D; Chlor-Trimeton Expectorant; Chlor-Trimeton Expectorant with Codeine; Coricidin; Coryban-D; Dimacol; Formula 44; Formula 44D; Hold (lozenge and liquid); Novahistine DH; Novahistine DMX; Novahistine Expectorant; Nyquil; Ornacol; Pediaquil; Pertussin 8-Hour; Robitussin; Robitussin A-C; Robitussin-CF; Robitussin-DM; Robitussin-DM Cough Calmers; Robitussin-PE; Romilar CF; Silence is Golden; terpin hydrate and codeine elixir; Triaminicol; Triaminic Expectorant; Triaminic Expectorant with Codeine; Trind; Trind-DM; 2/G; 2/G-DM; Vicks*
Rx analgesics—*Darvocet-N; Darvon; Darvon Compound-65; Demerol; Empirin Compound with Codeine; Equagesic; Fiorinal; Fiorinal with Codeine; Motrin; Norgesic; Parafon Forte; Percodan; Robaxin; Soma Compound; Synalgos-DC; Talwin; Tylenol with Codeine*
Rx expectorants—*Actifed-C; Ambenyl; Dimetane Expectorant-DC; Phenergan; Phenergan with Codeine; Phenergan VC; Phenergan VC with Codeine*
Rx cough suppressant—*Tussionex*
Rx sedatives and hypnotics—*Atarax; Ativan; Dalmane; Librium; meprobamate; Nembutal; phenobarbital; Quaalude; Tranxene; Valium*
Rx phenothiazines—*Compazine; Stelazine; Triavil*
Rx antibiotics—*amoxicillin; ampicillin; erythromycin; Keflex; Minocin; penicillin G; penicillin potassium phenoxymethyl; Terramycin; tetracycline hydrochloride; Vibramycin*

Health Care Accessories—*humidifier; vaporizer*

Related Topics—*Bronchitis; Pleurisy*

Tuberculosis

Since the earliest days of recorded history, tuberculosis has been considered one of the world's most feared diseases. Entire villages have been ravaged by this highly contagious and devastating disease. Until recently, patients with tuberculosis have been separated from the rest of the world and isolated in their own sanitoriums. But considerable progress has been made in the development of effective drugs for both treatment and prevention of tuberculosis, and many TB clinics in the United States have been closed.

Although less than 5 percent of the total American population will become affected, tuberculosis is still a major health problem in certain parts of the country. Worldwide, it is considered one of the leading causes of death.

Tuberculosis is caused by bacteria, and it is mainly transmitted by contamination of the air by coughs or sneezes from an infected person. It may also be transmitted by contaminated food.

Symptoms

Frequently there are no symptoms of tuberculosis, and the disease may go unnoticed for many years. If they do appear, symptoms include fever, chronic cough, thick sputum, weight loss, fatigue, and pleurisy. Spitting up blood is a frequent indication of tuberculosis. If the lungs of an individual with tuberculosis are examined after death, they can be seen to contain cysts. The body forms these cysts in an attempt to wall off the invading organism.

Treatment

Tuberculosis is most frequently treated with a combination of drugs, because treatment with a single drug allows the development of strains of bacteria resistant to that drug. Resistance does not develop as rapidly when the drugs are given in combination. Common antituberculosis drugs include isoniazid, rifampin, and streptomycin.

Drugs Used in Treatment

R_x antitubercular—*isoniazid*

Related Topic—*Pleurisy*

Whooping Cough

Whooping cough, or pertussis, is an extremely contagious infection of the respiratory tract caused by bacteria. Whooping cough can affect persons of all ages, but it most commonly affects children under the age of two, and it can be fatal. The disease is usually transmitted by airborne droplets from the sneezes or coughs of infected people. Its incubation period is about two weeks.

Symptoms

The onset of whooping cough is subtle: low-grade fever, runny nose and eyes, sneezing, tiredness, and loss of appetite. The initial symptoms resemble those of a cold with a persistent nighttime cough, and the disease is often not properly diagnosed or treated in its early stage when it is most contagious.

The cough gradually grows more severe for two to three weeks. If the infected person is unimmunized, or if his immunity has weakened, the cough eventually develops an unmistakable pattern: repeated attacks or spells (paroxysms), one severe cough following another so rapidly that the person is unable to draw breath. At the end of the coughing spasm, air is sucked deeply into the lungs, producing the characteristic "whoop." Vomiting of thick mucus usually follows.

These severe coughs persist for two to three weeks, then gradually subside over the next three to six weeks. A person with whooping cough is believed to be contagious for about six weeks after the onset of symptoms.

Treatment

Someone with whooping cough should be isolated for a few weeks, particularly from small children. Usual treatment includes several small, well-balanced feedings a day and plenty of fluids, especially when vomiting is severe. Cough suppressants or expectorants can be tried, but they are not usually very effective. A bulb suction syringe can be used to remove phlegm.

The doctor will prescribe antibiotics, including erythromycin and ampicillin, to treat whooping cough. Gamma globulin is recommended for children under the age of two to make the course of the disease milder.

In severe cases, tremors or convulsions may occur, in which case the use of oxygen may be necessary.

Immunization

The DPT vaccine is used to immunize against whooping cough. (The "P" stands for pertussis, the strain of bacteria which most commonly causes whooping cough.) It is usually recommended that infants receive three injections of the vaccine in their first six months—the first at two months, the second and third at two-month intervals. In very rare cases, the vaccine causes serious reactions, including encephalitis, fever, and coma, and may not always provide complete immunity. However the risk of the vaccine is considered minimal compared to the potential hazard of the disease itself.

Drugs Used in Treatment

Recommended treatment with OTC drugs—*For a codeine-containing cough syrup, we recommend Cheracol. For one that contains dextromethorphan, choose Cheracol D. Robitussin cough remedies are preferred for a brand of guaifenesin.*

OTC cough remedies—*Benylin DM; Breacol; Cheracol; Cheracol D; Chlor-Trimeton Expectorant; Chlor-Trimeton Expectorant with Codeine; Coricidin; Coryban-D; Dimacol; Formula 44; Formula 44D; Hold (lozenge and liquid); Novahistine DH; Novahistine DMX; Novahistine Expectorant; Nyquil; Ornacol; Pediaquil; Pertussin 8-Hour; Robitussin; Robitussin A-C; Robitussin-CF; Robitussin-DM; Robitussin-DM Cough Calmers; Robitussin-PE; Romilar CF; Silence is Golden; terpin hydrate and codeine elixir; Triaminicol; Triaminic Expectorant; Triaminic Expectorant with Codeine; Trind; Trind-DM; 2/G; 2/G-DM; Vicks*

℞ **antibiotics**—*amoxicillin; ampicillin; erythromycin; Keflex; Minocin; penicillin G; penicillin potassium phenoxymethyl; Terramycin; tetracycline hydrochloride; Vibramycin*

℞ **expectorants**—*Actifed-C; Ambenyl; Dimetane Expectorant-DC; Phenergan; Phenergan with Codeine; Phenergan VC; Phenergan VC with Codeine*

℞ **cough suppressant**—*Tussionex*

Health Care Accessory—*bulb syringe*

Cardiovascular System

The cardiovascular system nourishes every part of the body. Blood is the fluid that carries nourishment to the body's tissues. The heart is the pump that circulates the fluid, and the blood vessels are the tubes through which the nourishment flows.

Blood. Blood appears to be homogenous, but it is actually a mixture of different kinds of cells. It consists of formed elements (red blood cells, white blood cells, and platelets) and plasma, a straw-colored solution of protein and water that makes up more than half the volume of blood.

Red blood cells carry oxygen from the lungs to the body's tissues and carbon dioxide from the cells back to the lungs where it can be dispersed back into the air. There are about 27 million red blood cells in a teaspoon of blood. The oxygen is carried by hemoglobin, an iron-containing molecule in the red blood cells. Any reduction in hemoglobin or in the total number of red blood cells results in anemia.

White blood cells serve as scavengers and defenders. Whenever the body has a wound or damaged tissue or is fighting off an infection, white blood cells move in to destroy bacteria or any debris and to help the damaged area to regenerate. White blood cells also help produce the body's antibodies. One symptom of many diseases is a change in the number of white blood cells present in the body. The normal white blood cell count ranges from 25,000 to 50,000 per teaspoon. This number may rise greatly in persons with leukemia, while it may drop in some viral diseases.

The platelets help blood clot. There are 750,000 to 1,750,000 per teaspoon of blood.

Heart. The heart is a large, hollow, muscular organ containing four chambers. The heart lies between the lungs and directly behind the sternum. An average adult heart is about the size of a clenched fist, and it beats between 60 and 90 times per minute.

The right atrium receives blood from the veins of the body. From the right atrium, the blood is pumped into the right ventricle. The right ventricle circulates the blood through the lungs to exchange carbon dioxide for oxygen. This newly refreshed blood is then received into the left atrium, which pumps it into the left ventricle. The left ventricle has the responsibility for pumping blood through the aorta to the rest of the body.

Blood vessels. Blood vessels are classified according to their size, function, and physical makeup. Thus, we have the large or elastic arteries, the medium-sized or muscular arteries, the small arteries or arterioles, the capillaries, the small veins or venules, and the veins. Arteries receive the blood from the heart and take it to the various tissues of the body. Arteries usually subdivide into smaller vessels, and ultimately into numerous tiny vessels called capillaries. It is through the capillaries that blood's nutrients are transmitted to the tissues, and waste products from the tissues and cells are passed back into the blood. The venules and veins then carry this "used" blood back to the heart to be recirculated through the lungs for rejuvenation and subsequent recirculation through the body. Only in the pulmonary system (which carries used blood from the heart to the lungs and then back to the heart) does a vein carry fresh, oxygenated blood and an artery carry de-oxygenated blood.

Anemia

Anemia is a deficiency of the red blood cells either in number or hemoglobin content or both. At least 20 million Americans are believed to have some sort of anemia.

Anemia can be caused by an excessive blood loss, deficient red blood cell production, excessive red blood cell destruction, and by a condition of both decreased production and excessive destruction of red blood cells. Excessive blood loss is usually due to excessive menstrual flow or gastrointestinal bleeding, as from an ulcer. Deficiencies in red blood cell production may be due to deficiencies of certain vitamins or minerals—inadequate amounts of iron, copper, cobalt, vitamin B_{12}, and folic acid, as well as of various other substances such as vitamin B_6, vitamin B_2, protein, and possibly vitamin C. Excessive destruction of red blood cells may be due to allergy, defective blood cells, or deficiencies of enzymes. Anemias due to both decreased production and increased destruction of red blood cells include sickle cell anemia. Other causes of such anemias include chronic diseases such as infections, cancer, and rheumatoid arthritis; and various diseases of the liver, kidneys, adrenals, and bone marrow. Thus, most anemias are not caused by a dietary deficiency of iron, vitamin B_{12}, and folic acid. Therefore, "shot-gun" preparations containing iron and vitamins are not a cure-all to treat all anemias. Anyone who has anemia should not attempt to self-medicate, but should seek assistance from a doctor as soon as possible. Self-medication can obscure a diagnosis and may even contribute to an erroneous diagnosis.

Symptoms

In general, the symptoms of anemia include pallor, weakness, dizziness, ringing in the ears, spots before the eyes, headache, easy fatigability and drowsiness, irritability, and in some people, irregular mental behavior. People frequently report euphoric episodes in later stages of anemia. Additional symptoms may include loss of libido, mild fever, nausea, and vomiting. People with certain diseases may notice an increase in the symptoms of those diseases. For example, the senile individual's memory may be poorer than before, and someone with angina pectoris may find that their chest pains are worse than before. In general, the symptoms indicate an inability to circulate enough oxygen in the blood to meet the body's demands. If anemia is severe enough, heart disease may result.

Treatment

The different types of anemia are treated according to their specific cause. Part of the treatment for anemia is adequate bedrest—especially if symptoms involving the heart are present—and a diet rich in protein.

Types of Anemia

Iron-deficiency anemia. One of the most common types of anemia is due to a deficiency in iron (iron-deficiency anemia). Women are more likely than men to have iron-deficiency anemia. Many factors may contribute to a depletion of the body's iron stores. Chronic loss of blood—as described earlier—depletes the body of iron. Certain diseases of the intestinal tract, such as chronic diarrhea and hookworm infection, may decrease the absorption of iron. Pregnant women may become iron-deficient as their iron is diverted to the developing fetus.

Not surprisingly, treatment of iron-deficiency anemia is the administration of supplemental iron. Response is usually evident one to two weeks after treatment begins. Ferrous sulfate or ferrous gluconate taken orally is as effective as any other forms of iron, and they are the least expensive forms. Other forms of iron should be considered only if ferrous sulfate or ferrous gluconate causes severe stomach upset.

Pernicious anemia. Vitamin B_{12} is used in the formation of red blood cells. The daily requirement for vitamin B_{12} is very small—so small that a dietary deficiency is unlikely. However, some people are deficient in a specific substance known as the "intrinsic factor" which aids in the transport of vitamin B_{12} into the bloodstream. In these people, vitamin B_{12} will not be absorbed; this condition is known as pernicious anemia.

Symptoms of pernicious anemia are similar to the general symptoms of anemia already described. Onset is subtle. There may be sores around the mouth and tongue; the tongue usually appears smooth and beefy red. The skin may look yellowish. Diarrhea, attacks of abdominal pain, and weight loss are among the usual symptoms. There may be tingling in the fingers and toes and some loss of muscular coordination.

Pernicious anemia is treated with vitamin B_{12} given by injection. If the vitamin must be given orally, the intrinsic factor must be given at the same time. Folic acid given to people with pernicious anemia may mask symptoms of the disease; therefore, folic acid has been removed from many over-the-counter vitamin-mineral combination products. Bed rest is indicated during the severe part of the disease. Iron supplementation is not needed.

Folic acid deficiency. Like vitamin B_{12}, folic acid is essential to the formation of red blood cells. Folic acid is normally found in green, leafy vegetables, liver, mushrooms, and yeast. Deficiency of folic acid due to malnutrition is more common than might be thought. Adequate levels of vitamin C are necessary for the body to use folic acid, and alcohol interferes with its use. Thus, people living on marginal diets and alcoholics commonly have a folic acid deficiency which results in anemia.

Treatment is the oral administration of folic acid, either alone or combined with other vitamins.

Hemolytic anemia. Unlike the anemias discussed so far, hemolytic anemia is due to excessive destruction of red blood cells. The normal life span of a red blood cell is about 120 days. Hemolytic anemia is a condition in which the life span of the red blood cell is shortened and there is no compensating increase in the production of new red blood cells.

The symptoms of hemolytic anemia are similar to those of other anemias, but they are accompanied by signs of jaundice, spleen enlargement, and increased blood cell destruction. The condition may be inherited.

Hemolytic crises may occur: a sudden worsening of the condition indicated by chills, malaise, fever, pallor, shortness of breath, palpitations, dizziness, and weakness. The extremities, back, and abdomen ache. The individual may develop shock and experience severe abdominal pain and prostration. This condition can be an emergency, and it requires medical assistance and possibly hospitalization.

Hemolytic anemia is commonly caused by an allergy to a drug. Penicillin in large doses can produce hemolytic anemia, as can several other drugs, including methyldopa (Aldomet). An hereditary defect in the red blood cells can also cause hemolytic anemia.

Treatment should be directed toward the cause of the condition. Blood transfusions may modify the symptoms, but they will not cure the disorder. A corticosteroid, such as hydrocortisone, will reduce the inflammation due to allergy. If the anemia is due to some toxin (chemical, bacterial, blood parasite, or drug), the offending substance should be avoided. Treatment of the hereditary disorder often involves surgical removal of the spleen.

Sickle-cell anemia. Sickle-cell anemia is an inherited condition usually seen in blacks. The name of the disorder refers to the abnormal sickle shape taken by the red blood cells. These abnormal cells are not able to carry sufficient oxygen to the body's tissues.

Chronic symptoms of sickle-cell anemia are similar to those of other anemias, but the course of the disease is marked by crises during which the patient experiences disabling pain, especially in the bones and joints and/or the abdomen. Fever may also be present, and the crisis may last hours or days.

Complications of sickle-cell anemia can be fatal. They include blood clots, kidney damage, convulsions, osteomyelitis, enlarged heart, gallstones, and generalized infections.

Treatment is symptomatic. Analgesics may be used to control the pain, and antibiotics are given for infection. Oxygen may also be required for shortness of breath or similar symptoms.

Testing for sickle-cell anemia is a fairly simple and easy procedure because a diagnostic test (Sickledex, Ortho Pharmaceutical Corporation) is available by prescription.

Drugs Used in Treatment

Recommended treatment with OTC products—*Anemia is a serious condition and requires medical diagnosis. If your anemia is due to an iron deficiency, recommended treatment is with your pharmacy's generic brand of ferrous sulfate.*

OTC nutritional supplements—*see the list under Nutritional Disorders*

℞ **steroid hormones**—*Aristocort; Medrol; prednisone*

℞ **analgesics**—*Darvocet-N; Darvon; Darvon Compound-65; Demerol; Empirin Compound with Codeine; Equagesic; Fiorinal; Fiorinal with Codeine; Motrin; Norgesic; Parafon Forte; Percodan; Robaxin; Soma Compound; Synalgos-DC; Talwin; Tylenol with Codeine*

℞ **antibiotics**—*amoxicillin; ampicillin; erythromycin; Keflex; Minocin; penicillin G; penicillin potassium phenoxymethyl; Terramycin; tetracycline hydrochloride; Vibramycin*

Angina Pectoris

The term angina (pain) pectoris (chest) refers to chest pain caused by a heart condition. Angina pectoris occurs when the heart muscle does not receive enough blood. The pain is a signal to slow down to let the heart rest before it suffers permanent damage.

Angina pectoris is a syndrome, a set of symptoms. Its usual cause is atherosclerosis, a disease in which the blood vessels that supply the heart are blocked and the amount of blood reaching the heart is limited. A blood clot in one of these arteries may also cause angina.

Diagnosis

Angina pectoris is usually diagnosed by the patient's history and description of the pain. Classically, angina pectoris occurs as pain starting suddenly in the chest (sometimes at the breastbone) and radiating down along the left shoulder, arm, and wrist. It may be felt along the right arm, in the neck, or in the lower abdomen. It is usually brought on by exertion, but sometimes it occurs during rest or sleep. Most attacks last three to four minutes, and they increase in frequency with age.

The pain may not be described as "pain." It may feel like a burning, squeezing, choking, or aching sensation. It is sometimes described as a tightness or discomfort. The pain is sometimes attributed to gas or indigestion. The patient may also experience dizziness, shortness of breath, and ringing in the ears.

If an attack seems to differ from previous attacks in location or intensity, or if the attack is accompanied by sweating, nausea, diarrhea, and feelings of apprehension, a doctor should be contacted immediately. These may be symptoms of a heart attack rather than angina pectoris.

Treatment

To stop the pain once it appears, sublingual tablets of nitroglycerin or other medication, such as isosorbide, are taken. To prevent the pain from occurring, other drugs (nitroglycerin capsules, pentaerythritol tetranitrate, or propranolol) are taken daily.

Situations which bring on angina pectoris should be avoided. These include exercise such as walking up a flight of stairs or shoveling snow, emotional upsets, eating large meals, or cold weather. A cold weather mask will be helpful if exposure to the cold is unavoidable. The doctor will prescribe a diet and exercise program. Smoking is prohibited. Drugs may also be prescribed to treat underlying diseases such as high blood pressure.

Drugs Used in Treatment

℞ **antianginals**—*Isordil; Nitrobid; Nitrostat; Persantine*
℞ **beta blocker**—*Inderal*
℞ **smooth muscle relaxant**—*Pavabid*

Health Care Accessory—*cold weather mask*

Related Topics—*Atherosclerosis; Heart Attack; High Blood Pressure*

Atherosclerosis

Atherosclerosis is considered the primary cause of death among Americans. Atherosclerosis does not cause death directly, but the diseases caused by it—heart attack, stroke, and kidney disease—kill more Americans than cancer. Men are more likely to suffer the effects of atherosclerosis than women.

Atherosclerosis is a disease of the arteries. It is one type of arteriosclerosis, a group of diseases characterized by thickening and loss of elasticity of the arteries. Atherosclerosis is characterized by the accumulation of fats, cholesterol, sugars, and other substances on the arterial walls. The deposits of these substances are called "plaques." As plaques continue to accumulate over the years, the blood supply through the artery is decreased and the tissues and organs supplied by that artery may suffer from insufficient blood flow.

Symptoms

Atherosclerosis itself does not cause noticeable symptoms in its earlier stages. However, when the blood supply to the tissue becomes insufficient, symptoms may develop. For example, if the muscles of the heart are deprived of blood, chest pain (angina pectoris) may occur. If a kidney is deprived, blood pressure may increase and the kidney may eventually be damaged so that toxic chemicals accumulate in the blood. If blood supply to the brain is decreased, dizziness, light-headedness, disturbances of vision—even a stroke—may be experienced. Once symptoms have become apparent, little can be done to reverse the obstruction of the arteries. No drug will dissolve the plaques.

Prevention

The only treatments which have been tried are the surgical removal or scraping of the diseased arteries, and the use of artificial vessels. These are difficult procedures. Because there is no simple treatment for atherosclerosis and because the condition is so serious and prevalent in our society, everyone should know how to prevent the disease or decrease their risk of getting it.

Exercise. Exercise is effective at keeping blood levels of fat and cholesterol low, and vigorous daily exercise has been shown to delay or prevent plaque formation. It also encourages the development of new circulatory pathways so that if plaques do form, the heart has a better chance of surviving damage.

Smoking. Nicotine causes the blood vessels to constrict, depriving the body's tissues of blood; this adds to the effect of any plaques present. Studies have shown that a person with atherosclerosis who smokes a pack of cigarettes a day quadruples his chances of haveing a heart attack.

Diet. The role of diet in controlling atherosclerotic disease is not entirely clear. Restriction of fats and cholesterol in the diet may not reduce the likelihood of atherosclerosis, but neither will flooding the body with these substances be helpful. Limiting intake of these substances, maintaining a healthful weight, and avoiding large, heavy meals are generally considered beneficial in the prevention of atherosclerosis.

Drugs. There are several drugs (clofibrate, for example) which help keep fat and cholesterol levels in the blood low. The theory behind their use is that lowering the quantity of these substances in the blood will keep plaques from forming. This theory has never been proven.

Drugs Used in Prevention

R̵ antilipidemic—*Atromid-S*

Related Topics—*Angina Pectoris; Congestive Heart Failure; Heart Attack; High Blood Pressure; Stroke*

Blood Clots

Abnormal clotting of blood inside a vessel can lead to a limitation of the supply of blood into a particular area of the body, thus limiting the supply of oxygen and nutrients. Clots can cause severe effects, such as a stroke or heart attack, or they can result in nothing more serious than discomfort, tingling, or numbness in a finger or toe. If a clot forms in a vein, blood may not be able to pass through the vein, but will back up into other tissues, causing swelling and possible tissue destruction—a condition called hyperemia (congestion).

A clot attached to the wall of a vessel is called a thrombus. As long as it remains attached, the thrombus decreases the amount of blood that passes around it. This may cause damage to the tissues supposed to receive the blood—possibly resulting in a heart attack, stroke, or kidney disease. If the thrombus becomes detached from the wall and circulates through the body with the blood, it is known as an embolus. An embolus may become trapped in capillaries, blocking blood flow past that point. An embolus in the veins may reach the lungs (pulmonary embolism), a potentially fatal condition leading to partial or total destruction of the lung due to lack of blood supply.

Treatment

Anticoagulants are used in the treatment of blood clots. Heparin is an anticoagulant given by injection; Coumadin anticoagulant is given orally. Vasodilating drugs (Pavabid, Vasodilan) may be taken to dilate the blood vessels, but there is some doubt that these drugs actually help the condition. Analgesics might be used to relieve pain. Heat should never be applied to the area even though the skin may feel colder than normal, unless the doctor directs it.

Drugs Used in Treatment

R̟ anticoagulant—*Coumadin*
R̟ vasodilator—*Vasodilan*
R̟ smooth muscle relaxant—*Pavabid*
R̟ analgesics—*Darvocet-N; Darvon; Darvon Compound-65; Demerol; Empirin Compound with Codeine; Fiorinal; Fiorinal with Codeine; Motrin; Percodan; Synalgos-DC; Talwin; Tylenol with Codeine*

Related Topics—*Heart Attack; Stroke; Thrombophlebitis of the Deep Veins*

Buerger's Disease

Buerger's disease almost always occurs in men between the ages of 25 and 40 who smoke. It affects the extremities, and it is characterized by severe inflammation and blood clotting in the arteries and veins. In later stages of the disease, infection and tissue death (gangrene) may occur, necessitating amputation. The course of the disease is intermittent, meaning that it may suddenly appear and then disappear, reappearing at a much later date. The cause of Buerger's disease is unknown, although a relationship with tobacco smoking is apparent. Diabetes mellitus may be another predisposing factor.

Symptoms

All symptoms are related to lack of blood supply to the extremities. The feet and toes are the most commonly affected areas, although the hands and fingers are also sometimes affected. The affected area may feel cold or appear pale or (sometimes) red. Severe cramping pain is felt upon physical exertion and is relieved by rest. The area may feel numb and be highly sensitive to cold. If the pain becomes constant, and rest provides no relief, a physician should be called immediately because these symptoms may signal the beginning of gangrene.

Treatment

There is no specific treatment for the condition. The patient must give up smoking to keep the disease from worsening. Vasodilators or smooth muscle relaxants may be given to increase blood flow.

Symptomatic relief will be gained by avoiding use of the affected areas and applying heat (warm packs, hot water bottle, or heating pad) to the affected area to enhance blood flow. Aspirin or acetaminophen can be used to help reduce pain. Someone with Buerger's disease should sleep with the feet lower than the heart. An occasional drink of whiskey or another alcoholic beverage, taken with the approval of a doctor, may help dilate the blood vessels and further enhance blood flow.

Anyone with Buerger's disease should be tested for diabetes mellitus. If the affected area becomes infected, antibiotics will be given. Lack of blood supply to the feet and toes may contribute to the development of athlete's foot, and this should be treated with a topically-applied athlete's foot preparation (tolnaftate, for example).

Drugs Used in Treatment

OTC analgesics—*see the list under Pain and Fever*
OTC athlete's foot remedies—*see the list under Ringworm Infections*
℞ vasodilators—*Cyclospasmol; Vasodilan*
℞ smooth muscle relaxant—*Pavabid*
℞ antibiotics—*amoxicillin; ampicillin; erythromycin; Keflex; Minocin; penicillin G; penicillin potassium phenoxymethyl; Terramycin; tetracycline hydrochloride; Vibramycin*

Health Care Accessories—*heating pad; hot water bottle*

Related Topics—*Atherosclerosis; Diabetes Mellitus*

Congestive Heart Failure

Congestive heart failure is a condition in which the heart is not able to keep up with the body's demands for blood. The weakened heart is unable to pump enough blood to supply the body's tissues with the needed oxygen and other nutrients. A person with congestive heart failure usually has a history of obesity, high blood pressure, rheumatic heart disease, atherosclerosis, or kidney disease, but the disease may also occur suddenly without prior warning or known cause.

Congestive heart failure may affect the entire heart, or only one side. When the left atrium and ventricle are affected (left heart failure), blood and fluid collect in the lung. Right heart failure is characterized by swelling of the legs caused by a backup of blood and fluid.

Symptoms

Loss of energy, fatigue, and shortness of breath are typical symptoms of congestive heart failure. Inability to catch the breath after any physical activity, palpitations, and sweating are common. Because people with congestive heart failure often have a hard time breathing when lying down, they find it more comfortable to sleep propped up.

The edema (swelling) caused by right heart failure will be especially noticeable in the ankles and lower legs. The edema may be so severe that if the tissue is pressed, the imprint of the finger will remain visible for a few minutes after the pressure is released.

Treatment

Therapy for congestive heart failure involves identifying and curing the cause as well as treatment of the symptoms of the disease. In most cases, the drugs will have to be taken for the rest of the patient's lifetime.

The mainstay of therapy is a digitalis drug (Lanoxin, for example) and a diuretic. The digitalis drug is used to strengthen the heartbeat, helping the heart to pump blood more efficiently. The diuretic is used to relieve the edema; it helps the kidneys excrete fluid more efficiently, thereby preventing the collection of the fluid in the body's tissues. Meperidine or barbiturates may be given to aid in sleeping.

Oxygen may be necessary, perhaps continuously through the night. If oxygen is necessary for long-term use, it must be humidified to protect the breathing passages from drying out. Oxygen which has not been humidified should be used only in emergencies.

A strict diet must be maintained, and sodium intake should be restricted. Use of a salt substitute may be beneficial. Smoking is prohibited.

Someone with congestive heart failure may find a hospital-type bed that can be elevated more comfortably than the usual beds.

Drugs Used in Treatment

OTC salt substitute—*Co-Salt*
Rx heart drug—*Lanoxin*
Rx analgesic—*Demerol*
Rx diuretics—*Aldactazide; Aldactone; Diamox; Diuril; Dyazide; Enduron; hydrochlorothiazide; Hygroton; Lasix*
Rx potassium replacements (if using a diuretic that causes loss of potassium)—*K-Lyte; potassium chloride*

Related Topics—*Atherosclerosis; High Blood Pressure*

Edema

"Edema" (dropsy) is a general term that refers to a collection of fluid within the body's tissues. Swollen ankles, whether the swelling is caused by injury or prolonged standing, and the swelling around a bruise are examples of edema.

Edema is not really a disease, but it can be a symptom of several conditions. Some swelling is always present during any infection or inflammation. Edema is also caused by heart disease and kidney disease, and in these cases it is most likely to affect the ankles and lower legs. Certain types of blood vessel diseases are likely to cause edema. Being overweight and wearing tight garters or girdles, or rolled or elastic stockings can aggravate edema. It is also often present just prior to the onset of a menstrual period and is common during pregnancy.

Treatment

Edema is treated with diuretics such as HydroDIURIL and Lasix. Diuretics stimulate the kidneys to make more urine. The increase in urine output rids the body of excess fluid, eventually reversing the condition.

To prevent edema, a salt-free diet should be followed, and using a salt-substitute such as Co-Salt may be helpful.

Drugs Used in Treatment

OTC salt substitute—*Co-Salt*
Rx diuretics—*Aldactazide; Aldactone; Diamox; Diuril; Dyazide; Enduron; hydrochlorothiazide; Hygroton; Lasix*

Endocarditis

The endocardium is one of the membranes that line the heart (*endo-* means within; *-cardium* means heart). Endocarditis is an inflammation of the endocardium. Usually the inflammation is due to a bacterial infection, but it may also be caused by yeast or fungi.

The disease commonly occurs following the removal of teeth from a patient with infected gums, and it is because of the danger of endocarditis that a dentist will attempt to cure a gum infection with antibiotics before surgery.

Endocarditis may also occur after cardiac surgery, and it can be caused by certain infections of the blood.

Symptoms

There may be no symptoms of minor endocarditis, except for a slight fever. As the condition progresses, pain in the chest, anemia, loss of appetite, and fatigue will be noted. The fingertips become swollen and clubbed. Thin red streaks may appear under the fingernails and toenails. Nosebleeds and blood in the urine are also frequently seen.

Complications

Endocarditis can result in congestive heart failure, kidney failure, or other life-threatening diseases.

Treatment

Endocarditis caused by a bacterial infection is treated with penicillin. Restricted activity and bed rest are usually prescribed for several weeks until the doctor says it is safe to resume normal activities. The doctor may also prescribe vitamin-mineral supplements as needed to treat the anemia.

Drugs Used in Treatment

OTC nutritional supplements—*see the list under Nutritional Disorders*
Rx antibiotics—*amoxicillin; ampicillin; penicillin G; penicillin potassium phenoxymethyl*

Related Topics—*Anemia; Congestive Heart Failure*

Heart Attack

Heart attacks claim nearly 700,000 American lives each year. The disorder occurs when a coronary artery is blocked, usually by a blood clot (coronary thrombosis). Tissue death occurs in that part of the heart muscle which is not receiving blood and oxygen because of the blockage. This type of tissue death is known as myocardial infarction. The size of the lesion and the rate of scar formation determine many of the symptoms and signs as well as the rate of the patient's convalesence.

With special care for cardiac patients, the chances for surviving a heart attack are improving, although about a third of all people who have heart attacks die within a month. Sixty to 90 percent of those who also suffer shock or heart failure soon after their heart attack die within that first month. For those who recover without signs of heart failure, life expectancy is ten to 15 years. This statistic is less disheartening when we consider that most heart attacks occur in people in their mid to late 50's or early 60's. Life expectancy in patients with any degree of heart failure following the heart attack is only one to five years, however.

Symptoms

Classically, heart attacks cause crushing pain around the upper third of the breastbone. The pain is often accompanied by a cold sweat, restlessness, increased heart rate, and a feeling of impending doom. Other symptoms —wheezing, nausea, vomiting, coughing, and dizziness—have also been reported. The pain may be felt while at rest or during exertion. Interestingly, many heart attack patients are found in the bathroom, perhaps because of the nausea and vomiting, perhaps because the exertion of straining at stool precipitated the attack.

Some heart attack patients report no pain or minimal pain; some people do not realize they are having a heart attack. A mild attack may result in damage to only a small portion of the heart. The area may heal within a month or so, and perhaps there will be no other adverse effects, although the scar tissue may create other problems—such as arrhythmias or poor circulation—later on.

Some patients experience pain somewhat similar to that of angina, although more severe. This pain increases in intensity within a few minutes. It is not relieved by nitroglycerin and may become so severe that, unless relieved by narcotics, the patient will go into shock.

Treatment

Treatment *must* begin immediately. Emergency medical care must be obtained; the patient should be stabilized via the use of appropriate analgesics, antiarrhythmics, and oxygen before beginning the trip to the hospital. These same treatments will be continued enroute; meperidine, pentazocine, or lidocaine given by injection might be used. At the hospital the patient ideally should be put into a coronary care unit (CCU) where specially trained people are available to deal with life-threatening complications such as fatal arrhythmias. Such special care has been shown to prolong life among cardiac patients.

While in the coronary care unit, the heart patient should be at physical and mental rest. Medications useful to achieve that rest will include sedatives and tranquilizers such as barbiturates, Librium or Valium, or Dalmane for sleep at night. Stool softeners such as Colace laxative may make it easier for the patient to pass stools. Relief of pain can be achieved with narcotic analgesics.

Anticoagulants historically have been extensively used in myocardial infarction, but objective evidence to support their use is difficult to obtain. Surely in the short term, heparin by injection is indicated to prevent extension of the scar tissue or the formation of blood clots in the patient at rest. However, the long-term benefit of anticoagulants in myocardial infarction has not been shown.

An antiarrhythmic drug such as quinidine or procainamide will probably be given to keep the heartbeat strong and steady. The person may also be given a digitalis drug to strengthen the heartbeat, a diuretic to help the kidneys, and perhaps a nitroglycerin-like drug in case of recurrent chest pains.

Usually, after approximately one week, the patient will be moved to a "step-down unit" because less intensive monitoring is necessary.

Complications occur regularly with myocardial infarction, and often the major goal of treatment is the prevention of complications such as congestive heart failure, shock, pulmonary embolism, arrhythmias, stroke, extension of the infarction, and rupture of the heart.

Prevention

No formula has been proven to automatically insure against heart attack.

However, several factors seem to affect the incidence and severity of heart attacks. It is never too late to make healthful changes in one's lifestyle, although best results are achieved if these procedures are begun early in life.

Diet. A high-fat, high-calorie, high-cholesterol diet may promote the development of atherosclerotic plaques. These plaques may occlude blood flow into the coronary arteries, or they may break loose and form a lethal embolus. An embolus is a plug or clot moving in the bloodstream. It will stop moving and plug an artery when that artery gets small enough. This may be in the heart, brain, lungs, or other tissue. These plaques also aggravate hypertension, which, in turn, can cause heart attacks or heart failure.

To prevent heart attack, the diet should be tailored to keep the weight within tolerable limits. Excess poundage places an extra burden on the heart.

Stress. Stress may precipitate a heart attack or angina pectoris. Every attempt should be made to manage one's life-style to avoid stressful situations as much as possible, to get enough rest, and to learn to relax.

Exercise. Regular physical exercise strengthens the heart and blood vessels. A common finding among long-lived peoples is a life-long commitment to vigorous movement, either as exercise or as physical work. Tissues and functions that are not used waste away, and after only a short period of inactivity, cardiovascular deterioration begins.

Smoking. Studies have shown that smoking cigarettes increases the chances of having a heart attack.

Drugs Used in Treatment

OTC laxatives—*see the list under Constipation*
R_x **analgesics**—*Demerol; Talwin*
R_x **antiarrhythmics**—*Norpace; Pronestyl; quinidine sulfate*
R_x **beta blocker**—*Inderal*
R_x **sedatives and hypnotics**—*Atarax; Ativan; Dalmane; Librium; meprobamate; Nembutal; phenobarbital; Serax; Tranxene; Valium*
R_x **phenothiazine**—*Compazine*
R_x **smooth muscle relaxant**—*Pavabid*
R_x **anticoagulant**—*Coumadin*
R_x **heart drug**—*Lanoxin*
R_x **antianginals**—*Isordil; Nitrobid; Nitrostat; Persantine*
R_x **diuretics and antihypertensives**—*Aldactazide; Aldactone; Diamox; Diuril; Dyazide; Enduron; hydrochlorothiazide; Hygroton*
R_x **potassium replacements**—*K-Lyte; potassium chloride*

Related Topics—*Angina Pectoris; Atherosclerosis; Blood Clots; Congestive Heart Failure; Heartbeat Irregularities; High Blood Pressure; Thrombophlebitis of the Deep Veins*

Heartbeat Irregularities

The rhythmic beating of the heart is regulated by the action of several nerves. The heart's muscular contractions would continue without signals from these nerves, but the nervous impulses keep the heart beating at its proper rate.

If something damages these nerves or the heart muscle itself, the heartbeat may become irregular, a condition called arrhythmia. There are dozens of different kinds and many different causes of heartbeat irregularities. A heart attack may destroy some portion of the heart muscle, and the resulting scar tissue may interfere with the passage of nerve impulses. Smoking or ingesting caffeine in coffee, tea, chocolate, cocoa, or cola, may cause an abnormal heartbeat. Drugs, including drugs used to treat arrhythmias like digitalis and Inderal, may cause arrhythmias if taken in large amounts.

Symptoms

Arrhythmias may cause no symptoms; the patient may not even be aware of the irregular heartbeat. Some irregularity in the heartbeat is normal, and many arrhythmias are minor and not dangerous. Even a serious arrhythmia may cause no symptoms other than occasional palpitations or dizziness. On the other hand, some arrhythmias can cause fainting and angina.

Treatment

Arrhythmias which occur regularly, in someone elderly, or when other diseases of the heart (high blood pressure, congestive heart failure) are present, should be discussed with a doctor.

An occasional bothersome arrhythmia can sometimes be controlled by a decrease in the consumption of coffee, tea, or cola beverages or by a reduction or elimination of smoking. A regular exercise program may also be beneficial.

Drugs used to control irregular heartbeats include Inderal, quinidine sulfate, Pronestyl, and digitalis antiarrhythmics, but overdoses of these drugs can cause arrhythmias.

Drugs Used in Treatment

R antiarrhythmics— *Norpace; Pronestyl; quinidine sulfate*
R beta blocker—*Inderal*
R heart drug—*Lanoxin*

Hemorrhage

Hemorrhage is a term meaning bleeding. A hemorrhage occurs because of damage to some portion of the body in which blood vessels are torn or broken. A hemorrhage may be internal or external. If internal and slight, the loss of blood may be so gradual that the hemorrhage is not readily noticed or easily diagnosed. However, bleeding into the gastrointestinal tract, which may be due, for example, to a peptic ulcer, may cause black tarry stools. Bleeding in the stomach or esophagus may be indicated by the presence of blood in the vomitus.

An external hemorrhage may ooze if the injury is slight, or it may gush if the injury is severe.

Any hemorrhage serious enough to cause rapid loss of blood requires immediate attention, or it may result in death. Blood normally clots within seconds to minutes of injury to a blood vessel, thus checking the loss of blood and preventing death. If injury is severe, however, the clotting process may be inadequate to check the flow of blood.

Frequent hemorrhaging is always a cause for concern and requires a doctor's attention. Likewise, hemorrhage that doesn't stop within a reasonable period of time (minutes to hours, depending on the severity of the wound) should be seen by a doctor. Any evidence of blood in the stool should also be reported to a doctor at once. Internal bleeding may result from minor irritation to the gastrointestinal tract due to certain drugs (aspirin, Indocin, Butazolidin) or to hot foods or beverages. Or, it may be due to diseases ranging in severity from peptic ulcers to cancer of the colon. Products for testing stool for the presence of blood include Hematest Tablets (Ames Company) and Hemoccult Slides (Smith Kline Diagnostics), both of which are available without a prescription.

Treatment

Treatment of an internal hemorrhage involves correcting the cause of the hemorrhage. This may necessitate surgery.

An external hemorrhage is treated by applying pressure with a sterile gauze bandage. In an emergency situation, simply applying pressure on the wound may check the blood flow.

Health Care Accessories—*adhesive bandage; adhesive tape; gauze*

High Blood Pressure

Blood pressure is the amount of force with which the blood pushes against the walls of blood vessels as it circulates through the body. Blood pressure measurements are usually given as two numbers (120/80). The upper figure represents systolic pressure, the pressure attained as the heart pumps the blood into general circulation. The lower figure represents diastolic pressure, the pressure maintained in the arteries when the heart muscle relaxes.

Approximately one out of every ten Americans has blood pressure higher than it should be, or hypertension. There is no absolute figure which is considered normal blood pressure for everyone. However, if your systolic pressure is larger than 100 plus your age, it is too high. If your diastolic pressure is higher than 90, it is too high. Blood pressure readings may vary depending on a number of circumstances, including time of day, physical exertion, consumption of caffeine, or smoking cigarettes.

Symptoms

High blood pressure may not cause any apparent symptoms for many years. Therefore, it is important to have an annual physical and to have your blood pressure measured regularly.

Symptoms of high blood pressure which sometimes occur include: headache, especially when it appears early in the morning and is relieved as the day progresses; light-headedness; flushing of the face; ringing in the ears; loss of energy; and thumping in the chest. These symptoms may not be severe and may appear so gradually that the person may not suspect anything is wrong.

In advanced stages of hypertension, headaches become severe. Dizziness and visual disturbances may become common. Hemorrhages may appear in the eyes.

Complications

Few people die of high blood pressure, but the complications that develop because of high blood pressure are often fatal. Because high blood pressure makes the heart work harder, it may lead to heart disease. People with high blood pressure frequently develop kidney diseases and lung problems, and they are more likely to suffer strokes.

One serious form of high blood pressure is referred to as malignant hypertension. In malignant hypertension, the blood pressure rises rapidly—sometimes to alarming levels—necessitating hospitalization until the blood pressure is brought under control. Often the exact cause of this sudden rise is not known, although it may be due to tumors, kidney disease, or malfunction of an adrenal gland.

Treatment

Many drugs help to lower the blood pressure, including the thiazide diuretics, methyldopa, hydralazine, and reserpine. To gain the greatest benefit from such drugs, they must be taken exactly as prescribed and for as long as necessary—in some cases, for a lifetime. Each drug has side effects which may discourage the user from wanting to continue the drug but with continued use, people with hypertension can live longer and healthier lives.

People with high blood pressure must guard against overweight and restrict their use of salt. The doctor will prescribe a special diet and may prescribe anorexiants (drugs to reduce appetite). Salt substitutes and artificial sweeteners may also be helpful. Someone with hypertension should check the labels of all foods and OTC drug items. Some foods (tomato juice, for example) have a high sodium content, as do certain drugs (Alka-Seltzer antacid, for example).

Everyone who has hypertension should have a stethoscope and sphygmomanometer to measure blood pressure regularly.

Drugs Used in Treatment

℞ **antihypertensive and diuretic products**—*Aldactazide; Aldactone; Aldomet; Aldoril; Apresoline; Catapres; Diupres; Diuril; Dyazide; Enduron; hydrochlorothiazide; Hydropres; Hygroton; Minipress; Rauzide; Regroton; reserpine; Salutensin; Ser-Ap-Es*
℞ **beta blocker**—*Inderal*
℞ **potassium replacement**—*K-Lyte; potassium chloride*

Health Care Accessory—*blood pressure kit*

Related Topics—*Congestive Heart Failure; Heart Attack; Stroke*

Pericarditis

Pericarditis is an inflammation of the pericardial sac—one of the membrane sacs that surrounds the heart. It is usually caused by a viral or bacterial infection. The viral type is more frequent. Pericarditis may be caused by heart attacks, tumors, and bleeding into the pericardium due to injury. Pericarditis occasionally follows heart surgery.

Symptoms

The viral form of pericarditis occurs most commonly in men between the ages of 20 and 50, and it normally follows a viral respiratory infection. Pain appears suddenly in the chest area and radiates to the neck, shoulder, or back. Pain is worse when the patient lies down, and it may be accentuated by breathing or swallowing. Pain lessens when the patient stands upright or leans slightly forward. A fever (100° to 103° F or higher) is present. The chest is tender to the touch; the pulse may be rapid, weak, and irregular. The patient may be short of breath.

Treatment

Analgesics such as aspirin or acetaminophen are given to relieve the pain and fever. Aspirin and corticosteroids are useful in reducing inflammation. Antibiotics may be used if the inflammation is caused by bacteria. For severe pain, one of the narcotic analgesics may be needed.

Complete bed rest is recommended. Any fluid which has accumulated within the pericardial sac may be withdrawn by suction through a needle. If pericarditis is treated properly, the outlook is good. Most people recover in two weeks to three months. Although recurrences are uncommon, they do occur.

Drugs Used in Treatment

OTC analgesics—*see the list under Pain and Fever*
℞ steroid hormones—*Aristocort; Medrol; prednisone*
℞ antibiotics—*amoxicillin; ampicillin; erythromycin; Keflex; Minocin; penicillin G; penicillin potassium phenoxymethyl; Terramycin; tetracycline hydrochloride; Vibramycin*
℞ analgesics—*Darvocet-N; Darvon; Darvon Compound-65; Demerol; Empirin Compound with Codeine; Equagesic; Fiorinal; Fiorinal with Codeine; Motrin; Norgesic; Parafon Forte; Percodan; Robaxin; Soma Compound; Synalgos-DC; Talwin; Tylenol with Codeine.*

Raynaud's Disease

Raynaud's disease is a disorder of the blood vessels which occurs primarily in women between the ages of 15 and 45. When exposed to cold, the fingers and sometimes the toes blanch or turn bluish and get numb due to the constriction of the blood vessels. The same reaction is sometimes caused by emotional upset.

When the disease first becomes apparent, it usually affects only one or two fingers. As it progresses, however, all the fingers may become involved down to the palms. The thumbs are usually not affected.

Treatment

Recovery begins as soon as the extremity is placed in warm water or the individual enters a warm room. However, during the period of recovery, the digits may appear extremely red, and they may be throbbing and numb. They may appear swollen.

Prevention consists of avoiding the cold and protecting the extremities from exposure to cold by wearing warm gloves and stockings (if the toes are affected). People who have Raynaud's disease should be especially careful to protect the toes and fingers from injury and to treat infections in the fingers and toes quickly. Because there is insufficient blood flow into the area, the extremities will heal less readily.

The vasodilating drugs have been used to treat Raynaud's disease, but they are not of much benefit. They do increase blood flow, but they do not give complete relief.

Drugs Used in Treatment

℞ vasodilators—*Cyclospasmol; Vasodilan*

Rheumatic Fever

Rheumatic fever is the most common cause of heart disease in people under age 50. It occurs most frequently in people between the ages of 5 and 15. Caused by a bacterial infection, it often occurs several weeks after an attack of tonsillitis, a severe sore throat, or a middle ear infection.

Rheumatic fever usually affects the valves of the heart, although it may also involve other portions. The inflammation caused by the bacterial infection impairs the functioning of the valves and thereby impairs blood circulation. Complications of rheumatic fever can cause lifelong health problems including valve damage, heart failure, lung damage, and arrhythmias.

Symptoms

The major symptoms of rheumatic fever are fever and joint stiffness. The joints may feel hot, swollen, and tender. There may be a skin rash which lasts for days or months. Weight loss, sore throat, loss of appetite, abdominal pain, tiredness, and recurrent nosebleeds may also be present. Each of these symptoms is commonly associated with many other diseases, but if some of them occur within a few weeks after a severe sore throat or ear infection, they demand medical diagnosis.

Treatment

Streptococcal infections such as strep throat, tonsillitis, or ear infections should be treated promptly with penicillin to avoid rheumatic fever. Although the patient with one of these disorders is contagious and should be isolated, when the infection reaches the heart, isolation is no longer necessary.

Rheumatic fever will also be treated with penicillin, given in large doses by injection. After the disease has subsided, oral penicillin is continued on a daily basis, sometimes for several years, sometimes for the rest of the patient's life. Recurrences of rheumatic fever are common and dangerous; they may cause further heart damage. Therefore, anyone who has had rheumatic fever and develops a sore or scratchy throat should contact the doctor immediately. About 20 percent of all children who have had the disease will have a recurrence within five years.

Additional measures include the administration of aspirin to reduce fever and inflammation. Acetaminophen may also be used for fever, but it will have no effect on the inflammation. Glucocorticoid steroids such as prednisone may also be given to reduce inflammation.

Bed rest is usually necessary as long as symptoms are acute; this may take weeks or months. Then, normal activities may slowly be resumed, usually at least three months after onset of the disease. A nutritionally sound diet and plenty of fluids are indicated. Surgery is sometimes performed.

Drugs Used in Treatment

OTC analgesics—*see the list under Pain and Fever*
Rx antibiotics—*amoxicillin; ampicillin; penicillin G; penicillin potassium phenoxymethyl*
Rx steroid hormones—*Aristocort; Medrol; prednisone*

Health Care Accessory—*fever thermometer*

Related Topics—*Arthritis; Sore Throat*

Stroke

A stroke (also called cerebrovascular disease or cerebrovascular accident) is usually the culmination of an occlusive disorder in the arteries that carry blood to the brain. When an artery has been blocked and is unable to deliver blood carrying oxygen and nutrients to the brain, a portion of the brain dies. Permanent brain damage can occur if the brain cells are without oxygen and nutrients for as little as three to ten minutes. The plugged artery may be located within the brain or it may be outside the brain; frequently the major arteries leading from the heart to the brain become clogged in the area of the neck. Strokes may also occur because an artery ruptures or becomes spastic, i.e., it suddenly and violently contracts.

Usually, people who have strokes are over 40, but younger people sometimes have them as well. More than 80 percent of all stroke victims have had a previous history of high blood pressure. Most have also had some form of heart disease. Many have been obese, or have had atherosclerosis and/or diabetes.

Symptoms

A person having a stroke may have none of the usual symptoms, some of the usual symptoms, or all of the usual symptoms. Usual symptoms include dizziness, a failure of memory, falling, severe headache, visual disturbances, nausea, vomiting, emotional instability, and sometimes eventual unconsciousness followed by coma and perhaps convulsions. Breathing will be deep; it may sound like snoring.

After a stroke, those activities controlled by the damaged part of the brain may be adversely affected; the individual may lose use of an arm or leg or of an entire side of the body. Someone who has suffered a stroke may be unable to speak, or may find speaking and understanding language difficult. There may be blind spots in the vision.

One disorder that must be distinguished from stroke is referred to as a transient ischemic attack (TIA). TIAs are brief periods characterized by loss of memory, a weakness or numbness in an arm or leg, ringing in the ears, and a partial or complete loss of vision. An individual experiencing a TIA may be dizzy and may faint. Once the spell is past, usually within several minutes, there are no further symptoms and no residual effects. TIAs are believed by some people to be precursors to a stroke. Any individual experiencing TIAs should talk to a doctor and have tests to determine the likelihood of an eventual stroke. Surgery may be performed to help prevent a major stroke in persons who seem likely to have one.

Treatment

Numerous drugs have been described as beneficial in preventing stroke or in helping the patient who has had a stroke recover more quickly. These drugs include Pavabid smooth muscle relaxant, and Hydergine and Vasodilan vasodilators. The benefit claimed for these drugs is that of increasing the amount of blood coming into the brain, but this has never been shown to actually prevent strokes or to help speed recovery after a stroke.

Immediately after a stroke, oxygen should be administered to reduce further damage to the brain. Anticoagulant medication such as heparin or warfarin are given to help reduce the incidence of blood clot formation which would further hamper the delivery of blood to the brain.

Most people recover from strokes. There may be some impairment of movement or function in certain portions of the body, but with physical therapy, most functions can be restored.

Drugs Used in Treatment

℞ **smooth muscle relaxant**—*Pavabid*
℞ **vasodilators**—*Hydergine; Vasodilan*
℞ **anticoagulant**—*Coumadin*

Related Topics—*Atherosclerosis; Blood Clots; High Blood Pressure*

Thrombophlebitis of the Deep Veins

Thrombophlebitis is the partial or complete occlusion of a vein by a thrombus (blood clot) accompanied by a secondary inflammation of the venous wall. Thrombophlebitis of the deep leg and pelvis veins commonly occurs following surgery or childbirth, or heart attacks, stroke, or other conditions in which prolonged bed rest is required. It has been reported that from 30 to 60 percent of people undergoing surgery or having a major illness will develop a small thrombus. As many as 80 percent of all cases of thrombophlebitis involve the deep veins of the calf, although the process may occur anywhere deep in the legs or pelvis. If the thrombus becomes detached and is carried through the circulatory system, a potentially fatal pulmonary embolism (blood clot in the lung) may occur.

Predisposing factors include anemia, obesity, chronic infection, dehydration, malignancy, aging, and shock. A prolonged period in which the legs are not exercised—as when recuperating after surgery—is probably the single most frequent predisposing factor. Such periods without movement allow blood to accumulate in the elastic-walled veins. As circulation slows, blood clots begin to form. Pregnancy and oral contraceptives also predispose to thrombophlebitis, and a woman with a tendency to form clots or with a family history of thrombophlebitis should not take oral contraceptives.

Symptoms

Often, no symptoms become apparent until the disease is well advanced. If symptoms do occur, they include a tight feeling or pain in the calf or sometimes in the whole leg. Pain increases on walking. The leg usually looks white, feels heavy, and is extremely sensitive to the touch. When touched, the vein itself feels like a cord. A rapid pulse and a slight swelling around the calf will also be present.

Treatment

To prevent thrombophlebitis, care should be taken during and after surgery to keep blood from accumulating in the lower leg.

If thrombophlebitis develops, bed rest may be required for five to ten days during the period of severe inflammation. The legs should be raised 5 to 20 degrees above the trunk, which should be kept horizontal. Elastic bandages or stockings should be worn from the time the diagnosis is made. After inflammation has somewhat subsided, the patient can be allowed to walk for short periods, but not to stand or sit.

To decrease the incidence of blood clotting, anticoagulants are given. Relief from pain and inflammation may be obtained by using a hot water bottle over the area and administering analgesics.

Drugs Used in Treatment

OTC analgesics—*see the list under Pain and Fever*
℞ anticoagulant—*Coumadin*
℞ anti-inflammatory—*Butazolidin*
℞ analgesics—*Darvocet-N; Darvon Compound-65; Demerol; Empirin Compound with Codeine; Fiorinal; Fiorinal with Codeine; Motrin; Percodan; Synalgos-DC; Talwin; Tylenol with Codeine*

Health Care Accessories—*disposable hot packs; elastic bandage; elastic hosiery; gel hot and cold packs; heating pad; hot water bottle*

Unusual Internal Bleeding

The term "purpura" means bleeding into the skin. When large areas of skin are involved, another term, "ecchymosis," is used. "Petechiae" are tiny pinpoint hemorrhages under the skin.

Purpura may be a symptom of weakened blood vessels, blood diseases, or local damage to the blood supply as from insect bites or blows to the area. Some drugs cause the blood vessels to become sensitive and easily broken.

Various infections may cause bleeding, as will deficiencies of vitamin C (scurvy) or metabolic diseases (such as Cushing's syndrome, a disease of the adrenal gland). Bleeding into the skin is also a symptom of aging.

Whenever such bleeding becomes apparent and is unprovoked, medical attention is required, particularly if the purplish-red area persists or turns brown or black.

Varicose Veins

Veins are the blood vessels through which blood flows back to the heart. Venous flow from the upper part of the body is relatively easy; the distance is short and much of it is downhill. Venous flow from the legs, however, is literally "uphill" and against gravity. Valves in these veins normally prevent backflow of blood, but if they weaken and are not able to perform their job, blood may pool in the legs, causing the veins to bulge and dilate.

Varicose veins are dilated veins in the legs. The affected veins are close to the surface of the skin; deeper veins are protected by the surrounding muscles against massive dilation.

There may be a genetic predisposition to developing varicose veins; pregnancy and obesity also seem to contribute to their development. People whose occupations require that they stand for many hours at a time and those who must lift heavy objects seem to be more likely to have varicosities. The incidence of varicosities is much higher among women than among men.

Symptoms

Varicose veins appear as swollen, unsightly bluish cords. They may cause no other symptoms, or they may cause fatigue, itching, cramping, discomfort, and pain. The legs may swell with accumulated fluid.

Treatment

Anyone with varicose veins, or with a familial history of varicose veins, should wear elastic support stockings to provide additional support for the veins and to keep them from dilating abnormally. It is especially important to provide this support when standing for long periods or when lifting heavy objects. Whenever possible, the legs should be elevated to keep blood from pooling.

Varicose veins can be removed surgically, but new varicosities often appear at a later date. Another method of treatment is to inject a chemical into the dilated vein; this chemical (a sclerosing agent) closes off that area of the vein and forces the blood flow into the deeper venous system.

Health Care Accessory—*elastic hosiery*

Gastrointestinal Tract

The gastrointestinal tract processes food for use by the body and regulates the amount of food, water, and other substances that are absorbed into the bloodstream. It includes the digestive organs—the mouth, esophagus, stomach, intestines—and several accessory structures—the pancreas, liver, and gallbladder. A mucous membrane lines the entire digestive system and aids in the absorption of nutrients. The mucus secreted by the membrane lubricates the tract and protects it from caustic or irritating substances.

Mouth. The mouth is the beginning of the digestive tract, which is actually a tube over 30 feet long. More than simply an orifice, the mouth is where the digestive process starts. In the mouth food is chewed into smaller pieces and mixed with saliva. The saliva moistens the food, making it easier to swallow, and it contains an enzyme that helps to digest starches.

Esophagus. The esophagus transports food and liquid to the stomach. It is a muscular tube about nine inches long.

Stomach. The stomach serves mainly as a storage depot for substances entering the digestive system. In the stomach food is churned into smaller pieces and mixed with gastric juices.

Small intestine. From the stomach, food passes into the small intestine. In the first 12 inches or so of the small intestine (duodenum), the food is mixed with more digestive juices. Through the remainder of the small intestine (more than 20 feet), food is absorbed into the blood. Very little absorption of food occurs in either the stomach or large intestine.

Large intestine. The large intestine is approximately six feet long, and it is in the large intestine that the fecal mass is formed and water is reabsorbed to preserve the body's balance of fluids.

Colon. The colon, the lower portion of the large intestine, is the storehouse for fecal matter before it is transferred to the rectum. Finally the feces pass out of the body through the end of the digestive tube, the anus.

Liver. One of the accessory organs of the digestive system, the liver controls many of the body's physiological functions. It helps to detoxify and remove waste products from the blood and manufactures many different chemicals used by the body. The liver also destroys old and worn-out red blood cells. Although not directly concerned with the process of digestion, the liver does manufacture bile that contains materials required for the absorption of fat from the intestine.

Gallbladder. The gallbladder is a hollow organ located beneath the liver. Bile produced by the liver is stored in the gallbladder. When the bile is needed, the gallbladder contracts to release it into the small intestine.

Pancreas. The pancreas lies mostly behind the stomach. It has two primary functions. One portion, the exocrine portion, manufactures and secretes digestive enzymes that are delivered directly into the small intestine where they aid in digestion. The endocrine portion of the pancreas consists of the islets of Langerhans. These cells secrete the two hormones required for carbohydrate metabolism—insulin and glucagon—into the blood.

Alcoholic Hepatitis

Alcoholic hepatitis is the term used to describe the inflammatory condition of the liver that results from alcohol abuse. While alcoholic hepatitis does not develop in all who abuse alcohol, it is estimated that approximately one third of all excessive drinkers will be affected. Women are more commonly affected than men.

Although alcoholic hepatitis is often reversible, it is also the most common cause of cirrhosis of the liver in the United States, and cirrhosis of the liver is one of the most common causes of adult death in this country.

Symptoms

Alcoholic hepatitis usually occurs only after years of excessive drinking. In some people it may not develop after decades of alcohol abuse; in others, symptoms may appear after as little as a year.

Symptoms of alcoholic hepatitis are usually seen after an episode of heavy drinking. The individual complains of loss of appetite, abdominal pain and tenderness (particularly in the upper right quadrant), and nausea and vomiting. Fever, ascites (an abnormal accumulation of fluid in the abdominal cavity), spleen enlargement, and jaundice will be evident.

Treatment

Alcoholic hepatitis is treated with a diet high in calories and carbohydrates—usually in liquid formulas. During severe phases, intravenous feedings may be undertaken. Supplemental vitamins, particularly folic acid, will also be given. Corticosteroids are frequently given, but their benefits have remained partially unproven. A diuretic may be given to relieve ascites. The individual must give up alcohol or markedly reduce consumption.

Drugs Used in Treatment

OTC nutritional supplements—*see the list under Nutritional Disorders*
℞ **steroid hormones**—*Aristocort; Medrol; prednisone*
℞ **antihypertensives and diuretics**—*Aldactazide; Aldactone; Aldomet; Aldoril; Apresoline; Catapres; Diupres; Diuril; Dyazide; Enduron; hydrochlorothiazide; Hydropres; Hygroton; Minipres; Rauzide; Regroton; reserpine; Salutensin; Ser-Ap-Es*

Related Topics—*Cirrhosis; Jaundice*

Amebic Dysentery

Amebic dysentery (amebiasis) is an infection of the intestines caused by an ameba, a one-celled microorganism. The disease is transmitted through contamination of food and drink by fecal material from infected people. The microorganisms begin to develop in the large intestine. If left unchecked, they may work their way into the liver to cause possible abscesses leading to severe and fatal liver damage. Unless treated, the amebas may also travel to other parts of the body, causing infection and possibly permanent damage.

Although many people think that amebic dysentery occurs only in warm, tropical countries, it can occur anywhere and is common in parts of the United States—especially in the South. Fifty percent of the people who live in areas with poor sanitation may be carriers of these parasites. Anyone traveling in an area with poor sewerage and water treatment should take care to avoid eating poorly prepared food of any kind and should drink only bottled water.

Symptoms

Someone infected with these amebas may be asymptomatic, or they may experience only mild symptoms. However, if symptoms develop, they can become severe. The onset of abdominal pain and diarrhea may be slow. Sometimes, there are alternating periods of constipation and diarrhea. Eventually, there may be 20 or more brown, semi-fluid stools with a foul odor per day. Specks of blood (seen as black spots) and mucus may be visible on the stools. A fever may be present. As the disease progresses, weight loss and a decrease in appetite will be notable. Additional symptoms include headache, flatulence, nausea, fatigue, weakness, and abdominal cramping.

Treatment

Amebic dysentery is treated with complete bed rest (hospitalization may be required), plenty of fluids, and a diet rich in nutrients. Various amebicidal drugs may be used. Flagyl anti-infective is preferred as it kills the amebas and also protects the liver.

Drugs Used in Treatment

R anti-infective—*Flagyl*

Related Topics—*Constipation; Diarrhea*

Appendicitis

The appendix is a small strand of intestinal tissue that extends from the beginning of the large intestine. It is called a vestigial organ in that, while it probably served some function during early embryologic development, it has no known function in mature humans. Because of its location, the appendix can easily become obstructed and inflamed. When this occurs, the appendix swells. As the condition progresses, the appendix may become gangrenous, and it may perforate. Perforation results in an emptying of the intestinal contents into the body's abdominal cavity. Severe peritonitis develops, and unless it is treated immediately, death will result.

Symptoms

Appendicitis is most common between ages 5 and 30. The symptoms of appendicitis begin with pain in the area of the navel, followed by nausea, vomiting, and loss of appetite. Constipation is the usual symptom although diarrhea is present in one out of ten people. Constipation may lead people to seek relief through the use of cathartics. However, cathartics are always contraindicated for any type of abdominal pain. They may push the intestinal mass through the intestine at a more rapid rate and cause an inflamed appendix to rupture.

After several hours of nausea and vomiting, the pain usually shifts to the lower right part of the abdomen. It is made worse by sneezing, coughing, or movement. The area becomes extremely tender. A mild fever up to 102° F may be present, and the pulse is increased to about 100 beats per minute. If the fever increases even more and if the pain is very severe, rupture is almost certain. At this point the condition is a medical emergency.

146

Treatment

For appendicitis, surgery to remove the appendix is warranted. The surgical procedure is safe—much safer than risking the eventual infection and gangrene that would develop if the appendix perforated. Antibiotics such as penicillin or ampicillin are given to prevent further infection.

Anyone suffering severe abdominal pain should take no food, water, or drug until the doctor authorizes it.

Drugs Used in Treatment

℞ **antibiotics**—*amoxicillin; ampicillin; erythromycin; Keflex; Minocin; penicillin G; penicillin potassium phenoxymethyl; Terramycin; tetracycline hydrochloride; Vibramycin*

Black Stools

Black or dark red spots in the stools are a symptom of bleeding in the gastrointestinal system. Never treat such bleeding lightly, and do not attempt to take any medication. Avoid using aspirin and alcohol, and try not to smoke until after you have seen your doctor and found out what is causing the bleeding. The cause may be a small lesion that will heal spontaneously before you even see the doctor. On the other hand, the cause could be one of many serious diseases or a large lesion. Not treating such a problem could cause anemia and even death.

Cirrhosis

Cirrhosis is a chronic disease of the liver characterized by an accumulation of fibrous material, loss of liver cells, and impaired liver function. The most common cause is long-term alcoholism, but hepatitis, malnutrition, certain blood diseases, congestive heart failure, syphilis, and prolonged obstruction of the biliary tract may also cause cirrhosis. It is the fourth leading cause of death among Americans between the ages of 45 and 64. Only 35 percent of those whose liver function has been severely impaired by cirrhosis survive more than five years.

A liver damaged by cirrhosis may not be able to manufacture proteins or remove harmful substances from the blood. It may block blood flow, causing high blood pressure. Other complications include internal bleeding, abdominal distention due to fluid buildup, jaundice, and kidney failure. Eventually, stupor and coma develop. Patients with cirrhosis are extremely susceptible to infection and tend to develop severe infections. They are also more susceptible to liver cancer.

Symptoms

Symptoms of cirrhosis include nausea and vomiting, anorexia, weight loss, malaise, weakness, abdominal discomfort, loss of libido, bleeding tendencies (especially in the nose and as spots on the skin), and amenorrhea. Other symptoms sometimes reported include numbness or tingling in the fingers and toes, pancreatitis, inflammation of the tongue, and nutritional anemias; however, these latter symptoms are usually the direct effects of alcoholism.

More specific symptoms of cirrhosis include vascular "spiders" on the arms, face, and upper trunk. These appear as blood vessels in the form of the spokes of a wheel or of a spider. The ends of the fingers may be clubbed, and the liver will be enlarged and painful when pressed upon. As the disease progresses, massive edema, enlarged breasts (in men), and enlarged testicles will be present.

Treatment

Cirrhosis is treated with a rich, high-protein diet; rest; and strict abstinence from alcohol. Nutritional supplements containing high doses of vitamins and minerals are used. Prednisone or another glucocorticoid may be used when a high fever is present. A diuretic may be given to relieve fluid retention.

Drugs Used in Treatment

OTC nutritional supplements—*see the list under Nutritional Disorders*
R steroid hormones—*Aristocort; Medrol; prednisone*
R antihypertensives and diuretics—*Aldactazide; Aldactone; Aldomet; Aldoril; Apresoline; Catapres; Diupres; Diuril; Dyazide; Enduron; hydrochlorothiazide; Hydropres; Hygroton; Minipres; Rauzide; Regroton; reserpine; Salutensin; Ser-Ap-Es*

Colic

Colic is a condition common among infants less than three months of age. It is characterized by periods of intense, unexplained crying and apparent abdominal pain. Possible causes include overfeeding or underfeeding, an upset stomach from disagreeable foods, excessive burping, allergy, or tension.

Symptoms

Colic is identified by the child's prolonged crying, screaming, and fretfulness. There usually seems to be little the parent can do to relieve the child's distress. The infant may pass gas, have diarrhea, or vomit. The abdomen may feel firm and distended. Because of the pain, the infant often keeps the knees flexed and legs drawn up toward the abdomen.

Treatment

A doctor should be notified if colic persists. The doctor will determine whether anything serious is causing the infant's distress. In some cases, Bentyl antispasmodic is prescribed to be added to the formula. This drug reduces cramping by decreasing the motility of the intestinal muscles.

Treatment may call for a change of formula or a different feeding schedule. Feeding of a colicky child should be carried out in a quiet, relaxed atmosphere away from excessive noise or excitement. A pacifier may help, as will patting the baby's back to expel excess gas in some instances.

Drugs Used in Treatment

R antispasmodic—*Bentyl*

Constipation

Constipation in its true sense refers to abnormally difficult or infrequent passage of stools. Constipation is a symptom, not a disease. Bowel movements are motivated primarily by the nature of foods eaten, the time of day, and the proximity of and familiarity with a particular toilet, as well as by psychological factors. It is not necessary to have a bowel movement every day. Normal frequency may vary from three per day to three per week.

Constipation can be caused by both organic and functional disorders. Organic causes (those relating to changes in the structure of an organ) include obstruction of the intestine, weakness of the abdominal muscles, cancer, and diverticulitis. Functional disorders (those associated with impairment of function rather than change in structure) that can lead to constipation involve both local problems, such as lack of nervous stimulation of the bowel, and systemic disorders, such as infection or diseases of various endocrine glands.

Constipation can be caused by physical inactivity, and is commonly seen in bedridden, hospital, or nursing-home patients. It is also a relatively common side effect of drug therapy. Pregnant women are frequently constipated. Irregular eating habits, lack of fiber in the diet, and inadequate fluid intake may also lead to constipation.

In healthy individuals, the colon should be conditioned to expel feces in response to normal stimulation. Having a bowel movement at the same time every day is quite beneficial, although not necessary for good health. The best time is in the early morning, about 30 to 60 minutes after breakfast. The ingestion of food on an empty stomach activates and increases intestinal peristalsis. During the night, residue from the previous day's meals has moved to the rectal area and is ready to be eliminated. This is also the reason laxatives and cathartics work best if they are taken at night before bedtime. Their action is then ready for the morning.

Prevention

To prevent constipation, modify the diet to include adequate fiber, drink at least eight to ten glasses of water each day, exercise, and develop good bathroom habits. Laxatives should be used only when absolutely necessary; their prolonged use can impair normal bowel function. The use of laxatives to treat abdominal pain, vomiting, and other serious digestive tract symptoms can lead to life-threatening situations. Of course, there are legitimate medical uses for laxatives.

Laxatives are well used to treat persons poisoned with noncorrosive substances or those who have parasitic infestations. Laxatives are used routinely before surgery, delivery, and radiological examination of the gastrointestinal tract. Laxatives are also used to counteract the constipating effects of drugs such as the antacids, antispasmodics, iron medications, narcotics, phenothiazines, and tricyclic antidepressants. Stool softeners are quite useful after rectal surgery and to relieve the stress of passing stool in patients with congestive heart failure, high blood pressure, and hernias.

Laxatives

The basic types of laxatives include the stimulants, salines, bulk-forming, and lubricant or stool-softening agents. The terms laxative and cathartic are interchangeable in that all agents lead to the same result—that of facilitating bowel movements. Laxatives are usually thought of as agents that produce a mild passage of stools while cathartics are more forceful, producing a watery and sometimes explosive bowel movement.

Stimulant laxatives increase the movement of the intestines. Saline laxatives increase moisture in the intestine. Bulk-forming agents add fiber, and lubricants and stool-softeners add oil to lubricate or reduce the hardness of the material within the intestine.

Individual products within any category of laxatives (stimulant, saline, bulk-forming, or lubricant and stool softener) do not vary much. Some may be stronger than others, but this problem can be solved by adjusting dosage. Some may cause more cramping than others, but, in this case, a switch to another product will probably solve the problem.

Stimulant laxatives. Stimulants lead all other laxatives in sales; yet they are the least desirable. They irritate the walls of the intestines, and after prolonged use (one to two months), they may cause intense cramping, diarrhea, and fluid depletion. People who take stimulants repeatedly may come to depend on them to have a bowel movement, or they may develop ulcerative colitis or a nutritional disease. If a stimulant laxative must be taken, products such as Dulcolax tablets, Dorbane tablets, or Modane tablets should be chosen. These products have mild agents such as bisacodyl, casanthranol, or danthron. These mild agents produce less cramping than do stronger agents such as cascara sagrada and aloe.

When bisacodyl tablets are taken, the individual must be advised not to crush or chew them or take them with antacids or milk in order not to destroy the enteric coating of the tablets. If the enteric coating is destroyed, the bisacodyl will be prematurely released to irritate the esophagus and stomach, possibly causing intense cramping.

Castor oil, although it tastes terrible, is still considered to be one of the most thorough laxatives. It is also the fastest acting oral agent. Because castor oil is broken down to its active ingredient in the small intestine, it evacuates the contents of both the small and large intestines. It is therefore an excellent preparation for x-ray of the upper and lower gastrointestinal tract. It should not be used as a routine cathartic because it can lead to severe cramping, dehydration, and loss of nutrients.

Saline laxatives. Chemicals in saline laxatives dissolve in water but do not easily pass through the intestine into the bloodstream. When these products are taken with a full glass of water, the water stays in the intestine and lubricates the bowel. Because saline laxatives attract water molecules, they must be taken with at least one full glass of water to avoid pulling water out of the body into the intestine. Saline laxatives usually act within 30 to 60 minutes and produce a watery and somewhat explosive bowel movement. Therefore they must be taken only at a convenient time.

Bulk-forming laxatives. These laxatives have fibers from seed or other parts of plants that cannot be digested or absorbed by the body but do, however, have a high affinity for water. When they come in contact with water in the intestine, they swell, thus increasing the bulk of material in the intestine. They also produce a gel that lubricates the bowel.

Bulk-forming laxatives do not irritate the intestine as the stimulants do, and they cause less urgency than the saline laxatives do. For these reasons, they are the best choice for controlling long-term constipation. There is one precaution, however, about their use. Bulk-forming laxatives must be completely mixed with water before swallowing. If they are swallowed dry, they may swell in the throat and cause choking.

Lubricants and stool softeners. In the past, people have used vegetable, mineral, or other oils as laxatives. Some of these oils—including mineral oil—are absorbed into the body and produce serious side effects. Following repeated or prolonged use (one to two months), mineral oil may bring on an allergic reaction resembling pneumonia, or it may retard the body's absorption of vitamins A, D, and K.

While some people swear that "light" mineral oil is better than regular mineral oil, it has not been shown to provide any better laxative effect. Light mineral oil is usually more expensive than heavy (or regular) mineral oil and can cause rectal leakage which may stain undergarments.

Stool softeners have been used to prevent constipation or to treat long-term constipation. Stool-softening agents may take two to three days to produce any effect. But after that, their action is continuous. Liquid stool softeners can be mixed with milk, cola drinks, or fruit juice to disguise the taste of the stool softener. Mixing will not decrease the laxative effect. Capsules are more agreeable and less expensive; they should be taken by those who don't find it difficult to swallow capsules.

Drugs Used in Treatment

Recommended treatment with OTC drugs—*For a stimulant laxative, choose Dulcolax, Dorbane, or Modane. For a saline laxative, purchase a generic brand of epsom salts. Metamucil or Modane Bulk are the bulk-forming laxatives of choice. For a lubricant laxative, buy your pharmacy's generic brand of mineral oil. And for a stool softener, buy Colace, Surfak, or the pharmacy's generic brand of docusate (also called dioctyl sodium sulfosuccinate, or dioctyl calcium sulfosuccinate, or DSS). Peri-Colace contains a stimulant laxative along with a stool softener and is also recommended.*
OTC laxatives—*Agoral; Alophen; Carter's Little Pills; castor oil; Colace; Correctol; Dialose; Dialose Plus; Dorbane; Dorbantyl; Dorbantyl Forte; Doxidan; Dulcolax; Ex-Lax; Feen-A-Mint; Fleet Enema; Fletcher's Castoria; Haley's M-O; Metamucil; milk of magnesia; mineral oil; Modane; Modane Bulk; Modane Mild; Nature's Remedy; Neoloid; Nujol; Peri-Colace; Phillips' Milk of Magnesia; Regutol; Senokot; Serutan; Surfak*

Diarrhea

Diarrhea is an abnormal frequency and liquidity of bowel movements. It is usually considered an annoying, short-term occurrence, but it can be dangerous, resulting in dehydration and loss of essential salts, and it is a symptom of a health problem.

Diarrhea is usually an attempt by the body to rid itself of some irritating or toxic substance. This acute diarrhea is self-limiting, usually lasting one or two days, and never more than three. Acute diarrhea may be of toxic, infectious, or dietary origin. It could be the result of some acute illness or a response to emotional stress.

If diarrhea lasts more than three days, it is considered chronic diarrhea. Because it is usually the result of multiple causes, it is difficult to diagnose and treat. It may be a symptom of a serious organic disease such as cancer of the colon or rectum, chronic ulcerative colitis, amebic colitis, tuberculosis enteritis, sprue, or a host of other causes. Chronic diarrhea requires medical help.

Treatment

The best treatment for diarrhea is to rest and drink plenty of fluids. Heavy foods and rough vegetables should be avoided. Medical help should be sought if diarrhea persists for more than three days and/or the stool contains blood, pus, or mucus.

Several hundred OTC products are currently available to treat diarrhea. OTC antidiarrheal ingredients include adsorbents, paregoric, bacterial cultures, and anticholinergics.

Adsorbents. Kaolin, bismuth subgallate, pectin, activated charcoal, alumina gel, and attapulgite coat the walls of the stomach and intestine and absorb irritating materials by attracting irritants and keeping them from being absorbed into the bloodstream.

Paregoric. Paregoric slows the contraction of the intestines to reduce the number of bowel movements. Pure paregoric requires a prescription, but it is preferable to the OTC antidiarrheals combining paregoric with other ingredients. Only low doses of paregoric are available in OTC products such as Parepectolin diarrhea remedy. Contrary to popular belief, these low doses will not lead to abuse nor produce serious side effects. The prescription drugs codeine and Lomotil have similar actions. Paregoric and codeine are considered to be the agents of choice for the treatment of acute, short-term diarrhea. Using either of them to treat chronic diarrhea is irrational due to the increased chance for drug dependence. Because Lomotil also contains a subtherapeutic amount of atropine sulfate, abuse potential is limited, and it is currently considered to be an agent of choice for treating long-term, chronic diarrhea.

Bacterial cultures. Live bacteria, such as those in yogurt, supposedly restore bowel movement to normal. While many people swear by these products, little scientific evidence proves that they work. The same effect may be achieved by drinking milk or buttermilk or eating yogurt—and at less cost.

Anticholinergics. Atropine sulfate, hyoscyamine sulfate, homatropine methylbromide, and hyoscine hydrobromide reduce the movement of the intestine. However, to be effective, anticholinergics must be taken in high doses, and no OTC antidiarrheal product contains enough. The anticholinergics also can cause annoying side effects such as dry mouth, blurred vision, and thumping in the chest.

Antibacterials. Antibacterials have also been used to treat diarrhea. They require a prescription. Neomycin, long used as an antidiarrheal, is no longer indicated for this purpose because it may be absorbed into the body. In persons with renal malfunction, toxic levels may accumulate and lead to serious damage to the ear and possibly to irreversible deafness. Furazolidone (Furoxone) possesses toxicities similar to those of neomycin.

Drugs Used in Treatment

Recommended treatment with OTC drugs—*For those who insist on taking an antidiarrheal preparation, a combination of kaolin and pectin (for example, Kaopectate liquid diarrhea remedy), is recommended. A product that combines these ingredients with paregoric (e.g., Parepectolin) is also acceptable. Such products are the most economical and the safest. OTC products containing an anticholinergic should be avoided.*

OTC diarrhea remedies—*Donnagel; Donnagel-PG; Kaopectate; Kaopectate Concentrate; Lactinex; Parepectolin; Pepto-Bismol (liquid and tablet)*

R$_x$ **antidiarrheal**—*paregoric*

R$_x$ **anticholinergic and antispasmodic**—*Lomotil*

Diverticulitis of the Colon

A diverticulum is a small sac or pouch that projects out of the bowel wall. Although not usually found in the rectum, diverticula may occur throughout the intestinal tract, most frequently in the lower portion of the colon. Everyone has diverticula, and because the constant peristaltic activity of the bowel contributes to their formation, older people have more.

Diverticulitis is an inflammation of the diverticula, and it can cause serious problems. The condition is rare in persons under age 40, but the incidence increases to about 10 percent of those people over 60. Usually the inflammation results from infection of the diverticula. If the condition is left untreated, abscesses may form, resulting in further inflammation, a thickening of the tissue, and obstruction of the bowel. Within this thickened tissue mass, infection persists, causing further inflammation. This in turn may lead to extension of the abscesses to the point that they burst into the surrounding areas and organs. If the sterile peritoneal cavity is invaded by the infection, peritonitis results and death is probable in a matter of hours to days.

Symptoms

Symptoms of diverticulitis are similar to those of appendicitis: severe pain in the lower left part of the abdomen with nausea and vomiting; abdominal distention is also present. Constipation, or diarrhea, or both may be present. The individual develops chills and a fever. He becomes weak and the skin over the area becomes extremely tender. There may be blood in the stool.

Treatment

Diverticulitis must be treated with complete bed rest and antibiotics. Fluids are permitted, but food should not be given during the initial flareup. For severe pain, one of the narcotic-containing analgesics may be used. If constipation is present, laxatives are contraindicated. The antidiarrheal agent, Lomotil, is used to treat the diarrhea.

Drugs Used in Treatment

℞ antibiotics—*amoxicillin; ampicillin; erythromycin; Keflex; Minocin; penicillin G; penicillin potassium phenoxymethyl; Terramycin; tetracycline hydrochloride; Vibramycin*
℞ analgesics—*Darvocet-N; Darvon; Darvon Compound-65; Demerol; Empirin Compound with Codeine; Fiorinal with Codeine; Motrin; Percodan; Synalgos-DC; Talwin; Tylenol with Codeine*
℞ anticholinergic and antispasmodic—*Lomotil*

Related Topic—*Peritonitis*

Epigastric Pain

Pain in the upper abdomen below the ribs results from numerous conditions elsewhere in the body. The most common causes of pain in the epigastric region are peptic ulcer or the presence of some disagreeable substance in the stomach or intestine. If this pain is associated with nausea or vomiting, or perhaps with diarrhea, consider that the pain is from the intestine. If nausea and vomiting relieve the symptoms, the pain may be due to an ulcer, especially if it awakens the patient in the early morning and if it can be relieved by drinking milk or ingesting a light snack. However, the pain may also be due to angina pectoris (originating from the heart) and may even signify the beginning of a heart attack. If the pain occurs after you have been lying down for a few minutes and you can feel it in the chest, the pain may be from a hiatus hernia. Other conditions such as cancer or bleeding into the lower cavities may also cause epigastric pain.

Do not attempt to diagnose these conditions yourself, but seek the assistance of your doctor as soon as you realize that the pain recurs or causes severe discomfort.

Avoid taking any laxative product for a pain that occurs in the abdomen. If the pain is caused by appendicitis, the laxative could worsen the condition and cause severe infection throughout the body that may cause death.

Related Topics—*Angina Pectoris; Appendicitis; Heart Attack; Hiatus Hernia; Peptic Ulcer*

Esophagitis

The esophagus forms the passageway for food between the mouth and the stomach. It is also known as the gullet or food tube. Whenever the lining of the esophagus becomes inflamed, the condition is called esophagitis. Numerous factors may cause inflammation, including the ingestion of excessively hot or irritating foods or substances, smoking, severe vomiting, infections, and having a nasogastric tube inserted during surgery. One form of esophagitis, heartburn, occurs when gastric acid is regurgitated from the stomach into the lower portion of the esophagus.

Symptoms

Symptoms of esophagitis include burning pain in the chest and difficulty in swallowing. Someone with esophagitis may not want to eat for fear of choking or increasing the pain. Esophageal pain is frequently mistaken for heart attack.

Treatment

Treatment includes avoiding excessively hot or irritating foods and replacing them with bland substances. At least eight to ten glasses of fluids should be taken each day. Someone with esophagitis should avoid lying down for at least one to two hours after eating.

Drugs Used in Treatment

Recommended treatment with OTC drugs—*Antacids will reduce the acidity of irritating liquids as they are swallowed. It may be necessary to repeat the dosage quite often. There is little reason to recommend one OTC antacid over another. The product you choose should be one having an acceptable taste that does not cause you to be constipated or to have diarrhea. It may be just as well to purchase a nationally advertised brand such as Maalox or Mylanta, and then experiment with other brands to find the least expensive product acceptable to you.*
OTC antacids—*Alka-Seltzer; Alka-2; Amphojel; Di-Gel; Fizrin; Gaviscon; Gelusil; Gelusil II; Kolantyl; Maalox; Maalox #1; Maalox #2; Mylanta; Mylanta-II; Riopan; Rolaids; Tums*

Related Topics—*Heartburn; Peptic Ulcer*

Flatulence

Flatulence refers to excessive intestinal gas. Gas in the intestine is a result of air swallowed with food and water, of gases present in food, and of the action of bacteria in the intestines. Some of this gas is absorbed through the intestine, while that which is passed through the anus is called flatus.

Flatulence accompanied by other symptoms (chest pain, vomiting, diarrhea, change in color of urine or stool) may signal serious disease such as esophageal ulcer, hiatus hernia, gallstones, and various cancers.

Treatment

There is no specific treatment for flatulence. Anticholinergic and antispasmodic agents are used. If flatulence occurs because of anxiety, mild sedatives may be of value. The antiflatulent simethicone (Mylicon) may give temporary relief.

Foods—such as beans, dairy products, certain vegetables, and carbonated beverages—which lead to excessive flatulence should be avoided.

To avoid swallowing excess air, the patient should try to eat more slowly, keep the mouth shut while chewing, and avoid chewing gum.

Drugs Used in Treatment

OTC antiflatulent—*Mylicon*
R̥ anticholinergic—*Pro-Banthine*
R̥ anticholinergics and sedatives—*Donnatal; Librax*
R̥ anticholinergic and phenothiazine—*Combid*
R̥ antispasmodic—*Bentyl*

Food Poisoning

Staphylococcal Gastroenteritis. Food poisoning by toxins produced by staphylococcus bacteria ("staph") is the most common form of food poisoning in the United States. It frequently occurs after picnics and parties in warm weather. Whenever food has been allowed to sit unrefrigerated it can become infected. Contamination can occur in as little as four hours at a temperature above 80° F. Foods such as cheeses, processed meats, cream pies, custards, and salads (especially salads like potato or chicken salad) are among the foods most commonly contaminated.

Food can also be contaminated through handling by someone with a cut finger, a cold, or boils.

Symptoms

The abrupt onset of nausea, vomiting, diarrhea, and abdominal cramping and tenderness from two to four hours after eating may signal food poisoning. These symptoms may be accompanied by excessive sweating and salivation. Symptoms do not usually last longer than a day in adults. However, persons with diseases of the kidney or heart, and the very young and very old may be severely affected.

Treatment

Treatment consists of bed rest and avoidance of heavy foods. Light soups and water can be given if the patient is not nauseous or vomiting. No antibiotics or antidiarrheal medications should be taken. The antibiotics will be ineffective, and the condition of diarrhea is actually beneficial because it will help rid the system of the staphylococcal bacteria.

Botulism. Another type of food poisoning is caused by the toxin (poison) produced by the bacteria called *Clostridium botulinum*. Botulism can occur after the consumption of improperly processed home-canned food or by contaminated commercially prepared foods such as meats and vegetables. All cases of botulism are medical emergencies and must be treated by a doctor immediately. The toxin involved in botulism is one of the most dangerous substances known. It is absorbed by the small intestine and carried by the blood to the nerves, where it can cause a type of paralysis. The victim can die of suffocation.

Symptoms

The following become evident within one-and-a-half days after consuming contaminated foods: dizziness; difficulty in breathing, swallowing, and speaking; barking cough; dry mouth; and muscular weakness. Nausea, vomiting, abdominal cramps, and diarrhea are also sometimes present. The pupils become dilated.

Treatment

The disease must be treated immediately. It is treated with a botulinum anti-toxin injection.

Gallstones

A gallstone is a hardened mass formed in the gallbladder or the bile duct. The person most likely to have gallstones is a white, overweight woman over 40 years of age. The medical term for the condition is cholelithiasis, and its cause is not known, although it may be a metabolic disorder.

Symptoms

The condition may not cause any symptoms. If symptoms do appear, they commonly include flatulence, belching, indigestion, a feeling of fullness, constipation, and sometimes pain in the abdomen. If gallstones block the duct by which bile leaves the gallbladder, indigestion and constipation result. Jaundice may occur. If the stones push against the wall of the gallbladder or if one or more of them is passed through the bile duct, pain is the result.

Complications

Although the gallstones themselves may not cause any symptoms, serious complications may develop. The gallbladder may become inflamed, a condition called cholecystitis. When the gallbladder becomes inflamed, severe pain is usually felt within 30 to 60 minutes after eating. The pain is felt in the abdomen, and it may radiate to the sides, back, or shoulders. It often lasts for several hours. Frequently the person is thought to be experiencing a heart attack or severe complications of a peptic ulcer. Surgery is indicated. Narcotic analgesics will help control pain.

Other problems may also develop. If the gallstones block the flow of bile, jaundice may develop and severe damage to the liver may result. Occasionally, infection or damage to nearby organs results from pressure applied by the stone.

Treatment

Surgical removal of the gallbladder is common treatment. Persons with gallstones should not eat foods rich in fat or fried in grease. Gas-forming vegetables such as cucumbers, radishes, and turnips should be avoided. All foods should be tested in moderation before large quantities are consumed. A mild laxative is recommended if constipation is severe.

Drugs Used in Treatment

OTC laxatives—*see the list under Constipation*
R analgesics—*Darvocet-N; Darvon; Darvon Compound-65; Demerol; Empirin Compound with Codeine; Equagesic; Fiorinal; Fiorinal with Codeine; Motrin; Percodan; Synalgos-DC; Talwin; Tylenol with Codeine*

Related Topics—*Constipation; Jaundice*

Gastritis

The term "gastritis" refers to an inflammation of the mucous lining of the stomach. Both the cause of the inflammation and the symptoms produced by it are extremely variable. The condition may be caused by chemical, bacterial, or viral irritants, hot spicy foods or beverages, allergy, trauma, or stress, and it may range in severity from a slight irritation to complete debilitation. It may be acute or chronic.

Symptoms

Symptoms commonly include nausea, vomiting, abdominal pain, loss of appetite, a feeling of fullness, and diarrhea. If the condition is caused by infection, fever, chills, headache, fatigue, and cramping will be present.

Treatment

When gastritis is caused by the ingestion of an irritant (commonly alcohol, aspirin, Indocin, Butazolidin, or other medications), the condition will usually be relieved as soon as the irritant has been removed. If, however, the irritation is severe, the lining of the stomach may actually become deeply eroded and eventually ulcerated. Peptic ulcers may form.

Corrosive gastritis is seen after an individual accidentally or intentionally swallows concentrated acid or alkali. Severe irritation and hemorrhaging followed by intense scarring occurs. Gastric obstruction may ensue as the area of muscle between the stomach and intestine—known as the pylorus—becomes constricted and food cannot easily pass from the stomach into the intestine. In severe cases—usually by ingestion of acid—if the damage involves deep layers of the stomach wall, the stomach wall may become perforated.

Gastritis is often difficult to treat because its cause is not always known. Antinauseants, preferably the phenothiazines, are given for nausea. If pain is present, analgesics are employed. Aspirin may irritate the stomach and should not be used. Many individuals are placed on a bland diet and are told to avoid irritants such as coffee, tea, and other cola beverages. The use of tobacco should be avoided.

Antacids are given when hyperacidity or peptic ulcers are suspected. It is important to neutralize as much of the acid as possible. A paradox to keep in mind is that the actual quantity of gastric acid secreted in patients with gastritis may be less than normal. However, even these small amounts must be neutralized as much as possible to avoid further damage to the deeper layers of the stomach wall.

Drugs Used in Treatment

Recommended treatment with OTC drugs—*There is little reason to recommend one OTC antacid over another. The product you choose should be one having an acceptable taste that does not cause you to be constipated or to have diarrhea. It may be just as well to purchase a nationally advertised brand such as Maalox or Mylanta, and then experiment with other brands to find the least expensive product acceptable to you.*
OTC antacids—*Alka-Seltzer; Alka-2; Amphojel; Di-Gel; Fizrin; Gaviscon; Gelusil; Gelusil II; Kolantyl; Maalox; Maalox #1, Maalox #2; Mylanta; Mylanta-II; Riopan; Rolaids; Tums*
OTC analgesics—*Tempra; Tylenol; Tylenol Extra Strength (tablet, capsule, and liquid)*
Ŗ phenothiazine—*Compazine*

R̩ analgesics—*Darvocet-N; Darvon; Demerol; Talwin; Tylenol with Codeine*

Related Topics—*Food Poisoning; Nausea and Vomiting; Peptic Ulcer*

Gastroenteritis

Gastroenteritis is an inflammatory condition of the lining of the stomach and the intestine. It is caused by infections, food poisoning, parasites, allergies, bacteria, viruses, and toxins. The ingestion of extremely hot or irritating foods or fluids, alcohol, and drugs such as aspirin, Butazolidin and Indocin may cause it.

Symptoms

Symptoms include nausea, vomiting, abdominal cramping, and diarrhea. The symptoms appear suddenly and without prior warning. The individual may feel faint and weak. If an infection is present, a fever will occur. The skin may feel cold and clammy, and the individual will have a rapid pulse.

Treatment

The treatment of gastroenteritis includes bed rest and a restricted diet. No food or liquids should be given until the doctor directs it. When food is allowed, light and liquid meals should be taken, and heavier food should be avoided. Nausea and vomiting are treated appropriately.

Related Topics—*Diarrhea; Nausea and Vomiting*

Gingivitis

An inflammation of the gums is called gingivitis. It is usually caused by poor oral hygiene. The greatest single factor may be neglecting the removal of plaque and tartar. Infection, malocclusion, poor dental work, faulty dentures, and constantly breathing through the mouth may also incite gingivitis. It may likewise be a symptom of other diseases, including diabetes and scurvy.

Symptoms

The symptoms of gingivitis include an extremely sore mouth and gums. The gums become swollen and red or bluish purple. They bleed easily, and brushing the teeth becomes extremely painful.

Treatment

Although treatment of gingivitis can be carried out largely at home, complete treatment requires professional help in removing plaque and tartar. Additional dental work may also be required. A severe condition may necessitate antibiotic therapy to reduce further bacteria-induced inflammation.

Local pain can be treated by rinsing the mouth with a warm solution of one teaspoonful of salt in water or a solution of equal parts hydrogen peroxide and water. Most mouthwashes will provide temporary relief, although their use is not a treatment for the disorder.

Drugs Used in Treatment

Recommended treatment with OTC drugs—*Gly-Oxide gel releases oxygen in*

the mouth. When this product is used on or around the affected area of the gums, relief may be felt. Your pharmacy's generic brand of hydrogen peroxide, diluted with water and used to rinse the mouth, will also relieve the pain.
OTC canker sore and fever blister remedy—*Gly-Oxide*

Related Topic—*Trench Mouth*

Glossitis

Glossitis, inflammation of the tongue, may be a symptom of disease or the result of injury to the tongue. Diseases that can cause a sore tongue include cancer, syphilis, anemia, systemic infections, and nutritional deficiencies. The tongue may be injured by ill-fitting dentures, sharp teeth, mouth breathing, or irritants such as alcohol, tobacco, drugs, or hot or spicy foods.

Symptoms

The tongue may be extremely smooth and bright red, or it may be ulcerated. It will be painful and irritated, and may be swollen. There may be a foul taste in the mouth and bad breath.

Treatment

If the condition is due to disease, that disease must be treated. In general, however, no treatment is indicated for the damage usually heals quickly. If the condition recurs frequently or persists, a doctor should be consulted.

Drugs Used in Treatment

Recommended treatment with OTC drugs—*Gly-Oxide gel may bring temporary relief of the pain of glossitis.*
OTC canker sore and fever blister remedy—*Gly-Oxide*

Heartburn

Whenever the stomach's gastric juices push upward into the esophagus, a disagreeable burning pain is felt behind the sternum. This is termed heartburn or pyrosis, and it occurs because the gastric juices stimulate the nerve endings located in the esophagus. It is not a pain in the heart itself, although it is sometimes mistaken for a heart attack. Heartburn is common in pregnant women, and it usually disappears shortly after delivery. It may be a symptom of peptic ulcer disease, but heartburn does not automatically mean that the person has a peptic ulcer.

Treatment

Heartburn is best treated with OTC antacids. If the pain is severe, doses of antacid may need to be taken as frequently as every hour or two. Otherwise, a dose can be taken whenever the pain is felt. Pain relief will usually occur within a few minutes of taking the antacid.

Heartburn is relieved somewhat by sitting upright. Also, it can be reduced by eating small meals, losing weight, and avoiding tight-fitting clothing. Stress and certain substances (tobacco, alcohol, and caffeine) aggravate heartburn and should be avoided.

Avoid lying down after eating as this will allow the gastric juices to more readily enter the esophagus. If the condition is especially bothersome at night, elevate the head of the bed by about four to six inches with blocks or books placed under the legs. Do not eat or drink within one or two hours of going to bed.

Drugs Used in Treatment

Recommended treatment with OTC drugs—*There is little reason to recommend one OTC antacid over another. The product you choose should be one having an acceptable taste that does not cause you to be constipated or to have diarrhea. It may be advisable to purchase a nationally advertised brand such as Maalox or Mylanta, and then experiment with other brands to find the least expensive product acceptable to you. The antiflatulent simethicone (Mylicon) may help reduce excessive gas and relieve pain.*
OTC antacids—*Alka-Seltzer; Alka-2; Amphojel; Di-Gel; Fizrin; Gaviscon; Gelusil; Gelusil II; Kolantyl; Maalox; Maalox #1; Maalox #2; Mylanta; Mylanta-II; Riopan; Rolaids; Tums*
OTC antiflatulent—*Mylicon*
Rx anticholinergic—*Pro-Banthine*
Rx anticholinergic and sedative products—*Donnatal; Librax*
Rx anticholinergic and phenothiazine—*Combid*
Rx antispasmodic—*Bentyl*
Rx antisecretory—*Tagamet*

Related Topic—*Peptic Ulcer*

Hemorrhoids

Hemorrhoids (piles) often occur during pregnancy and among the obese, and are sometimes attributed to chronic constipation or straining at the stool. They are one of the most common disorders of the gastrointestinal tract.

Hemorrhoids are enlarged veins near the anus. The veins dilate and swell, causing severe inflammation. The inflammation can then lead to more swelling which causes intense itching and discomfort. Sometimes swelling continues until the veins protrude from the anus. When veins protrude they are called external hemorrhoids. Swollen veins that occur high in the anal canal are called internal hemorrhoids. External hemorrhoids are easy to diagnose, but only a doctor can determine how extensive internal hemorrhoids are.

Symptoms

Symptoms of hemorrhoids may be mild and remittent, but severe bleeding or itching call for quick medical intervention. Itching and pain are the most common symptoms. Additionally, there may be infection, bleeding, and even ulceration.

Treatment

Most hemorrhoids can be treated with OTC products. The most effective ingredient in most OTC hemorrhoid preparations is a local anesthetic. Local anesthetics relieve pain and itching, at least temporarily, although they do nothing to cure the underlying condition. The best local anesthetic found in OTC hemorrhoid preparations is benzocaine, though anesthetics like tetracaine, phenocaine hydrochloride, pramoxine hydrochloride, and dibucaine may provide some relief. Products containing local anesthetics should not be

160

used for longer than several days at a time. They may induce further irritation and increased itching. OTC products containing hydrocortisone are also effective but should not be used for more than several days without a doctor's approval.

Products containing antiseptics, astringents, or vasoconstrictors are not recommended unless they also contain a local anesthetic agent. No antiseptic, astringent, or vasoconstrictor has been shown to relieve the pain and itching of hemorrhoids as well as the local anesthetics.

OTC cream and ointment products are preferable to OTC suppositories. Suppositories normally are inserted past the site of pain or irritation and, therefore, do not provide effective pain relief.

For severe hemorrhoids that do not respond to OTC products, suppositories that contain the glucocorticoid, hydrocortisone, are available by prescription. When used exactly according to directions, these suppositories are effective. The hydrocortisone is released and diffuses to the site where it helps reduce the inflammation.

Sitting in a tub of warm water for 20 to 30 minutes or applying hot wet packs several times daily may help soothe irritated hemorrhoids. During an intense flare-up, taking a stool softener will reduce pain on defecation. Someone with hemorrhoids should avoid rough and irritating foods and should lose weight if obese. Hemorrhoids which develop during pregnancy will probably disappear following delivery. For severe hemorrhoids, the doctor may advise surgery.

Any hemorrhoids which do not improve within several days should be seen by a doctor.

Drugs Used in Treatment

Recommended treatment with OTC drugs—*Because hemorrhoids are swollen blood vessels and because drugs are absorbed into the bloodstream more readily whenever swelling is present, we suggest that you choose a product containing no more than 1 to 2 percent benzocaine (Wyanoid ointment, for example). A new product, Dermolate anal-itch ointment, contains hydrocortisone and is also effective, but should not be used for any extended period of time without a doctor's approval.*

OTC hemorrhoidal preparations—*Americaine; Anusol; Diothane; Gentz; Hazel-Balm; Lanacaine; Nupercainal (ointment and suppository); Preparation H; Tucks (cream, ointment, and pad); Wyanoid (ointment and suppository)*

OTC anal-itch ointment—*Dermolate*

℞ steroid hormone-containing anorectal product—*Anusol HC*

Related Topics—*Constipation; Pruritus Ani/Pruritus Vulvae*

Hepatitis

Hepatitis means inflammation of the liver. There are many possible causes and types of hepatitis; two of the most common are discussed here.

Hepatitis A. Formerly called infectious hepatitis or short-incubation hepatitis, hepatitis A is caused by a viral infection. The virus is usually transmitted in the stool or blood of an infected person or in contaminated food or water. The incubation period is relatively short, only 30 to 40 days. The infection is usually systemic; however the liver inflammation is usually the most severe manifestation. This form of hepatitis may occur in epidemics.

Hepatitis B. Hepatitis B (serum hepatitis or long-incubation hepatitis) is an infection of the liver caused by a virus usually transmitted by inoculation of infected blood or blood products. Transmission is also possible via shared razors or toothbrushes or by mouth-to-mouth contact. The incubation period is six weeks to six months.

Symptoms

Symptoms of hepatitis A and hepatitis B are similar, except that the onset of symptoms of hepatitis B is often more insidious. Symptoms usually appear in stages.

In the prodromal phase, general malaise, joint and muscle pain, and upper respiratory tract symptoms (nasal discharge, sore throat, etc.) appear. The patient is easily fatigued and suffers a loss of appetite out of proportion with the degree of illness. Nausea and vomiting follow, and diarrhea or constipation may occur. A low grade fever (103° F or less) is usually present, and chills occur. Pain in the abdomen is usually localized to the upper right quadrant and is made worse by jarring or hard work. The patient develops a distaste for smoking and usually loses weight.

The word icteric means relating to jaundice, and during the icteric phase jaundice usually appears five to ten days after the onset of symptoms, although it may also appear at onset. With the appearance of jaundice, the other symptoms are often intensified, although they then typically regress.

During the convalescent phase, the patient begins to feel better, and the jaundice, abdominal pain, and other symptoms disappear.

Treatment

While strict isolation of patients with viral hepatitis is not necessary, thorough washing of the hands after each bowel movement is required. The entire family should take care in washing their hands and thoroughly cleaning dishes, bedding, and clothing.

During the most acute phase, viral hepatitis is treated with strict bed rest. Hospitalization may be required. Although some believe that bed rest beyond the acute phase is necessary, it is usually not warranted. The patient can gradually return to normal activity as symptoms subside, but all strenuous physical exertion, alcohol, and other liver-damaging agents should be avoided. Complete recovery may take three to four months, although certain symptoms may persist beyond this period. Overall mortality is less than one percent, but it is higher among older people.

One variant of viral hepatitis is known as fulminant hepatitis, in which the patient's condition deteriorates rapidly. In such circumstances the patient must be closely guarded and blood transfusions may be tried.

Hiatus Hernia

The diaphragm is a muscular membrane that separates the abdominal organs from the organs of the chest. The esophagus penetrates the diaphragm above the stomach. Occasionally a small opening appears where the esophagus meets the diaphragm. The opening may be congenital. If a small part of the stomach extends upward into this opening, the condition is known as a hiatus hernia. It is most common in obese individuals and in women who have been pregnant.

Symptoms

A hiatal hernia may produce no symptoms, or it may produce pain in the chest that may radiate down across the abdomen. The pain occurs after eating, and is intensified when the individual lies down, coughs, or strains at stools. Someone with a hiatus hernia may belch frequently. Bleeding may result from a hernia, and the bleeding could lead to iron-deficiency anemia. It has been said that bleeding from a hiatus hernia is one of the major causes of blood loss in older people.

Treatment

Someone with a hiatus hernia should eat several small meals each day and should be careful to eat with the mouth shut to limit the amount of air swallowed. Foods that produce gas, such as cucumbers, radishes, and carbonated beverages, should be avoided. Additionally, tobacco, tea, coffee, and alcohol should be avoided. After meals the individual should not recline for at least two hours. If overweight, a weight-reduction diet should be maintained. When lifting heavy objects, someone with a hiatus hernia should avoid bending at the waist; rather, it is preferable to bend the knees and lift the object. People with hiatal hernias should elevate the heads of their beds four to six inches to relieve symptoms. Surgery may be advisable for some cases.

Drugs Used in Treatment

Recommended treatment with OTC drugs—*There is little reason to recommend one OTC antacid over another. The product you choose should be one having an acceptable taste that does not cause you to be constipated or to have diarrhea. It may be advisable to purchase a nationally advertised brand such as Maalox or Mylanta, and then experiment with other brands to find the least expensive product acceptable to you. The antiflatulent simethicone (Mylicon) may help reduce excessive gas and thus relieve pain.*
OTC antacids—*Alka-Seltzer; Alka-2; Amphojel; Di-Gel; Fizrin; Gaviscon; Gelusil; Gelusil II; Kolantyl; Maalox; Maalox #1; Maalox #2; Mylanta; Mylanta-II; Riopan; Rolaids; Tums*
OTC antiflatulent—*Mylicon*
R̩ₓ anticholinergic—*Pro-Banthine*
R̩ₓ anticholinergics and sedatives—*Donnatal; Librax*
R̩ₓ anticholinergic and phenothiazine—*Combid*
R̩ₓ antispasmodic—*Bentyl*
R̩ₓ antisecretory—*Tagamet*

Related Topics—*Heartburn; Peptic Ulcer*

Hiccups

A hiccup is an involuntary spasmodic contraction of the diaphragm. Hiccups are caused by irritation of the diaphragm. The diaphragm may be irritated by gas, excessive pressure, or from ingesting certain foods. The irritation causes a spasm, and the glottis (the vocal apparatus in the larynx) snaps shut to check the inflow of air, producing the characteristic "hiccup" sound.

Most people have had hiccups as a result of eating certain foods, laughing, or drinking. However, certain diseases may also cause hiccups. For example, certain nervous disorders and infectious diseases, such as encephalitis and other diseases of the brain, may cause hiccups. Disorders of the stomach, esophagus, bowel, pancreas, bladder, and liver may cause hiccups. Pregnancy can cause hiccups. Some people hiccup after drinking alcohol. The cause of persistent hiccuping (epidemic hiccups), is unknown.

Treatment

In most cases, hiccups are not significant. Any of the household remedies may provide relief. These include drinking a glass of water rapidly, swallowing sugar, placing an ice bag on the diaphragm below the rib cage, breathing into a paper (not plastic) bag and rebreathing the air, inducing vomiting, swallowing dry bread or crushed ice, applying slight pressure to the eyelids, applying a mustard plaster to the upper abdomen of course, and inducing mild fright in the individual. Most of these remedies work by increasing the carbon dioxide content of the lungs, thus stabilizing the breathing center, or by diverting the attention of the person with hiccups.

If hiccups occur for no apparent reason and do not respond to the usual household remedies, they may be a symptom of a more serious disease. In this case, they require medical attention. Several drugs have been used to treat hiccups, including the sedatives such as phenobarbital and chlorpromazine. Scopolamine, amphetamine, and the narcotics have been tried. None of these drugs produces consistent relief.

Drugs Used in Treatment

R̥ **phenothiazine**—*Thorazine*
R̥ **sedative and hypnotic**—*phenobarbital*

Ileitis

Ileitis, also called regional enteritis or Crohn's disease, is an inflammation of part of the alimentary canal, most frequently affecting the lower portion of the small intestine (ileum). The inflammation causes part of the intestine to become extremely thickened, and may block the passage of material through it.

Ileitis occurs most commonly among people with peptic ulcers or those who are extremely tense. It usually occurs between the ages of 20 and 30. Usually, it is not related to an infection.

Symptoms

Primary symptoms of ileitis include weight loss, anemia, and malnutrition. Diarrhea, mild fever, cramping in the lower abdomen, nausea, or vomiting may also be present.

Treatment

Treatment for ileitis includes strict bed rest and control of the symptoms of diarrhea and fever if present. Vitamin-mineral supplements are given to prevent malnutrition. A bland diet is followed, and lots of water (at least eight to ten glasses each day) is given. Occasionally antibiotics are given to prevent secondary infections, but these drugs are nonspecific and should only be given under close medical supervision.

Drugs Used in Treatment

OTC nutritional supplements—*see the list under Nutritional Disorders*
R̥ **antibiotics**—*amoxicillin; ampicillin; erythromycin; Keflex; Minocin; penicillin G; penicillin potassium phenoxymethyl; Terramycin; tetracycline hydrochloride; Vibramycin*

Indigestion

Indigestion, or dyspepsia, is defined as symptoms associated with not being able to properly absorb or use foods that are put in the stomach. Generally, dyspepsia produces mild pain in the stomach. It may also cause nausea, heartburn, flatulence, and bloating.

Commonly, indigestion is caused by eating during emotional upset, eating poorly cooked food, inadequately chewing food, eating too much or too rapidly, having bad teeth or bad eating habits, making poor dietary choices, or being in an unpleasant environment during meals. Constipation and smoking may predispose someone to indigestion. Foods with a high fat content or foods known to produce much gas may also cause indigestion.

Treatment

Indigestion caused by one of the factors mentioned above can usually be treated easily. It may be prevented by eating balanced meals in a relaxed environment and by eating moderate amounts of carefully chosen foods. Smoking before and immediately after meals should be avoided. Exercise and emotional upset following meals, should be avoided. Symptoms of heartburn, nausea, flatulence, etc., should be treated following guidelines explained elsewhere in this book. Antacids often bring general relief.

Symptom of Serious Disorder

Indigestion is one of those symptoms that "everyone gets," and many people ignore occasional indigestion. However, many serious disorders, including some that are not directly associated with the digestive tract, may cause indigestion. Therefore, if indigestion is not relieved by simple home measures, or if indigestion recurs frequently without identifiable relationship to food habits, medical diagnosis should be sought.

Heart attacks often cause pain mistaken for indigestion. Diabetes, Addison's disease, tuberculosis, hyperparathyroidism, uremia, and a variety of other generalized disorders may cause symptoms of mild indigestion. Indigestion may also be associated with cancer. Frequently, patients who are diagnosed as having cancer admit that they had occasional indigestion for several months prior to the diagnosis of their cancer. Less common causes of indigestion include certain diseases of the pancreas or intestine.

Because indigestion is associated with such a variety of diseases, diagnosis of its cause can be complicated. That is why a doctor ordering a barium enema to test for gastrointestinal disease may also give a chest x-ray to rule out tuberculosis or other diseases of the lungs. Many people who believe they have indigestion or some other vague symptom relating to a heart disorder frequently find that their symptom is caused by gallbladder disease or a hiatus hernia.

Drugs Used in Treatment

Recommended treatment with OTC drugs—*Antacids will bring relief whenever indigestion is caused by excess acid. There is little reason to recommend one OTC antacid over another. The product you choose should be one having an acceptable taste that does not cause you to be constipated or to have diarrhea. It may be advisable to purchase a nationally advertised brand such as Maalox or Mylanta, and then experiment with other brands to find the least expensive product acceptable to you.*
OTC antacids—*Alka-Seltzer; Alka-2; Amphojel; Di-Gel; Fizrin; Gaviscon; Gelusil; Gelusil II; Kolantyl; Maalox; Maalox #1; Maalox #2; Mylanta; Mylanta-II; Riopan; Rolaids; Tums*
OTC antiflatulent—*Mylicon*
R$_x$ anticholinergic—*Pro-Banthine*
R$_x$ antispasmodic—*Bentyl*
R$_x$ anticholinergic and phenothiazine—*Combid*
R$_x$ anticholinergics and sedatives—*Donnatal; Librax*
R$_x$ antisecretory—*Tagamet*

Irritable Colon

This very common disorder is known by many names: mucous colitis, spastic colon, irritable bowel syndrome, functional dyspepsia, nervous indigestion. It is responsible for at least half of all the disorders of the gastrointestinal system. It is usually caused by emotional upset or anxiety. Contributing factors include poor dietary habits and improper use of laxatives. The disorder is most commonly seen in young adults.

Symptoms

Symptoms are extremely variable. The appearance of symptoms often coincides with some emotional upset. The patient may have diarrhea or be constipated. A pain spreading across the abdomen and sometimes into the chest or shoulders is felt; occasionally the symptoms are mistaken for a heart attack or kidney stones. The abdomen will be bloated, and the patient may experience vomiting, headache, loss of appetite, fatigue, and anemia.

Treatment

The symptoms of diarrhea or constipation are treated. Mild tranquilizers may help alleviate the emotional state that caused the problem. Warm heat applied to the abdomen may relieve cramping. In severe cases, bed rest for several days to a week may be necessary. The diet should consist of small feedings of bland, nonirritating food.

Drugs Used in Treatment

℞ antidiarrheal—*Lomotil*
℞ sedatives and hypnotics—*Ativan; Librium; meprobamate; Nembutal; phenobarbital; Serax; Tranxene; Valium*
℞ phenothiazines—*Compazine; Stelazine*
℞ phenothiazine and antidepressant—*Triavil*
℞ sedative—*Atarax*
℞ anticholinergic—*Pro-Banthine*
℞ antispasmodic—*Bentyl*
℞ anticholinergic and sedative—*Librax*

Related Topics—*Constipation; Diarrhea; Nausea and Vomiting*

Jaundice

Jaundice is a yellowish tint on the skin and the whites of the eyes caused by an accumulation in the blood of a bile pigment called bilirubin. The tears and urine of someone with jaundice will be darker than they normally are. Jaundice is a common symptom associated with hepatitis.

Bilirubin is a dark yellow or red pigment derived from the breakdown of hemoglobin when red blood cells are destroyed. Bilirubin is concentrated in the liver and then conjugated with other substances to form bile, which is then released by the liver to the intestine.

166

Causes

The abnormality causing jaundice may be the overproduction of bilirubin (as is seen with an increased breakdown of red blood cells), the inability of the liver to transform bilirubin into bile (possibly due to an enzymatic deficiency), or an impairment in the excretion of bile.

One type of jaundice is seen in newborns who are deficient in one of the enzymes used to metabolize bilirubin. As a result bilirubin levels increase in the blood, giving the jaundiced appearance. If the concentration builds too high, a condition called kernicterus may result as bilirubin enters the brain and causes brain damage. Therefore, newborns are watched closely for signs of abnormal jaundice. Newborns normally have some degree of jaundice for a few days. This is usually harmless and disappears before the baby is two weeks old.

Jaundice is generally not considered a medical emergency. However, if obstruction of the liver persists for longer than four weeks, serious and permanent damage to the liver may develop.

Treatment

Treatment generally involves diagnosis and treatment of the cause of the condition.

Related Topics—*Cirrhosis; Gallstones; Hepatitis; Liver Disease, Drug-Induced*

Leukoplakia

Leukoplakia is a white or yellowish growth that occurs on the mucous lining of the oral membranes, especially around the cheeks and tongue. It usually occurs in middle-aged or elderly men, although anyone can develop it. Most frequently it is caused by irritation due to smoking or chewing tobacco, faulty dental work, alcohol, hot spicy foods, jagged teeth, ill-fitting dentures, or extremely hot foods. Occasionally it is caused by a deficiency of vitamin A or B, or by diseases such as syphilis. Occasionally leukoplakia may be precancerous, and any leukoplakia should be brought to the attention of a doctor so that cancer can be ruled out as a possible cause.

Symptoms

Usually, there are no symptoms other than the white or yellowish patches in the mouth. The patches may feel rough, and it is often this roughness which makes the patient aware of the patches. The patches may feel leathery or thickened; they may have fissures or be ulcerated. If the disease is not treated, severe pain may also be a symptom.

Treatment

Leukoplakia is treated by avoiding all irritants such as alcohol, nicotine, and hot or spicy foods. Loose or ill-fitting dentures should be corrected, and any necessary dental work should be performed. In some cases the patches are removed surgically. Vitamin supplements may be given.

Anyone who has had leukoplakia should be on the lookout for recurrences, particularly after the removal or correction of the causes listed above. If the growths do recur, a doctor should be contacted at once to rule out the possibility of mouth cancer.

Liver Disease, Drug-Induced

Certain drugs can cause liver damage that sometimes mimic symptoms of infectious hepatitis or obstructive jaundice. The disease appears to be largely an allergic reaction to the offending chemical. Diagnosis of such damage is often difficult and cannot be positive until after the drug has been taken for a long time.

Symptoms

When symptoms appear, they are similar to those of infectious hepatitis. In fact, drug-induced liver disease is sometimes called toxic hepatitis. There will be low-grade fever, nausea, malaise, and abdominal pain for four or five days. Severe itching may precede the appearance of jaundice. A mild loss of appetite may be experienced. There may or may not be tenderness in the upper right abdominal quadrant.

Treatment

Other than the elimination of the offending drug, there is no specific therapy. Glucocorticoids are sometimes administered, but they are not considered effective. Cholestyramine is sometimes effective in controlling itching.

Drugs Used in Treatment

R steroid hormones—*Aristocort; Medrol; prednisone*

Related Topics—*Hepatitis; Jaundice*

Loss of Appetite

"Anorexia" is the medical term for loss of appetite. Anorexia may occur temporarily with many diseases. Sometimes it signifies mild disorders such as a common cold or tiredness. However, anorexia may also be an important symptom of many severe diseases such as various cancers, infective disorders such as tuberculosis, endocrine disorders such as thyroid disease or Addison's disease, diseases of the kidneys, severe arthritis, or certain psychological disorders such as anxiety and hysteria. Anorexia is one of the nonspecific symptoms of almost all severe diseases. If loss of appetite persists for more than one day and there is no readily recognizable cause, such as a cold, medical attention should be sought.

Related Topic—*Anorexia Nervosa*

Morning Sickness

About 75 percent of all pregnant women have morning sickness. The condition consists of nausea with or without vomiting. It starts during the fifth or sixth week of pregnancy and may continue through the fourth or fifth month. Sometimes it lasts throughout the pregnancy.

Symptoms

Symptoms are most severe in the morning just after rising. The precise cause is not known, but it is believed that psychogenic factors are important. It is extremely important for a doctor to make sure that serious diseases, such as severe infections, cancer, gallbladder disease, and diabetes are not present.

Treatment

Many women respond to a modified diet. Dry foods eaten at frequent intervals may help. Highly spiced or odorous foods and items rich in fat should be avoided. Eating a light snack before getting out of bed in the morning may help. After all meals, a pregnant woman should lie down for 15 to 20 minutes.

Bendectin antinauseant is specifically indicated to reduce morning sickness symptoms. No other drug or treatment should be tried unless specifically recommended by the doctor.

Drugs Used in Treatment

R̞ antinauseant—*Bendectin*

Motion Sickness

Any type of motion can cause motion sickness; thus, we have air sickness, sea sickness, train sickness, and car sickness. Some people suffer motion sickness while moving backward, but not while moving forward. Some people begin to feel sick when they stand still and watch objects around them move. Ear or sinus infections or hot stuffy rooms can produce the same symptoms.

The condition is caused by a disturbance in the specialized receptors of the inner ear.Symptoms are caused by fluid shifts in the semicircular canals. These shifts cause confusing messages to be sent to the brain.

Symptoms

Motion sickness is characterized by nausea, with or without vomiting. Dizziness, loss of appetite, sweating, and difficulty in breathing may also be present.

Treatment

Long-term motion sickness can be exhausting. If vomiting occurs, persistent motion sickness can lead to dehydration. Motion sickness can be avoided by minimizing travel or rapid movements. For some people, keeping the eyes closed during travel may prevent the spells. During a trip, someone prone to motion sickness should lie still, if possible, and not move the head about. Alcoholic beverages should be avoided, although soft drinks may be consumed. Some people benefit from sucking on ice chips.

Drugs Used in Treatment

Recommended treatment with OTC drugs—*The medications dimenhydrinate, meclizine, or cyclizine (Bonine, Dramamine, Marezine) work fairly well in preventing motion sickness. To be most effective, a dose should be taken at least 30 to 60 minutes before a trip, with additional doses taken as directed on the labels.*
OTC antinauseants—*Bonine; Dramamine; Emetrol; Marezine*
R̞ antihistamine—*Benadryl*
R̞ antinauseant—*Antivert*
R̞ anticholinergic and sedative—*Donnatal*

Related Topic—*Nausea and Vomiting*

Nausea and Vomiting

Nausea is an unpleasant sensation difficult to describe precisely. Someone who is nauseous may evince pallor, chills, sweating, salivation, drowsiness, lassitude, headache, pupil dilation, and rapid heartbeat and respiration.

Vomiting, which may occur without nausea, is the forceful ejection of the contents of the stomach (and sometimes of the upper portion of intestines) through the mouth.

Numerous complex processes underlie the nausea and the vomiting process. Three hundred years ago it was written that "... 'tis profitable for man that his stomach should nauseate and reject things that have a loathsome taste or smell." Some argue that these mechanisms evolved to the individual's advantage, in that harmful substances can easily be rejected. However, few people recognize the condition as advantageous when they are experiencing it.

Causes

Nausea and vomiting may be induced by a wide variety of causes. Although some of these may be serious, most are not. Nausea and vomiting are common symptoms of food intolerance, motion sickness, and the morning sickness of early pregnancy. A sudden and severe pain, such as a blow to the testicles or hitting the thumb with a hammer, may also cause vomiting.

Vomiting is most often associated with a disease of the gastrointestinal tract. It may be caused by having lesions in the stomach or an obstruction in the intestines. It is a symptom of gastritis and peptic ulcers. One of the questions that doctors ask patients suspected of having peptic ulcers is whether vomiting is self-induced. People with peptic ulcers know that vomiting frequently relieves the pain, and self-induced vomiting is one of the symptoms that strongly suggests peptic ulcer disease. Poisonous or toxic substances in the stomach also may cause enough irritation to provoke vomiting.

Vomiting may also be caused by heart attacks, migraine headaches, Addison's disease, Ménière's syndrome, and diabetes. Vomiting not preceded by nausea is associated with brain tumors and with narrowing of the intestine due to peptic ulcer or to cancer of the gastrointestinal tract.

Treatment

Both nausea and vomiting usually subside once the causative factor has been removed or corrected. Vomiting that occurs after eating disagreeable foods or during morning sickness of pregnancy may require little or no treatment. Prolonged or repeated vomiting requires more attention. Serious loss of essential salts and fluids may result from continued vomiting. Persistent nausea may lead to nutritional imbalances.

Anyone who vomits regularly or frequently, anyone who vomits without being able to pinpoint a cause, and anyone who sees blood or red or dark brown spots in the vomitus, should seek medical assistance immediately. In such situations, the doctor will probably want to examine a sample of the vomitus.

Drugs called antinauseants or antiemetics are used to reduce the urge to vomit. The most effective antiemetics are phenothiazines such as Compazine. These can be taken by mouth, but the suppositories are preferable to treat vomiting. If vomiting is especially severe, the drugs may have to be injected.

Other drugs used as antiemetics include antihistamines, scopolamine, and a few miscellaneous substances. None of these items works as effectively as the phenothiazines. A product called Bendectin is promoted for nausea and vomiting of morning sickness. Bendectin is a mixture of an antihistamine and vitamin B_6. The antihistaminic component probably has a real antinauseant effect, but Vitamin B_6 has not been shown to be effective.

Emetrol antinauseant and Coke syrup, both of which can be purchased without a prescription, effectively treat mild nausea or vomiting caused by an irritant in the stomach. Both must be taken undiluted, and no other fluids should be taken for at least 15 minutes after taking a dose. Emetrol antinauseant and Coke syrup will taste better if chilled slightly before taking.

A vomit basin may be useful when treating a disease which causes frequent vomiting. A person who is vomiting needs to drink plenty of fluids. Tea and noncola beverages, especially ginger ale, are usually tolerated quite well. Solid food should not be taken, although soup or broth is usually prescribed. When vomiting has ceased, light foods such as crackers or toast should be tried before returning to a normal diet.

Drugs Used in Treatment

Recommended treatment with OTC drugs—*Bonine, Dramamine, and Marezine antinauseants contain drugs with antihistaminic properties; Emetrol antinauseant contains concentrated sugar. All will effectively relieve mild nausea.*
OTC antinauseants—*Bonine; Dramamine; Emetrol; Marezine*
Ŗ antinauseants—*Antivert; Bendectin; Tigan*
Ŗ phenothiazines—*Compazine; Thorazine*

Health Care Accessory—*vomit basin*

Related Topics—*Appendicitis; Diverticulitis; Food Poisoning; Gastritis; Headache; Ileitis; Indigestion; Irritable Colon; Morning Sickness; Motion Sickness; Pancreatitis; Peptic Ulcer; Peritonitis*

Pancreatitis

Pancreatitis is an inflammatory condition of the pancreas. The pancreas is composed of several kinds of tissue. One tissue secretes insulin, which controls blood glucose levels. Other tissues secrete enzymes that help the body digest food. Pancreatitis is an inflammation of the cells that secrete digestive enzymes. These enzymes may empty into the peritoneal cavity to cause severe peritonitis. If left untreated for several hours, death may result.

The disorder may be acute: a single episode causing severe pain. Chronic pancreatitis develops in about 10 percent of all persons who have suffered acute pancreatitis. Someone with chronic pancreatitis suffers recurring attacks that are not ordinarily as severe as an attack of acute pancreatitis.

The exact cause of pancreatitis is not known. It frequently occurs in alcoholics and persons with biliary tract disease. Pancreatitis may be related to an allergy to certain foods or drugs.

Symptoms

Pancreatitis causes severe steady pain and tenderness in the area of the stomach and intestine. The pain is frequently worse when lying down and less severe when sitting up and leaning forward. The abdomen may be distended. Also, nausea and vomiting, loss of appetite, and constipation are present. The patient may be sweating and extremely tense. Fever of 101° to 102° F is common. There may be palpitations, and the skin may feel cool and clammy. The person may go into shock. Oftentimes a heavy meal or an alcoholic binge precedes the attack. Attacks may last a few minutes to two weeks.

Treatment

Pancreatitis is a serious disorder and must be treated immediately. If left untreated, or if recurrent bouts occur frequently, the person can be left an invalid. Complications include diabetes mellitus, shock, and pancreatic insufficiency. A prescription analgesic such as Demerol or Talwin may be required to control the pain. Atropine should be given to control spasms. Complete bed rest is necessary, and hospitalization is required.

Shock may develop. To help prevent this, fluids will be given intravenously. Other drugs are used as the need arises. If the blood calcium levels fall, calcium injections are given.

During the first 48 to 72 hours no food or fluids are given by mouth. After this time, small quantities may be started and increased as tolerated.

Everyone with a history of pancreatitis or suspected pancreatitis should stick to a low-fat diet. Heavy meals and alcohol should be avoided.

Drugs Used in Treatment

℞ **analgesics**—*Darvocet-N; Darvon; Darvon Compound-65; Demerol; Empirin Compound with Codeine; Equagesic; Fiorinal; Fiorinal with Codeine; Motrin; Norgesic; Percodan; Synalgos-DC; Talwin; Tylenol with Codeine*
℞ **sedative and anticholinergic**—*Donnatal; Librax*
℞ **anticholinergic and phenothiazine**—*Combid*
℞ **anticholinergic**—*Pro-Banthine*
℞ **antispasmodic**—*Bentyl*

Related Topic—*Peritonitis*

Peptic Ulcer

About one out of every ten Americans suffers chronically with a peptic ulcer—an ulcer in the stomach or the duodenum, the first part of the small intestine. Ulcers in the duodenum are far more common than those in the stomach.

Ulcers are holes or erosions in the wall of the stomach or the intestine. They may occur alone or in multiples. They are usually produced when there is excess acid in the stomach or intestine. This acid, along with digestive enzymes, forms gastric juice that is powerful enough to erode intestinal tissue. Why some people seem to have excess acid is unknown. Suggested causes include stress, smoking, nervousness, tension, consumption of excessive coffee or tea, and taking certain drugs, but the only factor which has been identified for certain is heredity. People whose parents or other relatives had ulcers are more likely to have ulcers than are people who have no such history.

Symptoms

An ulcer, even several ulcers, may produce no symptoms at all. Sometimes, ulcers cause only vague discomfort or mild pain similar to that of indigestion or a pulled muscle. Sometimes ulcers cause pressure or a hungry, aching, or gnawing feeling. Someone with ulcers may have frequent heartburn. Ulcers may also produce a burning pain that radiates across the upper part of the body. Usually, the pain is most severe when no food is in the stomach—late morning, midafternoon, or during the night. Stress or overwork may cause a flare-up of pain. Bleeding ulcers produce blood in the stool or in the vomitus.

Characteristic ulcer pain begins about an hour after a meal, and it can be relieved by a light snack, antacids, or vomiting. The pain is the direct result of the contact of gastric juices with the nerve endings exposed within the ulcer crater. Prevention of this pain allows the ulcer to heal, and decrease in pain is a signal that the ulcer is healing.

Complications

Hemorrhage, perforation, and obstruction are the most commonly reported ulcer complications. Hemorrhage may occur as a rather simple and not very dangerous oozing of blood from the rich vascular tissue at the ulcer base. When hemorrhage occurs in the capillary bed, the blood will most likely clot, and no permanent damage results. However, a hemorrhage can also be massive and life-threatening if the bleeding is caused by erosion of the major deep-seated blood vessels. In this case, blood flow may not be checked by clotting, and the patient may die of shock.

Perforation, when the ulcer erodes through the stomach or intestinal wall, occurs in as many as 25 percent of patients with the disease. Severe perforation is the major cause of death associated with peptic ulcers. It can cause extreme loss of blood and it may allow the leakage of the nonsterile contents of the stomach or intestine into the sterile abdominal cavity. Peritonitis develops and may result in death.

Some obstruction of the outlet of the stomach or duodenum occurs in 20 to 25 percent of all ulcer patients. The obstruction may be due to scarring or to spasm and swelling. Symptoms of obstruction include the vomiting of a large volume of food, particularly if the food is undigested and from more than one meal.

Perforations and massive hemorrhage usually require surgery; obstruction may require surgery if due to scarring and if not relieved by medical therapy within a week.

Treatment

One of the best ways to treat a minor ulcer is to use an antacid. Many drugs used to treat ulcers require a prescription, but most of them are no better than the antacids that can be purchased over-the-counter.

Antacids are alkaline substances that combine with excessive stomach acid and neutralize it. They keep acid away from ulcer sites and from nerve endings in the stomach and intestinal walls. In so doing, they reduce the pain of an ulcer and allow it to heal naturally.

To be effective, large doses must be taken over a long period of time—sometimes two to three months or longer. Because most antacids leave a gritty feeling in the mouth, people tend to take them less often than they should, and, consequently, the ulcer does not heal as quickly as it should.

Hundreds of antacids are on the market. But most of them contain one or more of only four chemical compounds: sodium bicarbonate, calcium carbonate, magnesium salts, and aluminum salts.

Sodium bicarbonate, also known as baking soda and contained in Alka-Seltzer antacid tablets and Fizrin antacid, is the most powerful and the most dangerous of the antacid chemicals. Sodium bicarbonate forms carbon dioxide in the stomach. Too much carbon dioxide may stretch the stomach walls. Stretched stomach walls easily tear at the site of an ulcer. If the stomach wall tears, the contents of the stomach spill into the body, causing a severe infection or even death. Sodium bicarbonate also can be absorbed into the bloodstream and damage the heart or the kidneys. Sodium bicarbonate's action is short, and it must be taken more often than other antacid chemicals.

To relieve an attack of ulcer pain, one or more doses of baking soda or a sodium bicarbonate-containing antacid can be taken safely, but sodium bicarbonate should not be used for more than two or three consecutive days without consulting a doctor.

Calcium carbonate-containing products, like Alka-2 antacid tablets and Tums antacid, are quick-acting and potent, and they generate few side effects. The most severe side effect is "acid rebound." After one or two weeks of constant acid neutralization by calcium carbonate, the stomach responds by secreting more acid, and ulcer pain increases.

Magnesium salts products are not as potent as those with calcium carbonate, but they are effective. Their major drawback is their laxative effect. Antacids with magnesium salts can cause severe diarrhea if full doses are used regularly for more than one to two weeks. These antacids also can cause drowsiness or kidney problems in certain people. Anyone with kidney disease should talk to a doctor before taking any OTC product containing magnesium.

Aluminum salts are the least potent of all the antacid chemicals. Nevertheless, they have side effects. One side effect is constipation. To relieve constipation, drink plenty of water throughout the day or take a stool softener. Some products, like Gelusil II or Maalox antacids, contain both magnesium and aluminum salts. The laxative effect of the magnesium is balanced by the constipating effect of the aluminum. The use of antacids containing only magnesiusm or aluminum salts is not recommended; it is preferable to use products containing both.

Liquid antacids are far superior to tablets or wafers. Antacids neutralize stomach acid best when they have been ground into small particles, and antacid particles in liquids are much smaller than those in tablets of wafers. Tablets or wafers, however, may be more convenient to use during the day.

Many antacid products (Mylanta and Di-Gel tablets, for example) contain simethicone, a drug that reduces gas in the gastrointestinal tract. Such products—a combination antacid with antiflatulent—have been found to be safe and effective by the Food and Drug Administration's advisory review panel on antacids. However, it is generally advisable to purchase simethicone tablets instead of a combination product and thereby avoid taking simethicone except when needed to reduce excess gas.

The effectiveness of any antacid depends on how often it is taken. The dose of the antacid or the amount of acid in the stomach is not nearly as important. Follow the directions on the label. Don't take an antacid more often than directed, and don't miss any doses.

In addition to antacids, anticholinergics, antispasmodics, and a new drug called Tagamet are used to treat peptic ulcer disease. Anticholinergics slow the movement of the muscles that line the stomach and the intestine. This reduces the pain of peptic ulcers. They also decrease the secretion of hydrochloric acid. Antispasmodics (e.g., Bentyl) decrease the muscular movements only. Tagamet inhibits gastric acid secretion only. Its action is stronger than that of the anticholinergic drugs, and the drug has fewer annoying side effects.

People with ulcers should carefully watch their diet, try to refrain from highly seasoned or fried foods, and limit coffee, tea, and cola beverage intake. They should quit smoking and not drink alcoholic beverages. In general, anything that increases ulcer pain, such as stress, should be avoided. Antacids with magnesium should be avoided by people with kidney disease, and sodium bicarbonate should be avoided by people with heart disease.

Ulcer therapy should always begin with a doctor's examination. Anyone who finds blood in stools or vomitus should see a doctor immediately.

Drugs Used in Treatment

Recommended treatment with OTC drugs—*OTC antacids effectively relieve* the pain of a minor ulcer and allow it to heal. See the discussion above for some general guidelines on choosing an OTC antacid. There is little reason to recommend one OTC antacid over another. The product you choose should be one having an acceptable taste that does not cause you to be constipated or to have diarrhea. It may be advisable to purchase a nationally advertised brand such as Maalox or Mylanta, and then experiment with other brands to find the least expensive product acceptable to you.

OTC antacids—Alka-Seltzer; Alka-2; Amphojel; Di-Gel; Fizrin; Gaviscon; Gelusil; Gelusil II; Kolantyl; Maalox; Maalox #1; Maalox #2; Mylanta; Mylanta-II; Riopan; Rolaids; Tums

OTC antiflatulent—Mylicon

R anticholinergic—Pro-Banthine

R anticholinergic and phenothiazine—Combid

R anticholinergics and sedatives—Donnatal; Librax

R antispasmodic—Bentyl

R antisecretory—Tagamet

Related Topics—Heartburn; Peritonitis

Periodontal Disease

Periodontal disease is an inflammation of the membranes at the roots of the teeth, and it is always associated with an accumulation of bacterial plaque on the surfaces of the teeth. Periodontal disease begins when food particles and bacteria accumulate on the sides of the teeth, between the teeth, and on the gums at the base of the teeth. The gums become reddened, inflamed, and sensitive. If not treated, the gum tissue recedes from the tooth surface, forming a dental pocket, where more debris accumulates. If the condition is allowed to continue, the teeth will eventually loosen and may be lost, or they may move out of alignment with one another, causing difficulty in eating which may eventually lead to problems such as malnutrition.

Symptoms

In the early stages, periodontal disease may not cause symptoms perceived as significant. The gums may be slightly swollen and red, and they may bleed when the teeth are brushed. If pus develops the condition is called pyorrhea (pus flowing). If the pus does not drain, the condition will cause acute pain and swelling.

Treatment

Periodontal disease is best treated with a mouth rinse of 3 percent hydrogen peroxide diluted with an equal volume of warm water. It can also be effectively relieved with a product such as Gly-Oxide gel. If the condition is severe, antibiotics should be taken to reduce further bacteria-induced inflammation and formation of more dental pockets. If the disease is advanced, teeth may have to be removed, after which the area will be packed with antibiotics and cotton or gauze.

To prevent periodontal disease, follow a program of regular dental care: visit the dentist every six months, develop good brushing techniques, and use dental floss.

Drugs Used in Treatment

Recommended treatment with OTC drugs—Your pharmacy's generic brand of hydrogen peroxide, diluted with an equal part water, is recommended as a

mouth rinse. Gly-Oxide gel releases oxygen in the mouth and promotes healing.
OTC canker sore and fever blister remedy—*Gly-Oxide*
OTC miscellaneous—*hydrogen peroxide*
℞ antibiotics—*amoxicillin; ampicillin; erythromycin; Keflex; Minocin; penicillin G; penicillin potassium phenoxymethyl; Terramycin; tetracycline hydrochloride; Vibramycin*

Health Care Accessories—*dental floss; gauze; toothbrush*

Related Topics—*Gingivitis; Tooth Decay*

Peritonitis

The peritoneum is a membrane that lines the abdominal cavity. If an organ ruptures, or an injury such as a stab wound is received, or a blood vessel in the peritoneum breaks and material leaks out, the peritoneal membrane becomes inflamed. Bacterial infection may also cause such inflammation. This inflammation is termed peritonitis.

Symptoms

Symptoms include severe pain in the abdomen. Typical posture of someone with peritonitis is to lie still with knees drawn up. The slightest movement intensifies the pain. Nausea and vomiting may be present. Sometimes diarrhea, rapid heartbeat, fever, hiccuping, and extreme thirst occur.

Treatment

Peritonitis must be treated immediately. If not, shock may occur, resulting in death. The individual should not be given food or liquids until the doctor directs it.

In most cases, the cause of peritonitis must be surgically corrected. Morphine or other narcotic analgesics may be given for the pain. Antibiotics are given to alleviate infection. Other symptoms are treated as needed.

Drugs Used in Treatment

℞ analgesics—*Darvocet-N; Darvon; Darvon Compound-65; Demerol; Empirin Compound with Codeine; Fiorinal with Codeine; Percodan; Robaxin; Soma Compound; Synalgos-DC; Talwin; Tylenol with Codeine*
℞ antibiotics—*amoxicillin; ampicillin; erythromycin; Keflex; Minocin; penicillin G; penicillin potassium phenoxymethyl; Terramycin; tetracycline hydrochloride; Vibramycin*

Related Topic—*Appendicitis*

Toothache

A toothache is usually a signal that a tooth is infected (abscessed) or has a cavity that has reached the tooth pulp. Pain may be localized in the area of the affected tooth, or it may spread along various parts of the jaw or around the area of the eyes.

Treatment

Until a dentist can be reached to correct the problem, the pain can usually be treated with aspirin or acetaminophen. For more severe toothaches, the use of one of the stronger analgesics containing a narcotic may be necessary.

Many OTC toothache medications are available. Generally these contain a local anesthetic, such as benzocaine, or agents, such as clove oil that numb the nerve endings. The substance may be in either liquid or ointment form. It is best to put the agent on a pledget of cotton and insert the cotton into the cavity if one is present. The agent can also be rubbed onto the gums and surrounding area to help alleviate the pain. Recurrent toothache may signal that an infection is present. If the infection is not treated, the tooth and possibly parts of the gum may be completely destroyed.

Regular dental check-ups are advised to detect possible problems that may eventually lead to a cavity. The teeth should be brushed well after each meal and before going to bed. Dental floss should be gently worked in between each tooth where a toothbrush will not reach. Care should be taken to avoid injury to the gums when using dental floss.

Drugs Used in Treatment

Recommended treatment with OTC drugs—*Of the over-the-counter products containing local anesthetics, those containing benzocaine (Benzodent, for example) are the most economical and effective, and they produce the fewest side effects. Toothache remedies such as clove oil are also effective, but they are more likely to cause stinging on application.*
OTC analgesics—*see the list under Pain and Fever*
OTC toothache remedies—*Benzodent; Orajel; Pain-A-Lay*
R̥ analgesics—*Darvocet-N; Darvon; Darvon Compound-65; Demerol; Empirin Compound with Codeine; Equagesic; Fiorinal; Fiorinal with Codeine; Motrin; Percodan; Synalgos-DC; Talwin; Tylenol with Codeine*

Health Care Accessories—*dental floss; toothbrush*

Related Topic—*Tooth Decay*

Tooth Decay

Three factors are necessary to produce dental caries: bacteria, food for the bacteria, and a susceptible tooth. The bacteria change sugary, sticky food residues into acid which eats away at the tooth enamel. If allowed to continue, the decay reaches the layer of dentin beneath the enamel, and may eventually reach the pulp within the tooth, possibly forming an abscess. If an abscess is left untreated, the tooth will completely disintegrate.

Symptoms

Tooth decay is the most common cause of toothache, although a cavity may not cause pain in the early stages. The pain may be felt around the tooth itself, or it may radiate from the area of the tooth up across the area of the eye and into the temple. The pain may be sharp and stabbing or dull and chronic. Swelling may also be present. Severe decay, or decay affecting several teeth, may cause an unpleasant mouth odor.

Treatment

Dental caries must be treated by a dentist who will remove the decay and fill in the area with a suitable material.

Prevention

Prevention of tooth decay involves regular visits to the dentist, particularly during childhood when teeth are being formed, proper oral hygiene, dietary restraint, and the application or ingestion of fluoride.

Oral hygiene. The teeth should be brushed immediately after every meal, including snacks. If it is impossible to brush after eating, the mouth should at least be rinsed well, especially after eating sugary carbohydrate foods. Dental floss should be used to reach the places between teeth where bacteria may be residing. At your regular visit, your dentist will instruct you in proper cleaning techniques and will remove any plaque material. Dental plaque is a sticky, gummy, filmy substance that adheres to teeth, providing an ideal site for bacterial action. Its removal is an important part of a program of oral hygiene. Disclosing tablets can be purchased from your pharmacist; when they are chewed, they release a harmless dye that is swished around in the mouth. The dye stains any plaque which has not been removed by brushing. Any stained area indicates the need for more brushing.

Diet. Carbohydrate-containing foods (sugar, jams, cookies, pies, cakes, etc.) or any food that tends to adhere to the teeth should be avoided. The residue from these foods serves as food for bacteria to cause further acid production that leads to further decay. If these foods are not eliminated from the diet, their consumption should at least be limited to once a day. Snacking repeatedly with such foods exposes teeth to acidic attacks.

Fluoride. Teeth are less susceptible to decay if fluoride is ingested or applied to the teeth. Ingestion may be through the fluoridation of water or the use of a vitamin-mineral supplement containing fluoride. Dentists can apply a fluoride-containing preparation to the teeth. Fluoride-containing toothpastes and mouthwashes are also available and will help to form a more acid-resistant tooth.

Drugs Used in Treatment

℞ vitamin and fluoride supplement—*Poly-Vi-Flor*

Health Care Accessories—*dental floss; disclosing agents; toothbrush*

Related Topic—*Toothache*

Tooth Discoloration

Tooth discoloration is not a true symptom of disease. It usually results from bacteria, food stains, tobacco use, or poor oral hygiene. Excessive and vigorous brushing may destroy tooth enamel sufficiently to cause staining of the teeth. Discoloration is occasionally the result of the use of certain drugs, such as tetracycline, that can permanently discolor the teeth. Trauma to the teeth may result in discoloration.

Treatment

The best treatment for discolored teeth is to carefully brush them in a manner prescribed by a dentist. A good toothbrush and a mildly abrasive toothpaste should be used. Your teeth should be brushed after each meal or snack.

For severe discoloration, capping may be indicated. A dentist or doctor may also bleach the teeth, but if the discoloration is severe, the procedure may not whiten the teeth completely.

Health Care Accessory—*toothbrush*

Travelers' Diarrhea

Whenever an individual travels from one country to another and experiences climate, food, or sanitary conditions different from those he is accustomed to, diarrhea is likely to develop within two to ten days. Rarely will it continue as long as five to seven days, even if left untreated. However, it can produce weakness, dehydration, and a general feeling of tiredness.

Lomotil anticholinergic is recommended for travelers' diarrhea. Antibiotics are not recommended and may actually aggravate the diarrhea. Bottled water and only properly washed and prepared foods should be consumed during the trip if someone is particularly susceptible to travelers' diarrhea or is traveling in an area with poor sanitary conditions. For travel to some areas, the daily use of a tetracycline antibiotic may be indicated.

Drugs Used in Treatment

Recommended treatment with OTC drugs—*Pepto-Bismol diarrhea remedy has been effective in treating travelers' diarrhea.*
OTC diarrhea remedy—*Pepto-Bismol*
℞ anticholinergic and antispasmodic—*Lomotil*
℞ antibiotics—*Minocin; Terramycin; tetracycline hydrochloride; Vibramycin*

Related Topic—*Diarrhea*

Trench Mouth

Trench mouth (Vincent's infection) is an inflammatory disease of the gums. Factors believed to cause trench mouth include inadequate sleep and diet, stress, smoking, vitamin C deficiency, poor oral hygiene, diabetes, certain infections, and poisoning. Trench mouth is not communicable.

Symptoms

Trench mouth usually causes bleeding and pain. It may occur only in certain areas, or it may involve the entire mouth. The gums between the teeth die, and a dirty grayish appearance is noted. Ulcerous sores may appear. The teeth may loosen, resulting in serious jawbone damage. Talking, eating, and swallowing may be painful. A fever may be present, as well as a foul taste in the mouth, malaise, and loss of appetite.

Treatment

Treatment involves correction of precipitating factors. Hydrogen peroxide (3 percent) mixed in equal parts with warm water is useful as a mouthwash and gargle. For severe cases, systemic antibiotics (penicillin or tetracycline) and analgesics may be taken. Rest is indicated. A dentist should be consulted if the infection occurs often.

Drugs Used in Treatment

Recommended treatment with OTC drugs—*Choose your pharmacy's generic brand of hydrogen peroxide for use as a mouthwash.*
OTC miscellaneous—*hydrogen peroxide*
℞ antibiotics—*amoxicillin; ampicillin; erythromycin; Keflex; Minocin; penicillin G; penicillin potassium phenoxymethyl; Terramycin; tetracycline hydrochloride; Vibramycin*
℞ analgesics—*Darvocet-N; Darvon; Darvon Compound-65; Demerol; Empirin*

Compound with Codeine; Fiorinal; Fiorinal with Codeine; Motrin; Percodan; Synalgos-DC; Talwin; Tylenol with Codeine

Related Topic—*Gingivitis*

Ulcerative Colitis

Ulcerative colitis is a chronic inflammatory and ulcerative disease of the colon. Its causes are unknown, although allergic and psychological relationships have been shown. The condition can have an immediate onset, but most often it occurs slowly, starting with mild abdominal cramping, increased urgency to defecate, and bloody diarrhea. It is a condition that most often affects white persons under 50, usually between ages 18 and 35.

Symptoms

Cramping and bowel movements may occur 20 to 35 times daily or more. The stools are watery and contain little fecal material but much mucus, blood, and pus. A fever is present and may be high. In less severe cases patients experience alternating periods of remission and exacerbation. If the condition is acute, the patient becomes emaciated and may die due to hemorrhaging.

Treatment

The condition is serious and requires immediate medical supervision. Other diseases may occur if ulcerative colitis is not treated promptly. These include disorders of the liver, blood, and joints. Sexual development in children may be impaired. Cancer of the colon occurs more frequently in persons with ulcerative colitis.

Treatment of ulcerative colitis requires strict bed rest along with a very restricted diet. Treatment may last for many months. The diarrhea of a mild to moderate condition is treated with antiperistaltic agents, such as Lomotil. Anticholinergics, such as Librax or Donnatal, are given to reduce cramping. Sedatives, tranquilizers, and analgesics are given supportively if needed.

The sulfonamide, sulfasalazine, is the agent of choice for treating mild ulcerative colitis. It is effective during both the initial attack and relapses of the disease. Some doctors advise that drug treatment should be continued indefinitely as long as adverse reactions do not occur.

An enema containing the corticosteroid hydrocortisone is effective for treating acute flare-ups. However, these enemas are not effective in maintaining remission, and must be discontinued once the disease is controlled.

In severe cases of ulcerative colitis, a colostomy procedure may be done. This involves making an incision into the intestine so that fecal material drains from the intestine into a collection device called a colostomy bag. This allows the colon to rest as it is being treated. The colostomy is usually temporary and is closed after the colon has healed.

Drugs Used in Treatment

℞ **anticholinergics**—*Combid; Donnatal; Librax; Lomotil; Pro-Banthine*
℞ **antispasmodic**—*Bentyl*
℞ **steroid hormones**—*Aristocort; Medrol; prednisone*

Genitourinary Tract

The diseases, conditions, and symptoms discussed in this chapter affect the kidneys, the ureters, the urinary bladder, the urethra, and the prostate gland. The first four organs produce and excrete urine. The prostate gland is a male sex gland intimately connected with the urinary system.

Kidneys. The kidneys are bean-shaped organs that lie just below the diaphragm. They receive a rich supply of blood through the renal arteries. The kidneys have two functions: they filter waste materials from the blood and concentrate them into urine, and they reabsorb and return important nutrients to the blood. The total fluid outflow from both kidneys is about 125 ml per minute. Of this amount, 124 ml are reabsorbed. The reabsorption process assures that the body does not become depleted of nutrients such as glucose and substances such as sodium, potassium, and nitrogen.

Ureters. The ureters are two tubes that convey urine from the kidneys to the bladder.

Urinary bladder. The urinary bladder serves as a storage depot for urine before it is eliminated from the body.

Urethra. The urethra serves as the transport tubule from the bladder to the outside of the body. The male urethra is approximately nine inches long; the female urethra is about one and one-half inches in length. The male urethra passes through the prostate gland and penis and serves the dual function of transporting urine and semen from the body.

Prostate gland. The prostate gland is a male accessory sex gland that surrounds the juncture of the vas deferens and the urethra. In the prostate gland sperm are mixed with seminal fluid to produce semen.

Related Topics—*Female Reproductive Tract*

Acute Kidney Failure

Our kidneys filter wastes from the blood and concentrate them into urine to be excreted from the body. The kidneys also regulate and maintain the chemical balance of various substances in the body. Acute kidney failure (or acute renal failure) is a dangerous condition in which kidney function suddenly ceases. Kidney failure may be due to a variety of causes including the ingestion of various chemicals or drugs, injury, burns, infectious diseases, shock following surgery, heart attacks, transfusion with incompatible blood, severe water and electrolyte depletion, and complications of pregnancy.

Unless treated, someone with acute kidney failure may die within a week. Death results from the accumulation in the blood of toxic substances normally excreted by the kidneys. Acute kidney failure can also cause hemorrhage, pulmonary edema, and potassium intoxication.

Symptoms

A major symptom of acute renal failure is a sudden reduction in urine output. Urine flow may be decreased to as little as two tablespoons a day. Gradual loss of renal function may be signalled by loss of appetite, drowsiness, breathing disturbances, diarrhea, nausea, lethargy, and dry skin and mucous membranes. The breath may smell of urine. The rapid buildup of poisons in the body can also lead to confusion, disorientation, delirium, and eventually coma and death.

Treatment

Identification and treatment of the underlying cause of renal failure is essential. Shock must be prevented with intravenous fluids or drugs. An artificial kidney machine may be used to keep the patient alive until kidney function has returned. Complete bed rest is essential, and a low potassium, nitrogen, and protein diet must be followed. Diuretic drugs are contraindicated, and fluids must be restricted unless the patient is vomiting or has diarrhea.

Infection will be treated with antibiotics, and other symptoms will be treated as necessary.

Any trauma in the area of the kidneys must be brought to the attention of a physician immediately. Failure to do so may be fatal.

Drugs Used in Treatment

℞ antibiotics—*amoxicillin; ampicillin; penicillin G; penicillin potassium phenoxymethyl*

Related topics—*Glomerulonephritis; Urinary Tract Infections*

Bed-Wetting

Enuresis means regular, involuntary bed-wetting. About 10% of children over five are bed-wetters. Although most bed-wetting is functional (having no identifiable physical cause), it should be reported to the doctor because a small percentage of cases are due to abnormalities of the nervous system or bladder and must be treated. For example, urethral sphincters may not work properly. Also, some diseases—including juvenile diabetes, pinworms and epilepsy—may cause enuresis. Disease-related enuresis usually stops within weeks or a couple of months when the disease is treated.

For functional enuresis, parents can try a variety of measures—restricting evening fluids, reminding the child to urinate before retiring and waking the child to urinate. However, these measures are merely supportive and must not become a source of conflict. Probably the most important aids in resolving this problem are patience, a good supply of sheets and a hopeful attitude that the child will outgrow it.

Tofranil (imipramine) may be given at bedtime for its side effect of urine retention, or an anticholinergic drug such as Donnatal may be prescribed.

Drugs Used in Treatment

℞ anticholinergic—*Donnatal*
℞ antidepressants— *Tofranil*

Change in Urinary Habits

A change in urinary habits may be a symptom of many diseases. The change may occur in the frequency or timing of urination or in the volume or color of the urine itself.

Frequency. Increased frequency of urination commonly results from inflammation of the kidneys, bladder, or urethra produced by infection or from a decrease in the capacity of the bladder. Increased frequency of urination is usually accompanied by feelings of urgency.

Inflammation may affect any portion of the urinary tract. Severe infection may produce other symptoms such as fever and tiredness. Less severe urinary infections may not show any symptoms except an increased frequency of urination and occasional pain on urination. Increased frequency of urination is the earliest symptom in most cases of renal tuberculosis and diabetes. Either increased frequency of urination or pain on urination is a signal to see a doctor immediately.

The capacity of the bladder may be decreased by tumors or other pressures around the bladder itself, or by enlargement of the prostate gland. Whenever the capacity decreases, less urine can be held, causing more frequent urination. Whatever the cause, the help of a doctor must be sought immediately.

Timing. "Nocturia" means excessive nighttime urination. It is normal upon awakening during the night to have a desire to urinate. However, frequent awakening with the desire to urinate may be a symptom of inflammatory or infectious disease within the renal tract or of tumors or other disorders which cause pressure on the bladder and urinary system. Such illnesses usually cause other symptoms as well, including painful urination, a poor stream, or difficulty in starting. Anyone with these symptoms should see a doctor immediately.

Volume. "Polyuria" means the voiding of an excessive volume of urine. If an excessive volume of urine is produced during the night, and the bladder fills, pressure will be felt to awaken and void it. Thus, polyuria is one possible cause of nocturia.

Either polyuria or nocturia requires a doctor's diagnosis. Either can be a symptom of a disease of the endocrine glands, or of congestive heart failure, certain types of diabetes, or kidney disease.

Color. If urine appears to be darker than usual, it may have blood in it. In some cases, blood may be visible in the urine. Blood in the urine may indicate an infection or injury in the kidneys, leukemia, hemophilia, or kidney stones. The bleeding may be occurring in the kidneys, ureters, urinary bladder, or urethra. In males, the blood may arise from the prostate or seminal vesicles. In females, blood may appear due to disease in one of the neighboring organs, such as the uterus, vagina, or rectum, and may be mistaken as being in the urine. Any blood in the urine requires the immediate attention of a doctor.

Related Topics—*Acute Kidney Failure; Glomerulonephritis; Kidney Stones; Prostatitis; Urinary Tract Infections*

Glomerulonephritis

The nephron is the urine-forming unit of the kidney. The nephron contains the glomerulus, an intricately-woven cluster of capillaries where the blood is filtered and impurities are removed.

Glomerulonephritis (also called nephritis) is an inflammation of the glomeruli. It may have an abrupt onset (acute glomerulonephritis), or it may be characterized by slow progressive destruction of the kidneys (chronic glomerulonephritis). The disease affects both kidneys, and it is most commonly seen in children between the ages of three and ten, although 5 percent of the initial attacks of acute glomerulonephritis occur after the age of 50. The acute form frequently occurs after a streptococcal infection, although other strains of bacteria and certain drugs have also been implicated.

Glomerulonephritis is not a bacterial infection; bacteria are usually not found in the kidneys during glomerulonephritis. It is generally believed that the inflammation is an allergic response to a bacterial or other agent.

Symptoms

Symptoms of acute glomerulonephritis may appear about two weeks after a streptococcal infection. The symptoms of either form may be mild or severe. The patient develops a mild fever and will feel unwell, may have puffy eyes and face, pain along the flanks, headache, and reduced urine output. There may be blood in the urine, or the urine may appear dark brown. The person may feel short of breath. The blood pressure and heart rate may rise.

Complications

If complications develop, glomerulonephritis may be fatal. Because the kidneys are not functioning well, water, salt, and potentially toxic wastes will be retained, possibly resulting in cardiac failure. Severe hypertension may develop. Patients with glomerulonephritis are in particular danger if they develop an infection.

Treatment

There is no specific treatment for glomerulonephritis. Antibiotics will be given to eradicate the bacteria causing any infection, and other treatment is directed at relieving the symptoms and preventing complications. In some cases, steroids may be given. Strict bed rest is essential as long as symptoms persist. A diet low in protein is indicated. Carbohydrates are given liberally to provide calories and to reduce the breakdown of body proteins and prevent ketosis (a disturbance of the body's acid-alkali balance). Diuretic drugs are contraindicated, and salt must be restricted to avoid high blood pressure. Fluids should be restricted to amounts that the kidneys can handle.

Drugs Used in Treatment

℞ antibiotics—*amoxicillin; ampicillin; penicillin G; penicillin potassium phenoxymethyl*
℞ steroid hormones—*Aristocort; Medrol; prednisone*

Related Topic—*Acute Kidney Failure*

Kidney Stones

Kidney stones are among the most common of all kidney disorders. The condition occurs most commonly among middle-aged men, although stones can develop in any person. Some stones are as small as a grain of sand while others may grow as large as a walnut. They rarely form as a single stone; rather, many stones form.

Kidney stones usually result from abnormally high levels of calcium and phosphate in the urine. The minerals precipitate out as hardened masses in the kidneys. Certain disorders help to start this process. These include overactive parathyroid glands, gout, excess vitamin D, and excessive calcium intake (such as drinking too much milk). Drinking hard water does not predispose an individual to kidney stones. Even when treated, kidney stones can cause permanent kidney damage.

Symptoms

There may be no initial symptoms or only mild pain in the area of the kidney. Anemia may occur in a later stage. Occasionally blood may appear in the urine. The abdomen may become distended.

The symptoms become much more severe if the stone moves out of the kidney and into a ureter. Blockage of a ureter causes excruciating pain that begins in the area of the kidneys (the back) and radiates down across the abdomen and into the genitalia. The individual will be nauseous, vomiting, and sweating. Unless treated at once, he may become unconscious from the pain and go into shock.

A stone may be passed from the ureter into the bladder and through the urethra. The pain accompanying this movement is also severe. As the stone moves along, it may scratch the walls of the ureter and urethra, causing blood to appear in the urine. If a stone lodges in the ureter and blocks the passage of urine, permanent damage to the kidney may result. If a stone is passed, it should be retrieved and taken to the doctor for analysis of its content. If one stone was present, it is very likely that other stones are also present or will eventually form in the kidneys.

Treatment

Kidney stones are best treated by correcting the disorder that caused them. Three to four quarts of water per day should be consumed to help keep the stones from forming. Intake of foods rich in calcium should be limited.

There are no drugs to treat kidney stones directly. Thiazide diuretics decrease calcium excretion from the blood and thus help inhibit stone formation. Potassium supplements are sometimes given in conjunction with diuretics. If the stone is too large to pass, surgery may be required. With a doctor's approval, analgesics may be tried if a moving stone causes pain.

Sometimes kidney stones are caused by uric acid. If this is the case, the drug allopurinol will help reduce uric acid formation.

Drugs Used in Treatment

OTC analgesics—*see the list under Pain and Fever*
Rx analgesics—*Darvocet-N; Darvon; Darvon Compound-65; Demerol; Empirin Compound with Codeine; Fiorinal; Fiorinal with Codeine; Motrin; Percodan; Synalgos-DC; Talwin; Tylenol with Codeine*
Rx diuretics—*Aldactazide; Diuril; Dyazide; Enduron; hydrochlorothiazide; Hygroton*
Rx potassium replacements—*K-Lyte; potassium chloride*
Rx uricosuric—*Zyloprim*
Note: *Some of these products list kidney disease as a contraindication or warning; nevertheless, they are used in the treatment of certain kidney disorders. Your doctor will determine whether these drugs pose a hazard or will be beneficial to you.*

Prostatitis

Prostatitis is an inflammation of the prostate caused by an infection—often bacterial. It is usually associated with a kidney infection. It may be acute or chronic.

Symptoms

The symptoms of acute bacterial prostatitis include severe pain, fever, difficult urination, and a urethral discharge. The area over the prostate gland may feel extremely tender. If the inflammation is severe, the urethra may be blocked, preventing urine flow. Chronic prostatitis usually is not accompanied by fever, although there may be frequent need to urinate and a change in urine color.

Treatment

Prostatitis is treated with Septra or Bactrim, or with a tetracycline antibiotic for a minimum of two weeks. Bed rest is required during the acute phase. At least eight to ten glasses of water should be drunk each day. Aspirin or other analgesics can be taken for pain. Stool softeners should be used to avoid straining.

Drugs Used in Treatment

OTC analgesics—*see the list under Pain and Fever*
OTC laxatives—*see the list under Constipation*
R̽ antibacterial—*Bactrim*
R̽ antibiotics—*Minocin; Terramycin; tetracycline hydrochloride; Vibramycin*
R̽ analgesics—*Darvocet-N; Darvon; Darvon Compound-65; Demerol; Empirin Compound with Codeine; Fiorinal; Fiorinal with Codeine; Motrin; Percodan; Synalgos-DC; Talwin; Tylenol with Codeine*

Related Topic—*Urinary Tract Infections*

Urinary Tract Infections

The incidence of urinary tract infections is reported to be as high as 10 percent of the American population, depending on the age of the patient. Infections of the genitourinary tract are second only to those of the respiratory tract in frequency during childhood. Females have ten times the number of urinary tract infections than males.

The bacteria which cause urinary tract infections are inhabitants of the lower portions of the gastrointestinal tract. This may explain in part why women are more commonly affected than men. The female urethra is very short compared to that of the male, and the opening is relatively close to the anus. The infecting bacteria need not travel as far in the female as in the male, and, therefore, migration to the urethral opening is relatively easy.

Sites of Infection

Urinary tract infections are divided into those that affect the lower part of the urinary tract and those that involve the upper portions. Diseases of the lower portion include cystitis and urethritis. Infections of the upper urinary tract, pyelonephritis for example, are more severe and serious.

Urethritis. The urethra is the passageway from the bladder through which urine is carried to the outside. The female urethra averages an inch and a half in length. The male urethra passes from the bladder through the prostate gland and the shaft of the penis; its length averages nine inches. The male urethra, in addition to serving as the passageway for urine, carries reproductive materials.

Gonorrheal urethritis is the most common urethral infection in men, and it is characterized by discharge, pain on urination, and increased urgency to

186

urinate. The female urethra, more accessible to invading bacteria than that of the male, is more likely to be infected. Urethritis in the female is usually accompanied by a bladder infection (cystitis). Symptoms include pain on urination and urethral discharge.

Cystitis. Cystitis is an inflammation of the urinary bladder. It may follow an infection of the kidney, the prostate, or the urethra. People who are poorly nourished and generally run-down are predisposed to cystitis. It is more common among women than among men, probably because of the shorter female urethra.

The most common symptom is urgent, frequent, and painful urination. Urine output, though, is scanty. Blood may be apparent in the urine.

Pyelonephritis. Bacteria sometimes enter the upper urinary tract from the bladder and invade the kidney itself. The resulting infection, called pyelonephritis, may involve only one or both kidneys. Pyelonephritis is common among women—especially in childhood or during pregnancy.

Someone with pyelonephritis will be quite ill, with a fever of 104° to 105° F. Shaking chills, increased pulse rate, nausea, vomiting, and excruciating pain in the abdomen and back are also symptoms. The disorder must be treated immediately or severe, irreversible damage to the kidneys will result, possibly causing uremia and death. Treatment may require surgery and bed rest.

Treatment

The treatment of acute uncomplicated urinary tract infections is best performed with use of a sulfa drug such as sulfisoxazole or sulfamethazole. These drugs are effective against most of the bacteria that cause urinary tract infections. A combination product, sulfamethazole with trimethoprim (Bactrim or Septra), is also quite effective.

For people who are sensitive to sulfonamides or for those in whom the infection is not responding to therapy, a broad-spectrum antibiotic is the drug of choice. Ampicillin or amoxicillin are frequently chosen. Other therapy includes the cephalosporins and tetracycline. Erythromycin or an injectable aminoglycoside antibiotic may also be used.

Urinary tract infections are usually readily treated by drug therapy. However, all too often the infection reappears later or even becomes chronic—possibly in as many as 80 percent of the cases. Nearly all of these cases, other than those that were untreated or a result of poor patient compliance with therapy, are actually caused by a re-introduction of the infective organisms. Chronic infection may lead to serious health problems later in life such as cardiovascular disease (hypertension and congestive heart failure) or complete kidney failure. If the infection recurs and urinary flow is blocked by kidney stones, tumors, or an inflamed prostate gland, surgery is usually needed to correct the problem.

One of the major reasons for poor compliance with therapy is that in the overwhelming majority of urinary tract infections, the symptoms (painful or burning urination, more frequent or urgent urination, low back pain, blood or pus in the urine) disappear in a few days with or without drug treatment. Patients often stop taking drugs when they start feeling better. Therapy must be continued for the full course of treatment.

A person with a urinary tract infection should drink at least eight to ten glasses of water each day—and preferably more. If the condition is severe enough to cause dribbling, incontinence pants should be worn. It may be necessary to measure the quantity of urine with a urinal. Aspirin or acetaminophen and a thermometer may be necessary. An OTC product for testing the bacterial content of the urine is available.

Drugs Used in Treatment

OTC analgesics—*see the list under Pain and Fever*
R antibacterials—*Bactrim; Gantanol; Gantrisin; Macrodantin*
R antibacterial and analgesic combinations—*Azo Gantanol; Azo Gantrisin*
R antibiotics—*amoxicillin; ampicillin; erythromycin; Keflex; Minocin; Terramycin; tetracycline hydrochloride; Vibramycin*
R analgesic—*Pyridium*
Note: *Some of these products list kidney disease as a contraindication or warning; nevertheless, they are used in the treatment of certain kidney disorders. Your doctor will determine whether these drugs pose a hazard or will be beneficial to you.*

Health Care Accessory—*fever thermometer*

Related Topics—*Acute Kidney Failure; Prostatitis*

Female Reproductive Tract

The female reproductive organs include the vagina, cervix, uterus, Fallopian tubes, and ovaries.

Vagina. The vagina is the muscular passage leading from the outside of the body to the uterus. It measures four to five inches in length. Normally, the vaginal walls lie close together; however, during sexual intercourse they stretch easily to accommodate the male penis. During childbirth they extend even more to allow the baby to emerge.

The vagina has few nerve endings, and most of the nerve endings are located near the opening to the outside of the body. Within the vagina, little can be felt but pressure.

The vagina is naturally moist, although the quantity and quality of the vaginal secretions vary according to the woman's menstrual cycle and her emotional state. This natural, continuous lubrication is a self-cleansing process that makes vaginal douching normally unnecessary.

Cervix. The cervix is the narrow opening of the uterus. It projects into the upper end of the vagina. A tiny opening through the cervix leads to an inch-long canal connecting the vagina with the uterus. This is the canal traversed by sperm on their way into the uterus, and by menstrual discharge and babies leaving the uterus.

Uterus. The uterus is a muscular, pear-shaped hollow organ, about the size of a lemon normally. The uterine walls stretch considerably as a fetus develops within the uterus, and in late pregnancy the uterus may be as large as a medium-sized watermelon.

The rich, soft lining of the uterus, the endometrium, is renewed each month; it sloughs off and leaves the body as menstrual discharge.

Fallopian tubes. At the upper end of the uterus are two openings that lead to the Fallopian tubes. The Fallopian tubes extend back from the uterus to the ovaries. Conception occurs in the Fallopian tubes, and the inner environment of the tubes is conducive both to guiding the sperm in the right direction and to pushing the egg to the uterus.

Ovaries. The ovaries are small, firm, and roughly egg-shaped. Once a month, they produce an egg (two or more eggs may develop at the same time, but this occurs rarely). Ovulation occurs when the egg matures and passes from an ovary into a Fallopian tube. The ovaries also produce reproductive hormones.

Related Topics —*Genitourinary Tract; Sexually Transmitted Diseases*

Cervical Polyps

Cervical polyps are generally benign tumors that may appear at any time after the beginning of menstruation.

The polyps may occur at any site within the cervix, and they are usually less than one inch in length.

Symptoms

Abnormal vaginal bleeding and discharge are the most common symptoms. Polyps may also cause infertility and severe pain.

Treatment

Polyps may become infected or malignant and should therefore be removed, either by dilation and curettage or by surgery. The tissue removed is usually tested for malignancy. Warm acetic acid or saline douches for three to seven days after removal help control the inflammatory reaction. Antibiotics may also be indicated.

Drugs Used in Treatment

℞ antibiotics—*amoxicillin; ampicillin; erythromycin; Keflex; Minocin; penicillin G; penicillin potassium phenoxymethyl; Terramycin; tetracycline hydrochloride; Vibramycin*

Cervicitis

Among the most common of all female disorders, cervicitis is an inflammation of the cervix, the neck of the uterus. The inflammation may be caused by a specific infection (gonorrhea, syphilis) or it may be caused by a nonspecific bacterial infection. Pregnancy and childbirth may be predisposing factors; at least 60 percent of all women who have been pregnant have had cervicitis. Over 75 percent of all adult women have had the inflammation at some time.

Symptoms

Cervicitis causes the cervical mucus to become thin and clear; it may become streaked with pus and blood. The woman may experience low back pain, painful or heavy menstrual flow, painful urination, and abnormal vaginal discharge. The discomfort or pain may be made worse by intercourse.

Treatment

Mild cases may clear by themselves, or anti-infective vaginal ointments and creams may be given. More severe infections may require oral antibiotics or estrogen. A "D and C" (dilation and curettage) may be indicated in some cases. In this process, the cervix is expanded and its surface is scraped.

Mild cases may clear up within a few weeks; chronic cervicitis may require several months of active treatment.

Drugs Used in Treatment

℞ anti-infectives—*AVC; Sultrin*
℞ antibiotics—*amoxicillin; ampicillin; erythromycin; Keflex; Minocin; penicillin G; penicillin potassium phenoxymethyl; Terramycin; tetracycline hydrochloride; Vibramycin*
℞ estrogen hormone—*Premarin*

Contraception

Contraception is the voluntary prevention of pregnancy. While many contraceptive agents are available, there is no ideal method for preventing pregnancy. The "perfect" contraceptive would be effective, economical, reversible, and acceptable, safe, and simple to use. No single measure in use today possesses all of these qualities.

No matter what method is chosen, it must be used properly to be effective. Any method will be effective if it is used carefully enough, and even the most effective method will work only when it is used carefully and consistently. Below are listed reversible contraceptive methods in order of effectiveness, followed by a discussion of sterilization.

Oral Contraceptives

Oral contraceptive medications use the synthetic hormones progestin and estrogen either alone or in combination. The most common oral contraceptive is a combination of both estrogen and progestin given daily over a 21-day period. In this case, the hormones suppress the release of substances from the pituitary gland and thereby stop ovulation. On the other hand, if the egg by some chance does become fertilized, the medications render the endometrium less conducive to its implantation, thereby blocking pregnancy.

A combination product can be effective immediately when a cycle of oral contraceptive therapy is started on the fifth day after the beginning of menstruation. However, if the cycle is begun after childbirth, or if, for some reason, it was started later than the fifth day of the menstrual cycle, it cannot be relied on to prevent ovulation during that month. After oral contraceptives have been discontinued, ovulation will resume in most women within two or three cycles. If amenorrhea has resulted from their use, it may persist for another six months or longer.

Oral contraceptives have been associated with an increased risk of blood clots; cancer; depression; jaundice; hypertension; liver, kidney and gallbladder problems; and migraine headaches. Women taking any oral contraceptive should notify their doctor if they cough up blood or experience sudden shortness of breath or sharp chest pains. These signs may signify the presence of pulmonary blood clots. Sharp chest pains may also indicate that a heart attack has occurred or is about to occur. The warning signs of stroke include changes in vision, difficulty in speaking or moving the arms or legs, fainting spells, and severe headache. Patients should examine their breasts periodically for lump formation. Severe abdominal pain could indicate the presence of a ruptured liver tumor; and yellowing of the skin is a warning sign of jaundice. Estrogens may cause mental depression; any drastic change in mood should be reported to the doctor.

Intrauterine Devices (IUDs)

The exact mechanism for the action of the intrauterine device is unknown although it is known that IUDs are not contraceptives in the true sense of the word. They do not prevent ovulation, implantation, or fertilization of the egg. Rather, they cause a fertilized egg to be aborted.

IUDs consist of metal or plastic coils, rings, or spirals that are inserted by a doctor into the uterus. Their very physical presence probably initiates a minor inflammation that causes the egg to be sloughed off.

IUDs are sometimes difficult to insert. They may cause cramping, and occasionally the device is lost. Excessive bleeding and even perforation and infection may occur. Many women find the excessive or prolonged menses that occur with an IUD objectionable. Twenty percent of IUD users have the device removed within a year after the initial insertion.

Unlike the diaphragm and spermicidal jelly, foam, or cream, the IUD does not require that the user "prepare for" the sexual act. Also, none of the systemic side effects associated with oral contraceptives are noted with an IUD once it is in place. However, women with a history of frequent pelvic infections, blood clotting disorders, or severe menstrual problems (very heavy flow or severe cramps) may not be able to use the IUD.

Diaphragm and Spermicidal Agent

A diaphragm is a dome-shaped latex cup rimmed with a metal spring or band. It is designed to be inserted against the cervix prior to intercourse.

A diaphragm used with an appropriate spermicidal jelly or cream is an effective contraceptive agent. Diaphragms used alone are not effective; they are not stationary during intercourse. Their primary contraceptive action is to hold the spermicidal agent against the cervix. For extra protection a spermicidal preparation may be applied to the external facing of the diaphragm once it is inserted. A diaphragm must be fitted by a doctor, and a woman should be refitted if she gains or loses more than ten pounds, has surgery, delivers a child, or has a miscarriage.

Other than an allergic reaction (either the woman's or her partner's) to the latex or the spermicide, the diaphragm has few side effects. However, the woman must be highly motivated and very conscientious about its use to achieve a high rate of effectiveness.

Condoms

The condom is a sheath of rubber or animal membrane that fits around the penis to afford protection against pregnancy. It also protects against sexually transmitted disease. Other than sterilization, the condom is the only contraceptive method used by the male. The disadvantages of condoms include a psychological dulling of sensation and the danger of pregnancy should the condom be defective, i.e., should the sheath tear, split, or leak.

On the other hand, condoms have virtually no side effects and are easy to use and to obtain. When they are used carefully, they provide a high degree of protection against pregnancy.

Spermicidal Agents

Available over-the-counter, spermicidal foams, jellies, creams, and suppositories may be used with a diaphragm or alone. They act as physical barriers to the entry of sperm through the cervix, and their active ingredient destroys sperm on contact. To be effective, the preparation must remain in the vaginal tract for at least six to eight hours after intercourse. Premature removal by douching reduces the effectiveness. With any of these agents, if irritation to the vagina or penis occurs, the product should be discontinued.

Foams are considered by many to be the spermicidal agent of choice, because they are readily spread throughout the cervical area and are the least detectable agent during intercourse. The user must realize, however, that foam's effectiveness relies on even distribution of the spermicide in air bubbles. Therefore, the container must be well shaken before application.

Jellies are easy to remove because they are water-soluble, and the creams provide good lubrication. Neither is as effective a barrier as the foam or suppositories. The suppositories require that the users wait 15 to 20 minutes or more before intercourse. However, they are easy to insert and they provide a premeasured dose.

Natural Family Planning

Also called the rhythm method, natural family planning may incorporate calendar determination of a woman's fertile periods with careful measurement of her basal body temperature and with observation of her cervical mucus. The couple planning to use this method of contraception must be highly motivated and very conscientious in recording the woman's cycles. This method of contraception is more likely to be effective in women who have very regular menstrual periods.

The calendar method requires that a woman record her menstrual cycles for eight to twelve months. She then uses this record of past cycles to predict future cycles. When the fertile period has been determined, the couple abstains from intercourse for those days, or uses some other contraception.

To determine fertility by body temperature, a basal thermometer is needed and a basal temperature chart must be maintained on which body temperature is recorded carefully. The temperature should be taken immediately upon awakening before any other physical activity is attempted. The body temperature usually drops slightly one to one-and-one-half days prior to ovulation and will rise about 0.7° one to two days after ovulation. The higher temperature will continue throughout the remainder of the cycle. The third day after the initial rise marks the end of the fertile period.

The quality and quantity of cervical mucus is another determination of fertility. If using the cervical mucus method, a woman must become familiar with her pattern of discharge so that she can recognize the changes that signal ovulation. The problem with this method (and with the basal body temperature method) is that some women do not have clearly definable patterns of change. Also, douching, lubricants, or infection can change the discharge and mask the signals.

If couples are highly motivated and very careful, if they abstain from intercourse on fertile days or use a backup method of birth control, and if they fully understand the method, natural family planning can be very effective.

Sterilization

Sterilization is the permanent prevention of pregnancy. It is accomplished by surgery or the use of x-ray treatment on either sex.

The sterilization procedure for women is called tubal ligation. It involves severing or sealing off the fallopian tubes (the tubes that transport a fertilized egg from the ovaries to the uterus). When the tubes are cut, no organ is removed. Tubal ligation prevents impregnation because the egg cannot reach the uterus. Tubal sterilization does not cause a reduced sexual attractiveness or sexuality. It does not change the woman's appearance, and no adverse changes occur in sexual function. In fact, many women who previously feared pregnancy enjoy intercourse more thoroughly after sterilization.

Sterilization of the male partner, vasectomy, is often done in the doctor's office under local anesthesia. The tubes that transport sperm out of the testicles are cut and tied so that there are no sperm in the ejaculate. Impotence does not result. Occasionally, vasectomy may result in a spontaneous recanalization (although this happens in less than 1 percent of the cases). Vasectomy is sometimes reversible.

Drugs Used

Recommendations on the use of OTC contraceptive aids—*Personal considerations should determine which of the OTC contraceptives you want to use. Some people find certain products more aesthetically pleasing than others; other people may have an allergic reaction to certain products.*
OTC contraceptive products—*Conceptrol; Dalkon Kit; Delfen; Emko; Encare Oval; Ortho-Cream; Ortho-Gynol; Semicid*
℞ oral contraceptives

Health Care Accessories—*condoms; diaphragms; fever thermometers (basal thermometer only)*

Cystocele

A cystocele is a protrusion of the urinary bladder through the vaginal wall. The condition usually results from laceration, childbirth, or damage to the vaginal wall. The birth of a large baby increases the likelihood of cystocele.

Complications tend to affect the urinary tract. They include the presence of residual urine that may amount to two ounces or more, chronic recurrent cystitis, difficult urination, or stress incontinence.

Symptoms

Cystocele causes a feeling of vaginal fullness and looseness and the sensation of the presence of urine even after voiding. A slight bulge into the vagina may also be noted.

Treatment

Cystocele is surgically corrected. A rubber pessary inserted into the vagina may be necessary to reduce and support the cystocele in those patients who refuse or cannot undergo surgery. After menopause, estrogen will help control the condition. If infection is present, an appropriate antibiotic will be required.

Drugs Used in Treatment

℞ estrogen hormone—*Premarin*
℞ antibiotics—*amoxicillin; ampicillin; erythromycin; Keflex; Minocin; penicillin G; penicillin potassium phenoxymethyl; Terramycin; tetracycline hydrochloride; Vibramycin*

Endometriosis

Endometriosis is the aberrant growth of the uterine mucous membrane (endometrium) outside of the uterine cavity. It usually involves the visceral peritoneal surfaces and may cause severe pelvic pain, abnormal uterine bleeding, and possibly infertility. Seventy-five percent of all women with endometriosis are between 30 and 40 years old. It is most common in women who marry late and have no children. The ratio of white to black patients is two to one.

One theory suggests the cause of endometriosis is temporary closure of the cervix and menstrual blood flow into the abdominal cavity; some of the endometrium may implant there. Material may also be transferred through the vascular or lymphatic systems. Endometriosis may also develop following surgery in which some of the endometrium is sutured outside of the uterine cavity.

In the patient with endometriosis, endometrial material may be found in the ovaries, fallopian tubes, over the uterus, around the surface of the rectum, and even in the appendix. It is seen occasionally in the cervix, vulva, umbilicus, and sometimes within the vagina. Endometriosis rarely becomes malignant.

Symptoms

The symptoms include practically constant pelvic pain. The pain begins several days to a week before menses and increases in severity until menstrual flow has ceased. The more advanced the condition, the more severe the pain. There may also be pain due to local engorgement; this pain is reported to be of a "grinding" type that may be referred to the groin, hips, or the rectum depending upon the site of the endometriosis. However, one-third of all patients have no significant pain. When the rectum or bladder are involved, there may be bleeding from these sites. Infertility may result if the ovaries or tubes are involved, but this need not happen if the condition is treated.

Complications include obstruction of the urethra, bowel, and tubes. The ovaries may be completely destroyed. When large endometrium cysts rupture, they may lead to severe intra-abdominal bleeding with resultant peritonitis.

Treatment

Women with a suspected mild endometriosis should be examined every six months through the menopause. Pregnancy may inhibit the condition. Pain is relieved with prescription analgesics such as codeine or Demerol. Aspirin may work, but not when given alone. The drug danocrine, a weak synthetic androgen, suppresses endometriosis and is very effective, but it is also expensive. Large doses of estrogen may also be given. The tissue may also be removed by surgery or be destroyed by cauterization.

Drugs Used in Treatment

R oral contraceptives
R hormones—*Premarin; Provera*
R analgesics—*Darvocet-N; Darvon; Darvon Compound-65; Demerol; Empirin Compound with Codeine; Equagesic; Fiorinal; Fiorinal with Codeine; Motrin; Percodan; Synalgos-DC; Talwin; Tylenol with Codeine*

Infertility

Infertility is the inability to conceive. A couple is considered infertile if pregnancy does not occur after a year of normal sexual relations without contraceptives, if the woman conceives but aborts repeatedly, or if the woman repeatedly aborts after the first child. Ten percent of all couples are infertile.

Although there are many possible causes, male infertility is generally related to a deficiency in sperm count, to impaired sperm motility, or to abnormal sperm structure. The male is responsible in about 40 percent of all infertile couples. Female infertility is commonly due to a nutritional deficiency, hormonal imbalance, or some abnormality of the reproductive organs. Occasionally, tumors or infection will cause female infertility.

Infertility can be treated in many couples, but treatment generally takes three to four months of continual meeting with the physician. Both partners must be examined. When the cause of the infertility is determined, appropriate treatment can be initiated.

Treatment

If an endocrine imbalance is causing the fertility problem, treatment of that condition will generally restore full fertility. Hypo- or hyperthyroidism is one such common cause. When a physical abnormality is present, surgical correction (such as removal of a tumor) may restore full fertility. If failure to ovulate is the cause, Clomid synthetic estrogen may be given. However, the drug causes multiple births in about 20 percent of all pregnancies. While it has not been officially approved for this purpose, the drug has also been given to males to increase their sperm count. Corticosteroids and human menopausal gonadotropin (HMG) may also treat infertility.

When infertility occurs in the male, surgical correction of any abnormality of the penis or the testicles may improve fertility. Abnormal sperm structure is not treatable either by surgery or drugs.

If the cause of infertility is discovered and treated early, the prognosis for conception and normal pregnancy is good. Of course, there is no effective treatment of infertility caused by marked uterine underdevelopment or when other structures, such as the ovaries, are absent. If after a year of consultation and treatment the couple does not conceive, many physicians will recommend adoption.

Menopause

Menopause, that phase of life when menstruation ceases, is the end of a woman's reproductive cycle. It is a normal part of the change of life, or climacteric. It may be due to natural causes, or it may be premature or artificially induced.

Natural menopause occurs usually between ages 40 and 50 and results from a gradual decline in the function of the ovaries. As the ovaries become less functional, they cease to respond to hormonal stimulation and eventually stop secreting their own hormones and eggs. The entire process may take more than a year. Premature menopause usually occurs before the age of 40 and is due to premature attrition of the ovarian follicles. Artificial menopause occurs following surgical removal of the uterus or ovaries, surgical manipulation, or radiation therapy of the ovaries.

Regardless of its cause, the symptoms of menopause are similar and they may last from several months to several years. These may include nervousness; menstrual disturbances; lassitude; fatigability; flushes and chills; depression and crying spells; irritability; insomnia; alterations in libido; palpitations; headaches; numbness and tingling; muscular aches and pains, especially in the back; vertigo; edema; sweating; changes in urinary frequency; incontinence; nausea; and vomiting. Complaints of persistent lower back pain should always be investigated; the pain could be due to the deterioration of the spine that frequently occurs with aging. While it may occur at the same time, such deterioration is not a symptom of menopause.

Drug Therapy

If symptoms are severe, certain drugs may be prescribed. Estrogen replacement therapy is used to relieve hot flashes, vaginal dryness, or the acute symptoms of premature or artificial menopause. Generally, estrogen is given in cyclical doses. For example, it may be administered daily for 21 days, then withheld for seven days, after which the cycle is repeated. Therapy may continue only until the symptoms are brought under control or until menopause is complete, or it may be prolonged (generally the case with premature or artificial menopause). Estrogen therapy may have a beneficial effect on osteoporosis, the loss of bone density that often occurs with aging, but it may also cause an increased risk of cancer.

If emotional changes are especially troublesome, a mild sedative such as phenobarbital or diazepam or an antidepressant may be prescribed.

Drugs Used in Treatment

R̥ estrogen hormone—*Premarin*
R̥ sedative and hypnotic products—*Atarax; Ativan; Librium; meprobamate; Nembutal; phenobarbital; Serax; Tranxene; Valium*

℞ antidepressants—*Elavil; Sinequan; Tofranil*
℞ phenothiazines—*Compazine; Mellaril; Stelazine*
℞ phenothiazine and antidepressant—*Triavil*
℞ analgesics—*Darvocet-N; Darvon; Darvon Compound-65; Demerol; Empirin Compound with Codeine; Equagesic; Fiorinal; Fiorinal with Codeine; Motrin; Norgesic; Parafon Forte; Percodan; Robaxin; Soma Compound; Synalgos-DC; Talwin; Tylenol with Codeine*

Menstrual Disorders

Any disruption of the female hormone secretions can lead to a disturbance in the menstrual pattern. All of the following conditions can be symptoms of an underlying glandular disorder or of some other disease.

Amenorrhea

Amenorrhea is a complete lack of menses. Primary amenorrhea is a condition in which a woman has never menstruated and is at least 16 years old. Secondary amenorrhea is a condition in which menstruation ceases in a woman who has previously menstruated. Either condition can be caused by a number of factors including genetic defects or imbalances in female hormones. Amenorrhea may also result from the ingestion of certain drugs, travel to a strange environment, or psychological problems. The most common cause of secondary amenorrhea is pregnancy.

Treatment depends on the cause and therapeutic objective. Though pregnancy may not be sought, the patient usually wants regulation of her cycle. The doctor first attempts to determine what, if any, underlying condition is causing the lack of menses. Barring any serious underlying disease, the doctor may choose cyclic estrogen/progesterone therapy, perhaps with one of the oral products intended for contraception. Alternatively, the doctor may induce menstruation by giving an oral progesterone for five days. Menstrual flow should begin within a couple of days after the drug is withdrawn.

Oligomenorrhea

Oligomenorrhea is a condition in which the menses are infrequent and do not contain the normal amount of fluid. This condition is commonly seen in women who use oral contraceptives. If treatment is necessary it may be similar to that used to treat amenorrhea or it may involve switching to a different contraceptive combination.

Dysmenorrhea

Dysmenorrhea, or painful menses, is experienced to some degree by nearly all women. The symptoms consist of abdominal cramping (most common), low back pain, headache and, in some women, nausea and vomiting. The amount of difficulty caused by menstruation is related, to a great degree, to the pain threshold and emotional state of the woman. The pains usually start on the first day of menstruation and last about one-half day although some cramping may last into the next day or so. Primary dysmenorrhea occurs at the beginning of the menstrual age, usually without organic cause. Secondary dysmenorrhea occurs later in life, and there is invariably an underlying cause. Both types may be aggravated by psychic and emotional factors.

Primary dysmenorrhea is treated with analgesics, sedatives, and antispasmodics, but treatment of the secondary type includes diagnosing the underlying cause. Treatment may involve suppressing ovulation. Estrogens may be given for 21 days, then skipped for seven days. This pattern is repeated cyclically for three months. Another regimen of therapy is to give progesterone from day 5 to day 25 of the menstrual cycle. If these methods are not successful, the cause may be excessive estrogen production. If this is the case, administering methyltestosterone from day five to day ten may be effective through neutralization of endogenous estrogen. Using a hot water bottle or heating pad over the area may also bring relief.

Hypermenorrhea and Polymenorrhea

Hypermenorrhea is a condition characterized by menses that are excessively long or contain overly large amounts of fluid.

Polymenorrhea refers to menses that occur more often than 25 to 35 days apart. It is a relatively uncommon problem and when it does occur it is most likely to do so in the early or late years of menstruation.

These conditions can be caused by tumors, inflammation of the uterus, diseases affecting blood clotting, emotional disorders, or hormonal malfunction. If the result of the latter, the condition would be called functional uterine bleeding and may respond to progestin therapy. If due to the other causes, treating them along with supportive measures such as a more nutritious diet, rest, and hematinics would be indicated.

Premenstrual Tension

Premenstrual tension begins about a week to ten days prior to the beginning of menstruation and usually ceases when the flow begins. About half of all women suffer premenstrual tension to some degree.

The condition is characterized by headaches, nausea, nervousness and irritability, painful and tender breasts, and puffiness (edema) of the abdomen, feet, and ankles.

Premenstrual tension can be treated with aspirin or acetaminophen. If nervousness is severe, a tranquilizing agent such as phenobarbital may be beneficial.

Most OTC menstrual products contain a mild analgesic, caffeine or a mild diuretic (sometimes), or other ingredients. These combinations have never been shown to actually help relieve premenstrual tension. Aspirin taken with a cup of coffee, tea, or cola will provide the same relief. The mild diuretic contained in many OTC products is supposed to relieve puffiness and swelling, but no current study has shown that these diuretics actually work. Caffeine is also a mild diuretic, and a cup of coffee, tea, or cola will have the same effect.

Limiting salt intake for several days before menstruation may help avoid premenstrual tension. During this period, a salt substitute can be used.

Drugs Used in Treatment

Recommended treatment with OTC drugs—*If your menstrual disorder is related to an improper diet, we suggest you consult your doctor for guidelines on a nutritious diet and the possible need for supplements. Your needs will be better met that way than by supplementing your diet with OTC vitamin-mineral combinations. For relief of premenstrual tension, we suggest aspirin (or the OTC analgesic of your choice) taken with a cup of coffee.*
OTC nutritional supplements—*see the list under Nutritional Disorders*
OTC analgesics—*see the list under Pain and Fever*
OTC miscellaneous—*Co-Salt*
℞ oral contraceptives
℞ steroid hormone—*methyltestosterone*
℞ progesterone—*Provera*
℞ analgesics—*Darvocet-N; Darvon; Darvon Compound-65; Demerol; Empirin Compound with Codeine; Equagesic; Fiorinal; Fiorinal with Codeine; Motrin;*

198

Norgesic; Parafon Forte; Percodan; Robaxin; Soma Compound; Synalgos-DC; Talwin; Tylenol with Codeine
R̥ **analgesic and sedative combinations**—*Fiorinal; Fiorinal with Codeine*
R̥ **antispasmodic**—*Bentyl*
R̥ **antidepressants**—*Elavil; Sinequan; Tofranil*
R̥ **phenothiazines**—*Compazine; Mellaril; Stelazine*
R̥ **phenothiazine and antidepressant**—*Triavil*
R̥ **sedative and hypnotic products**—*Atarax; Ativan; Librium; meprobamate; Nembutal; phenobarbital; Serax; Tranxene; Valium*
R̥ **sedative and anticholinergic**—*Donnatal; Librax*
R̥ **anticholinergic and phenothiazine**—*Combid*
R̥ **anticholinergic**—*Pro-Banthine*

Health Care Accessories—*heating pad; hot water bottle*

Painful Coitus

Painful coitus, or dyspareunia, is frequently caused by a decrease in vaginal secretions, although it may be due to a variety of other causes. It may be primary (occurring early in marriage) or secondary (occurring later in marriage). The site of the pain may also be external (at the point of entry), or internal (deep within the genital canal or even beyond). Occasionally, some women describe both types of pain. An external dyspareunia may be associated with an occlusive or rigid hymen, or it may follow vaginal contracture due to inflammatory or traumatic disorders. Internal dyspareunia may be caused by severe cervicitis, prolapse or cancerous disease of the uterus, pelvic endometriosis, or severe vaginal infection.

Treatment

Functional painful coitus (that not caused by an organic disease) is best treated with psychotherapy and counseling. Both sexual partners must be counseled. Both partners must realize that foreplay is important. Additionally, when necessary, an appropriate vaginal lubricant may be useful. A patient should likewise not douche excessively.

When drug therapy is indicated, mild sedatives are indicated to reduce emotional tension. When the disorder is caused by constriction within the vagina, conical vaginal dilators of graduated sizes may be required. Local anesthetic ointments applied prior to coitus may bring temporary relief.

Drugs Used in Treatment

R̥ **sedatives and hypnotics**—*Atarax; Ativan; Librium; meprobamate; Nembutal; phenobarbital; Serax; Tranxene; Valium*
R̥ **phenothiazines**—*Compazine; Stelazine*

Postmenopausal Vaginal Bleeding

Vaginal bleeding after the cessation of menstrual function may be due to local or systemic causes. Cancer of the cervix or endometrium accounts for up to 50 percent of all cases of postmenopausal bleeding. Excessive or noncyclic administration of estrogen is the next most common cause. Trauma, polyps, hypertensive cardiovascular disease, atrophic vaginitis, blood dyscrasias, and tumors may also cause postmenopausal vaginal bleeding.

Symptoms

The discharge may vary from bright red to dark brown. There may be frank hemorrhage, and the bleeding may occur as a single episode of spotting or as a significant flow that persists for days or months.

Treatment

For any bleeding that persists, patients should be hospitalized for a definite diagnosis. Dilation and curettage will often cure the condition or will facilitate diagnosis. Withdrawal of all estrogen drugs will control many cases. In some cases, a total hysterectomy may be indicated.

Salpingitis

Salpingitis is an inflammation of the fallopian tubes. It is also referred to as pelvic inflammatory disease, or PID. It is directly or indirectly involved in about 20 percent of all gynecologic problems.

Women in the child-bearing years are most susceptible. It is always due to bacterial infection, usually with the same bacteria that cause gonorrhea.

Predisposing factors include infection following abortion, sexual contact, cervical or uterine cancers, operative delivery, and peritonitis.

Symptoms

The symptoms include severe cramping in the lower abdominal cavity. The cramps usually occur on both sides producing a nonradiating pain. Chills, fever, menstrual disturbances, abdominal tenderness, and discharge are also present. When occurring chronically, dysmenorrhea, infertility, recurrent low-grade fever, and tenderness in the pelvic area are noted.

Symptoms of salpingitis must be differentiated from other disorders that cause similar symptoms, such as acute appendicitis. With appendicitis, however, pain is generally localized to the right lower quadrant.

Treatment

Ampicillin is the antibiotic of choice. If the disorder is caused by the tuberculosis bacterium, streptomycin, along with isoniazid and other antitubercular agents are given. Pain is treated with prescription analgesics or sedative medications. Oral contraceptive therapy may be given to delay or prevent menstruation for one or two months.

When pelvic abcesses are large, surgery may be indicated for their removal.

The disorder generally subsides when the inflammation is confined to the uterine tubes and it is treated early and completely. If an abcess develops within or near one of the tubes, recurrent salpingitis may occur with infertility being the usual result.

Drugs Used in Treatment

℞ antibiotics—*amoxicillin; ampicillin; erythromycin; Keflex; Minocin; penicillin G; penicillin potassium phenoxymethyl; Terramycin; tetracycline hydrochloride; Vibramycin*

℞ analgesics—*Darvocet-N; Darvon; Darvon Compound-65; Demerol; Empirin Compound with Codeine; Equagesic; Fiorinal; Fiorinal with Codeine; Motrin; Percodan; Synalgos-DC; Talwin; Tylenol with Codeine*

℞ sedatives and hypnotics—*Atarax; Ativan; meprobamate; Nembutal; phenobarbital; Serax; Tranxene; Valium*

℞ oral contraceptives

Nervous System

Our nervous system is an intricate network of specialized tissue that controls our impulses, emotions, sensations, thought, and actions as well as all of the metabolic functions of living. The basic element of the nervous system is the neuron, or nerve cell. Individual neurons are among the largest cells in the body.

Central nervous system. The central nervous system consists of the brain and spinal cord. Approximately half of the neurons in the human nervous system are found in the brain, the largest portion of the central nervous system. An adult brain weighs more than three pounds and consists of billions of connecting nerve cells.The brain is an incredibly complex organ that controls more functions than have yet been catalogued. All our actions, sensations, and thoughts, whether awake or asleep, are mediated by the brain.

The spinal cord is fully continuous with the brain. It is protected by the vertebral column and the same membranes that protect the brain. Other than the cranial nerves(that connect directly with the brain),all the peripheral nerves arise from the spinal cord and branch out into the body through openings in the vertebrae. The spinal cord serves as a roadway to the brain for sensory impulses generated in the body and as a path for motor messages from the brain to control various body functions.

The spinal cord can generate certain reflex motor impulses, thus providing a protective fast circuit for the body. For example, the involuntary impulse to pull the hand away from a hot stove comes from the spinal cord, not the brain.

Peripheral nervous system. The peripheral nervous system includes the cranial nerves (those that branch directly from the brain) and the spinal nerves (those that branch out from the spinal cord). The peripheral nerves convey sensory messages to the central nervous system from receptor cells in the body. And they carry motor impulses from the central system to the muscles and glands that can act on those impulses.

Autonomic nervous system. The autonomic nervous system is a subsidiary system that governs smooth muscle tissue, i.e., the heart, digestive system, glands, lungs, and other organs not subject to willful control.

Alcoholism

Alcoholism is a major health problem in the United States. It is responsible for 30 to 40 thousand deaths and over 500 thousand injuries in traffic accidents each year. It has been estimated that alcoholism decreases the life span by 10 to 12 years.

Dependency on alcohol is similar to dependency on barbiturates, heroin, or other drugs. The true alcoholic is unable to go for a single day without drinking, or may have episodes of heavy drinking that last for three months or more interspersed with periods of relative sobriety.

Alcoholism is classified into three degrees or types. The first, episodic excessive drinking is described as intoxication that occurs as frequently as four times a year. The second, habitual excessive drinking is described as intoxication that occurs more than 12 times per year, or when an individual is recognized as being intoxicated more than once a week. The third stage is alcohol dependence, or addiction. This is shown by direct evidence (such as withdrawal symptoms) that suggests the individual is truly addicted.

It is known that the majority of alcoholics begin as "social" (moderate) drinkers who believe they can control their intake. However, over a period of time—often years—their intake gradually increases to the point that they become habitually excessive drinkers. Unless such a progression is arrested, true alcohol dependency usually follows soon after.

An alcoholic personality has not been clearly defined. Alcoholics may have periods of loneliness, shyness, isolation, hostility, self-destruction, sexual immaturity, depression, or schizoid tendencies. A familial, cultural, or genetic tendency to alcoholism seems to be apparent; the dependency is more common in certain families and ethnic groups than in the population at large.

Symptoms

The symptoms of acute intoxication are similar to those seen with an overdose of any central nervous system depressant (barbiturates, for example): inability to walk unsupported, drowsiness, sleepiness, errors in action and thinking, loss of inhibitions, poor muscle control, bloodshot eyes, and vomiting. One intoxicated person can never be compared exactly with another intoxicated person. Additionally, someone who is intoxicated may be inappropriately loud or abusive, or may act inappropriately for the situation. As the condition becomes more severe, there may be severe nervous and respiratory depression, stupor, shock, coma, and even death. Many deaths due to drug overdose are caused by a combination of drugs with alcohol —always a potentially lethal combination.

Symptoms of alcoholic withdrawal occur when an alcoholic suddenly stops drinking. These may range from anxiety and tremors to convulsions. Convulsions, if they occur, usually start within one to three days after the last drink, but they may not occur until one to one and one-half weeks later. During this period, the alcoholic will experience extreme wakefulness, exaggerated reflexes, gastrointestinal distress, tremors, and visual hallucinations (e.g., a feeling of being pursued by animals or bugs).

Alcoholic withdrawal is a serious situation and the individual should be hospitalized. Death can and has occurred during withdrawal when the alcoholic is not monitored carefully.

Complications

Complications of alcoholism include a variety of chronic brain syndromes, degeneration of the cerebellum, and damage to the peripheral nerves. Alcohol may permanently damage the liver and cause cirrhosis. Irritation of the esophagus may cause frequent bleeding. Alcoholism also affects metabolism and blood coagulation. Alcoholics frequently suffer from malnutrition.

Treatment

If alcoholism is detected before the age of 40 and the patient is fully cooperative, the chances for curing the dependency are excellent. The expectations for reversing alcoholism in older people or housewives with grown children is less promising. Much successful treatment is based on psychological, religious, or group counseling and support. Striking success has been obtained by the Alcoholics Anonymous organization in which alcoholics aid and support one another.

Withdrawal symptoms are usually treated by giving another sedative. Occasionally, anticonvulsant drugs may be required. A diet rich in calories, carbohydrates, and vitamins (particularly B complex) and minerals must be given.

Disulfiram (Antabuse tablets) is sometimes given each day to "dried-out" alcoholics to reduce the desire to consume alcohol. It causes an intensely uncomfortable feeling if the individual consumes any alcohol while taking the drug. In fact, the individual must be warned against using after-shave lotions, cough syrups, or any other item or cosmetic that contains even a trace of alcohol. When combined with alcohol, disulfiram causes severe nausea and vomiting, flushing of the face and neck, shortness of breath, weakness, palpitations, and headache. Anyone taking disulfiram should be warned of these effects and should be advised that individuals have died from coma and convulsions when large doses of alcohol and disulfiram have been mixed.

Drugs Used in Treatment

Recommended treatment with OTC drugs—*Alcoholic hangover headache may be treated with aspirin or acetaminophen. An antacid may help the nausea. One or two cups of salted tomato juice or a glass of fruit juice sipped slowly may also help.*
OTC analgesics—*see the list under Pain and Fever*
OTC antacids—*Alka-Seltzer; Alka-2; Amphojel; Di-Gel; Fizrin; Gaviscon; Gelusil; Gelusil II; Kolantyl; Maalox; Maalox #1; Maalox #2; Mylanta; Mylanta-II; Riopan; Rolaids; Tums*
OTC nutritional supplements—*see the list under Nutritional Disorders*
R̠ sedatives and hypnotics—*Atarax; Librium; Serax; Tranxene; Valium*
R̠ phenothiazine—*Mellaril*
R̠ anticonvulsant—*Dilantin*
R̠ diuretic and antihypertensive—*Aldactone*

Related Topics—*Alcoholic Hepatitis; Cirrhosis*

Anorexia Nervosa

Anorexia nervosa is a disorder characterized by an extreme aversion to food. Rarely is there an organic cause for the loss of appetite. Seven out of every eight patients with anorexia nervosa are female; most are teenagers.

Symptoms

People with anorexia nervosa have a morbid fear of gaining weight; the syndrome often starts with severe dieting. Some anorectics take huge doses of laxatives after eating in the belief that they will not absorb the food and gain weight. Others may exercise compulsively, perhaps for several strenuous hours a day to burn off calories.

Anorectics commonly refuse to eat and may make excuses that they are not hungry or that they are nauseated. Self-induced vomiting is common. Loss of weight may be drastic; some anorectics lose up to half their body weight. Loss of libido, cessation of menstruation, drying of skin, and symptoms of malnutrition occur. There may be fine, downy hair covering a large part of the body to the point that the person may appear hirsute. Anorectics frequently become tired, listless, and extremely weak. An anorectic may be unable to begin eating again even after the disease has been diagnosed.

Treatment

Treatment of anorexia nervosa is difficult, and therapy administered by a specialist in the field is recommended. Hospitalization to restore normal nutrition is often required, as is analysis by a psychiatrist. No drugs are used to treat the condition itself, although tranquilizers are sometimes given. Counseling will help the anorectic understand the disorder.

If anorexia nervosa is untreated, death may result due to malnutrition, severe infection, or suicide.

Anxiety

Anxiety is a word commonly used to mean tension or nervousness, and anxiety can be a normal reaction to a stressful situation. However, exaggerated anxiety out of proportion to the stimulus may be a symptom of disease, and severe, prolonged, or repeated anxiety attacks require medical help. Anxiety is generally experienced as feelings of terror, fright, panic, alarm, or apprehension, often without identifiable cause. Normally simple tasks and decision making become difficult. Anxiety may adversely affect sleep, appetite, digestion, and respiration.

Treatment

Anxiety may be a symptom of organic disease—diabetes, thyroid disease, high blood pressure, and various brain disorders, for example. Such causes should be ruled out before treatment is prescribed.

Once such diseases have been ruled out, the cause of the anxiety should be sought. All too often, the symptom is treated with drugs (such as Valium or phenobarbital) without attempting to treat the underlying cause of the anxiety. All antianxiety drugs should be used cautiously. They should be taken only when the symptom is present. However, many patients take these drugs routinely because of their pleasurable or relaxing effects.

One common cause of anxiety that is easily treated is over-consumption of caffeine. Reduction of caffeine consumption may relieve the symptoms completely.

Drugs Used in Treatment

R̴ **sedatives and hypnotics**—*Atarax; Ativan; Librium; meprobamate; Nembutal; phenobarbital; Serax; Tranxene; Valium*
R̴ **phenothiazines**—*Compazine; Stelazine*
R̴ **phenothiazine and antidepressant**—*Triavil*
R̴ **analgesics and sedatives**—*Fiorinal; Fiorinal with Codeine*

Depression

Depression is a normal reaction to common situations such as bereavement or marital upset. However, unremitting depression, depression that grows progressively worse, or depression without apparent cause demands medical concern. If such depression is evident, even if the individual denies being depressed, a doctor must be consulted. Depression left untreated may grow so severe that suicide is attempted. Up to 20 percent of people with this disorder commit suicide.

Depression may be caused by some situation in life as described above, and it may result from many illnesses, especially chronic disabling disorders. Depression that occurs independent of a person's life situation is that which causes the most medical concern.

Symptoms

Depressive illness may be of two types: recurrent depression, and cycles of depression and mania. Depression, whether recurrent or cyclical, is characterized by feelings of despondency, low self-esteem, apathy, and inertia. The patient may withdraw from social contacts and fail to respond emotionally to those closest to him or her. Job performance is often impaired, sleep patterns may be affected, and weight loss may be evident. Depressed patients often have a diminished sexual drive. Vague physical complaints (fatigue, a sense of heaviness) may verge on hypochondria. In severe cases, the patient may be deluded, focusing on evil and despair. Patients in this state are most likely to attempt suicide.

The manic phase may follow the depressive phase rapidly. The patient feels well, is confident and may become less inhibited, more talkative, and extremely active. However, this apparently positive mood may shift suddenly to hostility and resentment if the patient's view and plans are challenged or hindered. Actions may be inappropriate and tactless and may jeopardize the patient's career and personal relationships. Delusions are common in severe cases. Disrupted sleep, lessened food intake, and constant overactivity may lead to exhaustion.

Treatment

Manic-depressive patients should be hospitalized unless the disorder is very mild. The depressive phase may be treated with tricyclic antidepressants. The manic phase is usually controlled with lithium carbonate, and therapy with this drug may be continued for some time as it seems to prevent relapses. Psychotherapy is also beneficial. In severe cases, electroshock therapy may be necessary. It should be noted that not all cases of depression need to be treated either with drugs or electroshock therapy.

Drugs Used in Treatment

R antidepressants—*Elavil; Sinequan; Tofranil*
R phenothiazines—*Mellaril; Triavil*
R adrenergic—*Ritalin*

Dizziness and Vertigo

Dizziness and vertigo are symptoms similar to, and sometimes confused with, one another. Dizziness is a disturbed sense of relationship to one's spatial environment; it may be felt as a sensation of unsteadiness. Vertigo is a false sensation of movement; someone with vertigo may sense that the external world is moving around him or that he himself is moving.

Dizziness is a common symptom. It may be due to headache, anxiety, general debility, drug overdose, infectious diseases, or high or low blood pressure. There is no specific treatment for dizziness, other than identifying and treating the cause. The drug Antivert is frequently prescribed, but it has met with varying success.

Vertigo may result from diseases of the inner ear, middle ear infection, or tumors on the brain or nervous system. Severe infection may also cause vertigo, and vertigo sometimes occurs as a warning symptom of epilepsy or migraine headache. Severe or unexplained instances of vertigo should be reported to a doctor.

Drugs Used in Treatment

R antinauseant—*Antivert*

Drug Dependence

Drug dependence is a broad term used to include both habituation and addiction. Generally, dependence is classified into two types. Psychological dependence is a state of mind that craves continuous and repeated administration of the particular drug. Although psychological dependence may lead to compulsive use of a particular substance, abstinence may produce only feelings of discomfort, not the complex of symptoms known as withdrawal syndrome. Physical dependence is characterized by tolerance (the need to increase dosage of a substance in order to gain the desired effect) and withdrawal syndrome upon abstinence. Physical dependence does not occur with all types of drug dependence, and the symptoms and treatment of dependence differ according to the substance being abused.

Signs suggestive of drug abuse include sudden or dramatic alterations in job or school performance, emotional flare-ups, and deterioration of personal appearance (due to growing indifference with how one looks). More specific symptoms include wearing sunglasses at inappropriate times and places (to hide dilated or constricted pupils) and wearing long-sleeved shirts or blouses even on hot days to hide needle marks. Females may use makeup to conceal needle marks, and males may get tattooed at injection sites.

Sedatives

The effects of all central nervous system sedatives, including the barbiturates and alcohol, are basically the same. However, because the use of alcohol is more widespread and generally acceptable than the use of other sedatives, alcohol dependence is discussed elsewhere.

Dependence on the rapid- and intermediate-onset sedatives is more common than dependence on the longer-acting substances such as Librium. It is sometimes difficult to identify someone who has developed a dependency on these drugs. A general rule of thumb for many substances (most barbiturates and products such as Doriden, Miltown, Equanil, Quaalude) is that an individual who each day requires ten tablets or capsules of the usual dosage is physically dependent. It should also be noted that these substances are additive; that is, the effect of one of these drugs when taken in combination with other drugs of this type will be greater than if the drug were taken alone.

Symptoms of intoxication with sedatives include respiratory depression, drowsiness, sleep, slowness of speech, difficulty in thinking, impaired memory, narrowed attention range, abnormal eye movements, lack of coordination, and reduction of inhibitions. Overdosage can cause pupil dilation, stupor, shock, coma, and death.

The manifestations of sedative drug withdrawal include severe restlessness and anxiety, followed by gastrointestinal effects, twitching, severe drop in blood pressure, tremors, and weakness. Convulsions occasionally occur two to three days after withdrawal. Visual hallucinations, disorientation, and feelings of paranoia may persist for a week or more.

Treatment sometimes requires hospitalization. Frequently, dosages are "stepped down" (decreased gradually) to prevent withdrawal syndrome. The decrease in dosage may take several weeks before complete withdrawal of the drug can be considered. Social counseling is also beneficial.

Narcotics

Narcotics are used to relieve pain and induce sleep. Narcotics derived from opium include morphine, heroin (the most often abused narcotic), and codeine. Meperidine and methadone are synthetic narcotics. Propoxyphene and pentazocine, neither of which are classified as narcotics, have narcotic-like activity, especially when withdrawn after several months or more of administration. All produce similar effects.

Intoxication with these drugs produces euphoria and carefree relaxation, occasional restlessness with anxiety, drowsiness, mental cloudiness, mood changes, occasional vomiting, constricted pupils, and decreased gastrointestinal function. Severe overdosage causes depressed respiration, nausea and vomiting, deep sleep, coma, and flushing.

Symptoms of withdrawal may begin as soon as the first scheduled dose is missed. Initial symptoms include anxiety and craving for the drug. Within about four hours, symptoms become more severe; they reach their peak within 36 to 72 hours. Symptoms progress from yawning, tearing, perspiration, and nasal discharge to hot and cold flashes, tremors, and nausea. Then, vomiting, diarrhea, and abdominal discomfort ensue.

Narcotic overdose is treated with a specific antidote such as naloxone (Narcan) given intravenously. Hospitalization and close observation for a few days is necessary. Specific symptoms of withdrawal may be treated. Heroin dependence is sometimes treated with methadone maintenance, a program in which methadone is substituted for heroin. The dosage is controlled and gradually reduced. Chances for recovery are increased if the addict is given social counseling.

Stimulants

Cocaine and the amphetamines (diet pills) cause hyperactivity and an enhanced sense of mental and physical acuity when taken in moderation. High or rapidly repeated doses of cocaine produce high blood pressure, rapid heartbeat, hallucinations, sleeplessness, and nervousness. Paranoid delusions may develop, resulting in violent behavior. Overdose causes tremors, convulsions, delirium, and possible death. Tolerance to and physical dependence on cocaine do not develop, although psychological dependence is very likely.

The amphetamines cause symptoms similar to those of cocaine, but tolerance to the amphetamines does develop and a habitual user may consume staggering amounts of the drug in a single day. Continued high dosage of these drugs may produce anxiety, paranoia, and hallucinations. When the drug is withdrawn, the user develops an intense fatigue and need for sleep. Depression and suicidal tendencies may appear.

Close supervision and support help in discontinuing the use of stimulants. Symptoms of withdrawal are difficult to treat with other drugs.

Psychedelics

Psychedelics are drugs that intensify perception and may cause visual hallucinations. Mescaline, LSD, and phencyclidine (PCP, or angel dust) are psychedelics. Individual reactions differ, but initial symptoms of intoxication often include anxiety or tension followed by emotional release (laughing, crying). Shortly thereafter, distortions of perception (vision and hearing) and hallucinations occur, lasting for two to three hours. Occasionally fear of ego disintegration develops. Thereafter, a feeling of detachment and a sense of destiny and control are experienced. Some users remain disturbed after their "trip," and others experience "flashbacks," distortions of perception or sensation similar to that induced by the psychedelic and often precipitated by the use of alcohol, marijuana, or other drugs. Flashbacks may occur many months after use of the drug has stopped.

Psychological dependence on these drugs varies greatly, and there is no evidence of physical dependence. Withdrawal of the drug is often less difficult for the user than is dealing with the psychological problems associated with the drug's use. Counseling is helpful in maintaining social functioning.

Marijuana

Marijuana use is widespread. Chronic use often produces strong psychological dependence and possibly tolerance, but physical dependence on marijuana has not been proven. Marijuana produces mild euphoria, altered perception of time, emotional inhibition, and impairment of memory. These effects may be followed by depression, panic, fear of death, body image distortions, and hallucinations, particularly when marijuana is used with another drug. Usually no treatment is necessary but to allow the effects of the drug to wear off.

Volatile Solvents

Use of industrial solvents and aerosol sprays to achieve a "high" is a problem among juveniles. Partial tolerance to the fumes develops with daily use, but there is no withdrawal syndrome. Someone who is high from sniffing these substances will be dizzy; speech will be slurred; the gait, unsteady. Drowsiness, impulsiveness, excitement, and irritability may also be seen. Hallucinations may develop.

Inhalation of these solvents has led to death due to respiratory arrest, heart problems, and asphyxiation. Treatment involves counseling to improve the person's self-esteem and relationships with others.

Encephalitis

Encephalitis (also called sleeping sickness), is an inflammatory disease of the brain usually caused by a virus. Occasionally it occurs after chicken pox, smallpox, whooping cough, meningitis, measles, influenza, mumps, rubella, herpes, mononucleosis, and hepatitis. It may occur after vaccinations or may be due to drugs, toxins, or bacterial poisons.

The disease is highly contagious; people with encephalitis should be isolated. The very young and the very old are the most susceptible.

Symptoms

Symptoms occur suddenly. There may be a fever that, in infants, may go to 106° F. The fever usually lasts 10 to 12 days and may cause convulsions. Severe headache, vomiting, delirium, weakness of the eyes, persistent hiccups, and salivation are also symptoms. Sleepiness and a stiff neck are characteristic of encephalitis.

Treatment

Bed rest and quiet are mandatory treatment for encephalitis. Fever is controlled with aspirin or acetaminophen or, in severe cases, with phenobarbital. Cold compresses on the forehead may help bring the fever down. An antiviral drug, vidarabine, has been tried with some success. Hospitalization may be required.

Encephalitis has a high death rate, but even severely ill patients may recover completely.

Drugs Used in Treatment

OTC analgesics—*see the list under Pain and Fever*
Ŗ sedative and hypnotic—*phenobarbital*

Epileptic Seizures

Epilepsy is a brain disorder characterized by sudden and recurrent disruptions of consciousness with by changes in sensation or behavioral activity. A seizure is caused by a sudden release in the brain of a large burst of electrical energy. A number of underlying conditions (such as metabolic disorders, tumors, head injuries, and drug withdrawal) can cause seizures, and the tendency to have seizures can be inherited.

Epilepsy is more common among men, and most people have their first attack before age 30. Onset after this age suggests that the cause is an organic disease.

Classification

Not all epileptics convulse. A convulsion denotes involvement of the nerves that control movement; thus, during a convulsion, jerking, spastic movements occur. "Seizure," denoting simply an attack of epilepsy, is a more definitive term.

In the past, seizures were classified as grand mal (for big sickness), petit mal (little sickness), psychomotor, and focal. Although somewhat antiquated, this system is still in general use. A newer method lists seizures as partial or generalized, depending on the extent of involvement of the brain.

Simple partial. Simple partial seizures are confined to small areas of the brain. Symptoms may include seeing flashing lights; tingling in a finger, arm, or foot; perceiving bad odors; and speech impediment. Consciousness is retained.

Complex partial. This form is also called psychomotor epilepsy. The patient may remain motionless or display bizarre, repetitive, or inappropriate movements. Consciousness is maintained.

Generalized convulsive seizure. During this type of seizure (also called grand mal, or tonic-clonic seizure), the entire brain is swept over by a massive electrical discharge. This may cause the individual to cry out (from rapid expulsion of air from the lungs, not from pain). Then, the individual is likely to stiffen and fall to the ground, assuming the position directed by contraction of the strongest muscle mass. For example, if the biceps (flexor) is the strongest muscle in the arm, the arm bends inward. If the triceps (extensor) is the strongest muscle, the arm extends outward. Urinary and bowel control may be lost. Then, the massive spasm gives way to wild thrashing movements and the patient eventually slips into a period of deep sleep (postictal depression). Upon awakening, the individual may feel dazed and have a headache.

Generalized nonconvulsive seizures. These include "absence seizures" (new term for petit mal), and they usually occur in children. The only symptom may be repeated blinking or spells of "daydreaming." Consciousness is retained and many patients continue their normal activities completely unaware that they are experiencing a seizure.

Status epilepticus. This term refers to repeated seizures occurring at short intervals. Abrupt withdrawal of anticonvulsant drugs may precipitate an attack of status epilepticus. Such attacks may be fatal if not quickly terminated.

Treatment

The epileptic seizures of 70 to 80 percent of patients can be controlled by a variety of drugs. But a number of other factors also affect control of the disorder. Many patients have more seizures during periods of emotional stress, and patients who are particularly susceptible to stress-precipitated seizures often receive tranquilizers. Physical stress, such as lack of sleep, poor diet, and overexertion, may also precipitate seizures. Alcohol should be forbidden, but moderate exercise and social activities should not be curtailed. Driving is often permitted after seizures have been controlled for a period of time although state regulations differ. Except for protecting the patient from injury, most seizures do not require treatment.

Epilepsy is not a mental disease, but the epileptic is often subjected to the social and psychological stigmata that have become associated with epilepsy through misunderstanding and fear. It is often helpful to join a local branch of the Epilepsy Association of America (your doctor should have the local address). The Association helps the epileptic learn to cope with the condition and distributes information about new developments and research in the field.

Epileptics usually continue to take anticonvulsant therapy throughout their life. However, if seizures are controlled for three to five years, the doctor may slowly reduce the doses over a period of one to two years to see if the patient will remain seizure-free. Occasionally, all medication will be withdrawn.

Drugs Used in Treatment

R_x anticonvulsant—*Dilantin*
R_x sedative and hypnotic—*phenobarbital*
R_x diuretic—*Diamox*

Fainting

Fainting (syncope) is a temporary loss of consciousness. It is usually due to a reduction in the blood supply coming to the brain. Many factors may cause such a reduction, including emotional stress, physical exhaustion, starvation, and various drugs (such as certain high blood pressure medications). Certain diseases, such as anemia, hypoglycemia, diabetes, heart disease, atherosclerosis, bleeding peptic ulcers, and epilepsy may also cause fainting.

Fainting is, in fact, a normal and useful body reaction to a reduction of the brain's blood supply; it places the person in a position (head level with the heart) that ensures that the brain receives a sufficient amount of blood.

Fainting may be presaged by feelings of muscular weakness, nausea, perspiration, yawning, and sighing. The individual may feel nervous and lightheaded; the skin may be cold and moist; the vision, blurred. Fainting can often be prevented by sitting with the head bowed and placed between the knees. Spirits of ammonia or smelling salts may be inhaled, but this measure is not usually effective.

Treatment

To help someone recover from a faint, several steps should be taken. The individual should be lying down, preferably with the feet higher than the head. Clothing should be loosened; cool water may be splashed on the face. Increase ventilation, if possible. Recovery should occur within seconds of falling, although a sense of disorientation may prevent resumption of duties for several minutes.

Recurrent fainting spells should be discussed with a doctor.

Headaches

Headache is a common symptom suffered by everyone at some time. Headaches can be caused by emotional disorders, dental problems, eyestrain, muscle spasm, high fever, and nose, throat, or sinus problems. Certain types of headaches are associated with specific diseases—meningitis, brain tumors, and malignant hypertension, for example.

Headaches may be of any intensity and duration. A headache that can be relieved by an analgesic such as aspirin or acetaminophen should not cause undue concern. But persistent, intractable, or recurrent headaches, or headaches severe enough to interfere with one's daily routine should be reported to a doctor for diagnosis and treatment.

Headaches can generally be classified on the basis of their cause. Thus, we have vascular headaches, muscle spasm headaches, and sinus headaches.

Vascular Headaches

Vascular headaches are caused by the dilation of blood vessels in the head. The swollen vessels cause severe pressure on the nerves, resulting in intense pain. Vascular headache pain is throbbing; every time the heart beats, it forces more blood into the swollen vessels, increasing the pressure and pain. Vascular headaches sometimes last for many hours or days because once these blood vessels become engorged with blood, they are not easily shrunken.

The common or classic migraine is a vascular headache that results from constriction, followed by dilation, of the blood vessels. A migraine is often one-sided, but may occur on both sides of the head. The severe pain of a migraine is often preceded by an aura—premonitory symptoms that warn that a headache is on the way. These symptoms may include visual disturbances (seeing stars, lights, or zigzag lines), hearing noises, smelling certain fragrances, tingling in the arms or legs, or feeling generally depressed. Migraines are sometimes called "sick headaches" because they are often accompanied by symptoms of severe nausea and vomiting, and constipation or diarrhea.

Someone with a migraine looks and acts quite ill; the face is pale and sallow. The skin may be oily or sweaty. The migraine sufferer avoids light, activity, and noise because they intensify the pain. More women than men suffer migraines, and the headaches often occur cyclically—once a week, once a month, or more often. They are often associated with seasonal, environmental, occupational or other factors. Thus, we talk about the weekend migraine or the Monday migraine. For many women, migraine headaches are part of the premenstrual syndrome. Very often, migraine sufferers have a family history of the headaches.

Some people with migraines may be allergic to some food. The most common offenders are foods rich in animal fats, alcohol, chocolate, cheeses, cured meats, and certain seasonings.

Cluster headaches, or cluster migraines, occur more commonly among men than among women. These headaches cause intense, one-sided pain of short duration, but they may recur several times daily. The attacks often begin during sleep, and they are accompanied by symptoms of facial flushing, tearing, sweating, and nasal drainage.

Migraines may be prevented by taking ergotamine tartrate, but the drug must be taken exactly as directed at the first sign of an impending headache. Caffeine is sometimes included in the dosage, although there is no good evidence that it has any benefit.

Two other drugs, cyproheptadine and methysergide, are used on a routine basis to prevent migraine headaches. Methysergide has proven to be effective, but less data is available on cyproheptadine. Methysergide must also be taken as directed. Be sure to discuss the manufacturer's suggestion of a drug-free interval with your doctor. Following every six months of therapy with the drug, there must be a three-to-four week interval without the drug. If this schedule is not followed, severe toxicity may result.

The drug propranolol is useful to prevent migraine headache in severe cases. It is taken routinely to keep the blood vessels in the head from enlarging and to reduce the number of heartbeats per minute. A patient using propranolol must be closely supervised by a doctor.

When a migraine attack is coming on, sit quietly and avoid all excitement or noise. An ice pack may help to keep the pain reduced to tolerable levels. Some people also benefit from sitting in a tub of hot water or drinking a couple of cups of hot tea or water. These measures cause the blood vessels in the lower portions of the body to dilate, allowing some of the blood in the head to pool into lower areas, possibly resulting in less throbbing and less pain.

After the headache has been relieved, rest in bed for at least two hours. During this time, avoid all food, drink, and excitement. If these measures are followed, future attacks should be delayed.

Muscle Spasm Headaches

Muscle spasm headaches vary greatly in frequency and severity. They may persist for hours or days. Their onset is usually related to some specific stress that caused muscle tension and pressure.

Muscle spasm headaches usually cause steady, nonpulsating pain felt on one side of the head and in the area of the eyes. The scalp and neck area may be tender to the touch.

Sufferers of muscle spasm headache are usually in a constant state of anxiety. They appear tense, apprehensive, sensitive to the opinions of others, and are easily embarrassed and constantly worried. They frequently have trouble sleeping and are irritable and restless. Depression is a common finding.

This type of headache is treated with rest, relaxation, and avoidance of stress. Mild muscle relaxants are sometimes employed. Antianxiety agents are used to relax the individual. Heat (heating pads or hot baths) sometimes helps. Gentle massage to the painful area may reduce the pain. Analgesics such as aspirin and acetaminophen, while treating the pain do nothing for the underlying cause, and once the medicine wears off, the pain returns. It is important to identify the cause of the pain, and then correct it.

Sinus Headaches

Sinus headaches usually begin in the morning or early afternoon and improve or disappear by late in the day. The pain is usually dull and aching and seldom, if ever, associated with nausea or vomiting. It is caused by inflammation in the sinuses due to infection, allergy, or other irritation. Intensity is increased by shaking the head or bending forward. Also, coughing, wearing a tight collar, or straining at stool may increase the pain. And menstruation, cold air, sexual excitement, and alcohol, because they increase the amount of blood in the sinus tissues, may aggravate sinus headaches. A fall in the barometric pressure may also make a sinus headache worse.

Minor sinus headaches with muscle aches, fever, and malaise are best treated with aspirin or acetaminophen. In fact, most OTC pain-relief products contain one of these agents. If stronger analgesics are required, a serious condition such as a bad infection may be present and the assistance of a doctor should be sought.

Antihistamines and sympathomimetic amines (decongestants) are used, usually in the form of combination products that also contain either aspirin or acetaminophen. Antihistamines have little value in treating sinus headaches except that they dry respiratory secretions somewhat, which may exert some slight benefit on reducing sinus headache pain. The decongestant-containing products are more powerful drying agents, and by reducing the amount of secretions, they may alleviate the pressure and thus the pain. However, beware of using these products over a prolonged period of time as they have side effects of their own. Also, the prolonged drying effect, while perhaps beneficial at first in helping to reduce pain, may work against you over time, because the nasal mucus will be less able to ward off infections and irritation, thus the cause of the pain may persist and make conditions worse.

Other Headaches

Headaches may be caused by a number of other factors. Some causative factors are related to serious disease, but others are environmental and can be controlled by the individual. For example, many foods cause headaches in some people. Monosodium glutamate (often used in Chinese food), the nitrates and preservatives used in processed meat, and salt have all been known to cause headaches due to their effects on the vascular system. People accustomed to drinking a certain amount of coffee may get a headache if their consumption is reduced. Other people get headaches from skipping a meal or fasting. Working or lying in the sun for a long period of time can cause dehydration resulting in a headache. People living in older mobile homes may develop headaches from inhalation of the formaldehyde used in the home's construction. Others may develop a "rush hour headache" from breathing in the noxious fumes of mass transit vehicles. People who sleep with their heads under the bedding may wake up with a headache because the air breathed during the night contained decreased amount of oxygen. Allergies may cause headaches; people may be allergic to certain foods, or to something in the household environment, perhaps the pillows they sleep on. If you think you are allergic to something, try eliminating that item from your environment or diet or ask your doctor to arrange allergy tests for you.

Pressure or stress probably causes more headaches than any other single factor. Stress causes the muscles to tense up, resulting in increased pressure around the nerves in the back and neck. Some people subconsciously gnash or grind their teeth when under stress, and this may also cause a headache.

No doubt there are many other factors that may cause headaches, among them the ingestion of certain drugs, including oral contraceptives. The first order of headache treatment is to find and correct the cause. Symptomatic relief can usually be gained by taking aspirin or acetaminophen. If the headache is severe, one of the narcotic-containing analgesics may be necessary. A heating pad, water bottle, or ice pack may also be useful.

Drugs Used in Treatment

Recommended treatment with OTC drugs—*Aspirin or acetaminophen will relieve most minor headaches. The decongestant product we recommend for treating sinus headaches is Sudafed.*
OTC analgesics—*see the list under Pain and Fever*
OTC cold and allergy remedies—*Alka-Seltzer Plus; Allerest; A.R.M.; Bayer (children's and decongestant formulas); Chlor-Trimeton; Comtrex; Congespirin; Contac; Contac Jr.; Coricidin; Coricidin "D"; Coricidin Demilets; Coryban-D; Co Tylenol (regular and for children); Covangesic; Dristan (tablet and time capsule); 4-Way; Neo-Synephrine Compound; Ornade 2 for Children; Ornex; Sinarest; Sine-Off; Sinutab; Sinutab II; Sudafed; Sudafed Plus; Triaminicin; Viro-Med (liquid and tablet)*
OTC nasal decongestants—*Afrin; Allerest; Benzedrex; Coricidin; Dristan (in-*

haler and spray); Neo-Synephrine Intranasal; NTZ; Privine; Sine-Off Once-A-Day; Sinex; Sinex-L.A.; Sinutab; Triaminicin; Vicks

℞ **analgesics**—*Darvocet-N; Darvon; Darvon Compound-65; Demerol; Empirin Compound with Codeine; Equagesic; Fiorinal; Fiorinal with Codeine; Motrin; Norgesic; Parafon Forte; Percodan; Robaxin; Soma Compound; Synalgos-DC; Talwin; Tylenol with Codeine*

℞ **sedatives and hypnotics**—*Atarax; Ativan; Librium; meprobamate; Nembutal; phenobarbital; Serax; Tranxene; Valium*

℞ **phenothiazines**—*Compazine; Stelazine; Triavil*

℞ **migraine remedy**—*Cafergot*

℞ **beta blocker**—*Inderal*

℞ **antihistamine**—*Periactin*

Health Care Accessories—*disposable hot and cold packs; gel hot and cold packs; heating pad; hot water bottle; ice bag*

Hyperkinesis

The term hyperkinesis has been applied to a variety of hyperactivity states. The disorder is also known as hyperkinetic syndrome and minimal brain dysfunction. Typically, hyperkinesis affects children from less than one year in age to 16 years old. Boys are affected five times as often as girls.

An individual's level of activity is determined by two forces directed by the brain. One force directs stimulant activity, and the second is a counterbalancing, quieting force. It has been proposed that in hyperkinetic children, the quieting forces are not fully developed and the stimulating forces therefore take command of the child.

Symptoms

The hyperkinetic child is intensely restless, impulsive, has a short attention span, talks excessively, has poor impulse control, and is plagued with learning difficulties and emotional instability. These people have often been described as "motor-driven" in an attempt to symbolize their extremely active physical mannerisms. The child may even appear aggressive and destructive. Other persons often refer to these children as ill-mannered, spoiled, uncoordinated, or odd.

Treatment

Rarely is an actual lesion or damaged area in the brain identified when a hyperactive child is examined. The disorder is thus a biochemical deficiency that the child grows out of upon reaching adolescence. The goal of treatment for hyperkinesis is to alter the child's behavior so that he is better equipped to perform his daily tasks until the disorder is outgrown.

Paradoxically, hyperkinesis is best controlled with stimulating drugs such as the amphetamines and methylphenidate. These drugs preferentially stimulate the quieting part of the brain, and thereby calm the child. Other drugs, including the phenothiazines, Librium, meprobamate, and diphenhydramine have been used with some success. However, none are as effective as the stimulants. There are children who benefit immeasurably from such drug therapy. However, not all children displaying general symptoms of the hyperkinetic syndrome are candidates for these drugs. Likewise, children displaying these symptoms should never be given the drugs on a test basis in an attempt to diagnose the disorder. General symptoms of hyperkinesis may be indicative of more serious brain damage such as encephalitis or epilepsy, and a doctor should do a complete evaluation before prescribing drugs to treat hyperkinesis.

Alterations in diet have also been proposed as a method of treatment for hyperkinesis, and in some instances a special diet has been a successful control measure. Generally, all sugar is withheld, and only foods that do not contain artificial dyes or preservatives are allowed. Some hyperkinetic children benefit from drinking a cup of coffee two or three times a day. Consult your doctor for recommendations.

Drugs Used in Treatment

R phenothiazine—*Mellaril*
R adrenergic—*Ritalin*
R sedatives and hypnotics—*Librium; meprobamate*
R antihistamine—*Benadryl*

Impotence

Impotence is an inability in a male to obtain or keep an erection. Impotence may result from a physical abnormality of the genitalia that blocks the normal nerve impulses into the area. Diabetes mellitus, syphilis, alcoholism, drug dependence, multiple sclerosis, arteriosclerosis, and diseases of the nervous system could lead to impotence. However, most cases of impotence are psychological in origin; fear of causing pregnancy, religious inhibitions, emotional immaturity, guilt, and a negative self-concept may cause impotence. A man may be impotent with one sexual partner and not with another.

Treatment

Impotence due to a physical abnormality is treated by surgical or medical correction. Hormonal replacement therapy rarely may also be necessary. The patient frequently needs psychological counseling to help him cope with the situation.

Drugs Used in Treatment

R steroid hormone—*methyltestosterone*

Insomnia

Insomnia, or lack of sleep, affects people in two ways; the insomniac is either unable to fall asleep or has trouble remaining asleep. As a person ages, the amount of sleep required normally decreases, and individuals vary widely in their needs for sleep. However, if someone is repeatedly unable to fall asleep or repeatedly awakens early in the morning long before normal wakening time, a doctor's diagnosis should be sought.

Causes

Excitement, anxiety, stress, worry, or more serious psychological problems may keep someone from falling asleep. Environmental factors (a hot or stuffy room, a hard bed, noise, or unusual quiet) may make it difficult for some people to fall asleep. Indigestion, lack of exercise, the ingestion of mild stimulants (tea, coffee, or cola) before going to bed, or other minor problems (itching, shortness of breath, palpitations, or pain) may prevent sleep. Temporary insomnia is common at the onset of many illnesses.

Early awakening may be due to environmental factors; for example, the bed may face a window that lets in the early morning sun. Early morning noise, a need to urinate, or a cold room may also cause someone to wake early. A common cause of early awakening is depression. Nightmares may cause insomnia.

Treatment

Any repeated or distressing insomnia should be reported to a doctor for diagnosis and treatment. Insomnia may be cured by a change in habits—no more coffee past 6 P.M., for example. In some cases it may be necessary to prescribe sedatives and hypnotics.

Drugs Used in Treatment

Recommended treatment with OTC drugs—*OTC sleep aids are generally no more effective than plain aspirin, and those with anticholinergics and antihistamines may cause unpleasant side effects. If a minor ache or pain is keeping you awake, take aspirin or acetaminophen. Otherwise, try to identify and correct the cause of the insomnia.*
OTC analgesics—*see the list under Pain and Fever*
OTC sleeping aids—*Compoz; Nervine Nightime; Nytol; Sleep-Eze; Sominex*
R_x sedatives and hypnotics—*Atarax; Ativan; Dalmane; Librium; meprobamate; Nembutal; phenobarbital; Serax; Tranxene; Valium*

Meningitis

Meningitis is a bacterial or viral infection of the meninges, the membranes covering the brain and spinal cord. Bacterial meningitis is more common and dangerous. Meningitis is extremely communicable; the infection is transmitted by air-borne droplets that may be passed from person to person.

Symptoms

Onset may be sudden or gradual. Symptoms include chills and a high fever; a stiff neck; pains in the back, abdomen and head; nausea and vomiting. In some individuals, the back becomes rigid and a "heat" rash appears on the body. Breathing may become difficult and abnormal. Patients may become confused and delirious and may pass quickly into a coma. Occasionally, muscle twitching or convulsions may be noted.

Treatment

Because of its extreme communicability, epidemics of bacterial meningitis must be controlled by administering antibiotics. Penicillin and ampicillin may be used for this purpose. Persons with bacterial meningitis must receive one of these antibiotics quickly and without delay. Hospitalization is required.

Drugs Used in Treatment

R_x antibiotics—*amoxicillin; ampicillin; Keflex; penicillin G; penicillin potassium phenoxymethyl*

Multiple Sclerosis

Multiple sclerosis is a disease of unknown cause that attacks the brain and spinal cord. Possible causes include viral infection, inflammation, and degeneration of parts of the brain. The disease is characterized by patchy degeneration of the sheathlike covering of the nerves. The degeneration interferes with the normal function of the nerve pathways.

Symptoms

The symptoms of multiple sclerosis often begin following trauma, vaccination, pregnancy, certain injections, poisoning, or infection. Commonly seen symptoms include slurred speech, incontinence, spastic paralysis, abnormal eye movements, tremor, and spastic muscle responses. There is gradual decline in coordinated muscle movement. Later, there may be periods of euphoria and excitement. Vision may be lost in one or both eyes. The course of multiple sclerosis is characterized by periods of exacerbation followed by improvement. Unfortunately, as the disease progresses, the patient usually becomes more subject to other disorders. Although people usually do not die of multiple sclerosis per se, death may occur due to a complicating disease. Kidney and bladder infections are common complications.

Treatment

There is no specific treatment for persons with multiple sclerosis. Glucocorticoid steroids are sometimes used for acute relapses. Muscle relaxants are given to control spasticity.

It is most important to make sure the patient gets sufficient sleep and rest throughout the day. Sudden temperature changes should be avoided. Usually the person is uncomfortable in warm environments. Colder environments often make the patient feel temporarily better.

It is not uncommon for the disease to run 10 to 20 years. Remission periods may last for months or years. Survival after onset is usually less than 30 years.

Drugs Used in Treatment

℞ **steroid hormones**—*Aristocort; Medrol; prednisone*
℞ **analgesics**—*Darvocet-N; Darvon; Darvon Compound-65; Demerol; Empirin Compound with Codeine; Equagesic; Fiorinal; Fiorinal with Codeine; Motrin; Percodan; Synalgos-DC; Talwin; Tylenol with Codeine*
℞ **sedatives and hypnotics**—*Librium; Serax; Tranxene; Valium*

Myasthenia Gravis

Myasthenia gravis is a disease that causes extreme weakness and fatigability of the muscles. Any skeletal muscle may be involved but the ones chiefly affected include those of the lips, face, tongue, eyes, throat, and neck. The exact cause of myasthenia gravis is unknown, but it is known that there is decreased muscle response to nerve impulses. Some people believe that the disease is an allergic response to certain chemicals.

Symptoms

The primary symptom of myasthenia gravis is extreme fatigability of the muscles. The muscles eventually become weakened and may even become paralyzed to the point that the person is not able to move, talk, or breathe. Weakness of ocular muscles may lead to double vision and drooping eyelids. Talking and swallowing become difficult. Because control of the tongue is hampered, the voice may seem high-pitched and nasal. Myasthenia gravis appears most frequently in women from ages 20 to 30.

Treatment

Myasthenia gravis is treated with neostigmine. For severe conditions, the drug is given by injection. For less severe forms, tablets may be taken as directed. Other drugs used include pyridostigmine and ambenonium. Edrophonium is used in the diagnosis of myasthenia gravis. The drug is injected and if the patient suddenly improves, the diagnosis is considered positive.

Narcolepsy

Narcolepsy is a chronic condition characterized by the intense, uncontrollable desire to sleep. Its cause is unknown, and it usually persists throughout life. Males have the condition four times more often than females.

Symptoms

Recurrent sleep attacks occur daily in most people with narcolepsy. The attack may last for only minutes or for hours, and the sleep is similar to normal sleep except that it occurs at inappropriate times and in inappropriate places. Hazardous activities such as driving may be especially dangerous for the narcoleptic.

Treatment

Narcolepsy is treated with central nervous system stimulants such as dextroamphetamine sulfate and methylphenidate hydrochloride. Although these drugs may relieve the attacks, they do not eliminate the basic disorder and they do not prevent the attacks of muscular weakness that occur during emotional upset or elation.

Drugs Used in Treatment

R_x adrenergic—*Ritalin*

Neuritis

Neuritis is a general term for degenerative change in the nerve tissue. Despite the "itis" ending, it is generally noninflammatory. When it affects a single nerve, the condition is called mononeuritis. When several nerves are involved, the condition is called polyneuritis.

Mononeuritis is usually caused by trauma to the area, as from direct blows or from fractures. A prolonged, cramped posture (e.g., gardening) may be responsible. Occasionally, it may be due to an infection, poisoning with mercury, lead, or other toxins, or certain drugs such as isoniazid or sulfonamides. Polyneuritis is a symptom of diabetes and other disorders.

Symptoms

Neuritis causes a sensation of pins and needles, tingling, and stabbing pain. The pain is often worse at night and during temperature changes. Numbness and loss of sensation commonly occur. The individual may report weakness with diminished reflexes. Occasionally, sweating and dry skin are present.

Treatment

Because neuritis may be due to a variety of causes, its exact cause must be determined and corrected. For example, if drug-induced, neuritis is treated by discontinuing the drug or decreasing the dosage appropriately. When the cause is corrected, the individual usually recovers quickly although re-exposure to the causative agent may cause the symptoms to reappear. If the condition has persisted for some time, recovery may be incomplete. In this case, pain may be constant and muscle shrinkage may occur.

Acute neuritis is treated with complete rest. Mild analgesics may be required although narcotic analgesics should be avoided whenever possible.

Drugs Used in Treatment

OTC analgesics—*see the list under Pain and Fever*
R̵ analgesics—*Darvocet-N; Darvon; Darvon Compound-65; Demerol; Empirin Compound with Codeine; Equagesic; Fiorinal; Fiorinal with Codeine; Motrin; Norgesic; Percodan; Synalgos-DC; Talwin; Tylenol with Codeine*

Parkinson's Disease

Parkinson's disease is a disorder that affects the central nervous system. Its cause is not known; there may be several different causes. Generally, Parkinson's disease is attributed to a degeneration process in the brain. Once it begins, the symptoms can be controlled but the disease can never be reversed. Over a million Americans have the disease. It is not contagious and while it is not a killer, it can cause invalidism.

Symptoms

The disease usually comes on slowly. Usually it affects people in their late 50's and 60's. The major symptoms include muscular rigidity and weakness, involuntary tremors, a slow shuffling gait, salivation, and a "pill-rolling" motion of the hands. Initially, the individual may exhibit an altered masklike expression. A stolid facial musculature that does not express emotions such as joy or sorrow is characteristic of the disorder. The body movements gradually become slower. Walking becomes increasingly difficult. The legs begin to stiffen and feel heavy. The posture becomes stooped and a tremor begins. The tremor is usually worse when the individual is at rest, but not asleep, and working or moving the arms or legs frequently alleviates the tremor until rest is resumed.

Eventually, the individual experiences extreme difficulty in walking and getting out of chairs. Maneuvering the body around objects is difficult, and the individual may frequently stumble and fall. Minor movements such as buttoning a garment may become impossible. When attempting to walk, people with Parkinson's disease may run for a few steps to prevent falling forward. Once they have begun walking, their steps are generally slow and shuffling.

Treatment

A number of drugs have been found useful in alleviating symptoms of Parkinson's disease, including anticholinergics. These drugs must be taken regularly. Some of the antihistamines, especially Benadryl, may also prove useful in modifying the symptoms. To be effective, the antihistamine must have potent anticholinergic activity.

Levodopa (L-dopa) is another effective drug in treating Parkinson's patients. Other agents include amantadine hydrochloride and Sinemet. Surgery is effective in some cases.

Parkinson's disease is not cured by any drug. At most, the agents control the salivation and many of the tremors and unusual movements of the individual. Many patients can walk more freely and speak more coherently due to drug administration, but drugs may not be effective in every case.

Patients with Parkinson's disease should undergo regular physical therapy that includes massage and working the muscles. Daily exercise of the muscles, especially those of the fingers and hands, wrists, elbows, knees and neck, is helpful.

Drugs Used in Treatment

℞ antiparkinson drugs—*Artane; Sinemet*
℞ antihistamine—*Benadryl*

Polio

Polio (poliomyelitis, infantile paralysis) is an acute viral infection that may attack the nervous system, possibly causing paralysis in the part of the body controlled by the damaged portion of the brain or spinal cord. Paralysis and eventual death from respiratory depression occurs in 5 to 10 percent of all cases. Surprisingly, the polio virus is very prevalent and infects many people world-wide, but it causes clinical signs in less than 1 percent of those infected. The polio virus is spread by contaminated food and water and from insects.

Symptoms

Polio may cause symptoms so slight that the disease goes undiagnosed; there may be a slight fever, malaise, headache, sore throat, and possibly vomiting for one to three days. In more severe cases, there will be fever, severe headache, stiff neck and back, and muscle pain and weakness. The most dangerous form causes paralysis of the respiratory apparatus.

Prevention

Since the development of the Salk vaccine in 1955, the disease has all but disappeared in the industrialized nations of the world, although it is still a major problem in the underdeveloped countries. But an alarming percentage of American children have not been immunized against this dreaded disease, and some experts speculate that we may see a resurgence of the disease.

There are two types of polio vaccines. The Salk vaccine is an injectable preparation of inactivated (killed) viruses; the Sabin variety is the orally administered, live attenuated viruses form.

One recommended administration regimen for the Salk vaccine involves a series of four doses beginning when the child is between 6 and 12 weeks old. The next two injections are given at one-to-two month intervals with the fourth dose administered at age 8 to 16 months. A booster shot must be given every two to three years until adulthood.

The oral polio vaccine (Sabin) is first given at age 6 to 12 weeks, with a second dose 8 weeks later and a third dose in another 8 to 12 months. Just before the child begins to go to school, another dose is usually given, but no further boosters are needed. Adults need not be given either vaccine unless they are traveling to a part of the world where polio is common.

Treatment

If polio is suspected, the patient must be kept in bed until the disease has been ruled out, even if he feels better. Otherwise, he may relapse into a more serious form of polio. No drug will kill the virus or control its spread in the body.

Rabies

Rabies is an infectious viral disease that attacks the brain cells, causing central nervous system irritation. If left untreated, rabies can cause paralysis and death in less than a week.

Rabies is contracted from the bite of a rabid animal. The disease has been largely controlled in the United States through the vaccination of domestic pets, and most cases are now due to the bite of a wild animal. Any meat-eating animal can transmit the disease, and it is most often seen in bats, foxes, raccoons, skunks, and squirrels. According to the Public Health Service, even though thousands of people undergo the horrendous rabies treatment each year, only one to three cases of rabies are reported yearly.

Symptoms

Symptoms of rabies include pain, burning, and numbness at the bite site. The bite heals, but remains inflamed and tender. The patient becomes thirsty but cannot drink because it hurts to do so (hydrophobia—fear of water—is another name for the disease). The patient becomes irritable and salivates wildly. Symptoms gradually lead to convulsions, paralysis, coma, and death.

Treatment

The word "horrendous" describes the treatment regimen because the antirabies vaccine requires 24 injections—one daily for 21 days and booster shots on days 10, 20, and 30 after that. The antirabies vaccine can cause permanent paralysis or death, although these complications are rare. A newer, less dangerous vaccine that has an easier treatment regimen and fewer side effects is being developed.

All animal bites should be immediately and thoroughly washed with soap and water. A physician should be contacted and, if at all possible, the animal should be contained to determine its vaccination status, or whether rabies viruses can be isolated from its bloodstream. The physician must decide whether treatment should be initiated. Unprovoked attacks from domestic pets and bites resulting from stray dogs, cats, and wild animals or bats should be considered to be rabid, and treatment should be instituted at once.

Reye's Syndrome

Reye's syndrome was first recognized in 1963. It is a possibly infectious, possibly contagious disorder affecting children under the age of 18. It is characterized by swelling of the brain cells and infiltration of fat into the liver. It may follow a variety of common viral infections such as influenza, chicken pox, or herpes simplex. It occurs sporadically (a single case) and in minor outbreaks in specific areas. Without prompt, proper treatment, the disease can be fatal. Thirty to 40 percent of all children who contract the disease will die.

Symptoms

The initial symptoms of Reye's syndrome are similar to those of an upper respiratory tract infection. They also include mild gastrointestinal disturbances, spasticity, and hyperactivity. The child may be hypoglycemic. A symptom-free interval may follow, lasting for several hours or days, and then a period of constant vomiting ensues. Eventually delirium and coma develop. There may be convulsions. Breathing may be deep and irregular. The liver is enlarged and the abdomen tender if pressed around the area of the liver.

Marked swelling of the brain may be noted. Eighty percent of affected children who have convulsions die.

Treatment

Treatment is nonspecific, intensive, and symptomatic. The patient should be under close supervision. Corticosteroids are given.

Drugs Used in Treatment

℞ steroid hormones—*Aristocort; Medrol; prednisone*

St. Vitus' Dance

St. Vitus' Dance (Sydenham's chorea, rheumatic chorea, chorea minor) is seen mostly in younger people and is characterized by mild muscular weakness, emotional disturbance, and involuntary irregular movements. The disorder is usually (but not always) associated with rheumatic fever, and frequently develops with this disease. Other symptoms of rheumatic fever are apt to be present at the same time as St. Vitus' Dance. The disorder occurs more commonly in girls than in boys, and occurs more frequently in summer and early fall.

Symptoms

The primary symptoms include grimacing, clumsy movements, stumbling, irritability, excitability, and sleeplessness.The face, trunk, and extremities may involuntarily and dysrhythmically move. Movements are sudden, short, quick, and jerky. The person's walking and speech patterns may be affected. The arms and legs may become extremely weak and unresponsive to normal stimuli.

Treatment

There is no specific treatment for St. Vitus' Dance. The individual symptoms are treated as needed. For example, muscular twitching or irritability may be treated with sedatives or tranquilizers. The disease usually runs its course in two to three months, with no permanent damage being noted thereafter.

The disorder must be differentiated from normal tics or from side effects caused by certain drugs such as phenothiazines. The condition must also be differentiated from Huntington's chorea, a hereditary disease of the brain characterized by symptoms similar to those described above. This disease is nontreatable. Tranquilizers or phenothiazines and reserpine are used to manage the symptoms, which, nonetheless, continue throughout life.

Drugs Used in Treatment

℞ sedatives and hypnotics—*Atarax; Ativan; meprobamate; Nembutal; phenobarbital; Serax; Tranxene; Valium*
℞ phenothiazines—*Compazine; Stelazine*
℞ phenothiazine and antidepressant—*Triavil*
℞ anticholinergic and sedative—*Librium*
℞ analgesics and sedatives—*Fiorinal; Fiorinal with Codeine*

Schizophrenia

Schizophrenia is the name given to a group of syndromes characterized by disordered thoughts, moods, and behavior. The many different schizophrenic symptoms make a comprehensive classification system extremely difficult, if not impossible. Some people pass into and out of different types of schizophrenia quickly, displaying few easily recognized symptoms. Other schizophrenics suffer from a severe psychosis that results in permanent disability. Thus, schizophrenia is difficult to diagnose; a psychiatrist must usually make the final determination.

Schizophrenia usually begins in adolescence or early adult life. There are some childhood schizophrenics, but these are rare. The onset is usually gradual, and years often pass before the psychiatric disorder is finally recognized and medical attention is sought by family or friends of the patient.

Symptoms

The individual displays regressive intellectual functioning and bizarre behavior. A schizophrenic often hallucinates, experiences delusions, and withdraws from society. Thinking slows or shifts rapidly from topic to topic. The schizophrenic frequently appears autistic with frequent religious or sexual preoccupations. Moods shift quickly, regardless of environmental circumstances. The schizophrenic does not recognize these situations as symptoms of disease and rarely seeks medical help.

Treatment

Most types of schizophrenia are treated with antipsychotic medications such as the phenothiazines. These drugs have been responsible for reducing the number of patients in the country's mental wards, but they are not always completely effective. Schizophrenic patients often must take the drug throughout life, and periods of remission are common. In general, schizophrenia that comes on quickly is more effectively treated than is schizophrenic disease that appears slowly over years. Psychotherapy is also helpful.

Drugs Used in Treatment

Rx phenothiazines—*Compazine; Mellaril; Stelazine; Thorazine*
Rx antipsychotic agent—*Haldol*

Sciatica

Sciatica is an inflammation of the sciatic nerve, the longest nerve in the body. The sciatic nerve runs from the buttocks down to the feet.

Any condition that causes pressure on the sciatic nerve may cause sciatica. Such conditions include a slipped disc, arthritis, or tumors arising in the area of the spinal cord where the sciatic nerve branches out. Sciatica occurs most often in men aged 30 to 50; truck drivers and people who sit for long periods frequently develop the condition.

Symptoms

The symptoms include pain along the entire sciatic nerve. If the condition is caused by a slipped disc, the pain will be extremely severe. If it is caused by a strain such as coughing or a quick movement, the pain will be severe but not as excruciating as from a slipped disc. The skin along the course of the sciatic nerve will be extremely tender to the touch and whenever the leg is straightened, an additional pain may be felt in the area of the buttocks or along the distribution of the nerve.

Treatment

An individual with sciatica should avoid lifting heavy weights, assuming unusual positions, or making quick movements. A firm mattress should be used.

When sciatic pain is felt, application of moist heat may help to relieve the condition. Sitting in a tub of hot water is extremely beneficial. Aspirin may be all that is needed for the pain, although for severe pain, a narcotic-containing analgesic may be necessary.

Drugs Used in Treatment

OTC analgesics—*see the list under Pain and Fever*
℞ analgesics—*Darvocet-N; Darvon; Darvon Compound-65; Demerol; Empirin Compound with Codeine; Equagesic; Fiorinal; Fiorinal with Codeine; Motrin; Norgesic; Parafon Forte; Percodan; Robaxin; Soma Compound; Synalgos-DC; Talwin; Tylenol with Codeine*

Health Care Accessory— *heating pad*

Related Topics—*Arthritis; Backache*

Smoking

Cigarette smoking is one of the greatest public health problems in the United States. Its adverse effects range from mild physical complaints (bad breath, stained fingers and teeth) to a documented decrease in life span. Smoking is known to be a contributing, and perhaps the major, factor in various forms of heart and blood vessel disease, lung cancer, stroke, emphysema, and chronic bronchitis. Pregnant women who smoke are exposing the fetus to an increased risk of premature delivery, early abortion, stillbirth, and neonatal death. Infants born to women who smoke weigh an average of six ounces less than those born to nonsmokers. Smokers have a lowered resistance to infection and are more likely to develop ulcers. People who smoke increase their risk of developing severe gum disease, losing their teeth, and developing bad facial wrinkles. In addition to the hazards they impose upon themselves, cigarette smokers increase the respiratory irritation suffered by those in whose company they smoke. Parents who smoke are very likely to have smokers for children.

Nearly 1,000 constituents of tobacco smoke have been identified; many are irritants, toxic gases, or carcinogens. These particles are inhaled into the lungs, where they irritate the respiratory passages and increase the production of bronchial mucus, possibly initiating cancer.

One constituent of tobacco smoke, nicotine, is a stimulant to the central nervous system. Nicotine probably is the reason many people find smoking pleasurable and the reason many people become dependent on tobacco. Withdrawal from nicotine brings about unpleasant sensations likened to withdrawal from any drug.

Reducing the Risks

There is no way to treat the respiratory damage caused by cigarette smoking, but it is believed that the pathological process does not advance once the habit is given up. It is preferable, of course, never to start smoking in the first place. Although many people have stopped smoking over the past decade, it is believed that over 40 percent of all Americans still smoke, and the number of young people, teenagers, and women who smoke is increasing.

The best way to reduce the risk of tobacco-related illness is never to start smoking. If you already smoke, you should make every effort to stop. Clinics for people who want to stop smoking have been helpful to some. Hypnosis, aversion therapy, and group therapy have also been tried.

Several OTC products are designed as crutches to aid in helping to quit smoking. Most of these products contain the chemical lobeline, which serves as a substitute for nicotine. Lobeline has a stimulant action on the central nervous system similar to that of nicotine although less severe. Lobeline is available as a tablet or lozenge.

Most reports indicate that smoking pipes or cigars is not as hazardous as cigarette smoking. However, this hypothesis is still under investigation, although one thing is sure. Pipe and cigar smokers suffer higher incidence of cancer of the lip, mouth, larynx, and esophagus than do nonsmokers, although they have fewer cases of lung cancer than do cigarette smokers. Generally, pipe or cigar smokers do not inhale. Cigarette smokers have a higher incidence of mouth cancer than do pipe or cigar smokers.

Someone who finds it impossible to quit smoking entirely will still benefit from reducing the number of cigarettes smoked per day (preferably to five or less), smoking filter-tipped cigarettes, inhaling less, and leaving a longer stub, i.e., taking fewer puffs per cigarette.

Tetany

Tetany is a syndrome caused by hyperexcitation of the nervous system usually due to decreased calcium levels in the blood. The syndrome is usually the result of a deficiency of the parathyroid hormone. Parathyroid hormone is necessary for the body to reabsorb calcium in the kidneys and to maintain calcium blood levels at their proper concentration. When this hormone is decreased in concentration or activity, blood calcium levels fall and the individual becomes very excitable. A decrease in the hormone is usually related to accidental removal of the parathyroid glands during thyroid gland surgery. It may also be due to a lesion or some damage in a parathyroid gland which prohibits adequate production of the hormone.

Symptoms

Tetany causes numbness and tingling in the extremities, rhythmic cramping, spastic rigidity, wheezing, irritability, double vision, increased urinary frequency, nausea, fatigue, palpitations, weakness, and possible mental retardation. If allowed to persist, tetany causes lethargy, personality changes, and anxiety.

Treatment

Tetany is treated by giving calcium salts intravenously until the symptoms cease. Then calcium should be given orally to prevent the syndrome from returning. Other drugs used include dihydrotachysterol (Hytakerol) and calciferol. Parathyroid hormone injection is available, but the hormone cannot be given orally because it is destroyed in the intestines. A person with tetany should never take phenothiazine drugs because these drugs may cause Parkinson-like symptoms.

Tic Douloureux

Tic douloureux is a disease affecting the trigeminal nerve, a nerve in the side of the face. Its cause is unknown.

Symptoms

Tic douloureux causes sudden attacks of excruciating, jabbing pain. The attacks are often described as lightning-like jabs. They usually last only one to two minutes, but they may last as long as 15 minutes. Attacks may occur daily to only once a year or so.

The sharp pain is felt from the area of the ear down along the cheek through the area of the mouth. It may be brought on by a mere touch in the appropriate area, and people with tic douloureux may avoid talking, chewing, drinking cold water, and even shaving to avoid stimulating the onset of the pain. The incidence of the disease is higher in women, and it usually occurs in middle or late life. As the disease progresses, the periods between attacks become shorter. The attacks may be severe enough to render the patient suicidal.

Treatment

The drug of choice for treating tic douloureux is carbamazepine. Phenytoin and vitamin B₁₂ may help in some cases. Aspirin usually is not effective. Hot or cold packs may help. If drugs fail to help, surgery may be required.

Drugs Used in Treatment

℞ anticonvulsant—*Dilantin*

Health Care Accessories— *heating pad; ice bag*

Tics

A tic is any repetitive, purposeless movement of a muscle. Tics usually occur in children beginning between the ages of 5 and 14. However, they can occur at any age. A tic is basically an involuntary nervous twitch of a muscle group, and tics are usually without any serious consequences. However, tics sometimes develop following certain nervous system diseases such as encephalitis.

The tic may take any form: blinking of an eye, shaking the head, jerking the thigh, shrugging the shoulder, or grimacing. Tics frequently disappear as suddenly as they start. Tics are seen only when the individual is awake.

Treatment

Tics that persist should be seen by a doctor. The doctor will try to determine and treat the underlying cause, if possible. Tranquilizers are sometimes used, but these can only attempt to mask the symptoms, not treat the actual cause. Given enough time, the tic usually disappears spontaneously.

Joints, Bones, and Muscles

The skeleton, the bony framework of our bodies, comprises 206 bones. Bone, like the rest of the body, is living tissue. The red bone marrow in the center of the bone produces multitudes of red and white blood cells every minute. Bone is also the storehouse of calcium for the body—99 percent of the calcium in the body is found in the skeleton, and it is this calcium that keeps our bones firm and strong.

The skeleton enables us to stand erect and to move about, and it also protects our internal organs. The vertebral column encloses the major trunk of the nervous system, the spinal cord, and the skull protects the brain.

A joint is the juncture of two bones. Not all joints are movable; for example, the skull is composed of seven bones separated by cartilage. Most of the joints in our limbs are movable. They are held in place by ligaments attached to the bone. Cartilage lines the ends of the bones in a joint, and cartilage and fluid cushion and protect joints. Tendons attach muscles to bones. Movement occurs when a muscle contracts, pulling the tendon and thereby the bone to which it is attached.

Muscle comprises about 50 percent of our total body weight. It is composed of tissue that has the ability to contract, and it is classified into three types: striated, smooth, and cardiac.

Striated muscle is the muscle attached to the skeleton. It is under our conscious control. When we bend an arm, take a step, or sit down, our movements are made by contractions of striated muscle. Under a microscope striated muscle appears to be striped.

Smooth muscle is not striated; it lines most of the hollow organs of the body and its movements are governed by the autonomic nervous system. Smooth muscle aids in circulating blood and fluids through the body, it moves material through the digestive tract, it aids in respiration by moving the diaphragm, abdomen, and rib cage; in short, it is responsible for most of the metabolic functions of the body.

Cardiac muscle is the muscle that makes up the thick walls of the heart. Cardiac muscle is regulated by the autonomic nervous system, although it has the ability to contract without nervous impulses. It is striated like skeletal muscle.

Arthritis

Arthritis is one of the oldest known chronic illnesses. Some skeletons of prehistoric animals displayed in museums show signs of an arthritic condition. Rheumatoid arthritis cripples and disables more people than any other single disease. Arthritic patients may become so incapacitated that they are unable to perform even the most routine tasks. This incapacity, combined with the pain and deformity caused by the disease and with enforced idleness and dependency, often results in a sense of hopelessness and

227

depression on the part of the patient.

Arthritis is the name given to diseases involving principally the joints and is characterized by stiffness, pain, and inflammation. Rheumatism is a generic term used to refer to any of a variety of disorders affecting the connective tissue of the body that causes pain, stiffness, or limitation of motion.

As many as 90 to 100 different disease states have been defined as being types of arthritis; among the most common are osteoarthritis, rheumatoid arthritis, and bursitis.

Osteoarthritis

The most common form of arthritis is osteoarthritis, and this is what most laymen think of as arthritis. Many people over 40 have a mild, nonsymptomatic form of the disease due to normal wear and tear on the joints.

Osteoarthritis is a degenerative joint disease. It rarely affects the feet and ankles but may cause deformity in the knees and hips. The knees may become knobby and the patient with osteoarthritis may find it difficult to straighten the leg. Some patients become bow-legged and others, knock-kneed. Those who become knock-kneed have the most difficulty walking.

Osteoarthritis of the hip probably causes the most discomfort, and in advanced cases it can be crippling. The hip is a ball and socket joint, and wear and tear on it can greatly diminish mobility. Osteoarthritis of the hip can be very disabling, and is one of the more frequent reasons that older people must be cared for in extended care facilities rather than at home.

The patient with osteoarthritis should be careful to rest and protect the involved joints. Canes, crutches, and walkers relieve some of the pressure on affected joints, and weight reduction is also beneficial. Heat (electric heating pad or hot baths) is also effective in relieving pain. Carefully designed exercises help maintain joint mobility and muscle tone.

Osteoarthritis is also treated with aspirin, glucocorticoid steroids, gold salts, phenylbutazone, indomethacin, ibuprofen, and fenoprofen calcium.

Rheumatoid Arthritis

Rheumatoid arthritis is a progressively worsening disease of unknown cause. With rheumatoid arthritis the most common symptoms include morning stiffness, joint pain, and inflammation. Rheumatoid arthritis also causes cold, sweaty hands and feet, and painful swelling in one or more joints. Progressive loss of joint motion and eventual deformity of the joints occurs. Easy fatigability becomes prevalent. Some people develop anemia, and ulcers and nodules under the skin and at the affected joint. Many people have alternating cycles of remissions and flare-ups. Rheumatoid arthritis may cause total disability, and it often leaves the person extremely frustrated and severely depressed.

Rheumatoid arthritis can begin at any stage in life. In more than 70 percent of all cases, onset of the disease occurs between the ages of 30 and 70. Women are affected more frequently than men.

Rheumatoid arthritis usually begins without prior warning. The first symptoms are often nonspecific, such as a loss of appetite and easy fatigability. Later, morning stiffness and painful joints also occur, most often in the hands and feet, specifically the fingers and toes. Symptoms usually occur in both feet or both hands.

Severe disease often causes disabling and disturbing deformities of the hands, elbows, toes, and knees. The fingers may be displaced to the point that they no longer are in proper line with the arm and can even become distorted into positions that make normal manipulation quite difficult. Some patients are unable to perform simple tasks such as buttoning their clothes or picking up small objects. The elbows may become deformed to the point that they do not bend in the proper direction, and the patients can neither comb their hair, nor feed themselves. The toes may become so tender, sore, and deformed that the person is unable to stand or walk comfortably and specially designed shoes may be necessary. When the disease is severe enough, the knees may be painful unless elevated or bent. Unfortunately, when the knees are rested in a comfortable position (i.e., lying in bed with the knees resting on a pillow), they become stiff and the person is unable to walk.

In addition to drug therapy with the medications used for osteoarthritis, Naprosyn and Tolectin anti-inflammatories are used. Additional treatment includes at least eight to ten hours of sleep per night, with an extra hour or two of rest sometime during the day. Moist heat applied to the painful or stiffened joints will help to relieve the pain, and elastic support bandages, wristbands, or anklets will add support and lessen the pain.

Bursitis

Bursae are sacs located at the ends of the bones. They prevent damage to the bone during movement. They are lined with membranes that secrete lubricating fluid into the joints. The bursae are easily attacked by rheumatic diseases. "Housemaid's knee" is one example of bursitis.

When inflammation of the bursae (bursitis) occurs, it is usually localized and is the result of excessive pressure on that area. Most often, the condition can be adequately treated with local injections of glucocorticoid steroids, and recurrences can be minimized by avoiding the causative activity. For example, the baseball pitcher who develops bursitis in the shoulder or upper arm can continue pitching by resting the pitching arm adequately between starts. A person with a bunion, which is an inflamed bursae located at the point where the skin glides over the joint at the base of the big toe, can often obtain relief with better fitting shoes.

Bursitis is alleviated to some extent with rest, aspirin, and the application of heat. In severe cases or to speed healing in athletes, anti-inflammatory corticosteroids are injected directly into the painful area. Tranquilizing agents are given to reduce spasm. The affected joint is sometimes immobilized with a splint.

Drugs Used in Treatment

Recommended treatment with OTC drugs—*The best treatment for many arthritic disorders is aspirin in large doses. Aspirin reduces both pain and inflammation. Acetaminophen relieves pain, but it does not reduce inflammation, the underlying cause, and therefore it should not be used. Because such large doses are used, treatment may cause stomach distress. If so, ask your pharmacist for an enteric-coated product (we prefer Ecotrin) or one that has been buffered with antacids.*
OTC analgesics—*see the list under Pain and Fever*
OTC external analgesics—*Absorbine; Absorbine Jr.; Ben-Gay; Heet; Infra-Rub*
℞ steroid hormones—*Aristocort; Medrol; prednisone*
℞ anti-inflammatories—*Butazolidin; Clinoril; Indocin; Motrin; Nalfon; Naprosyn; Tolectin*
℞ sedatives and hypnotics—*Librium; Serax; Tranxene; Valium*

Health Care Accessories—*ambulation aids; disposable hot pads; elastic bandage; elastic hosiery; heating pad; hot water bottle*

Backache

Aside from headache, one of the most common complaints we humans experience is backache. Unfortunately, the causes of backache are multiple and varied. Pain that originates in the back from any cause is often transmitted to other areas of the body. Feeling this pain elsewhere frequently leads to an assumption that the pain is caused at that site rather than elsewhere. However, an experienced doctor can usually diagnose the cause of the pain correctly.

The following are among the most common factors that are known to induce backache.

Muscular Strain

Backache in one who gives a history of unusual activity in the recent past is likely to be due to a muscular strain, especially if the pain subsides in a short time.

The onset of pain may occur abruptly or slowly. In its severe form, a person will bend over or assume some position and not be able to straighten up. The pain itself may be felt as a stabbing or aching sensation.

The treatment is largely symptomatic. This includes the use of hot pads, avoidance of further strain, and using mild analgesics such as aspirin or acetaminophen. OTC items containing methyl salicylate in the form of a rub are used and recommended. They produce warmth at the site of application, and the rubbing is soothing and comforting.

Slipped Disc

If one of the cartilage discs found between the vertebrae becomes dislodged or injured, it may push against the spinal cord to inflict severe pain. These discs are composed of a soft gelatinous substance that is easily compressed to form a sort of shock absorber between the bones of the spinal column. When a disc becomes dislocated or if one ruptures, it may push against the nerves that branch from the spinal cord, causing severe pain. Additionally, numbness, tingling, or weakness may be referred to an arm or leg or some other part of the body.

Most people with this problem can give some history of past damage to the affected part of the back. The condition is usually caused by trauma, such as bending and straightening the back to lift heavy objects. Often the damage may not be felt for months or years after the injury.

The person will stand more upright than usual and curve the back toward the side opposite the pain. Tenderness may be felt along the path of the sciatic nerve, and there may be weakness in the foot or toe. There may also be weakness in the biceps and triceps muscles of the arm. The pain is often accentuated by motion, coughing, or straining in other ways.

Treatment must include strict bed rest with a firm mattress or with a board placed under the mattress. Also, hot packs and analgesics are useful. If aspirin or acetaminophen works, it should be used. Otherwise, the stronger narcotic-containing medications may be needed. Muscle relaxant drugs such as Valium are also given to reduce pain.

Back braces, supports, or belts may provide additional relief and prevent further damage. These should only be used on the advice of a doctor.

Surgery may be necessary to remove the ruptured disc. At that time the spine may also need to be fused. Drug treatment of the pain at best brings only temporary relief.

Never attempt any exercise program without having been instructed to do so by your doctor. Also, never submit yourself to surgery without first experiencing a long period of bed rest, aspirin, and moist heat. A second opinion on the necessity for surgery is also advisable.

Gynecological Causes

Premenstrual tension may cause a backache, and pain caused by a disorder of the female reproductive tract may be felt as a backache. Pregnancy also often causes severe backache that can sometimes be relieved by wearing a special girdle. Muscle strengthening exercises may prevent backaches due to pregnancy.

Degenerative Backache

As we age, our joint tissues also age. Therefore, this type of backache is more common in the older patient. It is related to osteoarthritic changes which occur normally with age.

Tension

Psychological tension related to the problems of life may cause a backache. Symptomatic relief can be obtained with applications of heat, use of a firm mattress, and analgesics such as aspirin or acetaminophen. Use of the more potent analgesics that contain narcotics is not recommended unless the milder agents do not work. Occasionally, antianxiety agents are useful.

Prevention and General Treatment

Correct posture is important to help prevent back pain. When picking up objects from the floor, be sure to lift with the legs, keeping the back straight. Avoid holding a telephone on the shoulder against the ear. Avoid sitting for long periods at a desk looking downward without moving the head. Avoid lying on the floor to watch television with the head jutted forward or lying on your back with your chin on your chest. Maintain proper posture whether sitting or standing.

Other factors must also be considered. The obese should lose weight. Persons leading a sedentary life should exercise to strengthen and stretch the back muscles.

For all types of back pain, bed rest is indicated to allow the muscles to rest. Applying hot, moist heat will help. Analgesics and muscle relaxants are beneficial. When inflammation is present, a glucocorticoid steroid is given.

Drugs Used in Treatment

Recommended treatment with OTC drugs—*If you want to use an OTC external analgesic, choose a product such as Ben-Gay ointment. These products contain methyl salicylate and can be rubbed into the skin vigorously without causing irritation. The vigorous rubbing will help to relieve pain.*
OTC analgesics—*see the list under Pain and Fever*
OTC external analgesics—*Absorbine; Absorbine Jr.; Ben-Gay; Heet; Infra-Rub*
R_X analgesics—*Darvocet-N; Darvon; Darvon Compound-65; Demerol; Empirin Compound with Codeine; Equagesic; Fiorinal; Fiorinal with Codeine; Motrin; Norgesic; Parafon Forte; Percodan; Robaxin; Soma Compound; Synalgos-DC; Talwin; Tylenol with Codeine*
R_X sedatives and hypnotics—*Librium; Serax; Tranxene; Valium*
R_X steroid hormones—*Aristocort; Medrol; prednisone*

Health Care Accessories—*disposable hot packs; gel hot and cold packs; heating pad; hot water bottle*

Cramps

Cramps are painful muscle contractions. They may result from excessive muscle fatigue, especially in sore or overworked muscles, or from a decreased blood supply to one part of the body. Cramps may also result from having abnormally low blood concentrations of salt, potassium, calcium, vitamin D, or other substances. Certain poisonous substances, including drugs and chemicals, may also cause cramps.

Cramps that occur upon movement or exertion and that are relieved by standing still are most likely caused by a disease that causes a decreased blood supply into the painful area. Cramps accompanied by dizziness, nausea, vomiting, or diarrhea are likely to indicate low blood levels of potassium, sodium, or some other substance. Periods of brief or extended unconsciousness or lapse of memory following cramps might be indicative of mild epilepsy or possibly a low concentration of vitamin D in the blood.

Cramps that occur regularly should not be neglected, but should be diagnosed by a doctor as soon as possible.

Gout

Gout is a special type of arthritis that is caused by excessive blood levels of uric acid due to either overproduction or underexcretion—and sometimes both. The uric acid precipitates in the tissues of the kidneys and in the joints to cause joint pain and deformity and kidney damage. Gout is most commonly seen in middle-aged men and is probably genetically controlled. Gout causes severe pain, and if left untreated or inadequately treated, it can cause severe kidney disease, possibly leading to other disorders such as high blood pressure and heart disease.

Symptoms

The most common symptom of gout is severe joint pain. This usually occurs first in the big toe, but other areas affected include the ankles, wrists, and thumbs. The toe appears red and shiny; it is swollen and extremely painful to the touch. The individual may have a fever and feel chilled.

Treatment

Gout can be treated by reducing the production of uric acid with the drug allopurinol. Or, levels of uric acid can be reduced by enhancing its secretion through the kidneys. The drug probenecid has this effect. Other drugs are used to decrease the inflammation in the joints to reduce the pain.

Colchicine is used for sudden attacks of gout pain. It works directly on the joints to reduce inflammation and relieve the pain. Colchicine should be taken only at the doctor's direction.

Additionally, the individual should drink at least eight to ten glasses of water per day. The gout patient should follow the diet prescribed by the doctor. A complete exercise program will help maintain joint mobility and promote a feeling of well-being.

Drugs Used in Treatment

R̨ uricosuric—*Benemid*
R̨ gout remedies—*colchicine; Zyloprim*
R̨ anti-inflammatory—*Butazolidin*

Related Topic—*Arthritis*

Muscular Dystrophy

Muscular dystrophy is the most common progressive muscular disease. Although its cause is not known, the disorder appears to be a hereditary condition affecting metabolism within the muscle cells. Onset most commonly occurs in people between the ages of 3 and 15. The primary danger with muscular dystrophy is that even though its symptoms are controlled, severe weakness with contractures of the muscles may lead to problems in movement. In addition, respiratory complications such as pneumonia are likely to occur. There is also a higher incidence of heart disease in persons with muscular dystrophy.

Symptoms

There are two primary types of muscular dystrophy, and their symptoms differ somewhat. The most common form, the Duchenne type, is marked by bulky calf and forearm muscles. This disorder usually occurs in males under three years of age. The thigh, hip, back, and shoulder muscles weaken progressively until, within a decade or so, the individual is unable to walk. Until that time, the gait is often waddling, and the patient finds it difficult to go up or down stairs. As the back muscles become weaker, curvature of the spine is noted. The individual falls frequently and has difficulty rising. There are cramping pains in the muscles. Respiratory infection occurs frequently and, especially in the second decade of life, cardiac failure may result.

In the second type, the facioscapulohumeral type, muscular atrophy begins early in life and affects the muscles of the face, shoulder, and upper arms. The muscles of the forearms are usually not involved. Persons of either sex may contract this type of muscular dystrophy. The eyelids become drooped and the upper lip thickens and overhangs the lower lip. The disease progresses slowly, with long periods of apparent arrest. Eventually, the face becomes expressionless and develops a mask-like appearance, and the individual is unable to raise the arms overhead.

Treatment

For either type, strict adherence to physical therapy measures must be followed. There is no specific drug therapy. Occasionally, muscle relaxant drugs are used to control the rigidity or the cramping pain associated with the disease. Aspirin and acetaminophen usually have little effect. The individual will eventually require the use of supportive means to walk or move about—such as canes, crutches, a walker, or (eventually) a wheelchair.

The disease is sometimes slow in its onset, and patients continue to grow progressively worse for many years. Death frequently occurs within ten years after the onset of the Duchenne type, while patients with facioscapulohumeral type may worsen for 20 to 50 years. Eventually, all patients are confined to chairs or beds.

Drugs Used in Treatment

℞ analgesics—*Darvocet-N; Darvon; Darvon Compound-65; Demerol; Empirin Compound with Codeine; Equagesic; Fiorinal; Fiorinal with Codeine; Motrin; Norgesic; Parafon Forte; Percodan; Robaxin; Soma Compound; Synalgos-DC; Talwin; Tylenol with Codeine*
℞ sedatives and hypnotics—*Librium; Serax; Tranxene; Valium*

Health Care Accessories—*ambulation aids*

Osteomyelitis

Osteomyelitis is an inflammation of the bone due to infection. It may be acute or chronic. It is due to direct implantation of microorganisms into bone (primary osteomyelitis) or by microorganisms that enter the bone through the blood vasculature (secondary osteomyelitis). The primary form is contracted mainly through fractures or wounds in which the bone is exposed. Nail wounds or other penetrating trauma into the bone may also cause the introduction of infective organisms into the area. Secondary osteomyelitis may result from infections elsewhere in the body that enter the bloodstream and then enter the bone.

Osteomyelitis may cause a loss of bone, soft tissue abscess formation, or a form of arthritis that may extend into the joints leading to severe pain and deformity.

Symptoms

The symptoms include deep pain in the area of the bone, severe fever, that may reach above 105° F, and profuse sweating. Movement may be extremely painful. The muscles over the area may be swollen, spastic, and extremely painful to the touch. When the infection is particularly severe, secondary infections may occur elsewhere in the body leading to a variety of symptoms dependent upon the target site.

Treatment

The condition is treated with wide-spectrum antibiotic therapy, but the dosage must be sufficiently high to assure that the drug enters the bone and fully destroys the microorganisms. Additionally, in severe cases an incision in the bone might be made to enable the doctor to aspirate pus or other debris. Pain can be controlled with prescription analgesics, but it is not usually adequately controlled with over-the-counter medications. Some authorities state that pain should not be completely abolished, because the intensity of the pain is one measure of the effectiveness of antibiotic treatment. Patients with chronic osteomyelitis should remain bedfast, preferably in a hospital, while the disease is being treated. It may take weeks to months for complete healing. Some doctors feel that all patients undergoing treatment for osteomyelitis should remain in bed. A rich diet and vitamin-mineral supplements should also be given.

Drugs Used in Treatment

OTC nutritional supplements—*see the list under Nutritional Disorders*
℞ antibiotics—*amoxicillin; ampicillin; erythromycin; Keflex; Minocin; penicillin G; penicillin potassium phenoxymethyl; Terramycin; tetracycline hydrochloride; Vibramycin*
℞ analgesics—*Darvocet-N; Darvon; Darvon Compound-65; Demerol; Empirin Compound with Codeine; Equagesic; Fiorinal; Fiorinal with Codeine; Motrin; Percodan; Synalgos-DC; Talwin; Tylenol with Codeine*

Osteoporosis

The most commonly encountered metabolic disease of the bone in Americans, osteoporosis is characterized by a decrease in the amount of bone present within the framework of the body. This disorder weakens bones and permits them to be easily broken. Unfortunately, the causes of osteoporosis are unknown. It is a disease most commonly seen in middle life or beyond. Women are more commonly affected than men.

One possible cause is a lack of estrogen. The disease most commonly occurs in women after the menopause. In fact, about one-third of all women over the age of 60 have some degree of osteoporosis. Some degree of osteoporosis may be present in cases of senility. Lack of physical activity is also thought to be a cause. Low intake or poor absorption of various nutrients is another possible cause.

Symptoms

The symptoms of osteoporosis include backache of varying severity. Women especially, following the menopause, may notice a shortening in their height. The bones become extremely brittle and even the slightest movement or activity may cause a bone to break. Osteoporotic people may break a vertebra by simply sneezing, coughing, or bending over to pick up an object.

Treatment

Osteoporosis is treated with estrogen and/or other steroids. Estrogens do appear to decrease bone loss. Testosterone may be used to stimulate protein buildup by the body. An adequate diet rich in nutrients and vitamin-mineral supplements are important. Sodium fluoride is sometimes given, but it must be cautiously administered. Calcium supplements and vitamin D appear to enhance bone formation.

Additionally, patients must be urged to exercise within their tolerance levels. For example, walking at least a mile a day will strengthen the bones. If analgesics are needed for the pain, aspirin, acetaminophen, or similar agents are usually satisfactory. Diets should be rich in protein, calcium and vitamin D. Milk and other milk products are ideal for this purpose. In advanced cases where the spine is weakened to the point that sitting or standing upright is difficult, the use of a back brace may be necessary. Canes, crutches, or a walker may be necessary for walking.

Drugs Used in Treatment

OTC analgesics—*see the list under Pain and Fever*
OTC nutritional supplements—*see the list under Nutritional Disorders*
Rx estrogen hormone—*Premarin*
Rx steroid hormone—*methyltestosterone*

Health Care Accessories—*ambulation aids*

Paget's Disease

Paget's disease, or osteitis deformans, is a bone disease of unknown cause. It commonly affects people over age 30, with up to 3 percent of all men and 2 percent of all women having some degree of Paget's disease. A familial relationship is apparent. Current research indicates that the disease may be due to viral infection or that it may be a benign form of cancer of the bone-forming cells.

Paget's disease is marked by excessive destruction and regrowth of bone. The regrowth occurs in an unorganized manner, and new bone structure may be bizarre.

Symptoms

Symptoms include severe deep bone pain that often becomes unbearable.

The bones soften, leading to bowing of the legs, loss of height, and easy fractures. The head may enlarge, headaches are common, and hearing is often impaired. Increased warmth is noted in the affected area because of the increased growth of blood vessels. Areas usually affected include the lower spine, legs, pelvis, and skull.

Treatment

Paget's disease is treated with a diet high in protein, vitamin C, calcium, and vitamin D. Additionally, estrogens and testosterone may be given. The current drug of choice for treating Paget's disease is Calcimar, a hormone extracted from salmon eggs. The use of Calcimar has greatly relieved the symptoms and increased the survival rate in patients with Paget's disease.

Persons with Paget's disease must avoid extreme exercise or trauma, or other situations that may cause increased burden or damage to the bones. Orthopedic devices to add support to the area may be required. The use of canes, walkers, crutches, or wheelchairs may help the individual move about and decrease pain.

While aspirin or acetaminophen may help relieve pain early in the disease process, these agents usually fail to bring relief later on. Using stronger analgesics is then necessary.

Drugs Used in Treatment

OTC analgesics—*see the list under Pain and Fever*
OTC nutritional supplements—*see the list under Nutritional Disorders*
Rx estrogen hormone—*Premarin*
Rx steroid hormone—*methyltestosterone*
Rx analgesics—*Darvocet-N; Darvon; Darvon Compound-65; Demerol; Empirin Compound with Codeine; Equagesic; Fiorinal; Fiorinal with Codeine; Motrin; Percodan; Synalgos-DC; Talwin; Tylenol with Codeine*

Health Care Accessories—*ambulation aids*

Rickets and Osteomalacia

In children, deficiency in vitamin D causes rickets, a bone disease. In adults, the same deficiency results in osteomalacia. The difference between the diseases is due to the difference between bones still growing and bones already formed.

Vitamin D is commonly found in eggs, liver, and fish liver oil. In the United States, milk is fortified with vitamin D. If exposed to sunlight, the body is able to make very small amounts of vitamin D.

Vitamin D is essential for proper utilization of calcium and phosphorus by the body. When a deficiency impairs the body's ability to use calcium and phosphorus, these minerals are not deposited in the bones. The bones then become soft and weak.

Symptoms

Children with rickets may be bowlegged or knock-kneed; the bones of their legs may not be strong enough to support their weight. Some children develop pigeon-breast; their teeth will be soft and poorly formed. They tire easily and may not be able to stand or walk unaided. If left untreated, a child with rickets may develop curvature of the spine and deformities of the limbs.

Osteomalacia causes pain in the limbs, pelvis, or spine, and progressive weakness of the limbs.

Treatment

Specific treatment includes administering vitamin D and calcium supplements. Improvement is usually rapid. Some people may also require pancreatic enzyme extracts and other vitamin-mineral supplements. Both disorders must be treated by a doctor.

Drugs Used in Treatment

OTC nutritional supplements—*see the list under Nutritional Disorders*

Related Topic—*Vitamin D Toxicity*

Sprained Ankle

A sprained ankle results when the ligaments around the ankle are torn. This may happen, for example, if weight is put on the foot when it is not firmly grounded. Severe pain and inflammation are the primary symptoms.

Treatment

An individual with a sprained ankle should not walk on the foot. The ankle should be covered with ice packs in the beginning to help keep the inflammation down. Analgesics may be used to reduce the pain. A cast may be necessary if the ligament is severely damaged. Crutches or a cane may be necessary to aid in walking once the ankle has started to heal. A day or two after the injury, application of warm, moist heat to the area should help in reducing the pain and inflammation.

Drugs Used in Treatment

OTC analgesics—*see the list under Pain and Fever*

Health Care Accessories—*disposable hot and cold packs; gel hot and cold packs; heating pad; hot water bottle; ice bag*

Sprained Wrist

A sprained wrist results from any undue strain on a muscle or tendon that causes stretching or tearing of the tissue. There may be bleeding into the wrist joint that causes further inflammation in the area. Severe pain and swelling are the primary symptoms.

Treatment

Every sprained wrist should be examined by a doctor. With the doctor's approval, the wrist should be tightly bound with an elastic bandage or a wrist support appliance. Initially, ice packs can be applied to the area to keep the swelling down. After the first day, ice packs can be replaced by hot water or hot, moist heat to reduce the pain and any further inflammation that does develop. Aspirin will relieve the pain and inflammation. Acetaminophen relieves the pain, but not the swelling. Additionally, the individual should rest the wrist.

Drugs Used in Treatment

OTC analgesics—*see the list under Pain and Fever*

Health Care Accessories—*disposable hot and cold packs; gel hot and cold packs; heating pad; hot water bottle; ice bag*

Systemic Lupus Erythematosus

Systemic lupus erythematosus (SLE) is an inflammatory autoimmune disorder that affects many body organs, especially the heart, lungs, spleen, and kidneys. About 85 percent of all patients are females, most of them between the ages of 10 and 50. Blacks are most often affected by this disorder. Although the cause of systemic lupus erythematosus is unknown, it is believed that people with the disorder manufacture antibodies that attack their own body tissues.

Onset is often seen during periods of emotional crisis or during severe exposure to sunlight or x-ray. Several drugs may cause the disorder as a side effect, including hydralazine, isoniazid, and certain anticonvulsive drugs. Viruses may also play a causative role.

Symptoms

The symptoms include loss of appetite, fever, malaise, and weight loss. Skin lesions may be present. A characteristic "butterfly" rash affects a few patients; it occurs over the nose and cheek area. Alopecia (loss of hair) is common. Severe pains affecting the joints are extremely common and may be falsely attributed to arthritis. Joint pain may be severe, but the condition rarely results in deformity. Additionally, photophobia, transient blindness, blurring of vision, and conjunctivitis are present. Pleurisy, leading to lung disease, is frequent. Pericarditis is common. Heart failure may eventually result.

Treatment

Systemic lupus erythematosus requires intense therapy. First of all, any possibly precipitating drug should be withdrawn. Corticosteroids are required to control the serious complications of the disorder including blood changes, pericarditis, myocarditis, convulsions, etc. Antimalarial drugs such as hydroxychloroquine may be used to reduce joint or skin inflammation. Other symptoms are treated as necessary.

Prognosis depends upon which organ systems have been involved. If the lung, kidney, or heart has been affected, the prospect is much worse than if the disease is limited to the skin and joints.

The individual may eventually become crippled. Orthopedic devices such as supports may be necessary, as well as canes, wheelchairs, crutches, or walkers.

Drugs Used in Treatment

R steroid hormones—*Aristocort; Medrol; prednisone*

Health Care Accessories—*ambulation aids*

Related Topics—*Allergy; Pericarditis*

Tennis Elbow

Tennis elbow is a form of bursitis that causes pain in the area of the elbow and possibly radiating down the arm. The condition is probably caused by repetitive grasping or rotating motions of the forearm that injure the tendons around the elbow. Middle-aged people usually develop this condition, although it is seen at all ages.

Treatment

The best treatment is simply to rest the arm. A cold pack applied to the area may reduce inflammation. Aspirin will relieve the pain and reduce inflammation. Corticosteroids may be given to control an acute attack of severe pain. An elastic bandage placed firmly over the forearm may also help reduce pain. In severe cases, a plaster cast or restrictive elbow brace may be required.

Drugs Used in Treatment

OTC analgesics—*see the list under Pain and Fever*
OTC external analgesics—*Absorbine; Absorbine Jr.; Ben-Gay; Heet; Infra-Rub*
℞ steroid hormones—*Aristocort; Medrol; prednisone*
℞ anti-inflammatories—*Butazolidin; Clinoril; Indocin; Motrin; Nalfon; Naprosyn; Tolectin*
℞ sedatives and hypnotics—*Librium; Serax; Tranxene; Valium*

Health Care Accessories—*disposable hot and cold packs; gel hot and cold packs; elastic bandage; elastic hosiery; heating pad; hot water bottle; ice bag*

Related Topic—*Arthritis*

Trick Knee

A "trick knee" results from damage to the cartilage around the knee. Damage is usually due to trauma to the knee. Severe pain and immobility of the knee are the major symptoms.

Treatment

Surgery may be necessary to repair damaged cartilage. Glucocorticoid steroids are given to help control the inflammation. Aspirin will help control the pain and prevent inflammation.

Drugs Used in Treatment

OTC analgesics—*see the list under Pain and Fever*
℞ steroid hormones—*Aristocort; Medrol; prednisone*

Miscellaneous Injuries

The topics covered in this section are, on the whole, the minor injuries likely to be encountered in most families. The guidelines given for treatment here are meant to allay anxiety and to indicate when medical treatment is probably necessary. This information is not a substitute for a comprehensive guide to first aid, and every family should have a first aid manual (for example, the one prepared by the American Red Cross) in its library. It is wise to learn about first-aid measures before emergencies occur. Therefore, it is also recommended that someone in every family take courses both in general first aid procedures and in cardiopulmonary resuscitation (CPR).

Animal Bites

Animal bites that break the skin are treated in basically the same way that other cuts, scrapes, or puncture wounds are treated. However, animal bites present the additional danger of rabies, and any animal bite that breaks the skin should be seen by a doctor.

Treatment

The wound should be thoroughly cleansed with soap and water. The animal should be observed for signs of illness. A wild animal should be captured and killed, if necessary. Contact a doctor at once.

Related Topics—*Cuts; Puncture Wounds; Rabies; Tetanus; Scrapes*

Bruises

A bruise is nothing more than a break in a blood vessel under the skin. Usually caused by a blow or a fall, a bruise is likely to be first red, and then black and blue. A black eye is an example of a typical bruise.

Minor bruises are little to worry about; extensive or severe bruising may indicate serious internal injury—see a doctor. Spontaneous bruises, i.e., those that appear without noticeable cause, should also be seen by a doctor.

Treatment

Apply cold to a minor bruise. The cold will limit discoloration and reduce pain, and limit swelling. After a day or so, apply heat. Heat will help hasten reabsorption of the bruise.

Health Care Accessories—*heating pad; ice bag*

Burns and Sunburn

The skin can be burned by flames, hot objects, the sun, or by electrical, radioactive, or chemical agents. Common chemical burns are caused by strong acid or alkali substances and by gas such as mustard gas or lewisite (an arsenic-containing gas).

Regardless of the cause, burns can result in severe damage. Someone severely burned may be in a state of shock due to fluid loss. There may be severe pain, fright, or anxiety. In addition, whenever the skin is broken, bacteria and other infective organisms may enter to cause internal infections.

Burn Classification

Burns are classified into three types. A first-degree burn damages the outer layer of skin, causing a sensation of increased warmth, tenderness, and pain. Redness and mild swelling occur. Most sunburns can be classified as a first-degree burn.

A second-degree burn involves the outer layer of skin and the layer immediately beneath it. Second-degree burns blister and are more painful than first-degree burns because nerve endings are affected.

A third-degree burn destroys all layers of skin and damages deeper tissues. Because the nerve endings are destroyed, a third-degree burn is painless once the initial damage is done. The skin may appear charred or white and lifeless. Someone with a third-degree burn usually goes into shock as evinced by lowered blood pressure, weak pulse, pale face, cold perspiration, increased respiration, restlessness, and confusion. The extremities feel cold and clammy.

Treatment

First-degree burns usually heal within two weeks without complications or scarring. Home remedies are sufficient for first-degree burns. Cold water soaks or milk compresses will relieve the pain and reduce swelling. Aspirin or acetaminophen will reduce pain. If pain is severe, a preparation containing codeine or another narcotic may be required.

A first-aid cream or ointment containing a local anesthetic may be used to reduce pain. Products containing benzocaine are the best, although other local anesthetics are also effective.

Second- or third-degree burns should be treated by a doctor. No cream or ointment should be applied to the burn area until after the doctor has examined it, because it will have to be removed before proper therapy can be performed. This can be painful and may cause further damage. Serious burns must be treated by systemic antibiotic therapy, such as penicillin. Hospitalization and bed rest are indicated for extensive burns. Skin grafts may be required for extensive second- and third-degree burns.

Drugs Used in Treatment

Recommended treatment with OTC drugs—*Americaine local anesthetic is recommended to relieve the pain of a first-degree burn. It contains 20 percent benzocaine.*
OTC analgesics—*see the list under Pain and Fever*
OTC local anesthetics—*Americaine; Nupercainal*
OTC antiseptics and burn remedies—*Bactine, Foille; Medi-Quik; Noxzema; Solarcaine*
R̞ analgesics—*Darvocet-N; Darvon; Darvon Compound-65; Demerol; Empirin Compound with Codeine; Equagesic; Fiorinal; Fiorinal with Codeine; Motrin;*

Norgesic; Parafon Forte; Percodan; Robaxin; Soma Compound; Synalgos-DC; Talwin; Tylenol with Codeine

Ŗ **antibiotics**—*amoxicillin; ampicillin; erythromycin; Keflex; Minocin; penicillin G; penicillin potassium phenoxymethyl; Terramycin; tetracycline hydrochloride; Vibramycin*

Related Topic—*Shock*

Concussion

A concussion is an injury to the brain resulting from a fall or a blow with a blunt object. A concussion may be mild or serious.

Symptoms

Someone who has suffered a head injury is likely to have a headache and feel sleepy, and may vomit and look pale. These symptoms do not indicate a concussion.

Symptoms that do indicate a concussion include unconsciousness, confusion, delirium, or amnesia. There may be repeated vomiting, disturbances in vision, balance or coordination, and a bloody or watery discharge from an ear or nostril. Pupils may not be equal in size (although some people's pupils are normally unequal). Someone who has had a concussion is not easy to awaken. There may be a stiff neck, slow pulse, or abnormal breathing.

Treatment

Any of the above symptoms of concussion signal a need for a doctor's attention. Someone who has suffered a head injury without displaying these symptoms should be watched carefully for 24 hours to make sure that no symptoms develop.

Treatment of a minor concussion is essentially bed rest, restriction of activity, and mild analgesics to treat headache. A serious concussion may require hospitalization and possibly surgery.

Drugs Used in Treatment

OTC analgesics—*see the list under Pain and Fever*

Cuts

Most cuts are only skin-deep, and they do not require a doctor's care. If, however, the wound is deep, there is a danger that underlying structures (muscles, tendons, nerves) may be damaged, and a doctor should be consulted. A cut with ragged edges, one embedded with dirt, or a serious cut on the face should also be seen by a doctor to minimize unsightly scarring and the danger of infection.

Treatment

Treat minor cuts as follows: apply pressure to the cut with sterile gauze (or clean cloth if gauze is not available) for five to ten minutes to stop bleeding. Once the bleeding has stopped, wash the wound thoroughly with soap and water. Make certain that no dirt remains within the cut. An antiseptic is usually not required. Dry the wound well, and close it with a nonsticking bandage or a butterfly. Keep a close watch for signs of infection over the next several days. Signs of infection include increased tenderness, swelling, pus, or red streaks radiating from the wound.

Major cuts require a doctor's attention to make sure no dirt remains in the wound. Stitches may be required to keep the wound closed. The doctor will advise if tetanus shots are needed.

Drugs Used in Treatment

Recommended treatment with OTC drugs—*Unless deep, cuts generally do not need to be treated with an antiseptic. If you want to apply a first-aid cream, choose Mycitracin, Neo-Polycin, Neosporin, or Polysporin.*
OTC external anti-infectives—*Baciguent; B.F.I.; Mercurochrome; Mycitracin; Neo-Polycin; Neosporin; Polysporin*

Health Care Accessories—*adhesive bandages; adhesive tape; dressings; gauze bandage*

Related Topics—*Puncture Wounds; Scrapes; Tetanus*

Electric Shock

Electric shock may cause a local, unpleasant tingling or fatal cardiac arrest depending on the amount of current, whether it is direct or alternating, the duration of exposure, and the current's pathway through the body.

Symptoms

Electric shock may cause temporary or prolonged unconsciousness. Pulse may be absent, blood pressure may fall, the skin may turn cold and blue, then eventually black. Breathing may stop or become rapid.

Treatment

The first concern is to free the victim from the current. Turning off the power, if it can be safely done, may be the most rapid way to free the victim. Otherwise, it may be necessary for the rescuers to move the victim away from the power source. When this is done, the rescuers must make sure that they are not grounded (standing on a dry board or dry newspapers, etc.) and should use a dry board, rope, or other non-metallic object to pull or push the victim free.

Once contact is broken, the victim should be given cardiopulmonary resuscitation until medical help arrives. Attempts at resuscitation should be continued for as long as necessary—breathing centers paralyzed by electric shock may take a long time to recover.

Fractures

It's often difficult to determine whether a bone is broken (fractured). Obvious deformity (an extra bend in a limb, for example) or pain that prevents use of an extremity usually indicates a fracture, but only x-rays can make the diagnosis certain. Other symptoms that may indicate a fracture include pain on movement, numbness, and swelling and blueness of the skin. If a seemingly minor accident causes pain that persists for three or four days, a doctor should be consulted. If the apparent injury is in the pelvis or thigh, or if the victim is sweating, pale, dizzy, or thirsty, medical attention should be sought immediately.

Treatment

If a fracture is suspected, movement of the injured limb should be limited. Splint the limb to give it support and immobilize it, and go to a doctor.

If the injury seems minor, apply cold packs to reduce pain and swelling. Aspirin or acetaminophen may be taken. Immobilize the limb with a splint, and rest and protect it. Test the limb frequently to see if pain persists. Pain 48 hours after the injury signals a need for a doctor's attention.

Drugs Used in Treatment

OTC analgesics—*see the list under Pain and Fever*

Health Care Accessory—*ice bag*

Frostbite

Frostbite is an injury caused by exposure to cold. Frostbite occurs when crystals form, either superficially or deeply, in the fluids and underlying soft tissue of the skin. Factors that contribute to the likelihood of suffering frostbite include dressing inadequately, the ingestion of alcohol, certain diseases of the vascular system, and exhaustion. The very young and the elderly are the most vulnerable.

Symptoms

Just before frostbite sets in, the affected skin may be slightly flushed; then hard, white, cold areas appear on the extremities or the face. The tissue may be insensitive; it will feel cold and numb. As the body part is rewarmed, the area becomes red and blotchy. It may be painful to the touch or there may be a sensation of "pins and needles" or of numbness. Small blisters may appear. Severe frostbite may cause gangrene (which, in some cases, may necessitate amputation).

Treatment

A traditional treatment of frostbite was to rub the area with snow. This method is contraindicated. Tissue damaged by frostbite is extremely tender, and any rubbing or friction can cause further damage.

Anyone suspected of having frostbite should get indoors as soon as possible. Rapid rewarming of the frostbitten part by immersion in warm (100° to 104° F) water is the preferred treatment. In the field, the frostbitten area can be rewarmed by contact with a warm body part. (Place frostbitten fingers in the armpit, for example.) Using water that is too hot can cause further damage to the skin. Try to keep the entire body warm. Warm drinks are helpful. Aspirin or acetaminophen help control the pain. Keep the area clean to prevent secondary infection.

Drugs Used in Treatment

OTC analgesics—*see the list under Pain and Fever*

Heatstroke

Heatstroke (also called heat collapse or sunstroke) is a grave emergency caused by exposure to excessive heat. Heatstroke occurs when the body's heat-regulating mechanism fails, as evidenced by an extremely high fever and lack of sweating. The individual collapses. If heatstroke is not treated, the condition may progress to convulsions, coma, and death.

Lack of water, alcoholism, excessive sweating, vomiting, and diarrhea increase susceptibility to heat disorders. Older people are most commonly affected although no one is immune.

Symptoms

Symptoms of oncoming prostration include a hot, dry, and flushed skin, dizziness, mental confusion, vertigo, headache, a fast and weak pulse, nausea, weakness, dim or blurred vision, mild muscular cramps, and irritability. The individual is listless or possibly unconscious. The body temperature is elevated and rises rapidly, possibly as high as 106° F or more. If the body temperature reaches 108° F and is not brought down immediately, severe and irreversible brain damage will occur.

Prevention

Persons working in hot climates should maintain a high fluid intake at all times. Light, loose-fitting, well ventilated clothing is generally advisable, although heavier clothing may be preferable in arid desert environments.

Treatment

Anyone who passes out should be given medical attention by a doctor. After a doctor or medical help has been summoned, the patient should be cooled rapidly. Place the individual in a tub of cold water and rub the skin until the temperature comes down. The individual may also be wrapped in a cold, wet sheet. Measure the body temperature with a rectal thermometer every eight to ten minutes. If the temperature goes below 98.6° F, then keep the patient warm. Keep massaging the skin to prevent the blood vessels from constricting. If the temperature again starts to go above normal, repeat the cold water soaks and rubbing.

Another condition, heat exhaustion, is similar to heatstroke, but less severe. The skin appears cold and clammy, but the pulse and body temperature seem normal. The person feels faint, but relaxation in the shade will relieve symptoms. Balanced fluids (such as Gatorade) are beneficial.

Health Care Accessory—*fever thermometer*

Puncture Wounds

A puncture is a wound whose depth is greater than its length and width. Most puncture wounds occur in the extremities and are caused by objects such as nails, needles, knives, pins, and splinters. Some puncture wounds actually perforate parts of the body—a nail, for example, might penetrate and pass through the foot.

Puncture wounds are ideal sites for developing tetanus (lockjaw), and they are prone to infection because they are hard to clean. If a puncture wound penetrates deeply, it may damage internal organs, particularly if the wound is on the chest or abdomen. In addition, punctures sometimes harbor foreign bodies (a broken needle, a piece of a splinter, etc.) that are difficult to detect.

Treatment

A puncture wound should be washed thoroughly with soap and water and inspected to make sure no objects remain in the wound. Surgery or x-rays may be required to determine that no foreign objects are present in the wound. Anyone with a puncture wound should consider having a tetanus booster. The wound should be covered with a sterile bandage and watched closely for signs of infection (redness, swelling, pus, increased tenderness).

If the wound is on the chest or abdomen, if part of the penetrating object remains in the wound, if tenderness persists for more than two days, or if signs of infection appear, the wound should be seen by a doctor.

Health Care Accessories—*adhesive tape; dressings; gauze bandage*

Related Topic—*Tetanus*

Scrapes

A scrape is a shallow break in the skin. Scrapes are distinguished from cuts and puncture wounds in that their depth is less than their surface length and width.

Some children seem to have scrapes every day. They are the most common and least dangerous of childhood injuries. Because most of them do not involve a full thickness of skin, they usually heal with little or no scarring.

Treatment

Apply pressure with a square of sterile gauze to stop the bleeding. Wash the wound with soap and water, and look carefully for any embedded dirt. Any dirt, sand, gravel, or blacktop left in the wound may be permanently sealed under the skin.

Once the wound is clean, a first-aid ointment may be applied. If the wound is likely to get dirty, cover it with a sterile, preferably nonsticky bandage. Otherwise, leave it open to the air and sun. Most scrapes scab rapidly. Watch for signs of infection until the scab falls off.

Drugs Used in Treatment

Recommended treatment with OTC drugs—*If you want to apply a first-aid cream, choose Mycitracin, Neo-Polycin, Neosporin, or Polysporin.*
OTC external anti-infectives—*Baciguent; B.F.I.; Mercurochrome; Mycitracin; Neo-Polycin; Neosporin; Polysporin*

Health Care Accessories—*adhesive bandages; adhesive tape; dressings; gauze bandage*

Shock

The term shock is used to describe a sudden decrease in blood pressure or a collapse of the circulation. Generally, shock occurs when a great deal of blood or fluid has been lost or when blood vessels dilate, causing blood to pool and not circulate effectively. Shock may occur with severe infection, burns, wounds and broken bones, hemorrhage, excessive vomiting, insect stings (in hypersensitive individuals), heart attacks, and certain drugs. Shock may happen in virtually every serious accident, burn, poisoning or injury.

If shock is not treated by a doctor, death usually results. Unfortunately, shock frequently does not occur until some time after the event when the individual is alone and no help is near.

Symptoms

Symptoms of shock include weakness, rapid but weak pulse, paleness, cold and clammy skin, sweating, chills, thirst, nausea, shallow breathing, and very low blood pressure. Unless treated, the person in shock will go into a coma.

Treatment

Shock should be considered in any emergency situation after immediate life-saving first aid is given, i.e., after bleeding has been stopped, after making sure that the victim's breathing passages are open, and after giving cardio-pulmonary resuscitation if necessary. The victim should lie flat, or with the head lower than the rest of the body (unless the head has been injured), and should be kept warm. Contact a doctor. A person in shock should be hospitalized as soon as possible. Do not give food or water until the doctor directs it.

There are no specific drugs used to treat shock. Epinephrine may be given to elevate blood pressure and re-establish circulation. Narcotics will ease pain and alleviate shock. Blood or plasma infusions may also be necessary. Massive doses of steroids are also used.

Tooth, Broken

A dentist should be notified whenever a tooth is broken, chipped, or damaged. If the damage is such that the soft pulp within the tooth is exposed, the tooth must be capped or filled. If the damage is great, the tooth may have to be removed. Otherwise bacteria may invade the soft tissues, causing an abscess at the tooth's root that may result in severe gum damage and possibly systemic infection.

Analgesics such as aspirin or acetaminophen may be taken to relieve any pain caused by the injury.

Drugs Used in Treatment

OTC analgesics—*see the list under Pain and Fever*
℞ analgesics—*Darvocet-N; Darvon; Darvon Compound-65; Demerol; Empirin Compound with Codeine; Equagesic; Fiorinal; Fiorinal with Codeine; Motrin; Percodan; Synalgos-DC; Talwin; Tylenol with Codeine*

Tooth, Knocked Out

If a tooth is knocked out in an accident, it should be carefully wrapped and taken—along with its owner—to a dentist immediately. It may be possible for the dentist to clean the tooth, sterilize it, and replant it in the gum. It will be fastened to surrounding teeth and held in place for a month or more. The tooth should eventually take hold and begin to grow again, although success is not guaranteed. Eventually the root of a replanted tooth will probably die away, and the tooth will come out. However, the replanting procedure may allow the use of the tooth for several years more than would be otherwise possible.

Analgesics such as aspirin or acetaminophen may be taken to help control any pain.

Drugs Used in Treatment

OTC analgesics—*see the list under Pain and Fever*
℞ analgesics—*Darvocet-N; Darvon; Darvon Compound-65; Demerol; Empirin Compound with Codeine; Equagesic; Fiorinal; Fiorinal with Codeine; Motrin; Percodan; Synalgos-DC; Talwin; Tylenol with Codeine*

Infectious Diseases

An infectious disease is one caused by the invasion and multiplication of microorganisms—bacteria, viruses, and protozoans for example. Each of us is susceptible to such invasion to a different degree; thus, some of us are able to tolerate and resist an infection such as the plague that wiped out enormous parts of the European population during the Middle Ages, and most of the people who are infected with the bacilli that cause leprosy never develop any symptoms. A break in the skin or being generally rundown can make us more susceptible to infection; inoculation with the appropriate vaccine can make us immune.

Common infectious diseases that principally affect one organ system are discussed in the appropriate section of this book. For example, amebic dysentery is discussed in the chapter on gastrointestinal tract disorders, and shingles (caused by a viral infection) is discussed with other disorders that affect the skin. The infectious diseases discussed here are generally those with symptoms that can be less specifically related to a single body system. Following is a description of the most common types of infectious diseases.

Bacterial infections. Bacteria are microscopic organisms, and are single-celled, that inhabit normal, healthy people by the billions. Most are harmless to humans; some, such as those that live in the intestinal tract, perform useful functions. Some disease-causing, or pathogenic, bacteria attack the body's tissues directly. Others secrete poisonous substances called toxins; botulism is an example of a disease caused by a bacterially produced toxin.

Bacteria can be transmitted from one person to another by skin contact (gonorrhea), by ingestion of food or drink (cholera), or by inhalation (tuberculosis). Bacterially-caused diseases are frequently curable; certain bacteria are killed by certain antibiotics. Other bacterial diseases are preventable by injection of an antitoxin or by vaccination.

Viral infections. A virus is the "bug" responsible for diseases as prevalent and relatively innocuous as the common cold and as life-threatening as rabies. Viruses are smaller than bacteria; some strains even infect bacteria. Viruses live and reproduce only within living cells, and only certain cells are vulnerable to a specific virus. We may be hosts to many viruses without suffering any adverse effects, but if enough vulnerable cells are attacked, we can become sick.

Viruses can be transmitted in the same ways that bacteria can. Animal or insect bites are another important mode of transmission.

There is no effective medical treatment for viruses. Because a virus lives inside a cell, any treatment designed to kill the virus is also likely to damage the cell. In addition, there are thousands of different viruses—each with different properties—and an agent effective against one virus probably would not stop the rest. Doctors can successfully immunize people against certain viruses by using a live but weakened virus or a strong serum from people previously infected by the virus. The efficacy of such immunization is evidenced by the eradication of smallpox. Until an effective treatment is developed, therapy for viral diseases aims for symptomatic relief.

Fungal infections. One example of a fungal infection is athlete's foot, an irritating but not dangerous disease. Another fungal infection is histoplasmosis, a possibly fatal disorder. Fungi are members of the vegetable kingdom that do not contain chlorophyll; most do not grow on humans but they are occasionally inhaled or picked up, and they can cause problems.

Protozoan infections. Protozoans are single-celled animals, some of which are serious parasites of man. Malaria, a disease caused by a blood protozoan, kills about a million people every year, and the protozoan that causes amebic dysentery may infect 10 percent of the population of the United States (although most will be asymptomatic). Malaria is transmitted by the bite of an infected mosquito. Intestinal protozoans are often contracted through ingesting food or water contaminated with cysts. Prevention of protozoan infections often hinges on good sanitation and hygiene.

Worm infections. The worms that infect man are multi-celled members of the animal kingdom that are often transmitted in contaminated food or drink or by the hand-to-mouth route. Hookworms gain entry to the body through the soles of the feet. Some worms remain in the intestine; others migrate through the body. Mild worm infestation may produce no symptoms, but severe infection with some worms can lead to anemia, to a form of pneumonia, and to other serious problems.

Candidiasis

Candidiasis is an infection caused by the fungus, *Candida albicans.* Usually it affects the skin and mucous membranes, although it may become systemic. This microorganism is normally found in the mouth and gastrointestinal tract; only when a debilitating disease or malnutrition occurs, or when a person starts taking a broad-spectrum antibiotic (such as ampicillin or tetracycline) that disrupts the normal balance of microorganisms, does an "overgrowth" of this fungus occur. Ill-fitting dentures may be a contributing factor to infections in the mouth.

The terms moniliasis and thrush are also used to describe this infection. Thrush is used almost exclusively to describe infections in the mouth.

Symptoms

Symptoms vary with the site of the infection. Thrush is characterized by creamy-white, curdlike patches in the mouth. The patches may cause pain, and if they are scraped away, a reddened bleeding surface is revealed. If the infection is in the anus or vagina, intense itching and burning will be primary symptoms. If vaginal, the infection may also cause a white or yellow discharge.

Treatment

Sometimes the infection spreads to other parts of the body, including the gastrointestinal tract and lungs. The infection is treated with antifungal drugs; nystatin is the agent of choice. The vehicle for administering the drug is chosen according to the site of the infection. The mouth may be rinsed with a nystatin wash three times a day before the medication is swallowed. Gentian violet solution (1 percent) may be painted on the affected area. Nystatin suppositories may be used for vaginal infections. Sometimes the use of a vaginal douche is also recommended. For serious infections, amphotericin B, miconazole, and clotrimazole are used.

Drugs Used in Treatment

℞ **antifungal agents**—*Lotrimin; Monistat 7; Mycostatin*

Chicken Pox

Chicken pox is caused by a virus; a similar virus causes shingles. Chicken pox is among the most communicable of all diseases. Epidemics occur during the winter and early spring every three to four years, with children between the ages of five and eight the most susceptible. People are susceptible until they have contracted the disease, but once they have contracted it, they have a lifetime immunity from further attacks.

Symptoms

Initial symptoms usually appear about two weeks after exposure and may include mild headache, low fever, and fatigue. Twenty-four hours after the initial symptoms (if they occur) the rash appears. The rash is generalized over the body except for the face and extremities, which are sometimes spared. It starts with redness and flushing but gradually (over a period of 24 to 48 hours) develops into raised blisters that finally crust. The person is contagious for six days after the rash appears. Symptoms are usually more severe among adults: and include high fever, stupor, and delirium.

Treatment

Someone with chicken pox should be isolated and should not share any personal items with others. The disease is transmitted by direct contact.

The milder forms require treatment only of the symptoms. The rash causes intense itching, and scratching may cause skin damage and infection. Application of calamine lotion or a product containing a local anesthetic to the blisters may be helpful.

Warm baths can also relieve the itching somewhat. After bathing, clean underclothing should be put on. The hands and nails should be kept clean, and the nails should be well trimmed to keep from spreading or introducing secondary infection by scratching.

Cyproheptadine, an antihistamine, is taken orally to help the itching. If any of the lesions become infected, application of an antibiotic ointment or cream will help. If the lesions are infected they will be surrounded by redness and may be draining pus.

Complications rarely develop from chicken pox. If any do, they may include infection of the blood, scarlet fever, and pneumonia. Encephalitis is a very rare complication.

Drugs Used in Treatment

Recommended treatment with OTC drugs—*To relieve itching, choose your pharmacy's generic brand of calamine lotion or the local anesthetic Americaine. Using a moisturizing oil in the bath water may also relieve the itching somewhat. Should the lesions become infected, apply Mycitracin, Neo-Polycin, Neosporin, or Polysporin.*

OTC miscellaneous— *calamine lotion*

OTC local anesthetics and burn remedies—*Americaine; Bactine; Foille; Medi-Quik; Noxzema; Nupercainal; Solarcaine*

OTC external anti-infectives—*Baciguent; B.F.I.; Mercurochrome; Mycitracin; Neo-Polycin; Neosporin; Polysporin*

R_x antihistamine—*Periactin*

Related Topic—*Shingles*

Cholera

Cholera is an infectious disease acquired by ingesting food or drink contaminated by feces from carriers of the cholera microorganism. Contaminated water supplies are the major source of infection. The microorganism lives in the intestine and secretes a powerful substance that in turn causes the symptoms.

Although cholera is rare in the United States today, travelers to other countries should take care to guard against cholera. If left untreated, the disease may be fatal in as many as 50 percent of all cases.

Symptoms

Initial symptoms of cholera include a slight fullness in the abdomen; stomach and leg cramps; cold, clammy, wrinkled skin; and loss of appetite. The hands and feet seem cold, and the individual may vomit. The characteristic and most dangerous symptom appears next—diarrhea with a large number of liquid stools that are first brown and then become clear and watery. The stools may contain small amounts of mucus or, because of the severity of the diarrhea, tiny shreds of intestinal tissue. These are sometimes referred to as "rice water" stools. Fluids must be replaced immediately; otherwise the person rapidly becomes dehydrated. Blood pressure goes down. The patient develops sunken eyes and subnormal body temperature. Breathing becomes rapid and shallow. Muscle cramps, diminished urination, shock, coma, and possible death follow.

Treatment

Cholera is treated with tetracycline, although tetracycline is not entirely effective. Fluids are given by intravenous injection. Electrolytes must be administered in order to maintain proper blood levels of the essential salts, especially potassium. The patient should be kept warm and should be given drinking water frequently.

Cholera is a self-limiting disease. Assuming that the patient receives adequate fluid and electrolyte replacement and that dehydration and shock do not occur, cholera runs its course in three to six days.

Drugs Used in Treatment

℞ antibiotics—*Minocin; Terramycin; tetracycline hydrochloride; Vibramycin*
℞ potassium replacements—*K-Lyte; potassium chloride*

Coccidioidomycosis

Coccidioidomycosis (Valley Fever, San Joaquin Fever, or Desert Fever) is most commonly seen in the southwestern United States and is caused by a fungus that grows in the soil in this area. The disease is most commonly seen among Mexicans, blacks, and Filipinos and is most serious among dark-skinned people. Pregnant women of any race are also more susceptible than the rest of the population.

The highest incidence of the disease is in areas, such as new housing developments, where the soil has been disturbed, thereby releasing the spores contained in the earth. Spores containing the fungus are carried by air currents and are inhaled by humans or by other animals. The animals release the spores in their droppings. Humans may pick up the fungus by handling the droppings in some way.

Symptoms

Over half of all infected persons do not have any demonstrable symptoms. Symptoms are primarily pulmonary. The individual may develop a fever, malaise, a slight dry cough, and chest pain. Night sweats and loss of appetite are common. Muscular aches, backache, and headache are present and may be severe. The individual may complain of weakness and weight loss. The knees and ankles frequently become swollen; the joints, painful. Breathing sounds become wheezy. The person may appear bluish, be short of breath, and may spit up blood.

Treatment

Coccidioidomycosis is treated with bed rest. The symptoms are treated as needed. All clothing and personal items of the patient should be thoroughly washed and dried before being used by other people. A possible complication is meningitis, which can be fatal.

Erysipelas

Erysipelas (St. Anthony's Fire) is an acute inflammation of the skin and underlying tissue caused by a bacterial infection.

Symptoms

The inflammation often starts at an open wound, classically on the nose or the cheek, although it can begin anywhere. The rash begins with a bright red spot which soon spreads to the surrounding skin. The area feels smooth, painful, and hot, and the dull red to scarlet rash gets larger from day to day. The area is tender and inflamed and can be pitted with a finger, showing that it is filled with fluid. There may be vesicles on the surface. As it spreads, the rash may advance to the eye area and cause the eyes to be swollen shut. The lymph nodes may be involved, becoming swollen and painful to the touch. The rash spreads for four to six days. Other symptoms include pain, fever, chills, and tiredness.

Treatment

Erysipelas has been recognized for over 2,000 years. At one time it was frequently fatal and was one of the most serious complications of surgical or bacterial wounds. The danger of the disease results from the possible complications—blood poisoning, pneumonia, and heart and kidney diseases (due to bacteria in the blood). Death may result.

Penicillin has lowered the incidence of fatalities due to this disease. Treatment with penicillin or ampicillin is usually satisfactory to completely eradicate erysipelas. Bed rest is a mandatory part of treatment, and the head of the bed should be elevated. Aspirin or acetaminophen should be taken for pain and fever. Cold compresses may also help relieve pain. All clothing and personal articles used by the infected person should be washed in hot, sudsy water before being reused or handled by other people.

Drugs Used in Treatment

OTC analgesics—*see the list under Pain and Fever*
℞ antibiotics—*amoxicillin; ampicillin; erythromycin; Keflex; Minocin; penicillin G; penicillin potassium phenoxymethyl; Terramycin; tetracycline hydrochloride; Vibramycin*

Histoplasmosis

Histoplasmosis is caused by a fungus found in the soil of many areas, including the central and eastern United States. The causative organism has been found in many animals, and it is believed that the most common introduction of the fungus to humans is through the contamination of soil from the droppings of chickens, bats, and pigeons. The spores may be picked up or inhaled. White middle-aged or older males are especially prone to the disease. Many people with histoplasmosis also have underlying chronic obstructive pulmonary disease (emphysema).

Symptoms

Symptoms of histoplasmosis may be mild or unrecognized. They may be mistaken for symptoms of a slight respiratory tract inflammation such as influenza or for those of tuberculosis. Histoplasmosis has been misdiagnosed as tuberculosis.

Mild flu symptoms may last three to four days. Some patients develop ulcerations on the tongue, palate, or other areas within the mouth. There may be a fever. Nausea, vomiting, and other gastrointestinal symptoms—including black, tarry stools—may be present. The individual may grow weak and emaciated. In later stages, more severe fever, cough, and chest pain develop. Liver and spleen enlargement may be noted. Lung x-rays reveal cavities similar to those caused by tuberculosis. Advanced, severe cases can be fatal due to respiratory damage.

Treatment

There is no specific therapy for the disease. Bed rest and treatment of the symptoms are indicated. Aspirin or acetaminophen may be given for fever and minor chest pain. The antifungal drug, amphotericin B, has proven useful in some patients with the disease. All of the patient's clothing and personal items should be thoroughly washed and dried before other people touch them.

Drugs Used in Treatment

OTC analgesics—*see the list under Pain and Fever*

Hookworm

Infection with hookworm is most common in warm climates where children go barefoot, such as in the southern United States. The hookworms penetrate the body through the soles of the feet and migrate through the body, eventually reaching the intestine where they attach to the intestinal wall and feed on blood. If the worms are not eliminated, anemia eventually results.

Symptoms

Symptoms include weakness, fatigue, hunger, shortness of breath upon exertion, and palpitations. There may be sores or small blisters on the soles of the feet where the worm entered. The sores itch profusely.

Treatment

Hookworm infestation is treated with anthelmintics. Without proper treatment, the worms may live for 10 to 20 years.

Drugs Used in Treatment

℞ anthelmintic—*Povan*

Infectious Mononucleosis

Mononucleosis is a viral infection that occurs mostly in young adults. It rarely occurs after age 35. Probably transmitted by respiratory droplets, the disease is often called the "kissing disease" although no one knows if kissing is actually a mode of transmission.

Symptoms

Symptoms of mononucleosis include fever; headache; sore throat; painful swelling of the lymph nodes in the neck, under the arms, and in the groin; weakness; fatigue; loss of appetite; and chills. Photophobia, eye pain, and jaundice may also be present. A rash may occur. Onset of mononucleosis is often gradual, and the symptoms may persist for as long as six months.

Treatment

Complete bed rest is indicated during the early stages of the disease. After the first week or so, the individual can walk about, but should avoid strenuous exercise or work for several months because of the danger of rupture of the spleen. Aspirin or acetaminophen will relieve pain and fever, and hot salt water gargles or OTC throat lozenges will soothe the sore throat. There is little danger from uncomplicated infectious mononucleosis.

Drugs Used in Treatment

OTC analgesics—*see the list under Pain and Fever*
OTC lozenges—*Cēpacol (anesthetic and regular); Chloraseptic; Listerine, Sucrets; Synthaloids; Throat Discs*

Leprosy

Leprosy (Hansen's Disease) is an infectious disease caused by a bacterium closely related to the organism that causes tuberculosis. Leprosy tends to occur in warm climates and economically underdeveloped countries. Most leprosy sufferers live in an equatorial band that includes Africa, Southeast Asia, and South America. Although it is no longer considered a scourge in America, it does occur in the southern states and Hawaii. Fewer than 150 new cases are diagnosed each year in the United States.

The method of transmission has not been positively identified, but it is believed that the disease is spread by bacilli-laden nasal discharges. Only a small percentage of a population seems to be susceptible; some people are infected and never develop symptoms.

Symptoms

Leprosy attacks the skin, mucous membranes, and nerves. Lesions appear on the skin and mucous membranes of the mouth. Depending on the type of leprosy, huge nodules may appear on the skin. The disease causes the skin to thicken and wrinkle, producing a massive overall disfigurement. Spontaneous amputation of the fingers (this may also occur with toes) may occur, producing the characteristic "claw" hand. The disfigurement has usually begun by the time the disease is diagnosed, and this cannot be reversed. As the disease progresses, nerve and bone tissues become diseased.

Treatment

Two drugs are used to treat leprosy—dapsone and sulfoxone. The disease can now be largely controlled, and most leprosy patients can now live at home as long as they are taking medication.

Malaria

Protozoan parasites cause malaria. They are usually transmitted by the bite of an infected anopheles mosquito, although the disease is also occasionally transmitted by the contaminated needles used by drug abusers.

Malaria is usually limited to the tropics and other warm countries. However, a significant number of new cases still appear every year in the United States. Usually the people who come down with malaria in this country have been bitten during travel outside the country.

Symptoms

An infected individual develops chills that usually last for 15 to 60 minutes. Nausea, vomiting, and headache follow. The succeeding "hot stage" may last for several hours and is usually accompanied by a spiking fever that may reach 104° F or higher. Shortly thereafter, the individual begins sweating profusely. The fever begins to subside and the patient frequently falls asleep to awake later feeling better. An entire cycle may take as long as 72 hours.

Serious complications of malaria include severe headache, convulsions, delirium, and coma. High fever may cause additional convulsions. In more advanced stages, jaundice and severe anemia may occur. Additionally, liver, spleen, and kidney damage occur. The mortality rate may be as high as 30 percent.

Treatment

Treatment for malaria includes many nonspecific modalities to control fever, headache, and other symptoms. Specific treatment includes the drugs chloroquine and primaquine. For certain strains, quinine sulfate is given, and for some people, sulfonamide therapy or antibiotics may be beneficial.

Drugs Used in Treatment

Recommended treatment with OTC drugs—*Quinine sulfate, available over the counter, is the treatment of choice for certain strains of malaria. Aspirin or acetaminophen will relieve fever and minor aching.*
OTC analgesics—*see the list under Pain and Fever*
Ŗ **antibiotics**—*amoxicillin; ampicillin; erythromycin; Keflex; Minocin; penicillin G; penicillin potassium phenoxymethyl; Terramycin; tetracycline hydrochloride; Vibramycin*
Ŗ **antibacterials**—*Gantanol; Gantrisin*

Mastoiditis

Mastoiditis is an inflammation of the small air spaces within the mastoid bone, the bone behind the ear. It is a complication of purulent acute middle ear infections, and it can result from chronic sinusitis, scarlet fever, measles, diphtheria, and other inflammatory diseases of the nose and throat. Modern antibiotic therapy for middle ear infections has made mastoiditis uncommon, but whenever middle ear infection is not adequately treated, mastoiditis is a potential complication.

Mastoiditis is characterized by the destruction of the bony structure surrounding the ear canal and middle ear. The extension of infection brings pus into the air spaces within the mastoid bone, and this pus softens and destroys the bone.

Symptoms

Symptoms usually begin with a sore throat and other symptoms parallel to those of a cold—including mild earache. One of the aforementioned disorders has usually been present.

The earache worsens; discharge from the ear develops; there may be fever; tenderness, redness, and swelling may be apparent around the mastoid process. There may be impairment of hearing.

Treatment

Mastoiditis is treated with penicillin or other antibiotics. Eardrops or oral analgesics will be used to relieve pain. Occasionally surgery is necessary; the surgeon drills into the mastoid bone and suctions out the pus and debris that has collected within the bone.

Any earache that lasts longer than two days, especially when accompanied by the other symptoms described above, requires diagnosis and treatment by a doctor.

Drugs Used in Treatment

OTC analgesics—*see the list under Pain and Fever*
R antibiotics—*amoxicillin; ampicillin; erythromycin; Keflex; Minocin; penicillin G; penicillin potassium phenoxymethyl; Terramycin; tetracycline hydrochloride; Vibramycin*
R otic solution—*Auralgan*
R analgesics—*Darvocet-N; Darvon Compound-65; Demerol; Empirin Compound with Codeine; Equagesic; Fiorinal; Fiorinal with Codeine; Motrin; Percodan; Synalgos-DC; Talwin; Tylenol with Codeine*

Related Topic—*Middle Ear Infection*

Measles (Rubeola)

Measles and chicken pox are two of the most easily transmitted infectious diseases. Measles is spread by droplets from infected persons. One bout with measles confers lifetime immunity, as does injection with the measles vaccine when given at the correct age (around 15 months). Children who were vaccinated before they were 15 months old should be revaccinated prior to entering school to assure full immunity. Serious complications may occur, including encephalitis, middle ear infection, mastoiditis, and pneumonia.

Symptoms

Symptoms include fever, runny nose, cough, and white eruptions on the mucous membranes of the cheeks (Koplik's spots). Within three days of the appearance of the fever, the rash begins. It appears first on the face and neck and then spreads over the body.

256

Treatment

There is no specific treatment for measles, although medications are given for relief of symptoms. Because the disease is very contagious, someone with measles should be kept in isolation for 10 to 14 days. The eyes will be red and sensitive to light, and the patient should stay in a dark room or wear sunglasses.

Drugs Used in Treatment

Recommended treatment with OTC drugs—*Your pharmacy's generic brand of calamine lotion will relieve the itching of the rash somewhat.*
OTC miscellaneous—*calamine lotion*

Mumps

Mumps is an acute, highly contagious disease caused by a virus. It is spread by airborne droplets from an infected person or by direct contact with an infected person. Mumps primarily affects the salivary glands, causing pain in the jaws while eating or swallowing. The pain is aggravated by acidic solutions such as vinegar.

The disease may, especially when contracted by people past puberty, affect other organs including the nervous system, pancreas, thyroid, kidneys, tear glands, prostate, and testes. About 25 to 30 percent of postpuberal males who contract mumps will experience swelling of the testes. The swelling may be severe and may even result in sterility, although this occurs rarely. If contracted during the first four months of pregnancy, mumps can cause birth defects.

Most people contract mumps between ages 5 and 15. Of these, a full 40 percent will not exhibit clinically significant symptoms. One attack usually confers lifelong immunity. Immunity is also passed on to a child from its mother. This immunity usually lasts for approximately one year. Mumps vaccine is not indicated until after a child is one year old because of the likelihood of inherited immunity. Anyone who has reached puberty and has not had mumps should be immunized.

Symptoms

Initial symptoms include fever and chills, headache, loss of appetite, and malaise. Chewing and swallowing will be painful as the glands begin to swell. Usually the area in front of and below the ear swells, but the swelling may extend farther onto the neck as well. The swelling may be unilateral.

Treatment

Treatment is nonspecific and symptomatic. The patient should be isolated until the swelling subsides. Bed rest is advisable while the fever lasts. Using a warm saline solution to rinse the mouth will alleviate mouth pain. The diet should consist of soups and soft, nonacidic foods.

If testicular swelling occurs, the testes may be supported by wearing a suspensory. Application of ice packs may help to keep pain and swelling to a minimum. Analgesics may be given to relieve pain and/or reduce fever.

Drugs Used in Treatment

OTC analgesics—*see the list under Pain and Fever*

Health Care Accessories—*ice bag; suspensory*

Pinworms

Pinworms are parasites one-fourth to one-half inch in length. In humans, they are found in the lower part of the small intestine, the upper part of the large intestine, and the rectum.

Pinworm infestation results when the eggs are picked up (from bedding, toys, or scratching) and transferred to the mouth by the hands. The eggs are swallowed; the worms develop and mature in the gastrointestinal tract, and the female emerges from the anus at night to lay eggs on the skin surface. This causes intense itching in the area.

Symptoms

Children are affected more often than adults, and the only symptom is often a complaint that the child cannot sleep well due to itching around the anus. Sleeplessness may lead to irritability and a loss of appetite.

Treatment

Pyrvinium pamoate is the drug of choice for treating pinworms. Gentian violet is a traditional remedy. However, prescription medication is more effective.

Someone with pinworms should take care to wash thoroughly at least once a day, paying particular attention to the rectal area. Children should be taught to scrub their hands thoroughly before meals and after going to the bathroom. Fingernails should be kept short and clean. Someone with pinworms should change underclothing and pajamas daily. These items should be washed daily with hot water and soap to remove eggs. It is usually necessary to treat the entire family for pinworm infestation.

Drugs Used in Treatment

℞ anthelmintic—*Povan*

Rocky Mountain Spotted Fever

Rocky Mountain spotted fever is caused by a microorganism that is transmitted to man by the bite of the woodtick. The tick picks up the microorganisms by biting infected rodents such as mice, rats, squirrels, or chipmunks. When an infected tick bites someone, the microorganism is transmitted. The disease was originally detected in the Rocky Mountains, but most cases now occur in an area along the Eastern Seaboard and extending as far west as the Mississippi River. Most cases occur in the late spring and summer.

Symptoms

The symptoms of Rocky Mountain spotted fever include a sudden onset of high fever, skin rash, headache, sore throat, loss of appetite and weight, and nausea. Eventually the fever becomes severe, and chills, aches in the bones and muscles, severe abdominal pain, and severe nausea and vomiting become evident. The person is restless, unable to sleep, and irritable. Later developments may include delirium, stupor, lethargy, and coma. The face will be severely flushed, the eyes will burn, and there may be a discharge from the eyes. The rash appears first on the wrists and ankles, and then spreads to the arms, legs, and trunk. Initially, the rash is small red spots, but the spots grow larger and become interspersed with blood spots (petechiae). The liver and spleen may be enlarged, and jaundice and gangrene may develop.

Treatment

Rocky Mountain spotted fever must be differentiated from measles, typhoid, and meningococcemia, all of which have similar symptoms. If left untreated, the disease has an extremely high mortality rate.

Once identified, the disease can be successfully treated with tetracycline or chloramphenicol antibiotics. Aspirin or acetaminophen may be used to control the fever. Bed rest is indicated during convalescence.

Anyone entering heavy brush or other areas where ticks may live should be examined for ticks at least two to three times a day. Several hours may elapse between the time the tick bites and the injection of the microorganism into the bloodstream. Early removal of the tick from the skin may prevent the injection of the microorganisms and the onset of the disease.

Ticks should never be touched with bare fingers, nor should they be crushed on the skin. They should be removed by placing a drop of gasoline, lighter fluid, kerosine, turpentine, grease, or a similar chemical directly on the tick. Then gently and carefully pull the tick off with tweezers, being certain not to crush the body. The area should then be thoroughly washed with soap and water and rubbing alcohol. Tincture of merthiolate or tincture of iodine should be applied to disinfect the area.

Drugs Used in Treatment

OTC analgesics—*see the list under Pain and Fever*
OTC miscellaneous— *iodine; merthiolate*
R antibiotics—*amoxicillin; ampicillin; erythromycin; Keflex; Minocin; penicillin G; penicillin potassium phenoxymethyl; Terramycin; tetracycline hydrochloride; Vibramycin*

Roundworm

Roundworm eggs reach the body through contaminated food or water. The larvae migrate through the body; the mature worm lives in the small intestine. They may be ten to twelve inches or more in length.

Symptoms

Infection with roundworms (ascariasis), if mild, may produce no obvious symptoms. The larval migration may produce respiratory symptoms such as fever, cough, and wheezing. Other possible symptoms include abdominal pains, loss of weight, and malnutrition. Due to malnutrition, fatigue and weakness may be present. There may be abdominal swelling and diarrhea. A skin rash is sometimes seen.

Treatment

Roundworm infection is best treated with piperazine or pyrantel pamoate.

Drugs Used in Treatment

R anthelmintic—*Povan*

Rubella

Rubella, also known as German or three-day measles, is a viral disease, that is usually milder and less contagious than other forms of measles. It is spread by droplets from the nose or mouth of people with the disease. The major danger of the disease is its effect on fetuses. If a pregnant woman contracts the disease—especially during the first trimester of pregnancy—abortion, stillbirth, or birth defects such as mental retardation could result. Therefore, the U.S. Public Health Service strongly recommends that all girls be vaccinated before they reach puberty. Better still, the combined rubella/rubeola vaccine can be given at 15 months to everyone. Vaccination or one attack of rubella confers lifelong immunity.

Symptoms

Initial symptoms of rubella are similar to those of a mild cold. Two to three weeks after direct contact with someone who has the disease, a low-grade fever and headache may be present. The rash will appear concurrently or within 24 hours of the appearance of these symptoms. The rash is rose colored and appears first on the face and neck and then spreads across the entire body. The lymph nodes will be swollen and tender; the muscles and joints may be painful. The rash lasts two to three days, and the patient is contagious from the time the symptoms start to at least four days later.

Treatment

Other than giving aspirin for relief of pain and fever, there is no treatment required for rubella, unless it is contracted by a pregnant woman.

If a woman is uncertain, she can have blood tests to determine whether she is susceptible to rubella. If she is susceptible and is not pregnant, she can receive the rubella vaccine. After vaccination, she must not become pregnant for at least three months.

If she is already pregnant, the vaccine must not be given as it could theoretically cause birth defects. If she has been exposed, gamma globulin injections can be given in the hope that they will modify the disease and prevent complications.

Drugs Used in Treatment

OTC analgesics—see the list under Pain and Fever

Health Care Accessory—fever thermometer

Scarlet Fever

Scarlet fever is an infectious disease caused by the streptococcal bacteria. The disease usually affects children and is highly contagious; it is spread by droplets from infected individuals.

Symptoms

Symptoms include a dark red rash over the entire body, a high fever, vomiting, and sore throat. The tongue will be inflamed and beefy red (raspberry or strawberry tongue). Small scarlet spots appear in the mouth. A grayish membrane appears over the back of the throat. The lymph nodes in the neck are enlarged. The face is flushed except around the mouth. After a week or so, the skin under the rash begins to peel. Without proper treatment, scarlet fever may result in severe inner-ear infections, rheumatic fever, encephalitis, and kidney disease.

Treatment

Penicillin is the treatment of choice. Aspirin or acetaminophen may be given to reduce the fever and ease the aches and pains. Bed rest is warranted during the early part of the disease. Hot or cold compresses applied to the lymph node area in the neck will also relieve the pain.

Drugs Used in Treatment

OTC analgesics—*see the list under Pain and Fever*
℞ antibiotics—*amoxicillin; ampicillin; erythromycin; Keflex; Minocin; penicillin G; penicillin potassium phenoxymethyl; Terramycin; tetracycline hydrochloride; Vibramycin*

Health Care Accessories— *fever thermometer; heating pad; ice bag*

Sexually Transmitted Diseases

The incidences of sexually transmitted diseases has increased to the point that many authorities now consider them to be at epidemic levels. It is now estimated that over 100 million cases of gonorrhea occur yearly worldwide, with over three million appearing in the United States. Three times as many men as women are diagnosed with the disease, owing in part to the large number of asymptomatic female carriers. More than half a million Americans contract syphilis yearly.

Although in most cases the following diseases are transmitted sexually, they may also be passed on to a new host by contamination of clothing, washcloths, furniture, or other inanimate objects. The diseases can also be transmitted to newborns during the birth process.

Genital herpes. Genital herpes is an infection of the lower genital tract caused by the herpes simplex virus, Type II. The disease is increasing in frequency; its incidence probably exceeds that of syphilis and equals that of gonorrhea in many social groups. The virus is believed to be a possible carcinogen, and if the infection occurs during pregnancy, it may cause stillbirth, spontaneous abortion, and neonatal death.

Genital herpes causes genital pain, a whitish vaginal discharge, painful urination, fever, malaise, loss of appetite, and vaginal bleeding. Multiple lesions appear in the genital area as low ulcerations filled with fluid.

The severe pain may be relieved with analgesic ointments. Because herpes genitalis is frequently accompanied by a fungal infection, nystatin vaginal suppositories may also be used. If the infection is present during pregnancy, delivery by cesarean section is usually performed to avoid transmitting the infection to the fetus. However, such measures are no guarantee that the child will not have the virus. Because no specific treatment is available for infants with genital herpes, those who contract the disease may die of viremia.

The infection frequently recurs, although the recurrent lesions are usually not as painful as the first ones and they do not last as long. Recurrence is more frequent during pregnancy, and the infection often recurs with the menses, or it may be provoked by emotional or physical stress, ultraviolet light, cold, or fever.

Symptomatic relief may be obtained with wet dressings and sitz baths. Antibiotic ointments may be useful to prevent secondary infection. An analgesic may be taken to relieve pain.

Gonorrhea. The only communicable disease reported more often than gonorrhea is the common cold.

Gonorrhea is a bacterial disease. The human is the only known natural host of the infection. The primary means of transmission is contact with infected individuals, usually through sexual activity. The most common points of entry into the body are the urethra and the endocervix, although the disease can also be passed between individuals through contact of the infected genitals with either the anal canal or mouth of the other sexual participant. Gonorrheal infections can also be passed from mother to child during delivery, possibly resulting in contamination of the baby's eyes, a condition known as ophthalmia neonatorium. If left untreated, it can lead to blindness. Because of this danger, most states have laws that require a few drops of 1 percent silver nitrate solution to be placed in the eyes of all newborns on delivery.

In adult males, the infection's point of entry is usually through the penis. About a week after the infection is contracted, a pus-filled discharge begins. As the infection spreads, the need to urinate becomes more frequent and urgent.

Fifty to 75 percent of the females who have contracted the disease may be asymptomatic. When symptoms do occur, they include increased vaginal discharge and frequent and painful urination. Rectal discomfort is common. When these symptoms occur, the disease has advanced beyond the urethra.

At this stage, the disease is uncomplicated gonorrhea. Left untreated, the infection may spread to surrounding tissues, causing complicated gonorrhea. In males the most frequent complication is the extension of the infection into the prostate, causing inflammation, tenderness, and urinary obstruction. Advancement into the seminal vesicles and urinary bladder may also occur. A type of arthritis affecting the hands, wrists, knees, and ankles caused by the bacteria is also seen. In the female the bacteria may invade the endometrium, causing inflammation. The infection can further advance into the fallopian tubes resulting in fever and lower abdominal pain, and eventually sterility.

Gonorrhea must be treated as quickly as possible. Penicillin or ampicillin are the drugs of choice. Many times, probenecid is given at the same time because it increases the activity of the antibiotic.

An estimated 2 to 5 percent of persons contracting gonorrhea become infected with syphilis at the same time. It is recommended that all individuals with suspected gonorrhea be tested for syphilis at the same time.

Syphilis. Syphilis is also caused by bacteria. About 10 to 90 days after infection occurs, an ulcer forms at the point where the bacteria entered the body (commonly in the genital area; on the penis, anus, rectum, vulva, cervix, or perineum). Sores may also form on the lips and tongue. This sore generally persists for two to six weeks and then heals spontaneously. Although the sores are open, they are painless. At times they are so small that they may go undetected. This stage is known as primary syphilis.

Syphilis is caused by bacteria that penetrate mucous membranes or damaged skin. Within a few hours these bacteria may enter the bloodstream, producing a systemic infection long before the appearance of the primary lesion. Additionally, the primary lesion, and even the more advanced skin eruptions are nonspecific—they resemble many other known skin diseases.

The systemic infection (secondary syphilis), caused by this invasion of the blood, usually becomes apparent four to six weeks after the healing of the primary ulcer. The symptoms include a flu-like syndrome of headache, sore throat, runny nose and eyes, joint pain, fever, and chills. The lymph nodes become enlarged and tender. There is a generalized skin rash, possibly punctuated by some purulent or scaly patches. On white skin, the rash appears as pale red blotches. On black skin, it may appear as darker patches. The spots are smaller than a half-inch in diameter.

A period of latent syphilis then occurs. During this stage, which may continue for the rest of the person's life, relapses of generalized or localized eruptions occur on the skin or mucous membranes.

A condition called tertiary or late syphilis can also emerge during this latent period. This is a progressive inflammatory condition affecting the heart, blood vessels, and/or the nervous system. In the cardiovascular disorder, large arteries (such as the aorta) weaken, bulge and may burst. Within the central nervous system (neurosyphilis) the spinal cord and brain are damaged, leading to brain damage, paralysis, loss of coordination, blindness, and other severe symptoms.

Syphilis can be transmitted from mother to fetus (congenital syphilis). The fetus is susceptible after the fourth month of pregnancy. The placenta is not a barrier to the syphilis bacterium. Once the bacteria infect the fetus, they grow and multiply rapidly, frequently resulting in malformation, interstitial keratitis, and (rarely) in death shortly after birth.

The treatment of choice for syphilis is penicillin injections. Tetracycline or erythromycin are also used.

Trichomoniasis. Trichomoniasis is an infectious sexually transmitted disease. The vagina, urethra, and prostate are all susceptible.

The symptoms in females include a persistent vaginal inflammation with itching, burning, and sometimes a profuse, yellowish discharge. Symptoms often become worse following menstruation.

Symptoms rarely occur in males. When they do occur, they are present as a urethral or prostatic inflammation, occasionally accompanied by a pus-filled discharge.

Trichomoniasis is treated with the drug metronidazole. Both sexual partners must be treated, even though symptoms may be present in only one. Partners should also avoid intercourse until several weeks after the infection has healed.

Venereal warts. Venereal warts are caused by a virus. The lesions occur in the genital area and are most likely to appear on sexually-active females. Coitus is the principle method of spreading the infection.

Venereal warts are characterized by a rough warty area on the perineum and the area around the vagina. The warts are quite small when they first appear, but they may develop to over an inch in size by the time the individual consults a doctor. In some cases, they become so large that they interfere with urination and defecation. If the warts break, secondary inflammation may occur, creating a foul-smelling, extremely tender, painful mass. At this point, the individual is no longer able to engage in intercourse. If the patient is pregnant, delivery will be by cesarean section.

The warts are treated with local application of 25 percent podophyllin or by surgical removal. The patient should be advised that touching the warts and then touching the area around the eyes may spread the infection.

If the patient is pregnant, treatment is extremely difficult and may be dangerous to the infant. In such cases, freezing of the tissues or their destruction by electrocauterization may be performed.

Contraceptive creams and foams appear to have both preventive and therapeutic effects on vaginal warts, as does improved vaginal hygiene.

Drugs Used in Treatment

R̥ **antibiotics**—*amoxicillin; ampicillin; erythromycin; Minocin; penicillin G; penicillin potassium phenoxymethyl; Terramycin; tetracycline hydrochloride*
R̥ **antibiotic potentiator**—*Benemid*
R̥ **anti-infective**—*Flagyl*

Smallpox

Smallpox, once a dreaded and highly contagious viral disease, has now been virtually eradicated. According to a bulletin issued by the Public Health Service in 1978, no new smallpox cases have been reported anywhere in the world since October, 1977. The Public Health Service no longer recommends routine immunization of children. In fact, it reports that the only time vaccination is necessary is for international travel. Some countries require evidence of smallpox vaccination as a condition of entry.

Tapeworm

Humans are infected with tapeworms by eating undercooked or raw meats or fish that contain worm cysts or eggs. The adult tapeworm lives in the human intestine, where it may grow to a length of 10 to 30 feet.

Symptoms

Tapeworm infestation may produce no symptoms, or the person may experience abdominal cramping, diarrhea, and loss of appetite. There may be nausea and vomiting. The individual may feel weak and exhausted.

Treatment

Tapeworm infestation is treated with niclosamide followed by a cathartic.

Tetanus

Tetanus (lockjaw) is a severe inflammation of the nerves within the central nervous system. Most cases of tetanus are caused by contamination of wounds through contact with soil or objects harboring the tetanus-causing bacteria. Drug addicts who use contaminated needles may also acquire the disease.

Tetanus is most likely to occur with a puncture wound or with a purulent necrotic lesion, but even small, seemingly well attended wounds may lead to tetanus because the causative microorganism is universally found. Newborns may acquire tetanus through the umbilicus.

The microorganism secretes a toxin which affects brain cells and the nerves within the spinal cord blocking the transmission of nerve impulses and thus causing muscular spasms and an inability to open the mouth (hence the term "lockjaw"). Eventually, the disease may affect the muscles of respiration, resulting in respiratory failure. In less severe cases, the muscles associated with swallowing may be hindered, possibly leading to choking.

Symptoms

Symptoms of tetanus include pain and tingling at the site where the bacteria entered, and spasticity of the surrounding muscles. The patient may be irritable and have a stiff neck and jaw. Difficulty in swallowing is common. Eventually the muscles of the jaw, face, abdomen, neck, and back become rigid and spasms may develop. Painful convulsions may occur. Respiration may be hampered, and the patient may find it difficult to breathe. The skin may become bluish. Fever is sometimes present. The primary complication is obstruction of the airway with depressed respiration. Eventually, urinary retention and severe constipation can occur due to spasms of the sphincters. Death may occur, usually through respiratory arrest and cardiac failure.

Treatment

Tetanus must be differentiated from other diseases and from certain drug reactions. It is treated by tetanus antitoxin. To treat possible complicating bacterial infections, penicillin or similar antibiotics may also be given. Aspirin or muscle relaxants may be used to alleviate the spasms and pain. Bed rest and avoidance of stimulation during convalescence is extremely important. Mild sedatives (phenobarbital, Valium, or even anticonvulsants such as phenytoin) are given in some cases.

Overall, the mortality rate for tetanus is about 40 percent; the death rate is higher in small children and old people. Areas of contamination around the head and neck are more serious than are wounds on other parts of the body. If the patient survives, recovery will be complete.

Active immunization against tetanus is advisable for everyone. It is especially important that patients who develop and recover from tetanus should undergo primary immunization for tetanus, with a series of tetanus toxoid injections. Patients who contract tetanus once may be predisposed to repeated infections in the future.

Drugs Used in Treatment

OTC analgesics—*see the list under Pain and Fever*
R̶ antibiotics—*amoxicillin; ampicillin; erythromycin; Keflex; Minocin; penicillin G; penicillin potassium phenoxymethyl; Terramycin; tetracycline hydrochloride; Vibramycin*
R̶ sedatives and hypnotics—*Atarax; Ativan; Librium; meprobamate; Nembutal; phenobarbital; Serax; Tranxene; Valium*
R̶ phenothiazines—*Compazine; Stelazine*
R̶ phenothiazine and antidepressant—*Triavil*
R̶ analgesics—*Fiorinal; Fiorinal with Codeine; Norgesic; Robaxin; Soma Compound*
R̶ anticonvulsant—*Dilantin*

Trichinosis

Trichinosis is an infection by a parasitic roundworm that is acquired by eating undercooked or raw meat, especially pork. The worms are barely visible to the naked eye, but when ingested they quickly mature and encase themselves within the muscles of the body.

Symptoms

Major symptoms include swelling in the face, especially around the eyes and forehead. Sweating and headaches are common. The individual may experience symptoms of gastric distress, such as nausea, vomiting, and diarrhea. If the organism invades the chest wall, the patient will experience extreme shortness of breath. If the infection is severe and if it does invade the chest wall, pneumonia can result. Other possible complications include heart failure and meningitis.

Treatment

Trichinosis is treated with any broad-spectrum anthelmintic. Glucocorticoid steroids are also given.

Trichinosis may be prevented by thoroughly cooking all pork products.

Drugs Used in Treatment

R̶ steroid hormones—*Aristocort; Medrol; prednisone*

Tularemia

Tularemia (rabbit fever, deerfly fever, tick fever) is an infection of wild rodents, especially of rabbits and muskrats. It is transmitted from animal to man by contact with infected animal tissue, for example, when skinning rabbits or trapping muskrats. Certain ticks and flies can also transmit the disease by biting. Eating improperly cooked infected meat or drinking contaminated water can spread the disease.

Symptoms

Symptoms include fever, headache, nausea, chills, vomiting, and weakness. Symptoms appear suddenly from one to ten days after transmission of the disease. A small blister appears at the site of inoculation. The lymph nodes in the area become enlarged and tender; they may seep. Pneumonia may develop if the organism spreads into the lungs. Eventually gastroenteritis, stupor, or delirium may occur. Generalized aches and rashes are common.

Treatment

Streptomycin is given along with tetracycline to treat tularemia. Chloramphenicol can be substituted for tetracycline. In addition, oxygen may be required, and an adequate fluid intake (eight to ten glasses) must be given each day. Aspirin or acetaminophen will help reduce fever and aches.

Drugs Used in Treatment

OTC analgesics—*see the list under Pain and Fever*
R̥ antibiotics—*amoxicillin; ampicillin; Minocin; Terramycin; tetracycline hydrochloride; Vibramycin*

Typhoid Fever

Typhoid fever (enteric fever) is caused by a microorganism named *Salmonella typhi*. It lives in human feces and is spread by flies and other insects. The incidence of typhoid fever in the United States has been falling steadily over the past few decades; however, it is still a serious illness when it occurs.

Symptoms

The disease usually has a gradual onset with initial symptoms similar to those of the flu. Over a period of a week to ten days (prodromal state), the patient develops a fever (which may reach 105° F or more). There may be chills and a dull, continuous headache. The patient suffers a general malaise and lethargy. Nosebleeds occur and a red rash appears on the trunk and abdomen. There may be a cough, a slow pulse, abdominal distention, and constipation or diarrhea. The tongue may be coated white or brown.

During the fastigium (severe, stage) the patient is extremely ill, and the fever stabilizes. Diarrhea or constipation and abdominal discomfort are severe. The patient appears generally wasted and exhausted.

Assuming that the patient survives the fastigium stage, the stage of defervescence occurs. The fever gradually declines to normal. The patient becomes more alert, and the abdominal symptoms disappear.

Complications

In about a third of all untreated cases, complications occur and account for 75 percent of all deaths due to typhoid fever. Possible complications include severe hemorrhage (accompanied by signs of shock), intestinal perforation, pneumonia, thrombophlebitis, myocarditis, psychosis, and kidney disease.

Treatment

Typhoid fever is treated with ampicillin or chloramphenicol, and when these drugs are used the prognosis is extremely good. Symptoms are treated appropriately; aspirin or acetaminophen is given for fever.

A patient with typhoid fever must be confined to bed, perhaps for a month or more. The patient should not be allowed to get up for any reason. A bed pan is required and lamb's wool should be used to help prevent bedsores. The patient's legs should be exercised to reduce the risk of thrombophlebitis.

It is important that all members of the family of a typhoid patient be immunized against the disease.

Drugs Used in Treatment

OTC analgesics—*see the list under Pain and Fever*
℞ antibiotics—*amoxicillin; ampicillin*

Health Care Accessories—*bedpan; fever thermometer; invalid cushion*

Typhus

Typhus is an infectious disease caused by a microorganism that infects lice. When a louse bites someone, it simultaneously defecates. If the person bitten scratches the bite, the infected fecal material of the louse is rubbed into the wound. The dried and highly infectious louse fecal material may also be inhaled into human lungs, possibly causing severe respiratory infections.

Symptoms

The symptoms of typhus include high fever, sometimes above 105° F, and severe, intractable headache. Additional symptoms include malaise, cough, and severe chest pain. Onset is abrupt—fever, chills, prostration, and other flu-like symptoms. Eventually symptoms progress to delirium and stupor.

A patient with typhus will be flushed, and the eyes will show signs of conjunctivitis. A severe rash may appear, beginning under the arms and spreading over the trunk and onto the extremities. It rarely spreads to the face, the palms, or the soles of the feet. In severe cases, the rash may cause bleeding that is sufficient to lower the blood pressure.

Possible complications of typhus include pneumonia and kidney damage.

Treatment

Typhus is treated with broad-spectrum antibiotics such as tetracycline. Penicillin alone is usually not sufficient. Chloramphenicol will be used in severe cases. Bed rest and isolation are indicated. Someone with typhus is highly contagious and should be kept away from other people to avoid spreading the disease. All clothing and objects handled by someone with typhus should be carefully cleaned. Aspirin or acetaminophen and sponge baths may be used to help control the fever.

Drugs Used in Treatment

OTC analgesics—*see the list under Pain and Fever*
℞ antibiotics—*amoxicillin; ampicillin; Minocin; Terramycin; tetracycline hydrochloride; Vibramycin*

Nutritional Disorders

The human body requires certain nutrients in order to maintain or restore health. Nutrients are chemical substances necessary for growth, normal body functioning, and the maintenance of life. Included as nutrients are proteins, fats, carbohydrates, vitamins, and minerals. Water is now also generally considered a nutrient.

Protein. Protein is the primary building block of cells and tissues; therefore a growing child needs a larger proportion of protein in the diet than does a healthy adult, who uses the protein mainly to repair cell damage.

Protein is made up of amino acids, and in the body protein is broken down into its component amino acids before being utilized. Because the human body can manufacture only 14 of the 23 essential amino acids, the diet must provide the other nine. Thus, protein foods are identified as complete (that is, containing all nine essential amino acids) or incomplete. Dairy products and eggs contain all essential amino acids and are of high biologic value to the body. Meat, poultry, fish, legumes, and potatoes have somewhat less value; cereal, breads, and root vegetables, still less. However, a combination of two incomplete proteins may provide high-quality complete protein—for example, rice and beans.

Carbohydrates. Carbohydrates (sugars and starches) are energy food. Cereals, fruits, vegetables, syrups, and sugars are rich in carbohydrates.

Carbohydrates should provide the bulk of the diet, 25 to 50 percent of the calories. In the United States, most people get about 50 percent of their calories in carbohydrates, a smaller percentage than that in many parts of the world where diets are heavily grain-based.

Fats. Fats provide certain essential acids for the body, as well as calories and flavor. They are a concentrated form of energy, and they are stored in the body to provide energy after the body's muscles have been depleted of glycogen. Fats are also necessary for the transportation of certain vitamins. Fats are found in meat, butter, margarine, oils, egg yolk, cream, avocados, and nuts.

In the average U.S. diet, fat provides about 40 percent of the calories. Many nutritionists feel that percentage is too high; in many parts of the world, half that consumption is normal and appears to be adequate.

Vitamins. The body cannot manufacture most vitamins, but they are required as catalysts for the utilization of the other nutrients in the diet. They are needed in very small quantities, although individual needs may vary widely, and can be readily obtained from a well-balanced varied diet.

Minerals. Trace amounts of certain minerals and large amounts of others (calcium, iron) are required by the body for the passage of nerve impulses, building bones and teeth, maintenance of the blood, and other metabolic functions. Relatively little is known about the role of and the need for many trace elements.

Dietary Guidelines

The key to maintaining a nutritious diet is to vary your food choices as much as possible and to be sure that you eat from each of the four primary food groups every day.

Fruits and vegetables. Fruits and vegetables provide minerals, vitamins, and carbohydrates. They are high in bulk, low in calories, and relatively inexpensive. It's recommended that four or more servings from this group be eaten every day, including a dark green or deep yellow vegetable and a citrus fruit.

Cereals and grains. Breads and other baked goods, pasta, rice, and cereals provide carbohydrates, protein, minerals, and vitamins. Four or more servings a day are suggested from this group. Try to choose products that are whole-grain or enriched.

High protein group. The high protein foods include meat, poultry, eggs, fish, legumes, and nuts. At least two servings a day from this group are recommended. Red meats contain the highest amount of saturated fat, and many authorities have suggested that Americans decrease their consumption of red meat in favor of other protein sources.

Dairy products. Milk, cheese, yogurt, and ice cream provide protein, calcium, and riboflavin, a B vitamin. Children, teenagers, and pregnant and nursing women require three to six or more cups of milk per day. Other adults need only two cups.

The Select Committee on Nutrition and Human Needs of the United States Senate has published its recommendations on dietary goals for Americans. In general, these goals include an increase in the consumption of fruits and vegetables, a decrease in the consumption of red meat and an increase in the consumption of poultry and fish, and a decrease in the consumption of high fat foods, sugar, and salt.

Need for Supplements

By choosing foods as suggested above and by following the recommended guidelines, most people's dietary needs will be met. However, certain groups with increased needs (pregnant and nursing women, infants, people with certain diseases) may benefit from dietary supplements. If you think you need extra vitamins, consult your doctor to see if a true deficiency exists. Taking large doses of certain vitamins can cause severe side effects.

OTC nutritional supplements—*Allbee; Chocks; Chocks Plus Iron; Femiron iron supplement; Femiron; Feosol iron supplement; Fergon iron supplement; Fer-In-Sol iron supplement; Geritol Junior (liquid and tablet); Geritol (liquid and tablet); Multicebrin; Myadec; One-A-Day; One-A-Day plus iron; One-A-Day plus minerals; Poly-Vi-Sol; Stresscaps; Stresstabs 600; Thera-Combex H-P; Theragran; Theragran-M; Unicap (capsule, chewable tablet, liquid); Unicap M; Unicap T; vitamin A; vitamin B_1; vitamin B_2; vitamin B_6; vitamin C; vitamin D; vitamin E*

Beriberi

Deficiency of vitamin B_1 (thiamine) is known as beriberi. Although rare in the United States, it does occur occasionally.

Beriberi results from any inadequate intake of vitamin B_1, as when the diet lacks foods containing the vitamin or when food is overly cooked or processed. Some diseases cause an increased need for thiamine, and others impair the body's ability to use it. Alcoholics sometimes exhibit beriberi; their intake of the vitamin is decreased while their need for it increases and their ability to absorb and utilize it is impaired.

Symptoms

Beriberi causes numbness or tingling in the fingers or toes, loss of appetite, fatigue, tenderness in the calves, muscle cramps, and hyperactivity. If the disease is allowed to progress, the skin becomes swollen, the extremities may become paralyzed, the heart rate and blood pressure increase, and shortness of breath develops. Someone with beriberi may have trouble walking or experience some loss in other motor functions.

Treatment

Supplementing the diet with vitamin B₁ usually reverses the disease rapidly. Improvement can be seen within 24 hours.

Drugs Used in Treatment

OTC nutritional supplements—*see the list under Nutritional Disorders*

Iron Toxicity

Iron is a common component of many vitamin-mineral combination products. It is used for its anti-anemic activity and is popularly known as a "blood tonic." Iron poisoning is the most frequently seen type of mineral poisoning.

Symptoms

Symptoms of iron toxicity appear 30 to 60 minutes following ingestion. Typical symptoms include black, tarry stools; nausea; vomiting; lethargy; diarrhea; fast, weak pulse; dehydration; low blood pressure; acidosis; and possibly coma. This first period is sometimes fatal. If the person survives this phase, symptoms subside in a few hours. However, 24 to 48 hours later, earlier symptoms return, in addition to edema, shock, convulsions, anuria (lack of urination), very high fever, and coma leading to death. Thus, iron toxicity is extremely dangerous, particularly so because the symptom-free period between the acute phases may lead someone to believe that the condition has corrected itself and further treatment is unnecessary.

Treatment

Iron toxicity is treated by giving ipecac syrup to cause vomiting, then, the victim should be taken to a hospital or doctor for further treatment. A person who has swallowed a large number of vitamin-mineral tablets containing iron or other iron preparations should be taken to the doctor without delay.

Drugs Used in Treatment

OTC miscellaneous—*ipecac syrup*

Obesity

It has been estimated that 40 to 50 percent of all adult Americans are obese; that is, they weigh at least 10 percent more than is healthful for them. It is difficult to define ideal weight because so many factors must be considered: muscular mass, genetic predisposition, age, and height, for example. However, the tables of ideal weights available from doctors give useful approximations, and a physician can appraise whether someone is significantly overweight.

Being overweight may cause fatigue, listlessness, achy muscles and joints, and shortness of breath, particularly after exertion. The obese are more likely to suffer high blood pressure, diabetes, gout, heart and gallbladder disease, and certain kinds of cancer than are the nonobese. Obesity complicates pregnancy and delivery. The obese tend to die earlier than people who are lean.

Causes

Obesity almost always results from ingesting more calories than are expended. The imbalance may be due to eating too much or exercising too little. Most often it is a combination of the two factors.

There are certain diseases in which the body does not properly use normal amounts of food and obesity occurs; for example, glandular disorders including deficiencies in the thyroid hormone or excessive insulin or adrenal steroid secretion may cause obesity. But these conditions are rare. Almost all cases of obesity are due to simple imbalance between caloric intake and expenditure.

Treatment

Prescription anorectics. Most prescription anorectics (drugs that will reduce the appetite) are derivatives of the stimulant dextroamphetamine. Examples include Dexedrine, Biphetamine, and Ionamin anorectics. These agents are indicated for short-term reduction of appetite (up to two weeks) and are ineffective if used for a longer period. Consequently, if these drugs are to be taken, they should be taken for only 10 to 14 days and then discontinued for the same period before drug therapy is resumed. In some states, the use of these drugs may be prohibited because they are relatively ineffective and have the potential for abuse.

For some years it was believed that thyroid hormone would speed up the metabolism sufficiently to cause weight loss. Digitalis was also used for similar reasons. This is a dangerous and inappropriate use of these drugs.

OTC diet aids. A wide variety of OTC items aim to depress the appetite and make it easier for a dieter to restrict caloric intake. Products containing phenylpropanolamine hydrochloride (Super Odrinex tablets, for example) reduce the appetite for a short period of time, but their effect wears off after a week or two of continuous use. It is recommended that such a product be taken from Monday through Friday with weekends "off," or that they be taken for periods of up to two weeks with one-week intervals between. These products may cause side effects such as nervousness, high blood pressure, or palpitations.

Some OTC diet aids contain benzocaine, a local anesthetic. Benzocaine numbs the nerves in the mouth to decrease the taste for food and the nerves in the stomach to eliminate the "hungry" feeling.

Some appetite suppressants provide vitamins. Not everyone who diets needs to take vitamins. If you want to take vitamins, buy them separately. You will save money.

When eaten before a meal, OTC diet candy (Ayds reducing candy, for example) is intended to reduce the appetite by providing sugar that will be absorbed into the bloodstream. The sugar signals the brain to direct the body to eat less. A piece of hard candy will provide the same effect as a piece of Ayds reducing candy and for less cost.

Dieting. No drug can take the place of limiting the amount of food consumed each day. A successful weight-loss program involves a nutritionally balanced diet that will help the dieter learn sound eating habits. Remember, before starting any diet, you should consult your doctor.

Drugs Used in Treatment

Recommended treatment with OTC drugs—*See the discussion of OTC diet aids on the previous page.*
OTC appetite suppressants—*Appedrine; Ayds; Slim-Line; Super Odrinex*
R anorectics—*Biphetamine; Fastin*

Pellagra

Pellagra is caused by niacin (vitamin B_3) deficiency. Niacin is a water-soluble B vitamin essential for cell metabolism. Deficiency is rare in the U.S. due to the enrichment of flours and grain products. It is sometimes seen in people with bizarre food habits or in areas where corn (maize) forms a large part of the diet.

Symptoms

Early symptoms include general malaise; red, rough skin; and a swollen and sore mouth and tongue. If the deficiency is not treated, the skin becomes redder, especially when exposed to light or when rubbed. Soreness and swelling of the mouth become worse. Diarrhea, headache, gastric disturbances, depression, mental disturbances, a scaly rash, rigidity of the extremities, and an uncontrollable sucking reaction may also develop.

Treatment

Pellagra usually responds completely to the administration of niacin (nicotinic acid). One form of niacin, nicotinamide (niacinamide), produces excellent results without affecting the cardiovascular system as do other forms. All vitamin supplements contain nicotinamide. A balanced diet is also an important part of treatment.

Drugs Used in Treatment

OTC nutritional supplements—*see the list under Nutritional Disorders*

Scurvy

Scurvy results from a deficiency of vitamin C (ascorbic acid). In the U.S., scurvy is sometimes seen in formula-fed infants who have not been fed fruits or juices or supplementary vitamin C. Infants born to mothers who took large doses (over 1000 mg per day) of vitamin C during pregnancy have been reported to develop scurvy after birth. Their bodies had adapted to the high levels of the vitamin and without it, they developed scurvy. Scurvy is also seen in the elderly on low incomes who have restricted their diets.

Symptoms

Vitamin C helps the body build and maintain cellular structures. Deficiency results in the breakdown of these structures as manifested by an increased bleeding tendency and poor healing of wounds. Other symptoms include weakness, irritability, bleeding of the gums and loosening of the teeth, anemia, swollen joints, and muscle changes. Infants deficient in vitamin C may lose their appetite and stop gaining weight.

Treatment

Scurvy is completely reversible if supplements of vitamin C are taken.

Drugs Used in Treatment

OTC nutritional supplements—*see the list under Nutritional Disorders*

Vitamin A Toxicity

Unlike most vitamins, surplus vitamin A is stored in the liver rather than eliminated by the body. Vitamin A toxicity may be acute (resulting from a single massive dose) or chronic (resulting from prolonged overdose).

Symptoms

Symptoms of excessive vitamin A ingestion include loss of appetite, loss of hair, irritability, headache, and painful joints. A skin rash, enlargement of the liver and spleen, anemia, and bone enlargement may also occur.

Treatment

Withdrawal of the dietary source of the excess vitamin A is the first step in treating the toxicity. Then, other symptoms are treated as necessary. Anyone suspected of having taken a very large dose of vitamin A should be taken to a doctor as soon as possible.

Vitamin D Toxicity

Of all the vitamins, vitamin D is the most toxic and the one likely to produce the most severe side effects. Given in large enough doses, vitamin D can be fatal.

Vitamin D helps the body reabsorb calcium and prevent it from being lost. Thus, blood levels of calcium are elevated by ingestion of vitamin D. Overdose of vitamin D causes blood levels of calcium to rise too high, possibly resulting in damage to the kidneys and heart. Over a long period of time, even slight overdoses of vitamin D indirectly cause calcification of soft tissue. If the high blood levels of calcium are maintained for a prolonged period of time, the calcium begins to deposit in the heart, kidneys, lungs, and other organs. These calcium deposits in the soft tissue can damage the organs.

Symptoms

The primary symptoms of ingestion of excess vitamin D are nausea, vomiting, loss of appetite and weight, excessive urination, weakness, and high blood pressure. Later developments include kidney failure and calcium deposits under the skin.

Treatment

Immediate removal of vitamin D from the diet or taking large doses of mineral oil will help treat the toxicity. Anyone suspected of having swallowed large amounts of preparations or tablets containing vitamin D should be taken to the doctor as soon as possible.

Drugs Used in Treatment

OTC laxative—*mineral oil*

Hormonal Disorders

Hormones are chemical messengers secreted by the endocrine glands into the bloodstream. They are carried by the bloodstream to various parts of the body where they influence cell activity.

The endocrine glands include the pituitary, the thyroid, the parathyroids, the pancreatic islet cells, the adrenals, and the gonads (the ovaries in the female, the testes in the male). The hormones that the endocrine glands produce are emptied directly into the bloodstream. Other glands, such as the sweat glands or the gastric glands, empty their secretions through tubes or ducts. Thus, the endocrine glands are also known as ductless glands.

Generally, hormones have three major functions. Their integrative function is to coordinate the activities of different tissue groups to act in a unified system in response to internal or external stimuli. Hormones serve a growth function in that they control the type and rate of growth. They also maintain the homeostatic condition of the body by maintaining its internal environment.

Pituitary gland. The pituitary gland is also known as the master gland because it oversees the activity of all of the other endocrine glands. The pituitary gland lies at the base of the brain. It secretes many different hormones that regulate the function of the other endocrine glands. The activity of the pituitary gland itself is partially regulated by the brain, but it also responds to the action of the other endocrine glands. Whenever an endocrine gland is not secreting sufficient hormone, the decrease in the blood concentration of that particular hormone automatically stimulates the pituitary gland to increase its output of the hormone that controls the other endocrine gland, thus directly stimulating the secretion of more hormone by the second gland. As the activity of the second endocrine gland increases, the concentration of its hormone in the blood increases, and a feedback system then signals the pituitary gland to slow its activity.

In addition to regulating other endocrine glands, the pituitary gland also produces several important endocrine hormones of its own. For example, it secretes a hormone called oxytocin that stimulates the uterus to contract at the time of childbirth. The pituitary also secretes a hormone called ADH (antidiuretic hormone, vasopressin). The most important action of antidiuretic hormone is its stimulating the distal renal tubules of the kidneys to permit water to leave the urine and remain in the body. Thus ADH conserves water.

Thyroid gland. The thyroid gland consists of two lobes, one lying on each side of the trachea. The two lobes are connected at the midline by a thin piece of tissue that extends over the trachea. The thyroid gland secretes thyroid hormone, and it is one of the most sensitive organs in the body. The thyroid hormone regulates the speed of virtually all of the basic cellular reactions of the body.

Parathyroid glands. The parathyroid glands are embedded within the tissue of the thyroid gland. They secrete parathyroid hormone that functions to regulate calcium levels in the blood.

Pancreatic islet cells. The pancreatic islet cells are scattered throughout the pancreas, and they produce the hormones insulin and glucagon. The function of insulin is to reduce the blood glucose content by stimulating its uptake by the cells of the body. Glucagon, on the other hand, stimulates the liver to release glucose into the blood to raise blood glucose levels. With insulin and glucagon working together, an individual's blood glucose level remains normal throughout life.

Adrenal glands. There are two adrenal glands, one lying on each kidney. The adrenal glands secrete steroid hormones that help to regulate the body's retention of sodium in the kidneys, thus regulating blood pressure. Other adrenal hormones, most importantly hydrocortisone (cortisol), control the metabolism of glucose, protein, and fat. Other adrenal hormones produce masculinization. In a male, this has little effect. If the glands are secreting too much hormone in a female, masculinization may occur.

Ovaries and testes. The ovaries are two small bodies located in the abdomen of the female. The testes are small ovoid glands in the scrotum of the male. The testes produce sperm and secrete male sex hormones. The male sex hormone, androgen, causes the appearance of the secondary male sex characteristics and helps to regulate the body's use of protein.

Two hormones, estrogen and progesterone, are secreted by the ovaries. These hormones are important in the reproductive process. Estrogen also controls the appearance of secondary female sex characteristics, causes water retention by the body, and maintains control over breast development and function. In addition to its effect during reproduction, progesterone is responsible for enlargement of the breasts during pregnancy and for development of the milk-secreting cells of the mammary glands. Both estrogen and progesterone aid in controlling menstruation. Decreases in either hormone will lead to irregularities in menstruation.

Abnormal Breast Enlargement

Breast enlargement is caused by various disorders of hormonal secretion, certain types of cancer, and certain drugs. Gynecomastia refers to a condition of enlarged breasts in the male. The condition may affect one breast or both. In the young male, it usually occurs in both breasts; in males over the age of 50, the condition may occur on only one side.

Once the cause has been identified and treated, the condition usually goes away within six months to one year. Abnormal breast enlargement is usually painless and without serious consequences. If the enlargement is accompanied by soreness or lumps, cancer may be the cause and the person should go to a doctor as soon as possible.

Adrenal Diseases

The adrenal glands are two small triangular bodies located on top of the kidneys. They secrete a number of hormones called steroids, the most important of which are hydrocortisone (or cortisol) and aldosterone. Hydrocortisone aids in the body's use of carbohydrates, fat, and protein and is known as a glucocorticoid steroid. Aldosterone causes the retention of sodium and water and the excretion of potassium. Because aldosterone affects the levels of sodium and potassium in the body, it is referred to as a mineralocorticoid.

Conn's syndrome. Conn's syndrome (or primary aldosteronism) is characterized by excessive secretion of aldosterone, resulting in excessive retention of sodium and fluid by the body, causing the blood pressure to go up. Symptoms include extreme thirst and increased urination. Numbness, tingling, muscle cramps, weakness, headache, and fatigue are common. Sometimes, transient paralysis occurs, usually in the lower extremities.

Conn's syndrome, if caused by an adrenal tumor, is treated by surgical removal of the tumor mass. Other cases may be adequately controlled by the administration of diuretics and antihypertensive drugs. The drug spironolactone is a direct antagonist to aldosterone and has proven to be useful in maintaining blood pressure at normal levels and keeping the disease from worsening.

Addison's disease. This rare disorder (1 in 25,000 people) results from insufficient secretion of steroids by the adrenal glands. The disease is serious, and unless adrenal steroids are taken, the patient will die of cardiovascular collapse.

Symptoms of Addison's disease include nausea, vomiting, sweating, abdominal pain, and loss of appetite. The person becomes irritable and depressed, and may develop a deep rash extending over the lips and gums. The patient is easily fatigued, craves salt, has low blood pressure and low blood glucose levels.

Treatment includes administration of both glucocorticoids and aldosterone. A patient taking steroids chronically is frequently advised to adjust the dosage should an upper respiratory infection, fever, or other illness develop. The patient should carry identification that indicates that the wearer has Addison's disease and is taking steroids.

Cushing's syndrome. Cushing's syndrome is a disease characterized by excessive secretion of glucocorticoids. It may be due to a tumor or abnormal cell growth in the adrenal glands. Symptoms include obesity of the face (often referred to as a "moon" face), shoulders ("buffalo hump" development), and trunk; high blood pressure; weakness; fatigability; and headache. The skin is thin and bruises easily; the bones become brittle. There are often purplish streaks on the abdomen. There may be increased hair growth. Females may develop amenorrhea; males, impotency.

If the disease is due to tumors, surgery is the treatment. Drug therapy and radiation treatment may also be used.

Drugs Used in Treatment

R steroid hormones—*Aristocort; Medrol; prednisone*

R antihypertensives and diuretics—*Aldactazide; Aldactone; Aldomet; Aldoril; Apresoline; Catapres; Diamox; Diupres; Diuril; Dyazide; Enduron; hydrochlorothiazide; Hydropres; Hygroton; Minipress; Rauzide; Regroton; reserpine; Salutensin; Ser-Ap-Es*

R beta blocker—*Inderal*

Health Care Accessory—*blood pressure kit*

Diabetes Insipidus

Diabetes insipidus is a disease that occurs most frequently among young males. The condition is usually caused by some insufficiency of the posterior pituitary gland to secrete the hormone, vasopressin. It may be due to a birth defect, head injury, or to surgical damage to the gland. In some cases, an adequate amount of the hormone is secreted, but the kidney fails to respond to the hormone. This condition is called nephrogenic diabetes insipidus.

Symptoms

The disease is characterized by excessive thirst and urination. Urine production may reach four gallons per day, but daily urine output of four or five quarts is most common. Patients with diabetes insipidus often crave ice water.

As long as the individual replaces fluids as they are lost, a normal physiological balance can be maintained fairly well. Problems arise should the patient become unconscious due to surgery or other causes. In such a case, dehydration may ensue within a short period of time. Whenever fluids are restricted, symptoms of irritability, headache, fatigue, hypothermia (lowered body temperature), muscular pains, weight loss, difficulty in swallowing, dehydration, insomnia, tachycardia, and shock may appear.

Treatment

A variety of products is available to treat symptoms of diabetes insipidus. These range from crude extracts of the entire posterior pituitary gland to synthetic preparations. In addition, several thiazide drugs and oral hypoglycemic agents are beneficial.

Such products do not modify the disorder; they treat only the symptoms. But, adequate control of symptoms and maintenance of fluid and electrolyte balance allows the patient with diabetes insipidus to live a full, comfortable life.

Drugs Used in Treatment

R_x **diuretics and antihypertensives**—*Aldactazide; Diuril; Dyazide; Enduron; hydrochlorothiazide; Hygroton*

Diabetes Mellitus

Diabetes mellitus is a disease of the pancreas. It is characterized by widespread disturbances in the metabolism that adversely affect the body's ability to supply and/or utilize insulin—a hormone used for the conversion of carbohydrates into energy.

Currently, there are an estimated five million diabetics in America. Another 325,000 diabetics are diagnosed each year. These figures indicate that one in every forty people is diabetic. More than half of all diabetics do not realize they have the disease. Diabetes-related diseases are the third leading cause of death in the United States; only heart disease and cancer cause more deaths.

Traditionally, the disease was classified by the time of onset—juvenile-onset diabetics display symptoms early in life, while adult-onset or maturity-onset diabetics may not show symptoms until after the fourth or fifth decade of life. Recently, these terms have been replaced by the terms insulin-dependent diabetes (which roughly replaces juvenile-onset) and noninsulin-dependent diabetes (roughly replacing maturity-onset).

Symptoms

The term diabetes, derived from a word meaning syphon, literally refers to any condition characterized by an excessive flow of urine. Mellitus denotes sweetness (mel is honey). Hence the diabetic is characterized as having a large urinary flow that would be sweet to the taste—the sweetness coming from glucose in the urine. Excessive production of urine with high glucose levels is often the first recognizable symptom of the disease. Additional symptoms include:

Increased thirst—the diabetic may have unquenchable thirst or may simply notice that more liquid is necessary to quench the thirst than was necessary in the past.

More frequent urination—the diabetic needs to urinate more often and may be woken during the night by the urge to void the bladder.

Feelings of fatigue or depression—the diabetic usually feels good early in the day, but becomes fatigued as the day progresses or after exertion.

Emotional instability—relatives of diabetics may note frequent flare-ups of emotion, although the diabetic may not be aware or may not admit that such flare-ups occur.

Prolonged wound healing—the diabetic may note that any wound or infection takes twice as long to heal. Gangrene is always a threat and amputation of the feet is more common in diabetics than in the rest of the population.

Increased hunger—this symptom usually occurs later in the disease, and the diabetic may notice it only after gaining 10 to 20 additional pounds.

Visual disturbances—blurring or other impairment of vision is often the only early symptom noted by the diabetic. Diabetics wearing corrective lenses may note the need for stronger lenses at shorter intervals. The number of diabetics first detected by eye doctors is reportedly very high. Diabetes is one of the major causes of blindness in the United States.

Itching—itching is especially common in the groin.

Neurological changes—the diabetic may notice tingling or dulled perception of vibration, pain, and temperature, especially in the lower extremities. Degeneration of some of the nerves may cause alternating diarrhea and constipation, urinary retention, and impotence.

Almost all chronic adverse conditions in the diabetic can be traced to inadequate blood supply. For example, diabetics frequently develop kidney failure, lesions of the eye, and atrophy of the nerves. Generally these processes occur because the walls of the capillaries that supply the areas with blood and nutrients become thickened, resulting in inadequate transfer of blood into the tissue's cells and poor exchange of waste products from these cells. Further, the diabetic has a higher susceptibility to atherosclerosis and damage to smaller arteries (referred to as microangiopathies), especially after age 40. Diabetics have a 20 times greater incidence of gangrene in the feet than nondiabetics.

Treatment

Although individual components of treatment plans vary widely among diabetic patients, the basic objective of all treatment is to reduce the incidence and severity of symptoms and complications, and to prolong life.

Diet. An appropriate diet and weight control is the treatment for most adult-onset diabetics. Drug therapy with insulin or with one of the oral hypoglycemic agents, in most cases, should never be instituted before the individual has been on a prescribed diet for at least three to four months to see

Dietary restraint as a sole treatment is not suitable for the insulin-dependent diabetic. While strict dietary control is mandated, regular insulin injections must always be given to diabetic children. While opinions differ regarding the constituents of an ideal diet for the diabetic, there are certain basic standards that prevail. For both young and old, the diet must conform with the eating habits of the rest of the family as well as satisfy the patient's tastes. The diet should be simple, at least in the initial stages. It must be easily adapted to any insulin regimen and the food should be ingested in quantities and at intervals that avoid a significant increase or decrease in blood sugar levels.

On the other hand, the basic nutritional requirements of the diabetic do not differ from those of the nondiabetic. Consequently, it is not necessary to purchase special foods or to cook meals differently for the diabetic family member. The doctor will have suggested diets to follow.

Insulin. Insulin is used for management of the diabetic. Although used by all ages, those persons who require insulin tend to be younger than 30 and are generally lean. The hormone is also occasionally used therapeutically in the nondiabetic for lowering serum potassium levels.

The major goal of treatment is to achieve maximum utilization of glucose throughout the day without inducing significant or prolonged hyper-or hypoglycemic episodes. To achieve this goal a careful schedule of insulin injections and dietary restraint is developed. In determining the type of insulin to be used, the physician carefully evaluates the patient's normal work-exercise schedule, the "stress" level at which the patient lives and works, and the types and timing of the family's meals. An intermediate-acting insulin is generally chosen for the first trial with a fast-acting or a long-acting insulin added to the regimen as needed. The fast-acting insulins should not be used alone since repeated doses will be required too frequently for assuring an entire day's control. Regular insulin is, however, the only insulin that can be given intravenously; it is the choice in treating emergency diabetic coma. The extremely long-acting insulins are likewise not normally used alone. In fact, their use should be discouraged in all but those patients who demonstrate a specific need for them. They may remain in the body for two or more days causing "overlapping" of insulin doses with subsequent hypoglycemia and possibly coma.

Many patients are excellent candidates for insulin therapy. A few, though, probably should not receive it, but should be managed by other means. Patients with psychiatric disorders, drug abusers, and alcoholics, as well as elderly people with poor eyesight, mental confusion, or cardiovascular or cerebrovascular disease are poor candidates unless they are hospitalized or in nursing homes or other situations where they can be closely supervised. Also, patients who refuse to adhere to rigid dietary time schedules or who frequently undereat or overindulge are not candidates for insulin injections.

Oral hypoglycemic agents. There are currently only a few orally administered drugs available for routine use in controlling diabetes. These include tolbutamide (Orinase), tolazamide (Tolinase), chlorpropamide (Diabinese), and acetohexamide (Dymelor). Although used in different dosage strengths, the drugs differ from each other mostly in their durations of action. The drugs all work by the same mechanism—they stimulate release of insulin from the pancreas. Thus, for these agents to be effective, the patient must have a functional pancreas capable of manufacturing insulin.

Each patient must be individually evaluated for response to drug administration. There are no fixed dosage rules. The ideal candidate for therapy with an oral drug requires fewer than 20 units of insulin daily. In these persons, all insulin can be discontinued once therapy is initiated. Patients requiring 20 to 40 units of insulin daily may be started on the oral drug and the insulin dose reduced by 50 percent. Those patients requiring daily insulin injections exceeding 40 units may generally receive the oral drug and reduce their insulin requirement by 20 percent. However, the chance for success in these patients is slim.

A wide variety of products and supplies is available to the diabetic. The urine can be checked for the presence of glucose, ketones, and other substances using urinalysis supplies which are available OTC. Syringes and needles are intended for repeated use or for disposal after a single use. Various equipment is used to help with the injections and to clean and protect injection supplies. Isopropyl alcohol and alcohol swabs are used to sterilize the skin before injecting insulin.

Drugs Used in Treatment

℞ oral antidiabetic drugs—*Diabinese; Orinase; Tolinase*
℞ antidiabetic—*insulin*

Health Care Accessories—*hypodermic syringes and needles; urine testing products (There are important differences among the various brands of OTC urine test products. Consult your pharmacist or doctor for recommendations on the product appropriate for you.)*

Hypoglycemia

Hypoglycemia is a symptom indicating a subnormal amount of glucose in the blood. Hypoglycemia causes hunger, anxiety, weakness, flushing and profuse sweating, headache, unsteadiness, confusion, apprehensiveness, vision disorders, lack of coordination, thick speech, rapid pulse, and palpitations. Symptoms may progress to lack of consciousness, convulsions, and coma. These manifestations of the condition are nonspecific—that is, they could be produced by a number of different disease states.

Medical literature has indicated a great deal of public confusion about hypoglycemia. Many people consult their doctors because they are convinced that they have hypoglycemia when, in fact, the condition is rarely present. Hypoglycemia does not cause depression, chronic fatigue, allergy, nervous breakdown, alcoholism, juvenile delinquency, childhood behavior problems, drug addiction, or inadequate sexual performance.

Causes

Hypoglycemia may be caused by hepatic damage resulting in the inability of the liver to store adequate amounts of glycogen; tumors on or overgrowth of the pancreatic islet cells (the islet cells produce insulin); Addison's disease; hypopituitarism; and cancer. Other causes include oversecretion of insulin due to excessive sugar intake; severe muscular exertion, or poor dietary habits during pregnancy or lactation. In many cases, the cause is unidentified—for some unknown reason, excessive amounts of glucose are transported from the bloodstream into the cells by an action of insulin. The glucose is then utilized and metabolized resulting in a lowered blood level of glucose (hypoglycemia). This type of functional disorder is thought to be the most common cause of hypoglycemia.

Treatment

Treatment may be attempted with drugs that either alter the absorption of glucose or reduce the release of insulin (phenytoin and diazoxide). Frequent meals rich in protein (20 percent or more) are the mainstay of therapy. A high-protein diet is an ideal tool for weight loss, and weight reduction often improves tolerance to glucose in patients in the early days of maturity-onset diabetes.

Drugs that slow intestinal motility (such as anticholinergics) or drugs that delay gastric emptying may be of value to some hypoglycemic patients. A drug called Proglycerin has been found useful in some hypoglycemic patients. Surgery may be performed if the condition results from tumors of the pancreas.

Patients with hypoglycemia should avoid tobacco and all beverages containing caffeine; both are known to aggravate the condition. Alcohol and aspirin should be used cautiously.

Drugs Used in Treatment

℞ anticholinergics and sedatives—*Donnatal; Librax*
℞ anticholinergic and phenothiazine—*Combid*
℞ anticholinergic—*Pro-Banthine*
℞ antispasmodic—*Bentyl*
℞ anticonvulsant—*Dilantin*

Related Topics—*Adrenal Diseases; Diabetes Mellitus*

Precocious Puberty

Precocious puberty is the abnormally early onset (before age ten in boys, age eight in girls) of gonadal or sexual function. True precocious puberty is characterized by early sperm production in boys and early ovulation in girls. A condition called pseudoprecocious puberty causes premature development of secondary sexual characteristics (pubic and axillary hair growth, penile enlargement, breast development) without sperm production or ovulation.

True precocious puberty is more commonly seen in girls than in boys. In most female cases, there is no identifiable cause and the outlook for a return to normal sexual development is good. However, in males, sexual precocity is usually associated with serious disease. In either sex, the condition may be caused by lesions in the hypothalamus, hypothyroidism, or brain tumors.

Symptoms

In both true and pseudoprecocious puberty, males develop hair on the face, under the arms, and in the pubic region, and have excessive penile growth, increased masculinity, and acne. Females show early breast development and pubic and axillary hair. In both sexes, the limbs begin to grow rapidly, but also tend to stop growing prematurely. Consequently, children with precocious puberty grow into adults of below average height and have arms and legs that are short in relation to the length of the trunk.

Treatment

Most cases may be treated by surgical removal of a causative tumor or surgical correction of a lesion, thus stopping the excessive secretion of sex hormones. Once the cause is corrected, children begin to grow at a normal rate and no further treatment may be necessary.

Thyroid Diseases

The thyroid gland is the largest of the pure endocrine glands. It lies in the neck in front of the trachea. Its major function is to synthesize, store, and secrete thyroid hormone. Thyroid hormone controls the body's metabolism; that is, it is responsible for the body's ability to generate heat. It also regulates the body's use of fat, cholesterol, sugars, and protein. It controls growth and enhances the development of tissues and bone. Thyroid hormone affects many of the body's organs, including the heart, gastrointestinal tract, and the brain and nerves.

Most thyroid diseases can be classified as the result of either an overactive thyroid gland (hyperthyroidism) or one that is functioning below its intended rate (hypothyroidism). The activity of the thyroid gland determines the basal metabolic rate (BMR), the quantity of oxygen consumed by the cells when the body is at rest. When large amounts of thyroid hormone are present, the BMR may increase well above normal. In the absence of the hormone the

BMR may drop to lower than normal value. Some people take thyroid hormone drugs to stimulate the body to use more oxygen and energy, believing that an increased rate of metabolism will burn off excess fat. Such use of these drugs is dangerous.

Goiter

A goiter is any enlargement of the thyroid gland. Goiters may result from hyperthyroidism or hypothyroidism, as well as from cancers of the thyroid gland. One type of goiter is the result of inadequate dietary consumption of iodine that is used by the thyroid gland to manufacture thyroid hormone. Today, iodized table salt ensures that most people get adequate iodine, making this type of goiter less common than it once was.

Hypothyroidism

Cretinism. Cretinism is the form of hypothyroid disease that appears in childhood. It may be due to either deficient embryonic development of the thyroid gland or to an inborn deficiency in iodine metabolism that makes the thyroid cells unable to "trap" iodine and manufacture thyroid hormone. In either case, the child's physical and mental development is retarded. If untreated, the condition results in dwarfism and mental retardation. The cretin will display delayed skeletal maturation, dry skin, and coarse, dry, brittle hair. The child will be constipated and slow in teething, and will have a poor appetite, a large tongue, protruding abdomen, and cold extremities. A yellowish skin is frequently seen. Sexual development is retarded, although maturation eventually occurs.

Cretinism is difficult to detect at birth because the fetus is supplied with thyroid hormone from the mother. If the condition is diagnosed and treated early, the cretin may develop normally. However, if several months elapse without treatment, severe mental retardation is inevitable. Cretinism causes a greater inhibition of bone growth than of soft tissue growth, and an untreated cretin will typically be short, stocky, and obese due to a disproportionate gain in body mass in relation to height.

Myxedema. Myxedema, or Gull's disease, is the maturity-onset form of hypothyroidism. It may result directly from thyroid dysfunction, or from overzealous use of radioactive iodine, ingestion of "goitrogen" drugs or chemicals, or from chronic thyroid infection. Or, it may occur secondary to a malfunctioning pituitary gland that fails to stimulate the thyroid. Whatever the cause, the condition is characterized by a weakening of muscle tone, easy fatigability, headache, cold intolerance, dry skin, slowed heart rate, decreased cardiac output, excessive sleepiness, increased weight, lowered voice in females, menstrual dysfunction, loss of hair, mental sluggishness, and generalized edema. The edema is due partly to fluid, and partly to an accumulation of a fatty substance between the cells of the skin.

In severe cases the edema may become excessive and the person develops a fixed stare, becomes apathetic, has speech and hearing difficulties, and experiences severe personality changes. Myxedematous patients are more susceptible to the action of central nervous system depressants, especially their effect on respiration. Severe complications are mostly of cardiac origin although severe infection is also common.

Hyperthyroidism

As many as 5 percent of all Americans will develop some degree of hyperthyroidism at some time in their life. It is about five times more common in women than men. When symptoms include eye protrusion, visual disturbances, and goiter, the condition is called Graves' disease.

282

Hyperthyroidism is usually caused by an interference with pituitary regulation of the thyroid gland. The interference leads to uncontrolled glandular activity. Contributory factors include extreme physical exertion, severe mental or emotional disturbances, cold climates, and heredity.

The increased activity generally causes an increase in the size of thyroid gland cells. The gland may grow to three or four times its normal size. The difference between hyperthyroidism and a simple goiter is that in the former, thyroid hormone is secreted at a 5 to 15 times greater rate than normal and numerous systemic effects are seen. In this instance, the enlarged gland is referred to as a "toxic goiter." Symptoms include intolerance to changes in temperature, gastrointestinal distress, muscle weakness, tremor, extreme impatience, nervousness, mental disturbances, insomnia, and exophthalmos—a condition in which the eyeballs bulge outward due to an accumulation of fluid, fat, and other substances behind the eyes. In severe cases of exophthalmos, ulceration of the cornea may occur because the eyeballs protrude so far that the patient cannot blink or close the eyes when sleeping. This leads to drying of the cornea with subsequent irritation and infection.

Thyroid crisis. Thyroid crisis (thyroid storm) is a life-threatening extension of hyperthyroidism in which massive quantities of thyroid hormone are released. Although rare, it is an extremely serious condition. The heart is especially vulnerable to the hormone and death may occur from arrhythmias. Thyroid storm frequently occurs immediately after removing part of the thyroid gland in hyperthyroid patients who were inadequately controlled prior to surgery. Other stressful situations such as trauma, hemorrhage, shock, or severe infection may also precipitate such a crisis.

Treatment

Goiter. If goiter is caused by ingesting an insufficient amount of iodine, adding trace quantities of iodine to the diet may be sufficient treatment. If a chemical in the diet is stimulating the thyroid (a goitrogen), eliminating the drug or foodstuff from the diet may suffice. Often, however, the cause cannot be found, so a thyroid hormone drug—either natural or synthetic—is utilized to suppress glandular activity. When therapy is successful, the thyroid gland will regress to normal size within three to six months.

Hypothyroidism. Hypothyroidism is treated with thyroid hormone supplementation, usually throughout life. Some doctors prefer synthetic products to natural desiccated thyroid for initiation of therapy, and although these newer agents are more potent, none is more effective than natural thyroid hormone extracted from the glands of animals slaughtered for food. In other words, when appropriate doses of the synthetic agents are given, they cause approximately the same activity as naturally-derived agents. Natural thyroid extract is the least expensive form of thyroid hormonal replacement therapy.

Hyperthyroidism. Hyperthyroidism is often treated surgically, but antithyroid drugs such as propylthiouracil may also be used. Other agents may also be given.

Drugs Used in Treatment

℞ **thyroid hormone replacements**—*Proloid; Synthroid; thyroid hormone*
℞ **beta blocker**—*Inderal*

Cancer

In the United States, one out of every four adult deaths is attributed to cancer. Only heart and blood vessel diseases cause more deaths than cancer. Cancer occurs most often in people over the age of 50, but it can occur at any age, and, in fact, certain types are the leading causes of death in children. Between the ages of 5 and 25, and in women between the ages of 25 and 50, cancer is the leading cause of death. Men get cancer more frequently than women, and blacks more frequently than people in other racial groups.

Cancer is a general term for a group of disorders characterized by abnormal growth of cells. Cancer cells grow uncontrollably into tumors (swollen or enlarged areas) which push on normal cells to destroy them, or cut off or compete for the normal cells' supply of blood and nutrients. Why these cells begin to grow uncontrollably is not known, nor is it known why cancerous tissue so frequently reappears after the initial growth has been surgically removed.

Cancers can occur anywhere on the body, and each may have a different appearance and cause different symptoms, but all cancers have several points in common: cancer cells do not remain within normal tissue boundaries. They grow faster than normal cells, and they spread to other parts of the body.

Cancer Terminology

The term tumor is sometimes used to designate a cancer, but all tumors are not cancerous. A tumor may be an abnormal growth from any cause. Warts and moles are tumors. Tumors may be benign or malignant (life-threatening). Cysts are differentiated from simple tumors in that they are not made up of living tissue. A cyst is a closed sac, frequently containing calcium, plasma, or pus.

The term metastasis refers to the spread of tumors from one tissue to another. A lung tumor can spread to the brain; a skin tumor may spread to the lung; breast tumors frequently spread to the bone. When a tumor spreads, it is said to have metastasized. Some tumors metastasize readily; others do not. Once a tumor has metastasized, removing the initial growth may prolong life, but it will not cure the disease.

Most Common Sites

The most common sites of cancerous growth include the rectum, breasts, sex organs, colon, lungs, skin, and bladder. In men, the skin, lungs, and large intestine are most frequently affected; in women, the most frequent sites are the breasts, skin, and large intestine.

Cancer Risk Factors

Genetic predisposition. A history of cancer in your family increases the likelihood that you will develop cancer. In this case, you should be especially aware of the warning signs of cancer and you should report any symptoms suggesting cancer to your doctor right away. But you should not be unduly worried; many other risk factors enter into the cancer equation and you may never develop the disease.

Environmental carcinogens. Potentially carcinogenic (cancer-producing) substances are being released into the environment in ever increasing amounts and diversity: exhaust emissions from automobiles, buses, trucks, trains, and planes; insecticide residues; industrial pollutants from smoke-stacks and sewerage; and fallout and waste materials from the testing of nuclear bombs and other articles of warfare. The introduction of these chemicals may have brought about the increase in the incidence of breast and lung cancer and possibly other types of cancer in the highly-industrialized areas of the country. Exposure to these substances was once believed to be localized and restricted to members of certain occupational groups. However, it is now recognized that all Americans are exposed to some extent, and that exposure may be lifelong and unavoidable.

Smoking. Most scientists have concluded that there is a definite rela-tionship between lung cancer and cigarette smoking. Nonsmokers have the lowest incidence of lung cancer, and statistics show that the more you smoke, the more likely you are to get lung cancer.

Because the incidence of lung cancer is consistently higher in urban areas than it is in rural areas, there has been some speculation on the rela-tionship between carcinogens in cigarettes and carcinogens in the environ-ment. Two interactions have been proposed: the carcinogens in cigarette tar may activate carcinogens absorbed from the atmosphere into the lungs, or the two substances may act together to promote the growth of tumors.

The Seven Warning Signals

Our best chance for curing cancer comes when we catch it in the early stages. Each person should be responsible for self-examination and con-sultation with the doctor when any symptom first appears. Memorize the seven warning signals of cancer:

1. A change in bowel or bladder habits.
2. A sore that does not heal.
3. Unusual bleeding or discharge.
4. A thickening or lump in the breast or elsewhere.
5. Indigestion or difficulty in swallowing.
6. An obvious change in a wart or a mole.
7. A nagging cough or hoarseness.

Regular check-ups are essential in detecting cancer at an early enough stage to successfully treat it. If you detect any of these seven warning signals, immediately seek your doctor's opinion.

Types of Cancer

Skin Cancer. Because their symptoms are usually readily apparent, skin cancers are usually discovered early, and most people consult their doctors early enough to assure a complete cure. Two of the three major skin cancers are easily and successfully treated with drugs (5-FU) if they are diagnosed in time. In some cases the cancerous growths can be removed in the doctor's office. The third common skin cancer, malignant myeloma, is more rare and more deadly than the other two. It usually causes death.

People who are frequently exposed to sunlight have a high susceptibility to skin cancer. Fair-skinned people are the most susceptible (especially blue-eyed blondes), while dark-skinned people rarely develop this type of cancer. Skin cancer develops more frequently in people past middle age.

More than 75 percent of all skin cancers are basal cell carcinomas. Although this type does not usually metastasize to other tissues, it may grow very deep into the area and destroy underlying tissues.

The symptoms of skin cancer include any change in the appearance of the skin, a sore that does not heal, or sudden unusual change in color, size, or shape of a wart, mole, or birthmark.

The symptoms of malignant myeloma may include a sudden increase in size or a darkening of a section of the skin. Anyone noticing such a change should contact a doctor immediately. Even as little as a day's delay may be sufficient to render treatment unsuccessful. The causes of malignant myeloma are unknown.

Malignant myeloma is treated by surgical removal of the tissue and surrounding areas as soon as it is discovered. X-ray treatment will be given. Additionally, several drugs, including actinomycin-D and BCNU may be used. However, even after treatment, a remission rate (five-year extended life span) of only 50 to 60 percent is expected.

Lung Cancer. Lung cancer is the most common fatal cancer. Symptoms may be subtle: a slight cough or wheezing that persists for many weeks and months, or a slight chest pain, or bad breath. In any event, symptoms are frequently so slight that the individual doesn't even recognize them as symptoms and consequently fails to have them checked by a doctor. But later, the symptoms become more severe. The coughing and wheezing increase. Shortness of breath develops. The minor chest pain may develop into a chronic intense dull feeling that doesn't go away. The individual becomes weaker, begins to lose weight, and may develop insomnia. In later stages, the individual may begin to cough up blood and be unable to move even a few steps without resting.

Lung cancer is difficult to treat. It usually requires the removal of a section of a lung (lobectomy) or even of a whole lung (pneumonectomy). However, by the time most lung cancers are detected, it is too late for surgery, and most patients must rely on radiation treatment or drugs. The drugs used include cyclophosphamide, 5-FU, and thiotepa.

Even with treatment, survival for more than five years after diagnosis is very rare. The American Cancer Society's recommendations for cancer screening no longer include an annual chest x-ray.

Breast Cancer. American women between the ages of 40 and 45 are at highest risk of developing breast cancer. However, it can strike at any age. One American woman dies every 15 minutes from breast cancer.

Your risks for developing breast cancer are greater: 1. if another family member has had cancer (especially breast cancer); 2. if you have had cysts within your breasts; 3. if you were pregnant or had your first child after the age of 30; 4. if you are overweight; 5. if you first menstruated before the age of 11; or 6. if you had a late menopause. Breast cancer also occurs infrequently in men. Thus, men should periodically examine their breasts. The correct method promoted by the American Cancer Society for examination of the breasts is presented in the section on keeping a personal health record.

Over 90 percent of all breast cancers are found by women during their home breast examinations. Breast self-examination should be performed at least once a month so that any change will be noticed as soon as it is detectable.

Several drugs cause an abnormal enlargement of the breasts as a side effect. Such enlargement is not cancerous and should not cause concern. Spironolactone (Aldactone and Aldactazide diuretics), isoniazid (INH antituberculosis drug), and chlorpromazine (Thorazine phenothiazine) are known to produce this effect.

Several drugs have been suspected of causing breast cancer, including reserpine, spironolactone, and thyroid hormone, but to date, no studies have shown a positive correlation. In fact, no widely used drug has been definitely shown to cause breast cancer.

If breast cancer is detected early, the chances of survival are great. Although some doctors believe that breast cancer should be treated with drugs, the majority believe that surgery is the best treatment. Most surgeons remove the entire breast (a simple mastectomy), although some will take just the lump and tissue immediately around it. This latter procedure is referred to as a lumpectomy. A lumpectomy is the more desirable treatment for the patient, although removal of the entire breast results in a higher absolute cure rate.

For years, a radical mastectomy was the most common treatment for breast cancer. In this procedure, the breast, the chain of lymph glands that leads from the breast to the armpit, and the chest muscles are removed.

Cancer of the breast may recur 15 to 20 years after surgical removal of a lump or of the entire breast. If one breast has been surgically removed because of cancer, the chances are greater that cancer will develop in the remaining breast. However, the use of the new cancer anti-tumor drugs has greatly reduced the incidence of secondary cancer.

Cancer of the Prostate. This is the second most common cancer among American men. American blacks have the highest prostatic cancer rate in the world. Most people with this type of cancer are elderly.

Many prostatic cancers produce no early warnings. Others may produce back pain or painful urination. Because prostatic cancer develops around the urethra, difficulties in urination (diminished stream, increased frequency, and sometimes an incomplete emptying of the bladder) may be major warning symptoms. There also may be blood in the urine.

Prostatic cancer is treated by surgical removal of the prostate and the administration of female sex hormones.

All men, especially those over age 50, are strongly urged to have an annual rectal examination. A doctor will palpate the prostate through the rectum to see if any lumps or abnormal growths are present. Early diagnosis and treatment produces a high cure rate.

Cancer of the Urinary Bladder. Bladder cancer is four times more common in men than in women. It is the fourth leading cause of cancer death among American men. It usually occurs after the age of 50, with most cases occurring in men in their seventies and eighties.

A major symptom is blood in the urine. Urination is usually urgent, frequent, and may be painful.

Surgical removal of the bladder is a common form of treatment, although radiation therapy and (occasionally) chemotherapy are also used. Treated early, over half the patients with bladder cancer will survive for more than three years.

Liver Cancer. Liver cancer is relatively uncommon, but dangerous. It is four times as common in men as in women. It is also most common after the age of 50. Persons with long-standing liver cirrhosis are at highest risk.

The symptoms of liver cancer mimic peptic ulcer disease and similar afflictions. Therefore, liver cancer is frequently not diagnosed until it is too late to be successfully treated.

If diagnosed early enough, the cancerous area can be removed surgically. But in over 75 percent of all cases, it is impossible to successfully remove all of the area. Therefore, chemotherapeutic drugs are used in most cases.

Stomach Cancer. Stomach cancer occurs mainly after the age of 50 and is twice as common in men as in women. Persons with a history of pernicious anemia or achlorhydria and persons with blood type A have a higher incidence of stomach cancer. It has been suggested that one of the factors which may promote stomach cancer is a diet rich in smoked or processed meats.

The early symptoms of peptic ulcer disease and stomach cancer are similar; someone with stomach cancer may believe the symptoms are due to a peptic ulcer. Symptoms include a vague sense of heaviness in the abdomen and pain resembling heartburn. Eventually, the individual feels tired, develops a dislike for food (especially meat), and loses weight. Later vomiting of blood or the appearance of blood in the stool occurs, but by this time, the condition is usually too advanced to be treated successfully. When treatment is possible, it involves removal of all or part of the stomach. Early treatment improves chances of survival. However, a five-year survival rate of only about 30 percent is the rule even with early diagnosis and treatment.

Pancreas Cancer. Pancreas cancer is one of the most dangerous kinds of cancers; it is nearly untreatable. Pancreatic cancer is usually undetectable until it is too late. Its symptoms are often vague: a deep gnawing pain within the body or extending to the back. X-rays will not detect the cancer easily. The mortality rate for cancer of the pancreas is nearly 100 percent.

A newer method of diagnosis has enabled doctors to diagnose pancreatic cancers earlier. This method involves a scanner referred to as a CAT scan (computerized axial tomography). The CAT scanner is also used for detecting brain tumors as well as for a wide variety of other diagnostic purposes.

Hodgkin's Disease. Hodgkin's disease invades the lymphatic tissue (lymph nodes). It is more common in men than in women and is responsible for approximately 3 percent of all cancers. Symptoms of Hodgkin's disease include soreness or tenderness around the lymph nodes, swelling of the legs, difficulty in breathing, and backache. Symptoms of advanced disease include severe itching, weight loss, weakness, and fever.

Hodgkin's disease is treated in some instances by removing the affected lymph gland, although x-ray treatment and chemotherapy usually provide a better cure rate.

Over half of all patients with early detected Hodgkin's disease will survive three years or longer. Survival chances improve in people less than 25 years of age, with about half of this age group generally living beyond five years.

Leukemia. Leukemia is a general term describing a variety of cancers of white blood cells. Leukemia causes the white blood cells to increase in number to the point that the other blood cells are crowded out. Anemia develops because of the decrease in red blood cells. With a decrease in the blood platelets, the blood cannot clot and bleeding disorders develop. Leukemia is more common in adults than in children, although it is the leading type of childhood cancer.

Symptoms of leukemia are wide and varied. In children, the symptoms usually appear to be identical to a cold, but they rapidly become more severe. The child complains of intense fatigue and appears white, both conditions due to anemia. Bleeding of the nose, or gums, or small purplish spots appearing on the skin may also be seen as a result of the decreased number of platelets. The child loses weight, may complain of a sore throat, and often develops severe night sweats.

Leukemia is treated by chemotherapeutic drugs and x-ray therapy. While survival longer than five years was relatively uncommon until recently, this may be achieved with controlled chemotherapy.

Bone Cancer. Bone cancer eats away at the bone to cause severe bone weakness and an increased chance of fracture. It also causes intense pain because of nerve damage. Bone cancer may originate in the bone itself or in other tissue and then spread to the bone. Large numbers of abnormal cells infiltrate into the bone marrow and reduce its production of blood cells. Rare in children, the disease is more commonly seen in men between ages 50 to 70.

Symptoms of bone cancer include severe pain in the bones. The pain is intense, aching, and deep; it is not relieved by the usual analgesics. Eventually, the pain may spread and progress to the point that the individual collapses from fatigue. Because of the pain, the individual loses his appetite and begins to lose weight, becomes extremely weakened, and develops anemia due to the inefficient production of red blood cells.

The outlook is grim. Most people die after the disease is diagnosed. X-ray treatment and chemotherapy are the treatments of choice. Surgery usually has no value.

Brain Cancer. Brain cancer is less common than other types of cancer, but it accounts for about 2 percent of all forms of cancer. It is more common in men than in women, and it occurs usually after mid-age. Survival depends on the extent of the tumor and its location, with about 20 percent of all patients surviving ten or more years beyond the diagnosis. The earlier the diagnosis, the better the chances of survival.

Symptoms of brain cancer are nonspecific. They may include headaches, nausea, vomiting, impaired vision, muscular weakness, loss of coordination, drowsiness, psychotic periods, or failing vision.

Brain cancer is treated primarily by surgical removal of the cancerous mass when possible. X-ray treatment and cancer chemotherapeutic agents may also be given.

Cancer of the Cervix and Uterus. Cancer of the uterus used to be the leading cause of death by cancer among women. It is now in approximately third place. Most uterine cancer occurs in the cervix, which is the narrow lower end of the uterus. Early diagnosis and detection using a Pap smear is a reliable method for detecting uterine cancer, and if caught early enough, the cancer is almost completely curable. The disease is most common in women past menopause. Sexually active women should have a Pap test at least every three years.

A Pap smear is an easy method for detection of cervical cancer. A Pap smear is done by inserting a cotton-tipped applicator around the opening of the cervix and removing some of the dead cells which normally slough off. If cervical cancer is present, some of these cells will appear abnormal when examined under the microscope. At an early stage, surgical removal of the cervix is almost 100 percent effective for treating the cancer.

Women who take estrogenic drugs have from 5 to 14 times greater risk of developing uterine cancer. Years ago, a synthetic estrogen named diethylstilbestrol (DES) was commonly used during pregnancy to reduce the incidence of threatened abortion. At the time, no danger was known. However, 20 years later, a higher incidence of uterine cancer has been detected in the daughters of women who used DES during pregnancy. The courts are currently debating the legal implications.

Twenty percent of all American women will develop cancer of the uterus. Five percent will die from it. It usually appears after menopause, and is closely related to previous x-ray treatment, prolonged estrogen stimulation, diabetes, obesity, hypertension, and childlessness. There is no relation to frequency of sexual intercourse.

Heavy menstrual flow in premenopausal women is the most common early symptom. Constipation is frequently seen. Additionally, a thin, watery vaginal discharge may also be seen, along with general pains in the lower back or abdomen.

Uterine cancer is best treated by surgically removing the uterus (hysterectomy). Radiation therapy is used as supplementary treatment. An annual Pap smear is the best way to detect uterine cancer at an early enough stage to be beneficially treated.

A recovery rate of 80 percent is suggested for those people whose cervical cancer is surgically removed following an early diagnosis. If this diagnosis is delayed so that the cancer has spread to the lymph nodes in the area, over half the cases will relapse after therapy.

Ovarian Cancer. Ovarian cancer accounts for about 5 percent of all cancer in women. It is most commonly seen between ages 45 and 74.

Ovarian tumors may become very large before causing any symptoms. Thus, at least 50 percent of all such cancers are considered inoperable by the time they are discovered. Symptoms include abnormal vaginal bleeding, pain in the lower abdomen and back, and enlarged abdomen. There may be pain in the area of the abdomen upon pressing. Such tumors are sometimes mistaken for pregnancy.

Ovarian cancers are treated by surgical removal if possible. Chemotherapy is also used. Little is known about the exact causes of ovarian cancers, and consequently little is known about prevention.

Thyroid Cancer. Cancer of the thyroid gland is frequently detected during a doctor's office examination. If a lump is detected, a sample may be taken for biopsy. Frequently the biopsy tissue is only a bit of normal thyroid tissue, and this is no cause for alarm. However, if the tissue is not normal, it may be malignant and should be removed surgically. Thyroid cancer is usually slow-growing and is curable by surgery. While it is still important to get your doctor's opinion concerning any lump in the throat, thyroid cancer present for as long as two to three years may be successfully treated by surgery.

Cancer of the Colon and Rectum. The colon and rectum are the second most common sites for cancer in women and the third most common sites in men. Persons with immune deficiencies or diseases of the digestive tract such as ulcerative colitis are more likely to develop these cancers. Persons with high bulk diets (bran, etc.) generally have a lower incidence of colon and rectal cancer.

Any change in bowel movements could be a symptom of cancer of the colon or rectum. Such symptoms may include discomfort that is not relieved by bowel movements, long thready stools, bleeding from the rectum, excessive diarrhea or even constipation. Weight loss, excessive gas, and pain are also seen.

To check for colon and rectal cancer, a doctor performs a rectal examination by pushing a finger through the anus into the rectum and feeling for the presence of protrusions or abnormal growths. By inserting the finger far enough, the prostate gland can also be examined for nodules or growths. In women, the cervix and parts of the uterus can be examined for similar protrusions.

A sigmoidoscope enables the doctor to examine farther into the rectum. Basically, it is a long, hollow tube with a light on the end of it. By examining the rectum and lower part of the intestine with the sigmoidoscope, rectal cancer and colon cancer can be readily detected. You should have a sigmoidoscope examination regularly after the age of 40. Consult your doctor.

If you have had symptoms such as blood or pus in your stool, or if someone in your family has had cancer of the colon, your doctor may request that you have a barium enema to check for abnormalities of the colon or large bowel.

Recently, do-it-yourself colon cancer detection kits have become available. These kits require that the consumer put a small specimen of a stool on a slide and mail it to a laboratory for analysis. Although not all cancers are detectable by this method, many cancers that may otherwise go undetected will probably be discovered. Consult your doctor or pharmacist.

When treated early enough, over half of all patients with cancer of the colon or rectum will survive longer than two years. Complete removal of the affected area by surgery is the best treatment. Treatment with drugs such as 5-FU may be undertaken. When the colon and/or rectum is removed surgically, a colostomy may be performed to enable the individual to maintain semi-normal bowel habits.

Treatment

There are three recognized effective treatments of cancer: surgical removal of diseased tissue, radiation to destroy malignant cells, and drug therapy (chemotherapy). In the past several decades many drugs have been developed which may be effective in treating the disease. Anticancer drugs in current use are very potent and possess only a moderate degree of selectivity and can produce severe toxicity. In other words, their side effects are often more severe than the symptoms of the disease they are used to treat.

Drug treatment of cancer presents certain problems not found in the treatment of infectious diseases. The only difference between a cancer cell and a regular cell is often its rate of growth. Therefore, cancerous cells are not always readily apparent. If a single cancerous cell survives chemotherapy, it may suffice to perpetuate the cancer, although symptoms may not reappear for several years.

Cancer patients may require a wide variety of medications and supplies for symptomatic relief in addition to those drugs used to treat their disease directly.

Pain. Not all cancer causes pain but many people fear cancer pain, and much pain is probably psychological in origin. Thus, analgesics should be available to the patient at all times. Sedatives may also be required to relax the overanxious patient.

Nutrition. Many cancer patients suffer from poor nutrition for numerous reasons, including a loss of appetite. A therapeutic formula of a vitamin-mineral supplement should be given regularly. For severely ill patients, one of the liquid food products that supplies extra calories should be given, in addition to regular meals.

Nausea and vomiting. Nausea and vomiting are common, due to the disease process itself as well as to side effects of many of the cancer-treating drugs. While most cancer patients will not respond to OTC anti-nauseant medication, some of the stronger medications (e.g., Compazine phenothiazine) will be beneficial.

Laetrile. Laetrile is a substance obtained from the dried seeds (pits) of various fruits such as apricots and peaches. Many articles and personal testimonies have claimed that laetrile is beneficial in the treatment of certain types of cancer. As yet, no sound scientific studies have proven or disproven the drug's benefits in cancer treatment. The FDA has given permission for studies to be done on humans using laetrile, but the results of these studies will probably not be available for several years. Some doctors have allowed their patients to take laetrile in addition to more orthodox cancer therapy or after conventional methods have failed. Others feel the drug is worthless. Until its benefits have been proven, laetrile should not be relied upon as the sole course of treatment for cancer. It should be noted that some patients have been poisoned by the cyanide content of incompletely processed laetrile.

Drugs Used in Treatment

OTC analgesics—*see the list under Pain and Fever*
OTC nutritional supplements—*see the list under Nutritional Disorders*
R̩ analgesics—*Darvocet-N; Darvon; Darvon Compound-65; Demerol; Empirin Compound with Codeine; Equagesic; Fiorinal; Fiorinal with Codeine; Motrin; Norgesic; Parafon Forte; Percodan; Robaxin; Soma Compound; Synalgos-DC; Talwin; Tylenol with Codeine*

Ŗ sedatives and hypnotics—*Ativan; Librium; meprobamate; Nembutal; phenobarbital; Serax; Tranxene; Valium*
Ŗ phenothiazines—*Compazine; Stelazine*
Ŗ phenothiazine and antidepressant—*Triavil*
Ŗ sedative—*Atarax*
Ŗ steroid hormones—*Aristocort; Medrol; prednisone*
Ŗ estrogen hormone—*Premarin*
Ŗ progesterone hormone—*Provera*
Ŗ uricosuric—*Zyloprim*

American Cancer Society Guidelines on Cancer Screening

Health counseling and cancer checkup (including examination for cancer of the thyroid, testicles, prostate, ovaries, lymph nodes, oral region, and skin) is recommended every three years for everyone over age 20, annually for those over 40.

Site of Cancer	Recommendation
Lung	An annual chest x-ray is no longer recommended.
Colon/Rectum	Everyone over age 40 should have an annual digital rectal examination; those over 50 should also have a stool guaiac slide test annually and a sigmoidoscopy every three years after having two negative examinations a year apart.
Uterus	Sexually active women should have a Pap test at least every three years after two Pap tests done a year apart are negative. High risk women should have Pap tests more frequently. Women under age 40 should have a pelvic examination every three years; those over 40 should have a pelvic exam annually. Women at menopause and those at high risk (who have a history of infertility, who are obese or fail to ovulate, who have experienced abnormal uterine bleeding, or those taking estrogen therapy) should have an endometrial tissue sample test.
Breast	Every woman over 20 should examine her own breasts every month. Those under 40 should have a doctor do a breast exam every three years; those over 40, every year. Those over 50 should have a breast x-ray taken yearly; those between 35 and 40 are advised to have a breast x-ray taken to use for comparison with those taken later. Women between 40 and 50 should have breast x-rays taken if their personal physician suggests it.

Part III
Drug Profiles

Drug Profiles

On the following pages you'll find more than five hundred drug profiles that provide information on more than 1200 drug products—both prescription and over-the-counter remedies. By studying the drug profiles, you learn what to expect from your medication, when to be concerned about possible side effects or drug interactions, and how to take the drug to achieve its maximum benefit. Each profile includes the following information:

Name. Most prescription drugs included in this section are listed according to their most popular trade names. Those products more commonly known by their generic names (insulin, for example) are listed generically. Certain very common OTC items are also treated generically (for example, calamine lotion). Note that generic drugs, unless they appear at the beginning of a sentence, are denoted by lowercase letters. The first letter of a trade name is always capitalized. The chemical or pharmacological classification for each trade-name product is listed after its name. To the left of the drug name we have indicated whether that product is ℞ (prescription) or OTC (over-the-counter).

It is common for a manufacturer to change the name of a product, or to remove or add certain ingredients to the product without changing the name. Thus, the name or ingredients of an item that you purchase may be different from that indicated in the profile.

Ingredients. The components of each drug product are itemized. Many drug products contain several active chemical components, and all are included in this category.

Equivalent Products. Many prescription drug products are available from more than one manufacturer, and this category includes other drugs that are chemically equivalent to the one profiled. Trademarked drugs in this category represent the most commonly known equivalents. Each entry in this category is followed by the manufacturer's name. If the drug is also available by its generic name, it is indicated in this category as well.

Dosage Forms: The most common forms (i.e., tablets, capsules, liquid, injectables, suppositories) of each profiled drug are listed, along with the color of the tablets or capsules. Colors for liquids, injectables, and suppositories are not included. Strengths or concentrations are also given.

Use: This category includes the most important and most common clinical uses for each profiled drug. Your doctor may prescribe a drug for a reason that does not appear in this category. This exclusion does not mean that your doctor has made an error. But if the use for which you are taking a drug does not appear in this category, and if you have any questions concerning the reason for which the drug was prescribed, consult your doctor.

Side Effects. OTC drugs list possible side effects; ℞ product profiles distinguish between major and minor side effects. The side effects of OTC drugs and the minor side effects of ℞ products are the most common and least serious reactions to a drug. Most of these side effects, if they occur, disappear in a day or two. Do not expect to experience these side effects, but if they occur and are particularly annoying, do not hesitate to seek the advice of your doctor or pharmacist. You may be advised to try an alternative drug.

Major side effects, should they occur, are signs that a prescription drug is not working properly for one reason or another. Your dosage may require adjustment; you may have an allergy that interferes with the drug's action within the body; or perhaps you should not be taking the drug at all. Major side effects are less common than minor side effects, and you will probably never experience them. But if you do, call your doctor immediately.

Contraindications. Some drugs are counterproductive in people with certain conditions, i.e., they should not be taken by people with these conditions. These conditions are outlined under "Contraindications." If the profiled drug has been prescribed for you and if you have a condition listed in this category, consult your doctor.

During the first trimester of pregnancy, almost all drugs are contraindicated. If you have any doubts about taking a drug during this period, consult your doctor at once.

Warnings. This category indicates when the profiled drug should be used with caution. For example, a close monitor is usually necessary if a drug is prescribed for people with liver or kidney disease. Many drugs, especially those containing narcotics, barbiturates, or hypnotic components, have the potential for abuse because tolerance (or decreased sensitivity) to the drug can develop. Certain drugs are perfectly safe when used alone but may cause serious reactions when taken with other drugs or chemicals. The "Warnings" category indicates which drugs may intensify or diminish the action of the profiled drug. Alcohol, for example, should never be taken with narcotics, barbiturates, or hypnotic compounds; a serious reaction may result. This category will guide you concerning the possible dangers of using the profiled drug.

Comments. Both vital and general information concerning the profiled drug are presented under "Comments." Here you will learn whether to take the drug at mealtime or before or after meals; what to do if dizziness or lightheadedness occurs; when a drug can mask some symptoms; how long the profiled drug takes to work; when to expect some side effects and which ones. Other information could concern the price of the drug, products with similar action, or methods of administering the drug. You will find this information helpful, especially if your doctor or pharmacist has failed to relate all the facts you should have.

The entries in the "Comments" section, combined with the other information included in the drug profiles, should guide you as to what to expect from the drug you are taking and when to seek medical advice. Never be reluctant to ask your doctor or pharmacist for further information about any drug you are taking.   If you wish to contact the manufacturer of a drug product, consult your pharmacist for the address.

OTC   A and D Ointment rash remedy

Manufacturer: Schering Corporation
Ingredients: anhydrous lanolin base; petrolatum
Dosage Form: Ointment (quantities of ingredients not specified)
Use: For treatment of abrasions; chafed skin; diaper rash; minor burns
Side Effects: Allergy; local irritation

OTC   Absorbine Arthritic external analgesic

Manufacturer: W. F. Young Inc.
Ingredients: menthol; methyl nicotinate; methyl salicylate
Dosage Form: Lotion (quantities of ingredients not specified)
Use: Used externally to temporarily relieve muscle ache and other pain
Side Effects: Allergic reactions (rash, itching, soreness); local irritation; local numbness

Warnings: Use this product externally only. • Do not use on broken or irritated skin or on large areas of the body; avoid contact with eyes. • When using this product avoid exposure to direct sunlight, heat lamp, or sunlamp. • If the condition persists, call your doctor.

Comments: This greaseless ointment smells good and may be attractive to a child. It should be stored safely out of the reach of children. • Be sure to rub this product well into the skin.

OTC Absorbine Jr. external analgesic and athlete's foot remedy

Manufacturer: W. F. Young Inc.
Ingredients: acetone; chloroxylenol; menthol; thymol; wormwood oil
Dosage Form: Lotion (quantities of ingredients not specified)
Use: Used externally to temporarily relieve pain in muscles and other areas
Side Effects: Allergic reactions (rash, itching, soreness); local irritation
Warnings: Use this product externally only. • Do not use on broken or irritated skin or on large areas of the body; avoid contact with eyes. • When using this product avoid exposure to direct sunlight, heat lamp, or sunlamp. • If the condition persists, call your doctor.
Comments: This product is probably more effective for athlete's foot than as an external analgesic.

Achromycin V antibiotic (Lederle Laboratories), see tetracycline hydrochloride antibiotic.

A-Cillin antibiotic (W. E. Hauck, Inc.), see ampicillin antibiotic.

OTC Acne-Aid acne preparation

Manufacturer: Stiefel Laboratories, Inc.
Ingredients: alcohol; chloroxylenol; resorcinol; sulfur
Dosage Forms: Cream: chloroxylenol, 0.375%; resorcinol, 1.25%; sulfur, 2.5%. Lotion: alcohol, 10%; sulfur, 10%
Use: Treatment of acne
Side Effects: Allergy; local irritation
Warnings: Do not get product in or near the eyes.
Comments: This preparation may stain the skin. • If the condition worsens, stop using this product and call your pharmacist.

OTC Acnomel Cake, Acnomel Cream acne preparations

Manufacturer: Menley & James Laboratories
Ingredients: resorcinol; sulfur; alcohol
Dosage Forms: Cake: resorcinol, 1%; sulfur, 4%. Cream: resorcinol, 2%; sulfur, 8%; alcohol, 11%
Use: Treatment of acne
Side Effects: Allergy; local irritation
Warnings: Do not get product in or near eyes.
Comments: If the condition worsens, stop using this product and call your pharmacist.

Actacin adrenergic and antihistamine (Vangard Laboratories), see Actifed adrenergic and antihistamine.

Actagen adrenergic and antihistamine (Generix Drug Corp.), see Actifed adrenergic and antihistamine.

Actamine adrenergic and antihistamine (H. L. Moore, Inc.), see Actifed adrenergic and antihistamine.

℞   **Actifed adrenergic and antihistamine**

Manufacturer: Burroughs Wellcome Company
Ingredients: pseudoephedrine hydrochloride; triprolidine hydrochloride
Equivalent Products: Actacin, Vangard Laboratories; Actagen, Generix Drug Corp.; Actamine, H. L. Moore, Inc.; Allerfrin, Rugby Laboratories; Allerphed, Spencer-Mead, Inc.; Corphed, Bell Pharmacal Corp.; Dri-Phed, Stayner Corp.; Eldefed, Elder Pharmaceuticals; Norafed, North American Pharmacal, Inc.; Sherafed, Sheraton Laboratories, Inc.; Sudahist, Upsher-Smith Laboratories, Inc.; Suda-Prol, Columbia Medical Co.; Tagafed, Tutag Pharmaceuticals, Inc.; Triafed, Henry Schein, Inc.; Triphed, Lemmon Pharmacal Co.
Dosage Forms: Liquid (content per 5 ml): pseudoephedrine hydrochloride, 30 mg; triprolidine hydrochloride, 1.25 mg. Tablet: pseudoephedrine hydrochloride, 60 mg; triprolidine hydrochloride, 2.5 mg (white)
Use: To relieve hay fever symptoms; respiratory congestion; middle ear congestion
Minor Side Effects: Blurred vision; confusion; constipation; diarrhea; difficult urination; dizziness; drowsiness; dry mouth; headache; heartburn; insomnia; loss of appetite; nasal congestion; nausea; palpitations; rash; reduced sweating; restlessness; vomiting; weakness
Major Side Effects: Chest pain; high blood pressure; low blood pressure; severe abdominal pain; sore throat
Contraindications: This drug should not be used to treat asthma. • This drug should not be taken by people allergic to it or to other antihistamines similar in chemical structure. • This drug should not be given to infants, or taken by nursing mothers. Consult your doctor immediately if this drug has been prescribed for you and you fit into any of these categories.
Warnings: This drug should be used cautiously by people who have glaucoma (certain types), ulcers (certain types), enlarged prostate, obstructed bladder, obstructed intestine, severe heart disease, diabetes, high blood pressure, asthma, thyroid disease, liver or kidney disease; and by those who are pregnant. Be sure your doctor knows if you have any of these conditions. • This drug should be used with caution in children and the elderly; follow your doctor's dosage instructions exactly. • This drug should not be used in conjunction with guanethidine or with monoamine oxidase inhibitors; if you are currently taking any drugs of this type, consult your doctor about their use. If you are unsure of the type or contents of your medications, ask your doctor or pharmacist. • While taking this drug, do not take any nonprescription item for cough, cold, or sinus problems without first checking with your doctor. • This drug may cause drowsiness; avoid tasks that require alertness. To prevent oversedation, avoid taking alcohol or other drugs that have sedative properties. • Because this drug reduces sweating, avoid excessive work or exercise in hot weather.
Comments: Chew gum or suck on ice chips or a piece of hard candy to reduce mouth dryness.

℞   **Actifed-C expectorant**

Manufacturer: Burroughs Wellcome Co.
Ingredients: codeine phosphate; guaifenesin; pseudoephedrine hydrochloride; triprolidine hydrochloride
Equivalent Products: Allerphed C expectorant, Spencer-Mead, Inc.; Dri-Phed-C expectorant, Stayner Corp.; Sherafed-C expectorant, Sheraton Laboratories, Inc.

Dosage Form: Liquid (content per 5 ml): codeine phosphate, 10 mg; guaifenesin, 100 mg; pseudoephedrine hydrochloride, 30 mg; triprolidine hydrochloride, 2 mg

Use: To suppress coughing, or provide symptomatic relief of cough in conditions such as common cold, acute bronchitis, allergic asthma, bronchiolitis, croup, emphysema, tracheobronchitis

Minor Side Effects: Blurred vision; confusion; constipation; diarrhea; difficult urination; dizziness; drowsiness; dry mouth; headache; heartburn; insomnia; loss of appetite; nasal congestion; nausea; palpitations; rash; reduced sweating; restlessness; vomiting; weakness

Major Side Effects: Chest pain; high blood pressure; low blood pressure; severe abdominal pain; sore throat

Warnings: This drug should not be used in conjunction with guanethidine, monoamine oxidase inhibitors, phenothiazines, or tricyclic antidepressants; if you are currently taking any drugs of these types, consult your doctor about their use. If you are unsure about the type or contents of your medications, ask your doctor or pharmacist. • This drug should be used cautiously by people who have high blood pressure and by those who are pregnant. Be sure your doctor knows if you have either of these conditions. • While taking this drug, do not take any nonprescription item for cough, cold, or sinus problems without first checking with your doctor. • This drug may cause drowsiness; avoid tasks that require alertness. To prevent oversedation, avoid taking alcohol or other drugs that have sedative properties. • Because this product contains codeine, it has the potential for abuse and must be used with caution. It usually should not be taken for more than ten days. Tolerance may develop quickly, but do not increase the dosage without consulting your doctor. An overdose usually sedates an adult but may cause excitation leading to convulsions and death in a child. • Because this drug reduces sweating, avoid excessive work or exercise in hot weather.

Comments: Chew gum or suck on ice chips or a piece of hard candy to reduce mouth dryness. • If you need an expectorant, you need more moisture in your environment. Drink nine to ten glasses of water daily. The use of a vaporizer or humidifier may also be beneficial. Consult your doctor.

OTC   **activated charcoal**

Manufacturer: various manufacturers
Ingredient: activated charcoal
Dosage Form: Black powder
Use: To counteract ingested poisons
Side Effects: None
Comments: This product works by binding with poisons in the stomach and intestine and preventing absorption of the poisons. • If using this product in addition to ipecac syrup, be sure to use the ipecac syrup first. Then wait at least 30 minutes before administering activated charcoal. (See the profile on ipecac syrup.) • This product stains the mouth, gums, and clothing. • See the discussion on poisoning in Part I.

Adapin antidepressant (Pennwalt Prescription Products), see Sinequan antidepressant.

Adipex-P anorectic (Lemmon Company), see Fastin anorectic.

Adsorbocarpine ophthalmic solution (Burton, Parsons & Company, Inc.), see Isopto Carpine ophthalmic solution.

OTC   **Afrin nasal decongestant**

Manufacturer: Schering Corporation
Ingredients: oxymetazoline hydrochloride; aminoacetic acid; sorbitol solution; phenylmercuric acetate; benzalkonium chloride; sodium hydroxide
Dosage Forms: Drop; Nasal spray (content per 1 ml): oxymetazoline hydrochloride, 0.5 mg; aminoacetic acid, 3.8 mg; sorbitol solution, 57.1 mg; phenylmercuric acetate, 0.02 mg; benzalkonium chloride, 0.2 mg; sodium hydroxide
Use: Temporary relief of nasal congestion due to colds, sinusitis, and hay
fever or other upper respiratory allergies
Side Effects: Blurred vision; burning, dryness of nasal mucosa; increased
nasal congestion or discharge; sneezing, and/or stinging; dizziness; drowsiness; headache; insomnia; nervousness; palpitations; slight increase in
blood pressure; stimulation
Contraindications: This product should not be used by persons who have
glaucoma (certain types).
Warnings: This product should be used with special caution by persons
who have diabetes, advanced hardening of the arteries, heart disease, high
blood pressure, or thyroid disease. If you have any of these conditions, consult your doctor before taking this product. • This product may interact with
monoamine oxidase inhibitors, thyroid preparations, and tricyclic antidepressants. If you are currently taking any drugs of these types, check with your
doctor before taking this product. If you are unsure of the type or contents of
your medications, ask your doctor or pharmacist. • To avoid side effects such
as burning, sneezing, or stinging, and a "rebound" increase in nasal congestion and discharge, do not exceed the recommended dosage and do not use
this product for more than three or four continuous days. • This product
should not be used by more than one person; sharing the dispenser may
spread infection.
Comments: This product has a duration of action of approximately 12
hours. Because it needs to be administered only twice per day, this product is
less likely to cause "rebound" congestion than nasal products containing different ingredients. • The spray form of this product, although slightly more
expensive than the drops, is preferred for adult use. The spray penetrates far
back into the nose, covering the nasal area more completely, and is more convenient to use. The drops are preferable for administration to children.

OTC   **Aftate athlete's foot remedy**

Manufacturer: Plough, Inc.
Ingredients: tolnaftate; alcohol
Dosage Forms: Aerosol liquid: tolnaftate, 1%; alcohol, 36%. Aerosol
powder: tolnaftate, 1%; alcohol, 14%. Gel: tolnaftate, 1%. Pump spray liquid:
tolnaftate, 1%; alcohol, 83%. Sprinkle powder: tolnaftate, 1%
Use: Prevention and treatment of athlete's foot and jock itch
Side Effects: Allergy; local irritation
Warnings: Do not apply this product to mucous membranes. • If your condition worsens, or if irritation occurs, stop using this product and consult
your pharmacist. • When using the aerosol form of this product, be careful
not to inhale any of the powder.
Comments: Some lesions take months to heal, so it is important not to
stop treatment too soon. • If foot lesions are consistently a problem, check
the fit of your shoes. • Wash your hands thoroughly after applying this product. • The gel and liquid forms of this product are preferable to the powders
for effectiveness; the best action of the powders may be in drying the infected area. • The aerosol sprays may be more expensive than the other
forms of this product; check prices before paying for convenience you do not
need.

OTC   **Agoral laxative**

Manufacturer: Parke-Davis
Ingredients: acacia; agar gel; egg albumin; glycerin; mineral oil; phenol-phthalein; tragacanth
Dosage Form: Emulsion (content per 100 ml): acacia; agar gel; egg albumin; glycerin; mineral oil, 27.7 g; phenolphthalein, 1.3 g; tragacanth
Use: Relief of constipation
Side Effects: Excess loss of fluid; griping (cramps); mucus in feces; pink to purple rash with blistering
Contraindications: Persons with high fever (100° F or more); black or tarry stools; nausea; vomiting; abdominal pain; or children under age six should not use this product unless directed by a doctor. • Do not use this product when constipation is caused by megacolon or other diseases of the intestine, or hypothyroidism. • Persons with a sensitivity to phenolphthalein should not use this product.
Warnings: Excessive use (daily for a month or more) of this product may cause diarrhea, vomiting, and loss of certain blood electrolytes. • Pregnant or nursing women, bedridden or aged patients should use this product only on the advice of their doctor. • A type of pneumonia may occur after prolonged (more than two months) and repeated (daily) use.
Comments: This product may discolor the urine and feces. • Evacuation may occur within 6 to 12 hours. Never self-medicate if constipation lasts longer than two weeks or if the medication does not produce a laxative effect within a week. • Limit use to seven days unless directed otherwise by a doctor since this product may cause laxative-dependence (addiction) if used for a longer time. • Mineral oil may interfere with the absorption of vitamins A and D, calcium, and phosphate. • This product is best taken at bedtime; it should not be taken at mealtime. • If this product leaks through the rectum, the dose should be reduced until this symptom disappears. • Do not take a stool softener product at the same time as you are taking this product.

℞   **Aldactazide diuretic and antihypertensive**

Manufacturer: Searle & Co.
Ingredients: spironolactone; hydrochlorothiazide
Dosage Form: Tablet: spironolactone, 25 mg; hydrochlorothiazide, 25 mg (ivory)
Use: Treatment of high blood pressure; congestive heart failure; cirrhosis of the liver accompanied by edema or ascites or both; removal of tissue fluid
Minor Side Effects: Diarrhea; dizziness; drowsiness; headache; increased urination; nausea; rash; restlessness; tingling in fingers and toes; vomiting
Major Side Effects: Blurred vision; breast enlargement (in both sexes); cancer; confusion; diabetes; difficulty in achieving erection; elevated blood sugar; elevated calcium; elevated potassium; elevated uric acid; gout; impotence; low potassium; low sodium; lupus erythematosus; muscle spasm; sore throat; weakness
Contraindications: This drug should not be taken by people who are allergic to either of its ingredients or to sulfa drugs. Consult your doctor immediately if this drug has been prescribed for you and you have such an allergy. • This drug should not be taken by people who have severe kidney disease, hyperkalemia (high blood levels of potassium), anuria (inability to urinate), or liver failure. Be sure your doctor knows if you have any of these conditions.
Warnings: Unlike many diuretics, Aldactazide diuretic rarely causes potassium loss. Hence the relatively high price of this drug is justified for persons with low potassium levels. Do not take potassium supplements

while taking this drug. • This drug should be used with caution by pregnant women and nursing mothers. • This drug interacts with colestipol hydrochloride, digitalis, lithium carbonate, oral antidiabetics, potassium salts, and steroids. If you are currently taking any drugs of these types, consult your doctor about their use. If you are unsure of the type or contents of your medications, ask your doctor or pharmacist. • Spironolactone has been shown to cause cancer in rats. This has not been shown to occur in people.

Comments: When taking this drug, as with many drugs that lower blood pressure, you should limit your consumption of alcoholic beverages in order to prevent dizziness or light-headedness. • Persons taking digitalis in addition to this drug should watch carefully for symptoms of increased toxicity (e.g., nausea, blurred vision, palpitations), and notify their doctor immediately if symptoms occur. • If you have high blood pressure, do not take any nonprescription item for cough, cold, or sinus problems without first checking with your doctor. • A doctor probably should not prescribe this drug or other "fixed dose" combination products as the first choice in the treatment of high blood pressure. The patient should receive each of the individual ingredients singly, and if the response is adequate to the fixed dose contained in this product, it can then be substituted. The advantage of a combination product such as this drug is based on increased convenience to the patient. • There are a few "generic brands" of spironolactone with hydrochlorothiazide. Consult your pharmacist; some of them are not generically equivalent to this drug.

R̥ₓ   **Aldactone diuretic and antihypertensive**

Manufacturer: Searle & Co.
Ingredient: spironolactone
Dosage Form: Tablet: 25 mg (light tan)
Use: Treatment of high blood pressure and hypokalemia (low blood levels of potassium); removal of fluid from the tissues
Minor Side Effects: Diarrhea; dizziness; drowsiness; nausea; rash; restlessness; vomiting; weakness
Major Side Effects: Confusion; difficulty in achieving an erection; enlarged breasts (in both sexes); impotence
Contraindications: This drug should not be used in persons with anuria (no urination), acute renal insufficiency, significant impairment of renal function, or hyperkalemia (high blood levels of potassium). Be sure your doctor knows if you have any of these conditions.
Warnings: This drug should be used with caution, since it may cause high potassium levels, and enlarged breasts. • This drug should be used with caution in patients with kidney disease. Be sure your doctor knows if you have such a condition. • This drug should be used with caution in pregnant women and in nursing mothers. • When this drug is taken with potassium salts, or other diuretics or antihypertensive agents, extreme caution should be taken. If you are currently taking any drugs of these types, consult your doctor about their use. If you are unsure of the type or contents of your medications, ask your doctor or pharmacist. Do not take potassium supplements while taking this drug, and ask your doctor how to avoid excess potassium in your diet.
Comments: Unlike many diuretics, this drug does not cause potassium loss. Hence, the relatively high price of this drug is justified for persons with low potassium levels. • This drug causes frequent urination. Expect this effect; it should not alarm you. • While taking this drug, as with many drugs that lower blood pressure, you should limit your consumption of alcoholic beverages in order to prevent dizziness or light-headedness. To avoid dizziness or light-headedness when you stand, contract and relax the muscles

of your legs for a few moments before rising. Do this by pushing one foot against the floor while raising the other foot slightly, alternating feet so that you are "pumping" your legs in a pedaling motion. • If you have high blood pressure, do not take any nonprescription item for cough, cold, or sinus problems without first checking with your doctor. • This drug causes cancer in rats, but it has not been shown to cause cancer in people. • There are a couple of "generic brands" of this drug. Consult your pharmacist about these items; some of them are not equivalent to this drug.

Rx Aldomet antihypertensive

Manufacturer: Merck Sharp & Dohme
Ingredient: methyldopa
Dosage Form: Tablet: 125 mg (yellow), 250 mg (yellow), 500 mg (yellow)
Use: Treatment of high blood pressure
Minor Side Effects: Constipation; diarrhea; dizziness; dry mouth; flatulence; headache; inflamed salivary glands; light-headedness; nasal congestion; nausea; sedation; sore tongue; vomiting; weakness
Major Side Effects: Anemia; slow pulse; breast enlargement; chest pain; darkening of urine; decreased libido; distention; edema; fever; impotence; jaundice; liver disorders; liver and urine test abnormalities; reduction in number of white blood cells
Contraindications: This drug should not be taken by people with active liver disease, such as acute cirrhosis or acute hepatitis. Be sure your doctor knows if you have such a condition. • This drug should not be taken by people who are allergic to it. Consult your doctor immediately if this drug has been prescribed for you and you have such an allergy.
Warnings: This drug should be used with extreme caution in persons with a history of previous liver disease or dysfunction, or stroke. Be sure your doctor knows if you have ever had such conditions. You should receive liver function tests periodically as long as you are taking this drug. • This drug should be used cautiously by women who may become pregnant, by pregnant women, and by nursing mothers. • This drug may interfere with the measurement of blood uric acid, so remind your doctor if you have or are being treated for gout. Also, many patients taking this drug react positively to the Coombs blood test, indicating destruction of red blood cells or allergy. Often the test is false positive, and no disorder is present, but you should have periodic blood tests as long as you are taking this drug. • This drug should be used with caution in conjunction with other antihypertensive drugs. • This drug should not be taken with amphetamines or decongestants. If you are currently taking any drugs of these types, consult your doctor about their use. Do not take any nonprescription item for cough, cold, or sinus problems without first checking with your doctor. If you are unsure of the type or contents of your medications, ask your doctor or pharmacist. • Do not discontinue taking this drug unless directed to do so by your doctor, because high blood pressure can return very quickly. • This drug may cause drowsiness, especially during the first few days of its use; avoid tasks that require alertness, such as driving or operating machinery.
Comments: Mild side effects (e.g., nasal congestion) are noticeable during the first two weeks of therapy and become less bothersome after this period. • To avoid dizziness or light-headedness when you stand, contract and relax the muscles of your legs for a few moments before rising. Do this by pushing one foot against the floor while raising the other foot slightly, alternating feet so that you are "pumping" your legs in a pedaling motion. • Notify your doctor of any unexplained, prolonged, general tiredness or if fever occurs. • Occasionally, tolerance to this drug may develop, usually between the second

and third month of therapy. Your doctor can deal with this circumstance. • Intake of alcoholic beverages should be limited while taking this drug.

℞ Aldoril diuretic and antihypertensive

Manufacturer: Merck Sharp & Dohme

Ingredients: hydrochlorothiazide; methyldopa

Dosage Forms: Tablet: hydrochlorothiazide, 15 mg; methyldopa, 250 mg (salmon); hydrochlorothiazide, 25 mg; methyldopa, 250 mg (white); hydrochlorothiazide, 30 mg; methyldopa, 500 mg (salmon); hydrochlorothiazide, 50 mg; methyldopa, 500 mg (white)

Use: Treatment of high blood pressure

Minor Side Effects: Constipation; diarrhea; dizziness; dry mouth; headache; increased urination; inflamed salivary glands; light-headedness; loss of appetite; nasal congestion; nausea; rash; sedation; tingling in fingers and toes; vomiting; weakness

Major Side Effects: Blurred vision; chest pain; elevated blood sugar; hyperuricemia (elevated uric acid in the blood); hypokalemia (low blood potassium); muscle spasm; sore throat; weakness

Contraindications: This drug should not be taken by people who are allergic to either of its components or to sulfa drugs. Consult your doctor immediately if this drug has been prescribed for you and you have such an allergy. • This drug should not be used by people with active liver disease (e.g., acute hepatitis or active cirrhosis) or severe kidney disease. Be sure your doctor knows if you have either of these conditions.

Warnings: This drug should be used with caution in persons with liver disease, anemia, allergies, asthma, or kidney diseases, or persons who are on kidney machines. Be sure your doctor knows if you have any of these conditions. • Use of this drug may cause fever, jaundice, liver disease, stroke, low blood levels of potassium and sodium, calcium retention, diabetes, and gout. This drug may affect urine tests, lab tests, and thyroid tests. Be sure your doctor knows you are taking this drug before you undergo any testing. • This drug should be used with caution in pregnant women and nursing mothers. • This drug should be used cautiously with other blood pressure drugs; it interacts with amphetamine, anesthetics, colestipol hydrochloride, curare, decongestants, digitalis, lithium carbonate, oral antidiabetics, and steroids. If you are currently taking any drugs of these types, consult your doctor about their use. If you are unsure about the type or contents of your medications, ask your doctor or pharmacist.

Comments: While taking this drug, do not take any nonprescription item for cough, cold, or sinus problems without first checking with your doctor. • Mild side effects (e.g., nasal congestion) are most noticeable during the first two weeks of therapy and become less bothersome after this period. • While taking this product (as with many drugs that lower blood pressure), you should limit your consumption of alcoholic beverages in order to prevent dizziness or light-headedness. • To avoid dizziness or light-headedness when you stand, contract and relax the muscles of your legs for a few moments before rising. Do this by pushing one foot against the floor while raising the other foot slightly, alternating feet so that you are "pumping" your legs in a pedaling motion. • This drug can cause potassium loss. To help avoid potassium loss, take this drug with a glass of fresh or frozen orange juice. You may also eat a banana each day. The use of a salt substitute helps prevent potassium loss. • Persons taking this product and digitalis should watch carefully for symptoms of increased toxicity (e.g., nausea, blurred vision, palpitations), and notify their doctors immediately if symptoms occur. • Remind your doctor if you have or are being treated for gout if he prescribes this drug. • This drug may interfere with the measurement of blood uric acid. Also, many patients react positively to the Coombs' test. The positive reaction usually indicates an allergy or destruction of red blood cells. Often, however, the test is false positive, and no disorder is present. Have periodic blood tests as long as you take this drug. • If you are allergic to a sulfa drug, you may likewise be allergic to this drug. • A doctor probably should not prescribe this drug or other "fixed dose" products as the first choice in the treatment of high blood pressure. The patient should receive each ingredient singly; and if the response is adequate to the fixed dose contained in this product, it can then be substituted. The advantage of a combination product is increased convenience to the patient.

OTC   **Alka-Seltzer analgesic and antacid**

Manufacturer: Miles Laboratories, Inc.
Ingredients: aspirin; sodium bicarbonate; citric acid
Dosage Form: Effervescent tablet: aspirin, 324 mg (5 grains); sodium bicarbonate, 1904 mg; citric acid, 1000 mg
Use: Relief of upset stomach, heartburn, or acid indigestion accompanied by headache or body aches and pains
Side Effects: Dizziness; mental confusion; nausea and vomiting; ringing in the ears; slight blood loss; sweating
Contraindications: This product may cause an increased bleeding tendency and should not be taken by persons with a history of bleeding, peptic ulcer, or stomach bleeding.
Warnings: Persons with asthma, hay fever, or other allergies should be extremely careful about using this product. The product may interfere with the treatment of gout. If you have any of these conditions, consult your doctor or pharmacist before using this medication. • Do not use this product if you are on a low-salt diet. • Do not use this product if you are currently taking alcohol, methotrexate, oral anticoagulants, oral antidiabetics, probenecid, steroids, and/or sulfinpyrazone; if you are unsure of the type or contents of your medications, ask your doctor or pharmacist. • The dosage instructions listed on the package should be followed carefully; toxicity may occur in adults or children with repeated doses.
Comments: These tablets must be completely dissolved in water before swallowing; three ounces of water per tablet is sufficient. • You can save money by taking aspirin instead of this product. Because it is taken in solution, this product does reach the bloodstream in less time and will give faster pain relief than plain aspirin. However, if you take your regular dose of aspirin, and follow it with a cup of hot water, the aspirin will reach your bloodstream almost as quickly as would this product.

OTC   **Alka-Seltzer antacid**

Manufacturer: Miles Laboratories, Inc.
Ingredients: citric acid; potassium bicarbonate; sodium bicarbonate
Dosage Form: Effervescent tablet: citric acid, 800 mg; potassium bicarbonate, 300 mg; sodium bicarbonate, 1008 g
Use: For relief from acid indigestion, heartburn and/or sour stomach
Side Effects: bloating; gas; gastric fullness
Contraindications: Persons with heart or kidney disease or those on a salt-free diet should not use this product.
Warnings: Long-term use (several weeks) may lead to increased calcium in the blood, renal insufficiency, and metabolic alkalosis (nausea, vomiting, mental confusion, loss of appetite).
Comments: This product must first be dissolved in water before taking • Self-treatment of severe or repeated attacks of heartburn, indigestion, or

upset stomach is not recommended. If you do self-treat, limit therapy to two weeks, then call your doctor if symptoms persist. Never self-medicate with this product if your symptoms occur regularly (two to three times or more a month); if they are particularly worse than normal; if you feel "tightness" in your chest, have chest pains, or are sweating; or if you are short of breath. Consult your doctor. • This product is safe and effective when used on an occasional basis only. Repeated administrations for longer than one to two weeks may cause "rebound acidity," resulting in increased gastric acid production. If this happens, your symptoms get worse. • This product works best when taken one hour after meals or at bedtime, unless directed otherwise by your doctor or pharmacist. • Do not take this product within two hours of a dose of a tetracycline antibiotic. Also, if you are taking iron, a vitamin-mineral product, chlorpromazine, phenytoin, digoxin, quinidine, or warfarin, remind your doctor or pharmacist that you are taking this product.

OTC Alka-Seltzer Plus cold remedy

Manufacturer: Miles Laboratories, Inc.

Ingredients: phenylpropanolamine bitartrate; chlorpheniramine maleate; aspirin

Dosage Form: Effervescent tablet: phenylpropanolamine bitartrate, 24.08 mg; chlorpheniramine maleate, 2 mg; aspirin, 324 mg (5 grains)

Use: Relief of symptoms of colds, "flu," sinus congestion, and hay fever

Side Effects: Anxiety; blurred vision; chest pain; confusion; constipation; difficult and painful urination; dizziness; headache; increased blood pressure; insomnia; loss of appetite; nausea; nervousness; palpitations; rash; ringing in the ears; slight blood loss; reduced sweating; tension; tremor; vomiting

Contraindications: This product should not be used by persons who have allergies, aspirin sensitivity, asthma, blood-clotting disease, gout, severe heart disease, severe high blood pressure, or vitamin-K deficiency. • This product should not be given to newborn or premature infants.

Warnings: This product should be used with special caution by the elderly or debilitated, persons on sodium-restricted diets, and by those who have diabetes, enlarged prostate, glaucoma (certain types), heart disease, high blood pressure, kidney disease, obstructed bladder, obstructed intestine, peptic ulcer, or thyroid disease. If you have any of these conditions, consult your doctor before taking this product. • This product may cause drowsiness. Do not take it if you must drive, operate heavy machinery, or perform other tasks requiring mental alertness. To prevent oversedation, avoid the use of alcohol or other drugs that have sedative properties. • This product interacts with alcohol, ammonium chloride, guanethidine, methotrexate, monoamine oxidase inhibitors, oral anticoagulants, oral antidiabetics, probenecid, sedative drugs, steroids, sulfinpyrazone, tricyclic antidepressants, and vitamin C. If you are currently taking any drugs of these types, check with your doctor before taking this product. If you are unsure of the type or contents of your medications, ask your doctor or pharmacist. • Because this product reduces sweating, avoid excessive work or exercise in hot weather.

Comments: Many other conditions (some serious) mimic the common cold. If symptoms persist beyond one week or if they occur regularly without regard to season, consult your doctor. • The effectiveness of this product may diminish after being taken regularly for seven to ten days; consult your pharmacist about substituting another product containing a different antihistamine if this product begins to lose its effectiveness for you. • Chew gum or suck on ice chips or a piece of hard candy to reduce mouth dryness. • Do not swallow these tablets whole; they must be completely dissolved in water before swallowing. Use approximately three ounces of water per tablet.

OTC   Alka-2 antacid

Manufacturer: Miles Laboratories, Inc.
Ingredient: calcium carbonate
Dosage Form: Chewable tablet: calcium carbonate, 500 mg
Use: For relief from acid indigestion, heartburn, and/or sour stomach
Side Effects: Constipation
Contraindications: Persons with kidney disease should not use this product.
Comments: Self-treatment of severe or repeated attacks of heartburn, indigestion, or upset stomach is not recommended. If you do self-treat, limit therapy to two weeks, then call your doctor if symptoms persist. Never self-medicate with this product if your symptoms occur regularly (two to three times or more a month); if they are particularly worse than normal; if you feel "tightness" in your chest, have chest pains, or are sweating; or if you are short of breath. Consult your doctor. • This product is safe and effective when used on an occasional basis only. Repeated administrations for longer than one to two weeks may cause "rebound acidity," resulting in increased gastric acid production. If this happens, your symptoms get worse. • This product works best when taken one hour after meals or at bedtime, unless otherwise directed by your doctor or pharmacist. • Do not take this product within two hours of a dose of a tetracycline antibiotic. Also, if you are taking iron, a vitamin-mineral product, chlorpromazine, phenytoin, digoxin, quinidine, or warfarin, remind your doctor or pharmacist that you are taking this product.

OTC   Allbee multivitamin

Manufacturer: A. H. Robins Company
Ingredients: ascorbic acid (vitamin C); thiamine mononitrate (vitamin B_1); riboflavin (vitamin B_2); niacinamide; pyridoxine hydrochloride (vitamin B_6); calcium pantothenate
Dosage Form: Capsule: ascorbic acid, 300 mg; thiamine mononitrate, 15 mg; riboflavin, 10.2 mg; niacinamide, 50 mg; pyridoxine hydrochloride, 5 mg; calcium pantothenate, 10 mg
Use: Dietary supplement
Warnings: This product contains vitamin B_6 in an amount great enough that it may interact with levodopa (L-dopa). If you are currently taking L-dopa, check with your doctor before taking this product.
Comments: If two or more capsules are taken daily, this product may interfere with the results of urine tests. Inform your doctor and pharmacist you are taking this product.

OTC   Allerest decongestant eyedrops

Manufacturer: Pharmacraft Division
Ingredients: benzalkonium chloride; boric acid; edetate disodium; methylcellulose; naphazoline chloride; sodium borate
Dosage Form: Drops: benzalkonium chloride, .01%; edetate disodium, .01%; naphazoline chloride, .012% (quantities of other ingredients not specified)
Use: Relief of minor eye irritation
Side Effects: Allergic reactions (rash, itching, soreness); local irritation; momentary blurred vision
Contraindications: Do not use this product if you have glaucoma.
Warnings: Do not use this product for more than two days without checking with your doctor.

306

Comments: A child who accidentally swallows this product is likely to become overstimulated. Call your doctor at once. • Do not touch the dropper or bottle top to the eye or other tissue because contamination of the solution will result. • This product contains boric acid which many medical authorities believe should not be used because it is toxic. Follow the directions on the package. • The use of more than one eye product at a time may cause severe irritation to the eye. Consult your pharmacist before doing so.

OTC   Allerest hay fever and allergy remedy

Manufacturer: Pharmacraft Division
Ingredients: phenylpropanolamine hydrochloride; chlorpheniramine maleate
Dosage Forms: Chewable tablet: phenylpropanolamine hydrochloride, 9.4 mg; chlorpheniramine maleate, 1 mg. Tablet: phenylpropanolamine hydrochloride, 18.7 mg; chlorpheniramine maleate, 2 mg. Timed-release capsule: phenylpropanolamine hydrochloride, 50 mg; chlorpheniramine maleate, 4 mg
Use: Relief of symptoms of hay fever, allergies, sinusitis, and nasal congestion
Side Effects: Anxiety; blurred vision; chest pain; confusion; constipation; difficult and painful urination; dizziness; headache; increased blood pressure; insomnia; loss of appetite; nausea; nervousness; palpitations; rash; reduced sweating; tension; tremor; vomiting
Warnings: This product should be used with special caution by the elderly or debilitated, and by persons who have asthma, diabetes, enlarged prostate, glaucoma (certain types), heart disease, high blood pressure, kidney disease, obstructed bladder, obstructed intestine, peptic ulcer, or thyroid disease. If you have any of these conditions, consult your doctor before taking this product. • This product may cause drowsiness. Do not take it if you must drive, operate heavy machinery, or perform other tasks requiring mental alertness. To prevent oversedation, avoid the use of alcohol or other drugs that have sedative properties. • This product interacts with alcohol, guanethidine, monamine oxidase inhibitors, sedative drugs, and tricyclic antidepressants; if you are currently taking any drugs of these types, check with your doctor before taking this product. If you are unsure of the type or contents of your medications, ask your doctor or pharmacist. • Because this product reduces sweating, avoid excessive work or exercise in hot weather. • The capsule form of this product has sustained action; never increase the recommended dose or take it more frequently than directed. A serious overdose could result.
Comments: Many other conditions (some serious) mimic the common cold. If symptoms persist beyond one week or if they occur regularly without regard to season, consult your doctor. • The effectiveness of this product may diminish after being taken regularly for seven to ten days; consult your pharmacist about substituting another product containing a different antihistamine if this product begins to lose its effectiveness for you. • Chew gum or suck on ice chips or a piece of hard candy to reduce mouth dryness. • The chewable tablet form of this product is intended for use by children.

OTC   Allerest nasal decongestant

Manufacturer: Pharmacraft Division
Ingredients: phenylephrine hydrochloride; benzalkonium chloride; edetate disodium; sodium bisulfate; saline phosphate buffer
Dosage Form: Nasal spray: phenylephrine hydrochloride, 0.5% (quantities of other ingredients not specified)
Use: Temporary relief of nasal congestion due to colds, sinusitis, hay fever,

307

or other upper respiratory allergies

Side Effects: Burning, dryness of nasal mucosa; increased nasal congestion or discharge; sneezing, and/or stinging; blurred vision; dizziness; drowsiness; headache; insomnia; nervousness; palpitations; slight increase in blood pressure; stimulation

Contraindications: This product should not be used by persons who have glaucoma (certain types).

Warnings: This product should be used with special caution by persons who have diabetes, advanced hardening of the arteries, heart disease, high blood pressure, or thyroid disease. If you have any of these conditions, consult your doctor before taking this product. • This product interacts with guanethidine, monoamine oxidase inhibitors, and thyroid preparations. If you are currently taking any drugs of these types, check with your doctor before taking this product. If you are unsure of the type or contents of your medications, ask your doctor or pharmacist. • To avoid side effects such as burning, sneezing, or stinging, and a "rebound" increase in nasal congestion and discharge, do not exceed the recommended dosage and do not use this product for more than three or four continuous days. • This product should not be used by more than one person; sharing the dispenser may spread infection.

Allerfrin adrenergic and antihistamine (Rugby Laboratories), see Actifed adrenergic and antihistamine.

Allernade antihistamine, anticholinergic, and adrenergic (Rugby Laboratories), see Ornade Spansule antihistamine, anticholinergic, and adrenergic.

Allerphed adrenergic and antihistamine (Spencer-Mead, Inc.), see Actifed adrenergic and antihistamine.

Allerphed C expectorant (Spencer-Mead, Inc.), see Actifed-C expectorant.

Almocarpine ophthalmic solution (Ayerst Laboratories), see Isopto Carpine ophthalmic solution.

OTC   Alophen laxative

Manufacturer: Parke-Davis
Ingredient: phenolphthalein
Dosage Form: Tablet: phenolphthalein, 60 mg
Use: Relief of constipation
Side Effects: Excess loss of fluid; griping (cramps); mucus in feces; pink to purple rash with blistering
Contraindications: Persons with high fever (100° F or more); black or tarry stools; nausea; vomiting; abdominal pain; or children under age three should not use this product unless directed by a doctor. • Do not use this product when constipation is caused by megacolon or other diseases of the intestine, or hypothyroidism. • Persons with a sensitivity to phenolphthalein should not use this product.
Warnings: Excessive use (daily for a month or more) of this product may cause diarrhea, vomiting, and loss of certain blood electrolytes.
Comments: This product may discolor the urine and feces. • Evacuation may occur within 6 to 12 hours. Never self-medicate if constipation lasts longer than two weeks or if the medication does not produce a laxative effect

within a week. • Limit use to seven days unless directed otherwise by a doctor since this product may cause laxative-dependence (addiction) if used for a longer time.

R̽   **Ambenyl expectorant**

Manufacturer: Marion Laboratories, Inc.

Ingredients: ammonium chloride; bromodiphenhydramine hydrochloride; codeine sulfate; diphenhydramine hydrochloride; potassium guaiacolsulfonate; menthol; alcohol

Dosage Form: Liquid (content per 5 ml, or one teaspoon): ammonium chloride, 80 mg; bromodiphenhydramine hydrochloride, 3.75 mg; codeine sulfate, 10 mg; diphenhydramine hydrochloride, 8.75 mg; potassium guaiacolsulfonate, 80 mg; menthol, 0.5 mg; alcohol, 5%

Use: Relief of coughing due to colds or allergy

Minor Side Effects: Blurred vision; confusion; constipation; diarrhea; difficult urination; dizziness; drowsiness; dry mouth; headache; insomnia; loss of appetite; nasal congestion; nausea; nervousness; palpitations; rash; reduced sweating; restlessness; vomiting; weakness

Major Side Effects: Low blood pressure; rash from exposure to sunlight; severe abdominal pain; sore throat

Contraindications: This drug should not be used in newborn or premature infants. • This drug should not be used in patients with asthma attacks, narrow-angle glaucoma, enlarged prostate, certain types of peptic ulcer, obstructed intestine, or bladder-neck obstruction. Be sure your doctor knows if you have any of these conditions. • This drug should not be used by people who are allergic to any of its ingredients. Consult your doctor immediately if this drug has been prescribed for you and you have such an allergy. • This drug should not be given to patients taking monoamine oxidase inhibitors. If you are currently taking any drugs of this type, consult your doctor about their use. If you are unsure of the type or contents of your medication, ask your doctor or pharmacist.

Warnings: Overdose or accidental ingestion of large quantities of this drug may produce convulsions or death, especially in infants and children. Follow dosage instructions carefully, and keep this drug out of the reach of children. • Patients using this drug should be aware of the probable additive effects with alcohol and other central nervous system depressants, including hypnotics, sedatives, and tranquilizers. Avoid the use of such drugs to prevent oversedation while taking this drug. If any such drugs are currently prescribed for you, consult your doctor about their use. • This drug should be used cautiously by persons engaged in activities requiring mental alertness, since the drug may cause drowsiness. Drive a car or operate machinery with caution when taking this drug. • This drug should be used cautiously by pregnant women and nursing mothers. This drug may inhibit production of breast milk. • This drug should be used with care in patients with a history of asthma. Be sure your doctor knows if you have such a history.

Comments: If you need an expectorant, you need more moisture in your environment. Drink nine to ten glasses of water each day. The use of a vaporizer or humidifier may also be beneficial. Consult your doctor. • While taking this drug, do not take any nonprescription item for cough, cold, or sinus problems without first checking with your doctor. • This drug may cause dryness of the mouth; chew gum or suck on ice chips or a piece of hard candy to reduce this feeling. • Because this drug reduces sweating, avoid excessive work or exercise in hot weather. • This product, like all products containing narcotics (e.g., codeine), are usually not used for more than seven to ten days. This drug has the potential for abuse and must be used with caution. Tolerance may develop quickly; do not increase the dose of this drug without first checking with your doctor. An overdose usually sedates an adult, but may cause excitation leading to convulsions and death in a child.

Amcill antibiotic (Parke-Davis), see ampicillin antibiotic.

Amen progesterone hormone (Carnrick Laboratories), see Provera progesterone hormone.

OTC   Americaine hemorrhoidal preparation

Manufacturer: Arnar-Stone Laboratories, Inc.
Ingredients: benzocaine; benzethonium chloride; polyethylene glycol base
Dosage Forms: Ointment: benzocaine, 20%; benzethonium chloride, 0.1%; polyethylene glycol base. Suppository: benzocaine, 280 mg; benzethonium chloride, 0.1%; polyethylene glycol base
Use: Relief of pain, burning, and itching of hemorrhoids
Warnings: Sensitization (continued itching and redness) may occur with long-term and repeated use.
Comments: Hemorrhoidal (pile) preparations relieve itching, reduce pain and inflammation, and check bleeding, but do not heal, dry up, or give lasting relief from hemorrhoids. • Certain ingredients in this product may cause an allergic reaction; do not use for longer than seven days at a time unless your doctor has advised you otherwise. • The suppository is not recommended for external hemorrhoids or bleeding internal hemorrhoids. Use the ointment form. Use caution when inserting applicator. • Never self-medicate for hemorrhoids if pain is continuous or throbbing, if bleeding or itching is excessive, or if you feel a large pressure within the rectum.

OTC   Americaine local anesthetic

Manufacturer: Arnar-Stone Laboratories, Inc.
Ingredients: benzocaine; benzethonium chloride; polyethylene glycols; water-dispersible base
Dosage Forms: Aerosol: benzocaine, 20%; water-dispersible base. Ointment: benzethonium chloride, 0.1%; benzocaine, 20%; polyethylene glycols
Use: First aid product for treatment of sunburn; minor cuts; scrapes; poison ivy; burns; and insect bites
Side Effects: Allergy; local irritation
Warnings: Do not use this product on broken skin. • This product should not be used on large areas of the body since enough of the medication can be absorbed to be toxic.
Comments: Remember that ointments that are put on serious (second- or third-degree) burns will have to be taken off before definitive treatment can be given. • Consult your doctor or pharmacist if you have any questions concerning the use of this product.

Ameri-EZP antibacterial and analgesic (W. E. Hauck, Inc.), see Azo Gantrisin antibacterial and analgesic.

Aminodur Dura-Tabs bronchodilator (Cooper Laboratories, Inc.), see aminophylline bronchodilator.

Rx   aminophylline bronchodilator

Manufacturer: various manufacturers

310

Ingredient: aminophylline

Equivalent Products: Aminodur Dura-Tabs, Cooper Laboratories, Inc.; Somophyllin, Fisons Corporation

Dosage Forms: Liquid (content per 15 ml): 270 mg. Suppository (content per suppository): 99 mg; 190 mg; 277 mg; 395 mg. Tablet: 100 mg; 200 mg (various colors)

Use: To relieve and/or prevent symptoms from bronchial asthma, pulmonary emphysema, and other lung diseases

Minor Side Effects: Gastrointestinal disturbances (stomach pain, vomiting); nervousness or restlessness

Major Side Effects: Convulsion; difficult breathing; palpitations

Contraindications: This drug should not be taken by people who are allergic to it, or who have an active peptic ulcer. Consult your doctor immediately if this drug has been prescribed for you and you have either of these conditions.

Warnings: Excessive doses of this drug are toxic, so follow your doctor's dosage instructions exactly. • This drug should be used cautiously by people who have heart disease, thyroid disease, high blood pressure, or a history of peptic ulcer; or by those who are pregnant. Be sure your doctor knows if you have any of these conditions. • Some children are unusually sensitive to aminophylline; this drug should be used cautiously in children. • This drug should not be used in conjunction with lithium carbonate, propranolol, or other xanthines; if you are currently taking any drugs of these types, consult your doctor about their use. If you are unsure of the type or contents of your medications, ask your doctor or pharmacist. • While taking this drug, do not use any nonprescription item for asthma without first checking with your doctor. • Avoid drinking coffee, tea, cola drinks, cocoa, or other beverages that contain caffeine. • Call your doctor if you have severe stomach pain, vomiting, or restlessness, because this drug may aggravate an ulcer.

Comments: While taking this drug, drink at least eight glasses of water daily. • Be sure to take your dose at exactly the right time. • Take this drug with food or milk. • If taking this drug causes you minor gastrointestinal distress, use a nonprescription antacid product, such as Maalox or Gelusil, for relief.

Amitril antidepressant (Parke-Davis), see Elavil antidepressant.

OTC   Ammens Medicated Powder rash remedy

Manufacturer: Bristol-Myers Products

Ingredients: aromatic oils; boric acid; 8-hydroxyquinoline; 8-hydroxyquinoline sulfate; starch; talc; zinc oxide

Dosage Form: Powder: aromatic oils, 0.14%; boric acid, 4.55%; 8-hydroxyquinoline, 0.1%; 8-hydroxyquinoline sulfate, 0.05%; starch, 41%; talc, 45.06%; zinc oxide, 9.1%

Use: For keeping baby skin dry; soothing diaper rash, prickly heat, and chafing

Side Effects: Allergy; local irritation

Comments: While using this product, be careful not to inhale any of the powder. • This product contains boric acid which many medical authorities believe should not be used because it is toxic. Follow the directions on the package carefully.

Rx   amoxicillin antibiotic

Manufacturer: various manufacturers

Ingredient: amoxicillin

Equivalent Products: Amoxil, Beecham Laboratories; Larotid, Roche Products, Inc.; Polymox, Bristol Laboratories; Robamox, A. H. Robins Company; Sumox, Reid-Provident Laboratories, Inc.; Trimox, E. R. Squibb & Sons, Inc.; Utimox, Parke-Davis; Van-Mox, Vanguard Laboratories; Wymox, Wyeth Laboratories

Dosage Forms: Capsule: 250 mg, 500 mg (various colors); Liquid (content per 5 ml): 125 mg, 250 mg

Use: Treatment of a wide variety of bacterial infections

Minor Side Effects: Diarrhea; nausea; vomiting

Major Side Effects: "Black tongue;" cough; mouth irritation; rash; rectal and vaginal itching; severe diarrhea; superinfection

Contraindications: This drug should not be taken by people who are allergic to penicillin. Consult your doctor immediately if this drug has been prescribed for you and you have such an allergy.

Warnings: This drug should be used cautiously by pregnant women and people who have asthma, severe hay fever, or other significant allergies. Be sure your doctor knows if you have any of these conditions. • Complete blood cell counts and liver and kidney function tests are advisable if you take this drug for an extended period of time. • This drug should not be used in conjunction with chloramphenicol, erythromycin, or tetracycline; if you are currently taking any drugs of these types, consult your doctor about their use. If you are unsure of the contents of your medications, ask your doctor or pharmacist.

Comments: This drug is almost identical in nature to penicillin and ampicillin. • Severe allergic reactions to this drug (indicated by breathing difficulties and a drop in blood pressure) have been reported, but are rare when the drug is taken orally. • This drug should be taken for at least ten full days, even if symptoms disappear within that time. • The liquid form of this drug should be stored in the refrigerator. • Diabetics using Clinitest urine test may get a false high sugar reading while taking this drug. Change to Clinistix or Tes-Tape urine test to avoid this problem.

Amoxil antibiotic (Beecham Laboratories), see amoxicillin antibiotic.

OTC   Amphojel antacid

Manufacturer: Wyeth Laboratories

Ingredient: aluminum hydroxide

Dosage Form: Suspension (content per teaspoon): aluminum hydroxide, 320 mg. Tablet: aluminum hydroxide, 300 mg or 600 mg

Use: For relief from acid indigestion, heartburn and/or sour stomach

Side Effects: Constipation

Warnings: Long-term (several weeks) use of this product may lead to intestinal obstruction and dehydration. • Phosphate depletion may occur leading to weakness, loss of appetite, and eventually bone pain. You can prevent this by drinking at least one glass of milk a day.

Comments: Self-treatment of severe or repeated attacks of heartburn, indigestion, or upset stomach is not recommended. If you do self-treat, limit therapy to two weeks, then call your doctor if symptoms persist. • Never self-medicate with this product if your symptoms occur regularly (two to three times or more a month); if they are particularly worse than normal; if you feel "tightness" in your chest, have chest pains, or are sweating; or if you are short of breath. Consult your doctor. • To prevent constipation, drink at least eight glasses of water a day. If constipation persists, consult your doctor or pharmacist. • This product works best when taken one hour after meals or at bedtime, unless otherwise directed by your doctor or pharmacist. The suspension form of this product is superior to the tablet form and should be used unless you have been specifically directed to use the tablet. • Do not take this product within two hours of a dose of a tetracycline antibiotic. Also, if you are taking iron, a vitamin-mineral product, chlorpromazine, phenytoin, digoxin, quinidine, or warfarin, remind your doctor or pharmacist that you are taking this product.

℞   ampicillin antibiotic

Manufacturer: various manufacturers
Ingredient: ampicillin
Equivalent Products: A-Cillin, W. E. Hauck, Inc.; Amcill, Parke-Davis; Ampico, Coastal Pharmaceutical Co., Inc.; Amplin, Winston Pharmaceuticals, Inc.; Omnipen, Wyeth Laboratories; Pen A, Pfipharmecs Division; Penbritin, Ayerst Laboratories; Pensyn, The Upjohn Company; Polycillin, Bristol Laboratories; Principen, E. R. Squibb & Sons; SK-Ampicillin, Smith Kline & French Laboratories; Supen, Reid-Provident Laboratories, Inc.; Totacillin, Beecham Laboratories
Dosage Forms: Capsule: 250 mg; 500 mg (various colors). Liquid (content per 5 ml): 100 mg; 125 mg; 250 mg; 500 mg
Use: Treatment of a wide variety of bacterial infections
Minor Side Effects: Diarrhea; nausea; vomiting
Major Side Effects: "Black tongue"; cough; mouth irritation; rash; rectal and vaginal itching; severe diarrhea; superinfection
Contraindications: This drug should not be taken by people who are allergic to penicillin. Consult your doctor immediately if this drug has been prescribed for you and you have such an allergy.
Warnings: This drug should not be used in conjunction with chloramphenicol, erythromycin, or tetracycline; if you are currently taking any drugs of these types, consult your doctor about their use. If you are unsure of the contents of your medications, ask your doctor or pharmacist. • This drug should be used cautiously by pregnant women and people who have asthma, severe hay fever, or other significant allergies. Be sure your doctor knows if you have any of these conditions. • Complete blood cell counts and liver and kidney function tests are advisable if you take this drug for an extended period of time.
Comments: This drug is almost identical in nature and action to penicillin and amoxicillin. • Severe allergic reactions to this drug (indicated by breathing difficulties and a drop in blood pressure) have been reported, but are rare when the drug is taken orally. • This drug should be taken for at least ten full days, even if symptoms disappear within that time. • The liquid form of this drug should be stored in the refrigerator. • Take the drug on an empty stomach (one hour before or two hours after a meal). • Diabetics using Clinitest urine test may get a false high sugar reading while taking this drug. Change to Clinistix or Tes-Tape urine test to avoid this problem.

Ampico antibiotic (Coastal Pharmaceutical Co., Inc.), see ampicillin antibiotic.

Amplin antibiotic (Winston Pharmaceuticals, Inc.), see ampicillin antibiotic.

Amtet antibiotic (Amid Laboratories, Inc.), see tetracycline hydrochloride antibiotic.

Anacin analgesic

Manufacturer: Whitehall Laboratories
Ingredients: aspirin; caffeine
Dosage Form: Tablet: aspirin, 400 mg; caffeine, 32 mg
Use: Relief of pain of headache, toothache, sprains, muscular aches, nerve inflammation, menstruation; relief of discomforts and fever of colds; temporary relief of minor aches and pains of arthritis and rheumatism
Side Effects: Dizziness; mental confusion; mild stimulation; nausea and vomiting; ringing in the ears; slight blood loss; sweating
Contraindications: This product may cause an increased bleeding tendency and should not be taken by persons with a history of bleeding, peptic ulcer, or stomach bleeding.
Warnings: Persons with asthma, hay fever, or other allergies should be extremely careful about using this product. The product may interfere with the treatment of gout. If you have any of these conditions, consult your doctor or pharmacist before using this medication. • Do not use this product if you are currently taking alcohol, methotrexate, oral anticoagulants, oral antidiabetics, probenecid, steroids, and/or sulfinpyrazone; if you are unsure of the type or contents of your medications, ask your doctor or pharmacist. • The dosage instructions listed on the package should be followed carefully; toxicity may occur in adults or children with repeated doses.
Comments: You can save money by taking plain aspirin instead of this product; there is no evidence that combinations of ingredients are more effective than similar doses of a single-ingredient product. The caffeine in this product may have a slight stimulant effect but has no pain-relieving value.

OTC   **Anacin, Maximum Strength analgesic**

Manufacturer: Whitehall Laboratories
Ingredients: aspirin; caffeine
Dosage Form: Tablet: aspirin, 500 mg; caffeine, 32 mg
Use: Relief of pain of headache, toothache, minor aches and pains, menstrual discomfort; relief of discomforts and fever of colds; temporary relief of minor aches and pains of arthritis and rheumatism
Side Effects: Dizziness; mental confusion; nausea and vomiting; ringing in the ears; slight blood loss; sweating
Contraindications: This product may cause an increased bleeding tendency and should not be taken by persons with a history of bleeding, peptic ulcer, or stomach bleeding.
Warnings: Persons with asthma, hay fever, or other allergies should be extremely careful about using this product. The product may interfere with the treatment of gout. If you have any of these conditions, consult your doctor or pharmacist before using this medication. • Do not use this product if you are currently taking alcohol, methotrexate, oral anticoagulants, oral antidiabetics, probenecid, steroids, and/or sulfinpyrazone; if you are unsure of the type or contents of your medications, ask your doctor or pharmacist. • The dosage instructions listed on the package should be followed carefully; toxicity may occur in adults or children with repeated doses.
Comments: The caffeine in this product may have a slight stimulant effect but has no pain-relieving value. • You can save money and get the same results by taking three plain aspirin tablets and drinking a cup of coffee at the same time instead of taking this product.

OTC   **Anacin-3 analgesic**

Manufacturer: Whitehall Laboratories

Ingredients: acetaminophen; caffeine
Dosage Form: Tablet: acetaminophen, 500 mg; caffeine, 32 mg
Use: Relief of pain of headache, toothache, sinusitis, muscular aches and strains, menstruation, colds or "flu"; temporary relief of minor arthritis pain; reduction of fever
Side Effects: When taken in overdose: blood disorders; rash; mild stimulation
Warnings: When taken in overdose, acetaminophen is more toxic than aspirin. The dosage instructions listed on the package should be followed carefully; toxicity may occur in adults or children with repeated doses.
Comments: You can save money by taking plain acetaminophen instead of this product; there is no evidence that combinations of ingredients are more effective than similar doses of a single-ingredient product. The caffeine in this product may have a slight stimulant effect but has no pain-relieving value.

Android steroid hormone (Brown Pharmaceutical Co., Inc.), see methyltestosterone steroid hormone.

Ang-O-Span antianginal (Scrip-Physician Supply Co.), see Nitro-Bid Plateau Caps antianginal.

Anoxine anorectic (Winston Pharmaceuticals, Inc.), see Fastin anorectic.

Antepar anthelmintic (Burroughs Wellcome), see Povan anthelmintic.

Antiminth anthelmintic (Roerig Pharmaceuticals), see Povan anthelmintic.

Antipress antidepressant (Lemmon Company), see Tofranil antidepressant.

℞   **Antivert antinauseant**

Manufacturer: Roerig
Ingredient: meclizine hydrochloride
Equivalent Products: Bonine, Pfizer Laboratories Division; Dizmiss, Bowman Pharmaceuticals; Eldezine, Paul B. Elder Co.; meclizine hydrochloride, various manufacturers; Wehvert, W. E. Hauck, Inc.
Dosage Forms: Chewable tablet: 25 mg (pink). Tablet: 12.5 mg (blue/white); 25 mg (yellow/white)
Use: To provide symptomatic relief of dizziness due to ear infections; or to relieve dizziness and nausea due to motion sickness
Minor Side Effects: Blurred vision; drowsiness; dry mouth
Contraindications: Do not take this drug if you are or may become pregnant. Experimental studies with rats have shown a high association of birth defects with the drug. Consult your doctor immediately if this drug has been prescribed for you and you are pregnant. • This drug should not be taken by people who are allergic to it. Consult your doctor immediately if this drug has been prescribed for you and you have such an allergy.
Warnings: This drug is not recommended for use by children. • This drug should not be used in conjunction with central nervous system depressants; if you are currently taking any drugs of this type, consult your doctor about

their use. If you are unsure of the type of your medications, ask your doctor or pharmacist. • This drug should be used cautiously by people who have liver or kidney disease. Be sure your doctor knows if you have such a condition. • This drug may cause drowsiness; avoid tasks that require alertness. To prevent oversedation, avoid the use of other sedative drugs or alcohol.

Comments: When used for motion sickness, take this drug one hour before travel, then one dose every 24 hours during travel. • Although most brands of this drug require a prescription, nonprescription forms are also available for purchase.

℞ Anusol-HC steroid-hormone-containing anorectal product

Manufacturer: Parke-Davis

Ingredients: benzyl benzoate; bismuth resorcin compound; bismuth subgallate; hydrocortisone acetate; Peruvian balsam; zinc oxide

Dosage Forms: Cream (content per gram): benzyl benzoate, 12 mg; bismuth resorcin compound, 17.5 mg; bismuth subgallate, 22.5 mg; hydrocortisone acetate, 5 mg; Peruvian balsam, 18 mg; zinc oxide, 110 mg. Suppository: benzyl benzoate, 1.2%; bismuth resorcin compound, 1.75%; bismuth subgallate, 2.25%; hydrocortisone acetate, 10 mg; Peruvian balsam, 1.8%; zinc oxide, 11%

Use: Relief of pain, itching, and discomfort arising from hemorrhoids and irritated anorectal tissues

Minor Side Effects: Burning sensation on application

Major Side Effects: None when used for short time only

Contraindications: This drug should not be used by people who are allergic to any of its ingredients. Consult your doctor immediately if this drug has been prescribed for you and you have such an allergy.

Warnings: This drug should be used with caution by pregnant women. Pregnant women should not use the product unnecessarily on extensive areas, in large amounts, or for prolonged periods. • If irritation develops, discontinue use of this drug, and notify your doctor. • This drug should be used with caution in children and infants. • Do not use this drug in the eyes.

Comments: This drug should not be used for more than seven consecutive days, unless your doctor specifically says to do so. • The suppository form of this drug should be stored in a cool, dry place.

OTC Anusol hemorrhoidal preparation

Manufacturer: Parke-Davis

Ingredients: Suppository: benzyl benzoate; bismuth resorcin compound; bismuth subgallate; Peruvian balsam; vegetable oil base; zinc oxide. Ointment: benzyl benzoate; Peruvian balsam; pramoxine hydrochloride; zinc oxide

Dosage Forms: Suppository: benzyl benzoate, 1.2%; bismuth resorcin compound, 1.75%; bismuth subgallate, 2.25%; Peruvian balsam, 1.8%; vegetable oil base; zinc oxide, 11%. Ointment (content per gram): benzyl benzoate, 12 mg; Peruvian balsam, 18 mg; pramoxine hydrochloride, 10 mg; zinc oxide, 110 mg

Use: Relief of pain, itching, and burning of hemorrhoids and other irritated anorectal tissues

Warnings: Sensitization (continued itching and redness) may occur with long-term repeated use.

Comments: Hemorrhoidal (pile) preparations relieve itching, reduce pain and inflammation, and check bleeding, but do not heal, dry up, or give lasting relief from hemorrhoids. • Certain ingredients in this product may cause an allergic reaction; do not use for longer than seven days at a time unless your doctor has advised you otherwise. • The suppository is less preferable for external hemorrhoids or bleeding internal hemorrhoids. Use the ointment form. Use caution when inserting applicator. • Never self-medicate for hemorrhoids if pain is continuous or throbbing, if bleeding or itching is excessive, or if you feel a large pressure within the rectum.

A.P.C. with Demerol analgesic (Winthrop Laboratories), see Demerol analgesic.

A-poxide sedative and hypnotic (Abbott Laboratories), see Librium sedative and hypnotic.

OTC   Appedrine Extra Strength appetite suppressant

Manufacturer: Thompson Medical Company, Inc.
Ingredients: ascorbic acid (vitamin C); caffeine; cyanocobalamin (vitamin B₁₂); d-calcium pantothenate; folic acid; niacinamide; phenylpropanolamine hydrochloride; pyridoxine hydrochloride (vitamin B₆); riboflavin (vitamin B₂); thiamine hydrochloride (vitamin B₁); vitamin A; vitamin D; vitamin E
Dosage Form: Tablet: ascorbic acid (vitamin C), 20 mg; caffeine, 100 mg; cyanocobalamin (vitamin B₁₂), 2 mcg; d-calcium pantothenate, 3.3 mg; folic acid, 0.133 mg; niacinamide, 6.6 mg; phenylpropanolamine hydrochloride, 35 mg; pyridoxine hydrochloride, (vitamin B₆), 0.66 mg; riboflavin (vitamin B₂), 0.57 mg; thiamine hydrochloride (vitamin B₁), 0.5 mg; vitamin A, 1667 IU; vitamin D, 133 IU; vitamin E, 10 IU
Use: Aid in diet control
Side Effects: Diarrhea; headache; insomnia; nervousness; increase in blood pressure, blood sugar, heart rate, and thyroid activity; in larger than the recommended dose: irregular heartbeat, upset stomach
Contraindications: Persons with heart disease, high blood pressure, diabetes, kidney or thyroid disease, pregnant or nursing women, and/or persons under 18 years of age should not use this product. Consult your doctor.
Comments: During the first week of taking this medication, expect increased frequency of urination. • Many medical authorities believe that the ingredient phenylpropanolamine does not help in weight loss programs. The FDA Review Panel has reported that it is effective. If you want to use this product, remember that you become tolerant to any beneficial effects after a couple of weeks. After each two weeks of use, stop for one week, then resume. • Take this product with a glass (eight ounces) of water. • The primary value in products of this nature is in following the caloric reduction plan that goes with them.

℞   Apresoline antihypertensive

Manufacturer: CIBA Pharmaceutical Company
Ingredient: hydralazine hydrochloride
Equivalent Products: Dralzine, Lemmon Pharmacal Company; hydralazine hydrochloride, various manufacturers; Nor-Pres, North American Pharmacal, Inc.; Rolazine, Robinson Laboratory, Inc.
Dosage Form: Tablet: 10 mg (yellow); 25 mg (deep blue); 50 mg (light blue); 100 mg (peach)
Use: Treatment of high blood pressure
Minor Side Effects: Diarrhea; dizziness; headache; loss of appetite; nasal congestion; nausea; numbness or tingling in fingers and toes; palpitations; vomiting
Major Side Effects: Fluid retention; rash; sore throat; tenderness in joints
Contraindications: This drug should not be taken by people who are allergic to it, or who have coronary heart disease or mitral valvular rheumatic heart disease. Consult your doctor immediately if this drug has been

prescribed for you and you have any of these conditions.

Warnings: This drug may cause angina and heart attacks and should be used cautiously by people in whom coronary heart disease is suspected. Pregnant women and people who have kidney disease should also use this drug with caution. Be sure your doctor knows if you have, or might have, any of these conditions. • This drug may cause lupus, stroke, nerve damage, or blood diseases; contact your doctor if any unexplained symptoms of tiredness, weakness, fever, aching joints, or chest pain (angina) occur. • Periodic blood tests are advisable while you are taking this drug. • This drug interacts with other antihypertensive drugs, amphetamines, decongestants, and monoamine oxidase inhibitors; if you are currently taking any drugs of these types, consult your doctor about their use. If you are unsure of the type of your medications, ask your doctor or pharmacist. • Do not stop taking this medication unless your doctor directs you to do so. • While taking this drug, do not take any nonprescription item for cough, cold, or sinus problems without first checking with your doctor. • This drug may affect your ability to perform tasks that require alertness; avoid driving or operating machinery if the drug makes you dizzy or otherwise impairs your concentration. • Limit your consumption of alcoholic beverages in order to prevent dizziness or light-headedness.

Comments: The effects of treatment with this drug may not be apparent for at least two weeks. • Mild side effects (e.g., headache or nasal congestion) are most noticeable during the first two weeks of drug therapy and become less bothersome after this period. • If you experience numbness or tingling in your fingers or toes while using this drug, your doctor may recommend that you take vitamin B$_6$ (pyridoxine) to relieve the symptoms. • To avoid dizziness or light-headedness when you stand, contract and relax the muscles of your legs for a few moments before rising. Do this by pushing one foot against the floor while raising the other foot slightly, alternating feet so that you are "pumping" your legs in a pedaling motion.

Aquaserp diuretic and antihypertensive (Spencer-Mead, Inc.), see Hydropres diuretic and antihypertensive.

Aquatensen diuretic and antihypertensive (Wallace Laboratories), see Enduron diuretic and antihypertensive.

R$_x$ **Aristocort steroid hormone (topical)**

Manufacturer: Lederle Laboratories
Ingredient: triamcinolone acetonide
Equivalent Products: Kenalog, E. R. Squibb & Sons; triamcinolone acetonide, various manufacturers
Dosage Forms: Cream: 0.025%; 0.1%; 0.5%. Ointment: 0.1%; 0.5%
Use: Symptomatic relief of skin inflammations caused by certain skin conditions such as eczema or poisoning
Minor Side Effects: Dryness; localized burning; irritation; itching; rash
Major Side Effects: Secondary infection
Contraindications: This drug should not be used by people allergic to it. Consult your doctor immediately if this drug has been prescribed for you and you have such an allergy.
Warnings: This drug should be used cautiously by pregnant women. Be sure your doctor knows if you are pregnant. • Do not use this drug in or

around the eyes. • Notify your doctor if irritation develops.

Comments: Apply this drug as thinly as possible to the skin. • The cream form of this drug is greaseless and will not stain your clothing. • The cream form is better than the ointment for use on the scalp or other hairy areas of the body. • The ointment form of the drug is preferable for people with dry skin. • If it is necessary for you to use this drug under a wrap, follow your doctor's instructions exactly; do not leave the wrap in place longer than specified. Do not use a wrap unless directed to do so by your doctor.

℞   **Aristocort steroid hormone (oral)**

Manufacturer: Lederle Laboratories

Ingredient: triamcinolone diacetate (syrup); or triamcinolone (tablet)

Equivalent Products: Kenacort, E. R. Squibb & Sons; Rocinolone, Robinson Laboratory, Inc.; SK-Triamcinolone, Smith Kline & French Laboratories; triamcinolone, various manufacturers

Dosage Forms: Syrup (content per 5 ml): 2 mg. Tablet: 1 mg (yellow); 2 mg (pink); 4 mg (white); 8 mg (yellow); 16 mg (white)

Use: Treatment of endocrine or rheumatic disorders; asthma; blood diseases; certain cancers; gastrointestinal disturbances such as ulcerative colitis; inflammations such as arthritis; dermatitis; poison ivy

Minor Side Effects: Dizziness; headache; increased sweating; increased susceptibility to infection; menstrual irregularities

Major Side Effects: Abdominal enlargement; cataracts; fluid retention; glaucoma; growth impairment in children; high blood pressure; impaired healing of wounds; peptic ulcer; potassium loss; weakness

Contraindications: This drug should not be taken by people who are allergic to it, or who have systemic fungal infections. Consult your doctor if this drug has been prescribed for you and you have either of these conditions.

Warnings: This drug should be used cautiously by people who have thyroid disease, cirrhosis, ulcerative colitis, kidney disease, high blood pressure, osteoporosis, myasthenia gravis, eye damage or disease, peptic ulcer, or tuberculosis; and by pregnant or nursing women. Be sure your doctor knows if you have any of these conditions. • This drug should be used cautiously in children and infants; their growth must be carefully observed if they receive prolonged treatment with the drug. • People using this drug should not be vaccinated against smallpox, and should not receive any other immunizations. This drug may cause sudden fluctuations in mood, personality changes, and can intensify psychotic tendencies and/or emotional instability. • This drug interacts with aspirin, barbiturates, diuretics, estrogens, indomethacin, oral anticoagulants, antidiabetics, and phenytoin; if you are currently taking any drugs of these types, consult your doctor about their use. If you are unsure of the type or contents of your medications, ask your doctor or pharmacist. • Blood pressure, body weight, and vision should be checked at regular intervals. Stomach x-rays are advised for persons with suspected or known peptic ulcers. • Do not stop taking this drug without your doctor's knowledge.

Comments: This drug is often taken on a decreasing-dosage schedule (four times a day for several days, then three times a day, etc.). A special packaging that arranges the tablets in this way, is available from Lederle Laboratories as Aristo-Pak steroid hormone. It is convenient but more expensive than buying loose tablets. • For long-term treatment, taking the drug every other day (e.g., 16 mg every other day rather than 8 mg daily) is preferred. Generally, taking the entire dose at one time (about 8:00 A.M.) gives the best results. Ask your doctor about alternate-day dosing and the best hour of the day to take this drug. • To help avoid potassium loss while using this drug, take your dose with a glass of fresh or frozen orange juice, and eat a banana each day. The use of Co-Salt salt substitute also helps prevent potassium loss. • If you are using this drug chronically, you should wear or carry a notice that you are taking a steroid.

Aristoderm steroid hormone (Lederle Laboratories), see Kenalog steroid hormone.

Aristogel steroid hormone (Lederle Laboratories), see Kenalog steroid hormone.

Aristo-Pak steroid hormone (Lederle Laboratories), see Aristocort steroid hormone (oral).

OTC | A.R.M. allergy remedy

Manufacturer: Menley & James Laboratories
Ingredients: chlorpheniramine maleate; phenylpropanolamine hydrochloride
Dosage Form: Tablet: chlorpheniramine maleate, 4 mg; phenylpropanolamine hydrochloride, 37.5 mg
Use: Relief of symptoms of hay fever, allergies, sinusitis, and nasal congestion
Side Effects: Anxiety; blurred vision; chest pain; confusion; constipation; difficult and painful urination; dizziness; headache; increased blood pressure; insomnia; loss of appetite; nausea; nervousness; palpitations; rash; reduced sweating; tension; tremor; vomiting
Warnings: This product should be used with special caution by the elderly or debilitated, and by persons who have asthma, diabetes, enlarged prostate, glaucoma (certain types), heart disease, high blood pressure, kidney disease, obstructed bladder, obstructed intestine, peptic ulcer, or thyroid disease. If you have any of these conditions, consult your doctor before taking this product. • This product may cause drowsiness. Do not take it if you must drive, operate heavy machinery, or perform other tasks requiring mental alertness. To prevent oversedation, avoid the use of alcohol or other drugs that have sedative properties. • This product interacts with alcohol, guanethidine, monoamine oxidase inhibitors, sedative drugs, and tricyclic antidepressants. If you are currently taking any drugs of these types, check with your doctor before taking this product. If you are unsure of the type or contents of your medications, ask your doctor or pharmacist. • Because this product reduces sweating, avoid excessive work or exercise in hot weather.
Comments: Many other conditions (some serious) mimic the common cold. If symptoms persist beyond one week or if they occur regularly without regard to season, consult your doctor. • The effectiveness of this product may diminish after being taken regularly for seven to ten days; consult your pharmacist about substituting another product containing a different antihistamine if this product begins to lose its effectiveness for you. • Chew gum or suck on ice chips or a piece of hard candy to reduce mouth dryness.

Rx | Artane antiparkinson drug

Manufacturer: Lederle Laboratories
Ingredient: trihexyphenidyl hydrochloride
Equivalent Products: Hexyphen, Robinson Laboratory, Inc.; T.H.P., Spencer-Mead, Inc.; Tremin, Schering Corporation; Trihexane, Rugby Laboratories; Trihexidyl, Henry Schein, Inc.; trihexyphenidyl HCL, various manufacturers

Dosage Forms: Sustained-release capsule: 5 mg (blue with white granules). Syrup (content per 5 ml): 2 mg. Tablet: 2 mg; 5 mg (both white)

Uses: Treatment of all forms of Parkinson's disease; prevention of tremors and other symptoms associated with central nervous system drugs such as Stelazine, Thorazine, and other similar phenothiazine drugs

Minor Side Effects: Blurred vision; constipation; difficult urination; dizziness; drowsiness; dry mouth; headache; mild nausea; nervousness; vomiting; weakness

Major Side Effects: None in most people. However, some people with arteriosclerosis or with a history of abnormal reactions to other drugs may exhibit symptoms of mental confusion, agitation, disturbed behavior, or nausea and vomiting; psychiatric disturbances can result from indiscriminate use leading to overdosage; narrow-angle glaucoma reported.

Warnings: People treated with this drug should have close monitoring of intraocular pressures at regular periodic intervals. • This drug should be used with caution by people with heart, liver, or kidney disorders, or with high blood pressure. People with any of these conditions should be under close medical observation. • Careful and constant long-term observation of people using this drug should be undertaken to avoid allergic and certain other reactions. • This drug should be used with caution in people with glaucoma, obstructive diseases of the gastrointestinal or genitourinary tract, and in elderly males with possible prostate gland problems. • Persons over 60 years of age require strict dosage regulation, since they frequently develop increased sensitivity to the action of this type of drug. • This drug should not be taken with antidepressants. If you are currently taking any drugs of this type, consult your doctor immediately about their use. If you are unsure of the type of your medications, consult your doctor or pharmacist.

Comments: This drug is frequently prescribed along with phenothiazine drugs such as Thorazine and Stelazine to reduce the tremors caused by phenothiazines. You should talk with your doctor about waiting before taking this drug to see if you really need it. Many people can take phenothiazine drugs successfully and may not need this drug. • The sustained-release capsule form of this drug is effective over a long time; never take it more frequently than prescribed by your doctor. A serious overdose may result. • Since this drug may cause dryness of the mouth, chew gum or suck on ice chips or a piece of hard candy to reduce this feeling. • Generic brands of this drug are available and vary widely in cost. Consult your doctor and pharmacist. • Certain other drugs, such as Cogentin (Merck Sharp & Dohme) and Kemadrin (Burroughs Wellcome) antiparkinson drugs, have similar actions to this drug.

OTC · Arthritis Pain Formula analgesic

Manufacturer: Whitehall Laboratories

Ingredients: aspirin (micronized); aluminum hydroxide gel; magnesium hydroxide

Dosage Form: Tablet: micronized aspirin, 486 mg (7.5 grains); aluminum hydroxide gel, 20 mg; magnesium hydroxide, 60 mg

Use: Temporary relief of minor aches and pain of arthritis and rheumatism, and of lower back pain; relief of pain of headache, nerve inflammation, toothache, menstruation; relief of discomforts and fever of colds

Side Effects: Dizziness; mental confusion; nausea and vomiting; ringing in the ears; slight blood loss; sweating

Contraindications: This product may cause an increased bleeding tendency and should not be taken by persons with a history of bleeding, peptic ulcer, or stomach bleeding.

321

Warnings: Persons with kidney disease, asthma, hay fever, or other allergies should be extremely careful about using this product. The product may interfere with the treatment of gout. If you have any of these conditions, consult your doctor or pharmacist before using this medication. • Do not use this product if you are currently taking alcohol, methotrexate, oral anti-coagulants, oral antidiabetics, probenecid, steroids, and/or sulfinpyrazone; if you are unsure of the type or contents of your medications, ask your doctor or pharmacist. • The dosage instructions listed on the package should be followed carefully; toxicity may occur in adults or children with repeated doses.

Comments: Magnesium interacts with tetracycline antibiotics. There may not be enough magnesium in this product to cause any problem, but if you are taking a tetracycline antibiotic in addition to this product, separate the dosages by at least two hours. • Pain-relief tablets, such as this product, that contain salts of magnesium or aluminum are known as buffered tablets. Such products dissolve faster than unbuffered products, but there is no evidence that they relieve pain faster or better than those products that do not contain buffers. Buffered tablets may be less likely to cause gastric upset in some people.

OTC   Arthritis Strength Bufferin analgesic

Manufacturer: Bristol-Myers Products
Ingredients: aspirin; aluminum glycinate; magnesium carbonate
Dosage Form: Tablet: aspirin, 486 mg (7.5 grains); aluminum glycinate, 72.9 mg (1.125 grains); magnesium carbonate, 145.8 mg (2.25 grains)
Use: Temporary relief from minor aches and pains, stiffness, swelling, and inflammation of arthritis and rheumatism; reduction of pain and fever of colds and "flu"; relief of pain of headache, muscular aches and strains, sinusitis, nerve inflammation, tooth extraction, menstruation
Side Effects: Dizziness; mental confusion; nausea and vomiting; ringing in the ears; slight blood loss; sweating
Contraindications: This product may cause an increased bleeding tendency and should not be taken by persons with a history of bleeding, peptic ulcer, or stomach bleeding.
Warnings: Persons with kidney disease, asthma, hay fever, or other allergies should be extremely careful about using this product. The product may interfere with the treatment of gout. If you have any of these conditions, consult your doctor or pharmacist before using this medication. • Do not use this product if you are currently taking alcohol, methotrexate, oral anti-coagulants, oral antidiabetics, probenecid, steroids, and/or sulfinpyrazone; if you are unsure of the type or contents of your medications, ask your doctor or pharmacist. • The dosage instructions listed on the package should be followed carefully; toxicity may occur in adults or children with repeated doses.
Comments: Magnesium interacts with tetracycline antibiotics. There may not be enough magnesium in this product to cause any problem, but if you are taking a tetracycline antibiotic in addition to this product, separate the dosages by at least two hours. • Pain-relief tablets, such as this product, that contain salts of magnesium or aluminum are known as buffered tablets. Such products dissolve faster than unbuffered products, but there is no evidence that they relieve pain faster or better than those products that do not contain buffers. Buffered tablets may be less likely to cause gastric upset in some people.

Asa-lief antiasthmatic (Columbia Medical Co.), see Tedral antiasthmatic.

OTC   **Ascriptin A/D analgesic**

Manufacturer: William H. Rorer, Inc.
Ingredients: aspirin; magnesium-aluminum hydroxide
Dosage Form: Tablet: aspirin, 325 mg (5 grains); magnesium-aluminum hydroxide, 300 mg
Use: Relief of pain, inflammation, and fever of rheumatoid arthritis, osteo-arthritis, and other arthritic conditions
Side Effects: Dizziness; mental confusion; nausea and vomiting; ringing in the ears; slight blood loss; sweating
Contraindications: This product may cause an increased bleeding tendency and should not be taken by persons with a history of bleeding, peptic ulcer, or stomach bleeding.
Warnings: Persons with kidney disease, asthma, hay fever, or other allergies should be extremely careful about using this product. The product may interfere with the treatment of gout. If you have any of these conditions, consult your doctor or pharmacist before using this medication. • Do not use this product if you are currently taking alcohol, methotrexate, oral anti-coagulants, oral antidiabetics, probenecid, steroids, and/or sulfinpyrazone; if you are unsure of the type or contents of your medications, ask your doctor or pharmacist. • The dosage instructions listed on the package should be followed carefully; toxicity may occur in adults or children with repeated doses.
Comments: Magnesium interacts with tetracycline antibiotics. There may not be enough magnesium in this product to cause any problem, but if you are taking a tetracycline antibiotic in addition to this product, separate the dosages by at least two hours. • Pain-relief tablets, such as this product, that contain salts of magnesium or aluminum are known as buffered tablets. Such products dissolve faster than unbuffered products, but there is no evidence that they relieve pain faster or better than those products that do not contain buffers. Buffered tablets may be less likely to cause gastric upset in some people.

OTC   **Ascriptin analgesic**

Manufacturer: William H. Rorer, Inc.
Ingredients: aspirin; magnesium-aluminum hydroxide
Dosage Form: Tablet: aspirin, 325 mg (5 grains); magnesium-aluminum hydroxide, 150 mg
Use: Relief of pain of headache, menstruation, minor injuries; relief of discomforts and fever of colds or "flu"; reduction of pain and inflammation of arthritis and other rheumatic diseases
Side Effects: Dizziness; mental confusion; nausea and vomiting; ringing in the ears; slight blood loss; sweating
Contraindications: This product may cause an increased bleeding tendency and should not be taken by persons with a history of bleeding, peptic ulcer, or stomach bleeding.
Warnings: Persons with kidney disease, asthma, hay fever, or other allergies should be extremely careful about using this product. The product may interfere with the treatment of gout. If you have any of these conditions, consult your doctor or pharmacist before using this medication. • Do not use this product if you are currently taking alcohol, methotrexate, oral anticoagu-lants, oral antidiabetics, probenecid, steroids, and/or sulfinpyrazone; if you are unsure of the type or contents of your medications, ask your doctor or pharmacist. • The dosage instructions listed on the package should be followed carefully; toxicity may occur in adults or children with repeated doses.
Comments: Magnesium interacts with tetracycline antibiotics. There may

not be enough magnesium in this product to cause any problem, but if you are taking a tetracycline antibiotic in addition to this product, separate the dosages by at least two hours. • Pain-relief tablets, such as this product, that contain salts of magnesium or aluminum are known as buffered tablets. Such products dissolve faster than unbuffered products, but there is no evidence that they relieve pain faster or better than those products that do not contain buffers. Buffered tablets may be less likely to cause gastric upset in some people.

Asminorel Improved adrenergic, sedative, and smooth muscle relaxant (Tutag Pharmaceuticals, Inc.), see Marax adrenergic, sedative, and smooth muscle relaxant.

OTC   Aspergum analgesic

Manufacturer: Plough, Inc.
Ingredient: aspirin
Dosage Form: Chewing gum tablet: aspirin, 227 mg (3.5 grains)
Use: Temporary relief of minor sore throat pain, simple headache, muscular aches and pains
Side Effects: Dizziness; mental confusion; nausea and vomiting; ringing in the ears; slight blood loss; sweating
Contraindications: This product may cause an increased bleeding tendency and should not be taken by persons with a history of bleeding, peptic ulcer, or stomach bleeding.
Warnings: Persons with asthma, hay fever, or other allergies should be extremely careful about using this product. The product may interfere with the treatment of gout. If you have any of these conditions, consult your doctor or pharmacist before using this medication. • Do not use this product if you are currently taking alcohol, methotrexate, oral anticoagulants, oral antidiabetics, probenecid, steroids, and/or sulfinpyrazone; if you are unsure of the type or contents of your medications, ask your doctor or pharmacist. • The dosage instructions listed on the package should be followed carefully; toxicity may occur in adults or children with repeated doses.
Comments: There is no apparent advantage to the dosage form of this product.

Rx   Atarax sedative

Manufacturer: Roerig
Ingredient: hydroxyzine hydrochloride
Equivalent Products: hydroxyzine hydrochloride, various manufacturers; Vistaril (see Comments), Pfizer Laboratories Division
Dosage Forms: Syrup (content per ml): 10 mg. Tablet: 10 mg (orange); 25 mg (green); 50 mg (yellow); 100 mg (red)
Use: Symptomatic relief of anxiety and tension; treatment of pruritus caused by allergic conditions
Minor Side Effects: Drowsiness; dry mouth
Major Side Effects: Convulsions; tremors
Contraindications: Do not take this drug if you are allergic to it or are pregnant. Consult your doctor immediately if the drug has been prescribed for you and you have either of these conditions.
Warnings: This drug should be used cautiously by people who have liver or

kidney disease. Be sure your doctor knows if you have either of these conditions. • This drug should not be used in conjunction with central nervous system depressants, alcohol, or other drugs that have sedative properties; if you are currently taking any drugs of these types, consult your doctor about their use. If you are unsure of the type or contents of your medications, ask your doctor or pharmacist. • This drug may cause drowsiness; avoid tasks that require alertness.

Comments: The generic name for Vistaril sedative is hydroxyzine pamoate; although not generically identical, Vistaril is equivalent to Atarax sedative and other hydroxyzine hydrochloride products. • Chew gum or suck on ice chips or a piece of hard candy to reduce mouth dryness.

R̲x   **Ativan sedative and hypnotic**

Manufacturer: Wyeth Laboratories
Ingredient: lorazepam
Dosage Form: Tablet: 0.5 mg; 1 mg; 2 mg (all are white)
Use: Relief of anxiety, tension, agitation, irritability, and insomnia
Minor Side Effects: Change in appetite; depression; dizziness; drowsiness; dry mouth; headache; nausea; rash; unsteadiness; weakness
Major Side Effects: Eye function disturbance
Contraindications: This drug should not be used by people who are allergic to it. Consult your doctor immediately if this drug has been prescribed for you and you have such an allergy. • This drug should not be used by people with acute narrow-angle glaucoma. Be sure your doctor knows if you have this condition.
Warnings: This drug is not recommended for use in patients with a primary depressive disorder or psychosis. • Patients using this drug should not operate dangerous machinery or drive motor vehicles. • Use of this drug will decrease a person's tolerance for alcohol and other central nervous system depressants. While taking this drug, do not take such drugs. • Use of this drug may cause physical and psychological dependence. Withdrawal symptoms, not unlike those noted with withdrawal from alcohol and barbiturates, have occurred following abrupt discontinuation of this drug. Such abrupt stoppage may also result in quick return of symptoms for which the patient is being treated. Do not stop taking this drug without informing your doctor. If you have been taking the drug regularly, and wish to discontinue the drug's use, you must decrease the dose gradually, following your doctor's instructions. • This drug has the potential for abuse and must be used with caution. Tolerance may develop quickly; do not increase the dose without first consulting your doctor. Patients with depression accompanying anxiety should use this drug with extreme caution, since this drug may strengthen any suicidal tendencies. • Dosage of this drug for elderly and debilitated persons should not initially exceed 2 mg daily in order to avoid oversedation and other adverse reactions. This drug should be used cautiously in persons with impaired liver and kidney function. Be sure your doctor knows if you have such a condition. • This drug has not been shown to be effective in persons with anxiety coupled with heart or stomach disease. Be sure your doctor knows if you have either of these conditions. This drug should be used with caution in children under 12 years of age, in pregnant women, and in nursing mothers. This drug is safe when used alone. When it is combined with other sedative drugs or alcohol, serious adverse reactions may develop.
Comments: This drug is currently used by many people to relieve nervousness. It is effective for this purpose, but it is important to try to remove the cause of the anxiety as well. Phenobarbital is also effective for this purpose, and it is less expensive. Consult your doctor. • This drug may cause

dryness of the mouth. To reduce this feeling, chew gum or suck on ice chips or a piece of hard candy.

℞   Atromid-S antilipidemic

Manufacturer: Ayerst Laboratories
Ingredient: clofibrate
Dosage Form: Capsule: 500 mg (orange-red)
Use: Reduction of fat or cholesterol in the blood in atherosclerosis (arteriosclerosis or hardening of the arteries), and certain kinds of skin lesions caused by excessive fat levels in the blood
Minor Side Effects: Abdominal cramps; bloating; decreased libido; diarrhea; dizziness; dry and falling hair; fatigue; flu-like symptoms; gas; headache; impotence; muscle cramps; nausea; palpitations; rash; vomiting; weakness; weight gain
Major Side Effects: Anemia; arrhythmias; blood clots; chest pains; enlarged liver
Contraindications: This drug should not be used by pregnant women or nursing mothers. • This drug should not be used by people with liver or kidney disease. Be sure your doctor knows if you have either of these conditions.
Warnings: Use of this drug should be discontinued if the desired fat-reduction results are not obtained after three months, since this drug may cause liver tumors. • This drug should be used cautiously by people with heart disease, ulcer, or a history of jaundice or liver disease. Be sure your doctor knows if you have any of these conditions. • Since this drug can cause "flu-like symptoms," your doctor will have to differentiate this from actual viral and/or bacterial disease. • This drug is likely to interact with anticoagulants. If you are currently taking any drugs of this type, consult your doctor about their use. If you are unsure of the type or contents of your medication, ask your doctor or pharmacist. • Because of the long-term nature of therapy with this drug, frequent lab tests concerning the liver should be performed, especially during the first few months of treatment. Complete blood counts should be performed periodically, since anemia and leukopenia have been reported in patients taking this drug. • Before initiating therapy with this drug, attempts should be made to control serum fat levels with diet, weight loss in obese patients, control of diabetes, etc. This drug should be used with caution in young children.
Comments: This drug effectively lowers cholesterol and fats in the blood, but whether this drug actually prevents a heart attack or other diseases associated with hardening of the arteries is not known. • Before taking any nonprescription item for treatment of aches of a cold, check with your doctor. Your aches may be a side effect of using this drug.

OTC   A-200 Pyrinate antilouse preparation

Manufacturer: Norcliff Thayer, Inc.
Ingredients: deodorized kerosene; piperonyl butoxide technical; pyrethrins
Dosage Form; Liquid: deodorized kerosene, 5%; piperonyl butoxide technical, 2%; pyrethrins, 0.165%
Use: Controls body lice; head lice; pubic lice; and their eggs
Side Effects: If swallowed: coma; convulsions; nausea; restlessness; vomiting
Contraindications: Persons with asthma or those sensitive to ragweed should not use this product.
Warnings: Avoid contact with mucous membranes. • Do not get this product into eyes. Flush eyes with copious amounts of water if eyes are acciden-

tally contaminated. • If skin irritation or signs of infection are present, call your doctor. • Consult your doctor if infestation of eyebrows or eyelashes occurs. • This product is harmful if swallowed. Do not inhale.

Comments: Follow directions. Do not exceed recommended dosage. • In order to prevent reinfestation with lice, all clothing and bedding must be sterilized or treated at the same time as using this product.

Rx   Auralgan otic solution

Manufacturer: Ayerst Laboratories
Ingredients: antipyrine; benzocaine; dehydrated glycerin
Equivalent Products: Aurasol, Bowman Pharmaceuticals; Eardro, Jenkins Laboratories, Inc.; Oto, North American Pharmacal, Inc.
Dosage Form: Drops (content per ml): antipyrine, 54.0 mg; benzocaine, 14.0 mg; dehydrated glycerin, 1.0 ml
Use: Removal of earwax; relief of pain and swelling due to middle ear infections or "swimmer's ear"
Comments: To administer eardrops, tilt your head to one side with the affected ear turned upward. Grasp the earlobe and pull it upward and back to straighten the ear canal. (If administering eardrops to a child, gently pull the earlobe downward and back.) Fill the dropper and place the prescribed number of drops in the ear. Be careful not to touch the dropper to the ear canal as the dropper can easily become contaminated this way. Keep the ear tilted upward for five to ten seconds, then gently insert a small piece of cotton into the ear to prevent the drops from escaping. • Water greatly reduces the effectiveness of this drug, so do not wash or wipe the dropper after use. Close the bottle tightly to keep out moisture. Discard any remaining medicine after treatment has been completed so that you will not be tempted to use the medication for a subsequent ear problem without consulting a doctor. Middle ear disorders are serious and should be treated only according to a doctor's advice.

Aurasol otic solution (Bowman Pharmaceuticals), see Auralgan otic solution.

OTC   Auro eardrops

Manufacturer: Commerce Drug Co.
Ingredients: camphor; propylene glycol; thymol
Dosage Form: Drop (quantities of ingredients not specified)
Use: Earwax removal
Side Effects: Allergic reactions (rash, itching, soreness); local irritation
Contraindications: Do not use product if your eardrum is punctured.
Warnings: Stop using eardrops if a rash or redness occurs.
Comments: Do not rinse dropper or touch to ear. To do so may contaminate the dropper and consequently the solution. • To warm eardrops to room temperature, hold bottle in your hands or rotate it between your palms before use. • If you do not feel better in two days, call your doctor. • Keep the bottle tightly capped between uses.

Rx   AVC anti-infective

Manufacturer: Merrell-National Laboratories
Ingredients: allantoin; aminacrine hydrochloride; sulfanilamide
Dosage Forms: Cream: allantoin, 2%; aminacrine hydrochloride, 0.2%; sulfanilamide, 15%. Vaginal suppository: allantoin, 0.14 g; aminacrine hydrochloride, 0.014 g; sulfanilamide, 1.05 g
Use: Treatment of vaginal infections

Minor Side Effects: Burning sensation; discomfort; itching; mild rash

Contraindications: This drug should not be used by people who are allergic to sulfa drugs. Consult your doctor immediately if this drug has been prescribed for you and you have such an allergy.

Warning: Patients should be on guard for manifestations such as skin rash, which could be an indication of systemic poisoning. If such manifestations develop, this drug's use should be discontinued and your doctor contacted.

Comments: Use this drug until the prescribed amount of medication is gone. Improvements in symptoms should occur within a few days, but treatment should be continued through one complete menstrual cycle unless definite diagnosis is made and specific therapy initiated. If there is no response within a few days or if symptoms recur, this drug should be discontinued and another attempt made by appropriate lab methods to isolate the organism responsible and therapy started. • Refrain from sexual intercourse, or ask your partner to use a condom, until treatment is finished, to avoid reinfection. • Douching with a suitable solution before insertion of the suppository may be recommended for hygienic purposes. • A sanitary napkin may be used to prevent staining of clothing.

Aveeno Bar skin cleanser (Cooper Dermatology Division), see Aveeno Colloidal Oatmeal bath product.

OTC Aveeno Colloidal Oatmeal bath product

Manufacturer: Cooper Dermatology Division
Ingredients: oatmeal derivatives
Dosage Form: Powder
Use: To soothe and cleanse sensitive skin; to help protect against diaper rash in infants
Side Effects: Rash; itching (occasional; associated with allergy to product)
Comments: To use this product, place the powder directly in the bathtub and soak in the bath water. • Two other products containing Aveeno Colloidal Oatmeal are available for people with sensitive skin. Aveeno Bar, a skin cleanser, contains Aveeno Colloidal Oatmeal, 50%; a mild, soap-free sudsing agent; and lanolin. Aveeno Lotion, a moisturizer applied directly to irritated skin, contains Aveeno Colloidal Oatmeal, 10%; nonionic surfactants; and emollients.

Aveeno Lotion moisturizer (Cooper Dermatology Division), see Aveeno Colloidal Oatmeal bath product.

OTC Ayds appetite suppressant

Manufacturer: Campana Corporation
Ingredients: benzocaine; candy-flavored base
Dosage Form: Candy cube: benzocaine, 5 mg; candy-flavored base
Use: Aid in dietary control
Comments: The primary value in products of this nature is in following the calorie-reduction plan that goes with it.

Azodine analgesic (North American Pharmacal), see Pyridium analgesic.

Rx Azo Gantanol antibacterial and analgesic

Manufacturer: Roche Products Inc.
Ingredients: phenazopyridine hydrochloride; sulfamethoxazole
Dosage Form: Tablet: phenazopyridine hydrochloride, 100 mg; sulfamethoxazole, 0.5 g (red)

Use: Treatment of a variety of painful infections of the urinary tract

Minor Side Effects: Abdominal pain; change in urine color; depression; diarrhea; headache; nausea; vomiting

Major Side Effects: Blood disorders; chills; convulsions; drug fever; fluid retention; hallucinations; increased sensitivity to sunlight; insomnia; itching; jaundice; rash; ringing in the ears; sore throat; toxic nephrosis

Contraindications: This drug should not be taken by children under age 12, pregnant women at term, nursing mothers, or people with liver or kidney disease. This drug should not be taken by people who are allergic to either of its ingredients. Consult your doctor immediately if this drug has been prescribed for you and you have any of these conditions or such an allergy.

Warnings: This drug should be used with caution during pregnancy. • This drug should be given with caution to people with impaired kidney or liver function and to those with blood diseases, severe hay fever or other allergies, or bronchial asthma. Be sure your doctor knows if you have any of these conditions. • Adequate fluid intake must be maintained when taking this drug. • Complete blood counts and urinalysis should be done frequently when receiving this drug. Report any symptoms of fever or sore throat to your doctor at once; these are early signs of blood disorders. • This drug interacts with barbiturates, methenamine hippurate, methenamine mandelate, methotrexate, oral antidiabetics, oxacillin, para-aminobenzoic acid, or phenytoin. If you are currently taking any drugs of these types, consult your doctor about their use. If you are unsure of the type or contents of your medications, ask your doctor or pharmacist. • This drug may cause you to be especially sensitive to the sun. Avoid exposure to sunlight as much as possible while taking this medication.

Comments: This drug should be taken for at least ten full days, even if symptoms have disappeared within that time. • This drug should be taken with at least a full glass of water. Drink at least nine glasses of water each day. • This drug may color your urine reddish-orange soon after ingestion. Do not be alarmed. • Diabetics may get a false reading for sugar or ketones while using this product.

℞   **Azo Gantrisin antibacterial and analgesic**

Manufacturer: Roche Products, Inc.

Ingredients: phenazopyridine hydrochloride; sulfisoxazole

Equivalent Products: Ameri-EZP, W. E. Hauck, Inc.; Azo-Soxazole, Columbia Medical Co.; Azosul, Reid-Provident Laboratories, Inc.; Suldiazo, Kay Pharmacal Company, Inc.

Dosage Form: Tablet: phenazopyridine hydrochloride, 50 mg; sulfisoxazole, 0.5 g (red)

Use: Treatment of a variety of bacterial infections of the urinary tract, and relief of the pain of urination caused by infection

Minor Side Effects: Abdominal pain; change in urine color; depression; diarrhea; headache; nausea; vomiting

Major Side Effects: Fluid retention; hallucinations; itching; jaundice; rash; ringing in the ears; sore throat

Contraindications: This drug should not be taken by people who are allergic to it, or who have certain liver or kidney diseases. The drug should not be used by those who are pregnant or nursing. Consult your doctor immediately if this drug has been prescribed for you and you have any of these conditions. • This drug should not be taken by children under age 12.

Warnings: This drug may cause allergic reactions and should, therefore, be used cautiously by people who have asthma, severe hay fever, or other significant allergies. The drug should be used cautiously by people who have liver or kidney disease. Be sure your doctor knows if you have any of these conditions. • This drug can cause blood diseases; notify your doctor immediately if you experience fever, sore throat, or skin discoloration, as these can be early signs of blood disorders. • This drug should not be used in conjunction with barbiturates, local anesthetics, methenamine hippurate, methenamine mandelate, methotrexate, oral antidiabetics, oxacillin, para-aminobenzoic acid, or phenytoin; if you are currently taking any drugs of these types, consult your doctor about their use. If you are unsure of the type or contents of your medications, ask your doctor or pharmacist.

Comments: This drug should be taken for at least ten full days, even if symptoms disappear within that time. • Take this drug with at least a full glass of water. Drink at least nine to ten glasses of water each day. • This drug will cause your urine to become orange-red in color. Do not be alarmed by this side effect. The urine will return to its normal color soon after the drug has been discontinued. • This drug may cause you to be especially sensitive to the sun, so avoid exposure to the sun as much as possible and use an effective sunscreen that does not contain para-aminobenzoic acid (PABA). • Diabetics may get a false reading for sugar or ketones while using this drug.

Azolid anti-inflammatory (USV [P.R.] Development Corp.), see Butazolidin anti-inflammatory.

Azo-100 analgesic (Scruggs Pharmacal Company, Inc.), see Pyridium analgesic.

Azo-Soxazole antibacterial and analgesic (Columbia Medical Co.), see Azo Gantrisin antibacterial and analgesic.

Azo-Standard analgesic (Webcon Pharmaceuticals), see Pyridium analgesic.

Azo-Stat analgesic (O'Neal, Jones & Feldman), see Pyridium analgesic.

Azosul antibacterial and analgesic (Reid-Provident Laboratories, Inc.), see Azo Gantrisin antibacterial and analgesic.

OTC   **Baby Magic Lotion rash remedy**

Manufacturer: The Mennen Co.
Ingredients: benzalkonium chloride; lanolin; refined sterols
Dosage Form: Lotion (quantity of ingredients not specified)
Use: For keeping baby skin dry; soothing diaper rash, prickly heat, and chafing
Side Effects: Allergy; local irritation

OTC   **Baby Magic Oil rash remedy**

Manufacturer: The Mennen Co.
Ingredients: lanolin; mineral oil
Dosage Form: Oil (quantities of ingredients not specified)
Use: To prevent or relieve irritation or rash of baby's skin
Side Effects: Allergy; local irritation

OTC   **Baby Magic Powder rash remedy**

Manufacturer: The Mennen Co.
Ingredient: methylbenzethonium chloride
Dosage Form: Powder (quantity of ingredient not specified)

Use: For keeping baby skin dry; soothing diaper rash, prickly heat, and chafing

Side Effects: Allergy; local irritation

Comments: While using this product, be careful not to inhale any of the powder.

OTC   Baciguent external anti-infective

Manufacturer: The Upjohn Company

Ingredient: bacitracin

Dosage Form: Ointment (content per gram): bacitracin, 500 units

Use: Prevents infection from cuts and abrasions; treats impetigo

Side Effects: Allergic reactions (rash, itching, soreness); local irritation

Comments: Apply this product at least three times daily to maintain effectiveness. • If the infection does not clear in two to three weeks, consult your doctor or pharmacist.

OTC   Bactine antiseptic

Manufacturer: Miles Laboratories, Inc.

Ingredients: alcohol; benzalkonium chloride

Dosage Forms: Aerosol spray; Liquid spray: alcohol, 3.17%; benzalkonium chloride, 0.13%

Use: First aid product to clean superficial wounds

Side Effects: Allergy; local irritation

Contraindications: Do not use this product on animal bites or puncture wounds.

Warnings: This product should not be used on large areas of the body since enough of the medication can be absorbed to be toxic. • Do not use this product for more than ten days.

R_x   Bactrim antibacterial

Manufacturer: Roche Products, Inc.

Ingredients: sulfamethoxazole; trimethoprim

Equivalent Product: Septra, Burroughs Wellcome Co.

Dosage Forms: Liquid (content per 5 ml): trimethoprim, 40 mg; sulfamethoxazole, 200 mg. Tablet: trimethoprim, 80 mg; sulfamethoxazole, 400 mg (yellowish green). Double-strength tablet: trimethoprim, 160 mg; sulfamethoxazole, 800 mg (white)

Use: Treatment of chronic urinary tract infections; certain respiratory infections, or middle-ear infections

Minor Side Effects: Abdominal pain; depression; diarrhea; headache; nausea; vomiting

Major Side Effects: Fluid retention; hallucinations; itching; jaundice; rash; ringing in the ears; sore throat

Contraindications: This drug should not be used to treat strep throat. • This drug should not be taken by people who are allergic to sulfonamides, or by those who are pregnant or nursing. Consult your doctor immediately if this drug has been prescribed for you and you have any of these conditions. • This drug should not be used by infants under two months old.

Warnings: This drug should be used cautiously by elderly patients who also take diuretics. • This drug may cause allergic reactions and should, therefore, be used cautiously by people who have asthma, severe hay fever, or other significant allergies. People who have certain vitamin deficiencies or liver or kidney disease should also use this drug with caution. Be sure your doctor knows if you have any of these conditions. • This drug can cause blood diseases; notify your doctor immediately if you experience fever, sore throat, or skin discoloration, as these can be early signs of blood disorders. • This drug should not be used in conjunction with barbiturates, local anesthetics, methenamine hippurate, methenamine mandelate, methotrexate, oral antidiabetics, oxacillin, para-aminobenzoic acid, or phenytoin; if you are currently taking any drugs of these types, consult your doctor or pharmacist. • If you are taking an anticoagulant drug in addition to this drug, remind your doctor.

Comments: This drug should be taken for at least ten full days, even if symptoms disappear within that time. • Take this drug with at least one full glass of water. Drink at least nine to ten glasses of water each day. • This drug may cause you to be especially sensitive to the sun, so avoid exposure to the sun as much as possible and use an effective sunscreen that does not contain para-aminobenzoic acid (PABA).

Bamate sedative and hypnotic (Century Pharmaceuticals, Inc.), see meprobamate sedative and hypnotic.

Bamo sedative and hypnotic (Misemer Pharmaceuticals), see meprobamate sedative and hypnotic.

Barbita sedative and hypnotic (North American Pharmacal, Inc.), see phenobarbital sedative and hypnotic.

OTC   Bayer Aspirin analgesic

Manufacturer: Glenbrook Laboratories
Ingredient: aspirin
Dosage Form: Tablet: aspirin, 325 mg (5 grains)
Use: Relief of pain of headache, toothache, sprains, muscular aches, nerve inflammation, menstruation; relief of discomforts and fever of colds or "flu," or following immunizations; temporary relief of minor pains of arthritis and rheumatism
Side Effects: Dizziness; mental confusion; nausea and vomiting; ringing in the ears; slight blood loss; sweating
Contraindications: This product may cause an increased bleeding tendency and should not be taken by persons with a history of bleeding, peptic ulcer, or stomach bleeding.
Warnings: Persons with asthma, hay fever, or other allergies should be extremely careful about using this product. The product may interfere with the treatment of gout. If you have any of these conditions, consult your doctor or pharmacist before using this medication. • Do not use this product if you are currently taking alcohol, methotrexate, oral anticoagulants, oral antidiabetics, probenecid, steroids, and/or sulfinpyrazone; if you are unsure of the type or contents of your medications, ask your doctor or pharmacist. • The dosage instructions listed on the package should be followed carefully; toxicity may occur in adults or children with repeated doses.

OTC   Bayer Children's Chewable Aspirin analgesic

Manufacturer: Glenbrook Laboratories
Ingredient: aspirin
Dosage Form: Chewable tablet; aspirin, 81 mg (1.25 grains)
Use: Relief of pain of headache, toothache, sprains, muscular aches; relief of discomforts and fever of colds or "flu," or following immunizations; temporary relief of minor pains of arthritis and rheumatism
Side Effects: Dizziness; mental confusion; nausea and vomiting; ringing in the ears; slight blood loss; sweating

Contraindications: This product may cause an increased bleeding tendency and should not be taken by persons with a history of bleeding, peptic ulcer, or stomach bleeding.

Warnings: Persons with asthma, hay fever, or other allergies should be extremely careful about using this product. The product may interfere with the treatment of gout. If you (or your child) have any of these conditions, consult your doctor or pharmacist before using this medication. • Do not use this product if you are currently taking alcohol, methotrexate, oral anticoagulants, oral antidiabetics, probenecid, steroids, and/or sulfinpyrazone; if you are unsure of the type or contents of your medications, ask your doctor or pharmacist. • The dosage instructions listed on the package should be followed carefully; toxicity may occur in adults or children with repeated doses.

Comments: These tablets should be chewed, not swallowed whole.

OTC — Bayer children's cold remedy

Manufacturer: Glenbrook Laboratories
Ingredients: phenylpropanolamine hydrochloride; aspirin
Dosage Form: Chewable tablet: phenylpropanolamine hydrochloride, 3.125 mg; aspirin, 81 mg (1¼ grains)
Use: To reduce fever, relieve nasal congestion and minor aches and pains due to colds and "flu"
Side Effects: Dizziness; mental confusion; mild to moderate stimulation; nausea and vomiting; ringing in the ears; slight blood loss; sweating
Contraindications: This product should not be used by persons who have allergies, aspirin sensitivity, asthma, blood-clotting disease, gout, or vitamin-K deficiency.
Warnings: This product should be used with special caution by persons who have diabetes, heart disease, high blood pressure, or thyroid disease. If your child has any of these conditions, consult your doctor before administering this product. • This product interacts with alcohol, ammonium chloride, guanethidine, methotrexate, monoamine oxidase inhibitors, oral anticoagulants, oral antidiabetics, probenecid, sedative drugs, steroids, sulfinpyrazone, tricyclic antidepressants, and vitamin C. If your child is currently taking any drugs of these types, check with your doctor before administering this product. If you are unsure of the type or contents of your child's medications, ask your doctor or pharmacist.
Comments: Many other conditions (some serious) mimic the common cold. If symptoms persist beyond one week or if they occur regularly without regard to season, consult your doctor. • Have your child chew gum or suck on ice chips or a piece of hard candy to reduce the sensation of mouth dryness.

OTC — Bayer Decongestant cold and allergy remedy

Manufacturer: Glenbrook Laboratories
Ingredients: phenylpropanolamine hydrochloride; chlorpheniramine maleate; aspirin
Dosage Form: Tablet: phenylpropanolamine hydrochloride, 12.5 mg; chlorpheniramine maleate, 2 mg; aspirin, 325 mg (5 grains)
Use: Relief of symptoms of colds, "flu," sinus congestion, and hay fever
Side Effects: Anxiety; blurred vision; chest pain; confusion; constipation; difficult and painful urination; dizziness; drowsiness; headache; increased blood pressure; insomnia; loss of appetite; nausea; nervousness; palpitations; rash; ringing in the ears; slight blood loss; reduced sweating; tension; tremor; vomiting

Contraindications: This product should not be used by persons who have significant drug or food allergies, aspirin sensitivity, asthma, blood-clotting disease, gout, severe heart disease, severe high blood pressure, or vitamin-K deficiency. • This product should not be given to newborn or premature infants.

Warnings: This product should be used with special caution by the elderly or debilitated, and by persons who have diabetes, enlarged prostate, glaucoma (certain types), heart disease, high blood pressure, kidney disease, obstructed bladder, obstructed intestine, peptic ulcer, or thyroid disease. If you have any of these conditions, consult your doctor before taking this product. • This product may cause drowsiness. Do not take it if you must drive, operate heavy machinery, or perform other tasks requiring mental alertness. To prevent oversedation, avoid the use of alcohol or other drugs that have sedative properties. • This product interacts with alcohol, ammonium chloride, guanethidine, methotrexate, monoamine oxidase inhibitors, oral anticoagulants, oral antidiabetics, probenecid, sedative drugs, steroids, sulfinpyrazone, tyricyclic antidepressants, and vitamin C. If you are currently taking any drugs of these types, check with your doctor before taking this product. If you are unsure of the type or contents of your medications, ask your doctor or pharmacist. • Because this product reduces sweating, avoid excessive work or exercise in hot weather.

Comments: Many other conditions (some serious) mimic the common cold. If symptoms persist beyond one week or if they occur regularly without regard to season, consult your doctor. • The effectiveness of this product may diminish after being taken regularly for seven to ten days; consult your pharmacist about substituting another product containing a different antihistamine if this product begins to lose its effectiveness for you. • Chew gum or suck on ice chips or a piece of hard candy to reduce mouth dryness.

OTC　　　　Bayer Non-Aspirin analgesic

Manufacturer: Glenbrook Laboratories
Ingredient: acetaminophen
Dosage Form: Tablet: acetaminophen, 325 mg (5 grains)
Use: Relief of pain of headache, toothache, muscular aches and strains, menstruation, colds or "flu"; temporary relief of minor arthritis pain; reduction of fever
Side Effects: When taken in overdose: blood disorders, rash
Warnings: When taken in overdose, acetaminophen is more toxic than aspirin. The dosage instructions listed on the package should be followed carefully; toxicity may occur in adults or children with repeated doses.

OTC　　　　Bayer Timed-Release Aspirin analgesic

Manufacturer: Glenbrook Laboratories
Ingredient: aspirin
Dosage Form: Time-release tablet: aspirin, 650 mg (10 grains)
Use: Temporary relief of low-grade pain in conditions such as rheumatoid arthritis, osteoarthritis, bursitis; or other prolonged aches and pains such as from minor injuries or menstruation; relief of pain of headache, colds, and similar conditions
Side Effects: Dizziness; mental confusion; nausea and vomiting; ringing in the ears; slight blood loss; sweating
Contraindications: This product may cause an increased bleeding tendency and should not be taken by persons with a history of bleeding, peptic ulcer, or stomach bleeding.

Warnings: Persons with asthma, hay fever, or other allergies should be extremely careful about using this product. The product may interfere with the treatment of gout. If you have any of these conditions, consult your doctor or pharmacist before using this medication. • Do not use this product if you are currently taking alcohol, methotrexate, oral anticoagulants, oral antidiabetics, probenecid, steroids, and/or sulfinpyrazone; if you are unsure of the type or contents of your medications, ask your doctor or pharmacist. • This product has sustained action; never take it more frequently than directed. The dosage instructions listed on the package should be followed carefully; toxicity may occur in adults or children with repeated doses.

Rx   **Benadryl antihistamine**

Manufacturer: Parke-Davis
Ingredient: diphenhydramine hydrochloride
Equivalent Products: Bendylate, Tutag Pharmaceuticals, Inc.; diphenhydramine hydrochloride, various manufacturers; Fenylhist, Mallard Incorporated; Habdryl, Bowman Pharmaceuticals; Nordryl, North American Pharmacal, Inc.; Phen-Amin, Scrip-Physician Supply Co.; SK-Diphenhydramine, Smith Kline & French Laboratories; Valdrene, The Vale Chemical Co., Inc.
Dosage Forms: Capsule: 25 mg; 50 mg (both pink/white). Liquid (content per 5 ml): 12.5 mg
Use: Treatment of motion sickness; Parkinson's disease; insomnia; cough; or allergy-related itching and swelling
Minor Side Effects: Blurred vision; confusion; constipation; diarrhea; difficult urination; dizziness; drowsiness; dry mouth; headache; insomnia; loss of appetite; nasal congestion; nausea; nervousness; palpitations; rash; reduced sweating; restlessness; vomiting; weakness
Major Side Effects: Low blood pressure; rash from exposure to sunlight; severe abdominal pain; sore throat
Contraindications: This drug should not be given to infants, or taken by nursing mothers. People who are allergic to this drug or similar antihistamines should not use this drug. Consult your doctor immediately if this drug has been prescribed for you and any of these statements apply to you. • This drug should not be used to treat asthma or other symptoms of the lower respiratory tract.
Warnings: This drug should be used cautiously by people who have asthma, glaucoma (certain types), ulcers (certain types), enlarged prostate, obstructed bladder, obstructed intestine, thyroid disease, heart disease, or high blood pressure; and by those who are pregnant. Be sure your doctor knows if you have any of these conditions. • Elderly people are more likely than others to experience side effects, especially sedation, with this drug, and should use the drug with caution. • This drug should not be used in conjunction with central nervous system depressants or monoamine oxidase inhibitors; if you are currently taking any drugs of these types, consult your doctor about their use. If you are unsure of the type of your medications, ask your doctor or pharmacist. • While taking this drug, do not take any nonprescription item for cough, cold, or sinus problems without first checking with your doctor. • This drug may cause drowsiness; avoid tasks that require alertness. To prevent oversedation, avoid taking alcohol or other drugs that have sedative properties. • Take only the prescribed amount of this drug. An overdose usually sedates an adult but can cause excitation leading to convulsions and death in a child. • Because this drug reduces sweating, avoid excessive work or exercise in hot weather.
Comments: Chew gum or suck on ice chips or a piece of hard candy to reduce mouth dryness.

OTC   Benadryl Cream local anesthetic

Manufacturer: Parke-Davis
Ingredient: diphenhydramine hydrochloride
Dosage Form: Cream: diphenhydramine hydrochloride, 2% in a water miscible base
Use: Symptomatic relief of itching due to eczema, hives, insect bites, poison ivy and oak, sunburn, and other minor skin conditions
Side Effects: Allergic rash; local irritation; stinging
Contraindications: This product should not be used on broken, blistered, raw, or oozing areas of the skin.
Warnings: Do not use this product on large areas of the body because enough of the medication could be absorbed to be toxic. • Do not get this product in the eyes or use on mucous membranes. • If irritation develops, discontinue use of this product.

Rx   Bendectin antinauseant

Manufacturer: Merrell-National Laboratories
Ingredients: doxylamine succinate; pyridoxine hydrochloride (vitamin B₆)
Dosage Form: Tablet: doxylamine succinate, 10 mg; pyridoxine hydrochloride, 10 mg (white)
Use: Treatment of nausea and vomiting due to pregnancy ("morning sickness")
Minor Side Effects: Blurred vision; confusion; constipation; diarrhea; dizziness; drowsiness; headache; irritability; nausea; nervousness; palpitations; rash; restlessness; vomiting
Major Side Effects: Abdominal pain; disorientation; low blood pressure; rash from exposure to sunlight; sore throat
Warnings: Like all drugs considered for use during pregnancy, this drug should be used only when clearly needed, particularly during the first trimester. There is a controversy over this drug's side effects. • Because this drug may cause drowsiness, it should be taken with caution by people driving motor vehicles or operating machinery. • This drug may add to the effects of alcohol and sedatives. Consult your doctor before taking any such drugs.
Comments: This drug should not be chewed or crushed, but swallowed whole. • This drug has a sustained action and, therefore, should never be taken more frequently than prescribed by your doctor. A serious overdose may result.

Bendylate antihistamine (Tutag Pharmaceuticals, Inc.), see Benadryl antihistamine.

Rx   Benemid uricosuric

Manufacturer: Merck Sharp & Dohme
Ingredient: probenecid
Equivalent Products: Probalan, The Lannett Company, Inc.; probenecid, various manufacturers; Probenimead, Spencer-Mead, Inc.; Robenecid, Robinson Laboratory, Inc.
Dosage Form: Tablet: 500 mg (yellow)
Use: Prevention of gout attacks; also used with penicillin to prolong blood levels of penicillin
Minor Side Effects: Dizziness; headache; loss of appetite; nausea; rash; vomiting
Major Side Effects: Fatigue; flushing; kidney disease
Contraindications: Treatment with this drug should not be started during an acute attack of gout. • This drug should not be taken by people who have

kidney stones, blood diseases, or by those who are allergic to it. Consult your doctor immediately if this drug has been prescribed for you and you have any of these conditions. • This drug should not be used by children under two years of age.

Warnings: This drug should be used cautiously by people who have peptic ulcer, or liver or kidney disease; or by those who are pregnant. Be sure your doctor knows if you have any of these conditions. • This drug should not be used in conjunction with indomethacin, para-aminosalicylic acid, salicylates, or sulfinpyrazone; if you are currently taking any drugs of these types, consult your doctor about their use. If you are unsure of the type or contents of your medications, ask your doctor or pharmacist. • If you are taking methotrexate, penicillin, or ampicillin in addition to probenecid, remind your doctor. • Do not take aspirin or alcohol without first consulting your doctor. • Probenecid may affect the results of some urine tests, so remind your doctor that you are taking this drug if you are asked to provide a urine sample.

Comments: The effects of treatment with this drug may not be apparent for at least two weeks. At the beginning of probenecid therapy, gout attacks may increase in number and severity. To control the attacks, your doctor may prescribe colchicine to be taken in addition to the probenecid. If both these drugs are prescribed for you, you may save some money by taking ColBENE-MID uricosuric, a combination product that contains probenecid and colchicine in one tablet. Consult your doctor. • Take this drug with at least one full glass of water. Drink at least nine glasses of water each day. • Diabetics using Clinitest urine test may get a false high sugar reading while taking this drug. Change to Clinistix or Tes-Tape urine test to avoid this problem.

OTC   Ben-Gay external analgesic

Manufacturer: Leeming Division
Ingredients: menthol; methyl salicylate
Dosage Forms: Lotion: menthol, 7%; methyl salicylate, 15%. Ointment: menthol, 10%; methyl salicylate, 15%
Use: Temporary relief of pain in muscles and other areas
Side Effects: Allergic reactions (rash, itching, soreness); local irritation; local numbness
Warnings: Use this product externally only. • Do not use on broken or irritated skin or on large areas of the body; avoid contact with eyes. • When using this product avoid exposure to direct sunlight, heat lamp, or sunlamp. • Before using this product on children under 12 years of age, consult your doctor. • If the condition persists, call your doctor.
Comments: This product is greaseless, smells good, and may be attractive to a child. It should be stored safely out of the reach of children. • Be sure to rub this product well into the skin.

Rx   Bentyl antispasmodic

Manufacturer: Merrell-National Laboratories
Ingredient: dicyclomine hydrochloride
Equivalent Products: Dibent, W. E. Hauck, Inc.; dicyclomine hydrochloride, various manufacturers; Di-Spaz, North American Pharmacal, Inc.; Spastyl, Vangard Laboratories
Dosage Forms: Capsule: 10 mg (blue). Liquid (content per 5 ml): 10 mg. Tablet: 20 mg (blue)
Use: Treatment of gastrointestinal disorders, including peptic ulcer, irritable colon, mucous colitis, acute enterocolitis, and neurogenic colon
Minor Side Effects: Blurred vision; constipation; difficult urination; dizziness; drowsiness; dry mouth; increased sensitivity to light; headache; insom-

nia; loss of taste; nervousness; palpitations; reduced sweating

Major Side Effects: Impotence; rapid heartbeat; rash

Contraindications: This drug should not be taken by people who have severe ulcerative colitis, severe hemorrhage, obstructed bladder, obstructed intestine, heart disease (certain types), or myasthenia gravis. Consult your doctor immediately if this drug has been prescribed for you and you have any of these conditions.

Warnings: This drug should be used cautiously by people who have glaucoma, enlarged prostate, high blood pressure, thyroid disease, liver or kidney disease, or heart disease; or by those who are pregnant. Be sure your doctor knows if you have any of these conditions. • People who have ulcerative colitis should be especially careful about taking this drug, and should never increase the dosage unless told to do so by their doctor. • This drug should not be used in conjunction with amantadine, haloperidol, phenothiazines, or antacids; if you are currently taking any drugs of these types, consult your doctor about their use. If you are unsure of the type or contents of your medications, ask your doctor or pharmacist. • This drug always produces certain side effects, which may include dry mouth, blurred vision, reduced sweating, drowsiness, difficult urination, constipation, increased sensitivity to light, and palpitations. • Avoid tasks that require alertness. • Avoid excessive work or exercise in hot weather. • To prevent oversedation, avoid taking other drugs that have sedative properties or alcohol. • Call your doctor if you notice a rash, flushing, or pain in the eye.

Comments: This drug is best taken one-half to one hour before meals. • This drug does not cure ulcers, but may help them improve. • Chew gum or suck on ice chips or a piece of hard candy to reduce mouth dryness. • A product combining Bentyl antispasmodic with phenobarbital is available for persons who are especially nervous or anxious. Despite the phenobarbital content, Bentyl antispasmodic with phenobarbital has not been shown to have high potential for abuse.

Bentyl antispasmodic with phenobarbital (Merrell-National Laboratories), see Bentyl antispasmodic.

OTC   Benylin DM cough remedy

Manufacturer: Parke-Davis

Ingredients: dextromethorphan hydrobromide; alcohol; ammonium chloride; sodium citrate

Dosage Form; Liquid (content per 5 ml, or one teaspoon): dextromethorphan hydrobromide, 10 mg; alcohol, 5%; ammonium chloride; sodium citrate

Use: Temporary relief of coughs due to minor throat and bronchial irritation

Side Effects: Drowsiness; nausea; vomiting

Warnings: This product interacts with monoamine oxidase inhibitors. If you are currently taking any drugs of this type, check with your doctor before taking this product. If you are unsure of the type or contents of your medications, ask your doctor or pharmacist.

Comments: Do not use this product to treat chronic coughs, such as those from smoking or asthma. • Do not use this product to treat productive (hacking) coughs that produce phlegm.

OTC   Benzedrex nasal decongestant

Manufacturer: Menley & James Laboratories

Ingredients: propylhexedrine; menthol; aromatics

Dosage Form: Inhaler: propylhexedrine, 250 mg; menthol, 12.5 mg; aromatics

Use: Temporary relief of nasal congestion due to colds, sinusitis, hay fever, or other upper respiratory allergies; temporary relief of ear block and pressure pain due to air travel

Side Effects: Blurred vision; burning, dryness of nasal mucosa; increased nasal congestion or discharge; sneezing, and/or stinging; dizziness; drowsiness; headache; insomnia; nervousness; palpitations; slight increase in blood pressure; stimulation

Contraindications: This product should not be used by persons who have glaucoma (certain types).

Warnings: This product should be used with special caution by persons who have diabetes, advanced hardening of the arteries, heart disease, high blood pressure, or thyroid disease. If you have any of these conditions, consult your doctor before using this product. • This product interacts with monoamine oxidase inhibitors, thyroid preparations, and tricyclic antidepressants. If you are currently taking any drugs of these types, check with your doctor before taking this product. If you are unsure of the type or contents of your medications, ask your doctor or pharmacist. • To avoid side effects such as burning, sneezing, or stinging, and a "rebound" increase in nasal congestion and discharge, do not exceed the recommended dosage and do not use this product for more than three or four continuous days. • This product should not be used by more than one person; sharing the dispenser may spread infection.

OTC   Benzodent toothache and sore gums remedy

Manufacturer: Vicks Toiletry Products Division

Ingredients: benzocaine; denture adhesive-like base; eugenol; hydroxyquinoline sulfate

Dosage Forms: Cream: benzocaine, 20%; denture adhesive-like base; eugenol, 0.4%; hydroxyquinoline sulfate, 0.1%

Use: Relieves pain of toothache and sore gums

Side Effects: Allergic reactions (rash, itching, soreness)

Warnings: If you have an oral ulcer which does not heal within three weeks, see your dentist.

Comments: This product is useful for a toothache only when the nerve is exposed. • Teething lotions and toothache preparations are similar.

Betapen-VK antibiotic (Bristol Laboratories), see penicillin potassium phenoxymethyl antibiotic.

Bexophene analgesic (Mallard Incorporated), see Darvon Compound-65 analgesic.

OTC   B.F.I. Powder external anti-infective

Manufacturer: Beecham Products

Ingredients: aluminum potassium sulfate; bismuth subgallate; bismuth formic iodide; boric acid; eucalyptol; menthol; thymol; zinc phenolsulfonate

Dosage Form: Powder: bismuth formic iodide, 16.1% (quantities of other ingredients not specified)

Use: Promotes the healing of cuts; abrasions; minor burns; poison ivy and oak; skin irritations

Side Effects: Allergic reactions (rash, itching, soreness); eye irritation; local irritation

Warnings: Do not apply this powder to broken skin or raw areas, particularly on infants and children.

Comments: Apply this product at least three times daily to maintain effectiveness. • If the infection does not clear in two to three weeks, consult your doctor or pharmacist. • This product contains boric acid which many medical authorities believe should not be used because it is toxic; follow directions on the package carefully. • This product has a low order of effectiveness. For serious skin infections another product should be chosen; consult your pharmacist.

Bio-Tetra antibiotic (General Pharmaceutical Prods., Inc.), see tetracycline hydrochloride antibiotic.

Rx   **Biphetamine anorectic**

Manufacturer: Pennwalt Pharmaceutical Division
Ingredients: amphetamine; dextroamphetamine resin
Dosage Form: Capsule: amphetamine, 3.75 mg; dextroamphetamine resin, 3.75 mg (white). Amphetamine, 6.25 mg; dextroamphetamine resin, 6.25 mg (black/white). Amphetamine, 10 mg; dextroamphetamine resin, 10 mg (black)
Use: Short-term treatment of obesity
Minor Side Effects: Diarrhea; dizziness; dry mouth; headache; insomnia; nausea; restlessness; unpleasant taste in the mouth; vomiting
Major Side Effects: Elevation of blood pressure; euphoria; overstimulated nerves; rapid heartbeat; tremor
Contraindications: This drug should not be taken by people with certain types of heart disease, high blood pressure, hyperthyroidism, or severe hardening of the arteries; or in an agitated state.
Warnings: This drug should be taken cautiously by women who are pregnant and by people with diabetes or high blood pressure. Be sure your doctor knows if you are pregnant or if you have either of these conditions. • This drug has the potential for abuse and should be taken cautiously. Tolerance develops quickly; do not increase the dose without consulting your doctor. • This drug should not be taken with acetazolamide, guanethidine, monoamine oxidase inhibitors, insulin, phenothiazines, sodium bicarbonate, or tricyclic antidepressants. If you are currently taking any drugs of these types, consult your doctor about their use. If you are unsure about the types or contents of your medications, ask your doctor or pharmacist. • This drug is not recommended for use as an anorectic agent in children under 12.
Comments: The effects of this drug on appetite control wear off; do not take it for more than three weeks at a time. One way to get full benefit from this drug is to take the drug for three weeks, stop for three weeks, then resume taking it. Consult your doctor about this regimen. • Weight loss is greatest during the first three weeks of taking this drug; it decreases after that. • To be effective, therapy with this drug must be accompanied by a low-calorie diet. • This drug has sustained action; so never take it more frequently than your doctor prescribes. A serious overdose may result. • This drug may mask symptoms of fatigue and pose serious danger; it may decrease your ability to perform potentially dangerous or hazardous tasks, such as driving or operating machinery. Never take this drug as a stimulant to keep you awake. • Do not take this drug later than 3:00 P.M. to avoid sleeplessness. • While taking this drug, do not take any nonprescription item for cough, cold, or sinus problems without first checking with your doctor. • Dexedrine (Smith Kline & French Laboratories) has approximately the same effects as this drug.

Birth control pills, see oral contraceptives.

OTC   Blistex Ointment canker sore and fever blister remedy

Manufacturer: Blistex, Inc.

Ingredients: alcohol; ammonia; ammonium carbonate; beeswax; camphor; diisostearate; fragrance; lanolin; mineral oil; paraffin; peppermint oil; petrolatum; phenol; polyglyceryl-3; sodium borate

Dosage Form: Ointment: camphor, 1%; phenol, 0.4% (quantities of other ingredients not specified)

Use: Local treatment of minor oral inflammations such as canker sores and fever blisters

Comments: If you have an oral ulcer which does not heal within three weeks, see your dentist.

OTC   Blis-To-Sol athlete's foot remedy

Manufacturer: Chattem Laboratories

Ingredients: benzoic acid; salicylic acid; undecylenic acid; zinc stearate

Dosage Forms: Aerosol powder (content per gram): zinc stearate, 10 mg; salicylic acid, 10 mg; benzoic acid, 10 mg. Gel: undecylenic acid, 5%. Liquid (content per gram): undecylenic acid, 50 mg; salicylic acid, 90 mg. Powder (content per gram): zinc stearate, 10 mg; salicylic acid, 19 mg; benzoic acid, 19 mg

Use: Treatment of athlete's foot

Side Effects: Allergy; local irritation

Warnings: Do not apply this product to mucous membranes, scraped skin, or to large areas of skin. • If your condition worsens, or if irritation occurs, stop using this product and consult your pharmacist. • When using the aerosol form of this product, be careful not to inhale any of the powder.

Comments: Some lesions take months to heal, so it is important not to stop treatment too soon. • If foot lesions are consistently a problem, check the fit of your shoes. • Wash your hands thoroughly after applying this product. • When using the liquid form of this product, avoid contaminating the contents of the bottle by pouring some of the liquid into a separate container for each use. • The gel and liquid forms of this product are preferable to the powders for effectiveness; the best action of the powders may be in drying the infected area. • The aerosol powder may be more expensive than the other forms of this product; check prices before paying for convenience you do not need.

Blupav smooth muscle relaxant (Bluco Incorporated), see Pavabid Plateau Caps smooth muscle relaxant.

OTC   Bonine antinauseant

Manufacturer: Pfipharmecs Division

Ingredient: meclizine hydrochloride

Dosage Form: Chewable tablet: meclizine hydrochloride, 25 mg

Use: For prevention or treatment of motion sickness

Side Effects: blurred vision; drowsiness; dry mouth; children may react with primary symptoms of excitement (nervousness, uncoordinated movements, twitching of muscles, flushed skin, tremors, and convulsions)

Contraindications: Children under 12 years of age and pregnant women should not take this medication.

Comments: Vomiting is one of the body's defense mechanisms to rid itself of toxic or poisonous substances. Do not self-medicate with this product if vomiting has occurred for two or more days. Call your doctor. • Nausea and vomiting in women, especially early in the day, are early symptoms of pregnancy. Never take this product, or any other drug, until pregnancy has been ruled out. • If your vomitus has blood in it, or if you have headache or abdominal pain, call your doctor. • This product is recommended only for nausea or vomiting caused by motion sickness. It is less effective for other disorders. • For best results, take this product one hour before departure. • While taking this drug, avoid tasks that require alertness and the excessive use of alcohol, tranquilizers, or any drug that sedates the nervous system.

OTC   Borofax rash remedy

Manufacturer: Burroughs Wellcome Co.
Ingredients: boric acid; lanolin
Dosage Form: Ointment: boric acid, 5%; lanolin
Use: Treatment of abrasions and minor burns; chafed skin; diaper rash
Side Effects: Allergy; local irritation
Comments: This product contains boric acid, which many medical authorities believe should not be used because it is toxic. Follow the directions on the package carefully.

OTC   Brasivol acne preparation

Manufacturer: Stiefel Laboratories, Inc.
Ingredients: aluminum oxide; detergents; neutral soap
Dosage Form: Cream (fine, medium, or rough) (quantities of ingredients not specified)
Use: Treatment of acne
Side Effects: Allergy, local irritation
Warnings: Do not get product in or near eyes.
Comments: If the condition worsens, stop using this product and call your pharmacist. • Wash area gently with warm water and pat dry before applying this acne preparation. • Avoid exposure to heat lamps, sunlamps, or direct sunlight when using this product.

OTC   Breacol cough remedy

Manufacturer: Glenbrook Laboratories
Ingredients: dextromethorphan hydrobromide; phenylpropanolamine hydrochloride; chlorpheniramine maleate; alcohol
Dosage Form: Liquid (content per 5 ml, or one teaspoon): dextromethorphan hydrobromide, 10 mg; phenylpropanolamine hydrochloride, 37.5 mg; chlorpheniramine maleate, 4 mg; alcohol, 10%
Use: Temporary relief of cough, nasal congestion, and other symptoms of colds
Side Effects: Anxiety; blurred vision; chest pain; confusion; constipation; difficult and painful urination; dizziness; drowsiness; headache; increased blood pressure; insomnia; loss of appetite; mild stimulation; nausea; nervousness; palpitations; rash; reduced sweating; tension; tremor; vomiting
Contraindications: This product should not be used by persons who have severe heart disease or severe high blood pressure. • This product should not be given to newborn or premature infants.
Warnings: This product should be used with special caution by the elderly or debilitated, and by persons who have asthma, diabetes, enlarged prostate, glaucoma (certain types), heart disease, high blood pressure, kidney disease, obstructed bladder, obstructed intestine, peptic ulcer, or thyroid disease. If you have any of these conditions, consult your doctor before taking this product. • This product may cause drowsiness. Do not take it if you must drive, operate heavy machinery, or perform other tasks requiring mental alertness.

To prevent oversedation, avoid the use of alcohol or other drugs that have sedative properties. • This product interacts with alcohol, guanethidine, monoamine oxidase inhibitors, sedative drugs, and tricyclic antidepressants. If you are currently taking any drugs of these types, check with your doctor before taking this product. If you are unsure of the type or contents of your medications, ask your doctor or pharmacist. • Because this product reduces sweating, avoid excessive work or exercise in hot weather.

Comments: Many other conditions (some serious) mimic the common cold. If symptoms persist beyond one week or if they occur regularly without regard to season, consult your doctor. • Do not use this product to treat chronic coughs, such as from smoking or asthma. • Do not use this product to treat productive (hacking) coughs that produce phlegm. • Chew gum or suck on ice chips or a piece of hard candy to reduce mouth dryness.

R_x   **Brethine bronchodilator**

Manufacturer: Geigy Pharmaceuticals
Ingredient: terbutaline sulfate
Equivalent Product: Bricanyl, Astra Pharmaceutical Products
Dosage Form: Tablet: 2.5 mg; 5 mg (white)
Use: Relief of bronchial asthma and bronchospasm associated with bronchitis and emphysema
Minor Side Effects: Headache; increased heart rate; muscle cramps; nausea; nervousness; palpitations; sweating; tremors; vomiting
Contraindications: This drug should not be taken by people who are allergic to any sympathomimetic amine drug. Consult your doctor immediately if this drug has been prescribed for you and you have an allergy of this type.
Warnings: This drug should be used cautiously by people who have diabetes, high blood pressure, hyperthyroidism, heart disease (certain types), or epilepsy. Be sure your doctor knows if you have any of these conditions. • This drug is not recommended for use by children under age 12. • This drug should not be used in conjunction with guanethidine or with monoamine oxidase inhibitors; if you are currently taking any drugs of these types, consult your doctor about their use. If you are unsure of the type or contents of your medications, ask your doctor or pharmacist. • While taking this drug, do not take any nonprescription item for cough, cold, or sinus problems without first checking with your doctor. Do not take any other drug containing a sympathomimetic amine without consulting your doctor.
Comments: While taking this drug, drink at least eight glasses of water daily.

Bricanyl bronchodilator (Astra Pharmaceutical Products), see Brethine bronchodilator.

Bristacycline antibiotic (Bristol Laboratories), see tetracycline hydrochloride antibiotic.

Bristamycin antibiotic (Bristol Laboratories), see erythromycin antibiotic.

Brocon antihistamine (Forest Laboratories, Inc.), see Dimetapp antihistamine.

Bromatapp antihistamine (Henry Schein, Inc.), see Dimetapp antihistamine.

Bromepaph antihistamine (Columbia Medical Co.), see Dimetapp antihistamine.

Bromophen antihistamine (Rugby Laboratories), see Dimetapp antihistamine.

OTC   **Bromo-Seltzer analgesic**

Manufacturer: Warner-Lambert Company
Ingredients: acetaminophen; sodium bicarbonate; citric acid
Dosage Form: Granules (content per capful): acetaminophen, 325 mg; sodium bicarbonate and citric acid to yield 2.8 g sodium citrate
Use: Relief of upset stomach, acid indigestion, or heartburn accompanied by headache or body aches and pains
Side Effects: Abdominal cramping; blood disorders; liver disease (jaundice); nausea and vomiting; rash (all occur only when overdose is taken or in hypersensitive persons)
Warnings: Do not use this product if you are on a low-salt diet. • Persons with kidney disease should use this product with caution. If you have such a condition, consult your doctor or pharmacist before using this medication. • When taken in overdose, acetaminophen is more toxic than aspirin; the dosage instructions listed on the package should be followed carefully.
Comments: The granules must be dissolved in water before being swallowed. When taken as directed, this product rarely causes side effects, and any that occur are usually mild. • You can save money by taking plain acetaminophen instead of this product; there is no evidence that the ingredients in this product that make it fizz make it more effective than similar doses of a non-fizzy product. • This product has recently been reformulated, but it is still marketed in the same way.

OTC   **Bronitin asthma remedy**

Manufacturer: Whitehall Laboratories
Ingredients: ephedrine; guaifenesin; pyrilamine maleate; theophylline
Dosage Form: Tablet: ephedrine, 24 mg; guaifenesin, 100 mg; pyrilamine maleate, 16.6 mg; theophylline, 120 mg
Use: For control of bronchial asthma
Side Effects: Anxiety; blurred vision; chest pain; confusion; constipation; dizziness; drowsiness; dry mouth and respiratory passages; headache; increased blood pressure; increased frequency of urination; insomnia; loss of appetite; nausea; nervousness; palpitations; rash; restlessness; sweating; tension; tremor; vomiting. Children may react with primary symptoms of excitement (convulsions, flushed skin, nervousness, tremor, twitching of muscles, and uncoordinated movements).
Warnings: Persons with glaucoma should use this product with caution. Consult your doctor or pharmacist if you have any questions concerning the use of this product. • Overdose may result in convulsions, coma, and cardiovascular collapse. • While taking this product, avoid the use of sedative drugs or alcohol, guanethidine, monoamine oxidase inhibitors, or tricyclic antidepressants. If you are taking any medication of these types, or if you are unsure of the type of medication you are taking, consult your doctor.
Comments: If you require an expectorant, you need more moisture in your environment. Drink eight to ten glasses of water each day. The use of a vaporizer or humidifier may also be beneficial. Consult your doctor.

OTC   Bronkaid asthma remedy

Manufacturer: Winthrop Laboratories
Ingredients: ephedrine sulfate; guaifenesin; theophylline anhydrous
Dosage Form: Tablet: ephedrine sulfate, 24 mg; guaifenesin, 100 mg; theophylline anhydrous, 100 mg
Use: For control of bronchial asthma
Side Effects: Anxiety; blurred vision; chest pain; confusion; constipation; dizziness; drowsiness; dry mouth and respiratory passages; increased blood pressure; increased frequency of urination; insomnia; loss of appetite; nausea; nervousness; palpitations; rash; restlessness; sweating; tension; tremor; urinary retention; vomiting. Children may react with primary symptoms of excitement (convulsions, flushed skin, nervousness, tremor, twitching of muscles, and uncoordinated movements).
Warnings: Persons with persistent coughs, high blood pressure, diabetes, heart, or thyroid disease should consult a doctor before using this product. • Repeated use of this product may cause nausea and vomiting, depressed reflexes, and breathing difficulties in persons with kidney disease. • Overdose may result in convulsions, coma, and cardiovascular collapse.
Comments: If you require an expectorant, you need more moisture in your environment. Drink eight to ten glasses of water each day. The use of a vaporizer or humidifier may also be beneficial. Consult your doctor. • While taking this product, avoid the use of guanethidine, monoamine oxidase inhibitors, or tricyclic antidepressants. If you are taking any medication of these types, or if you are unsure of the type of medication you are taking, consult your doctor. • If fever is present, consult your doctor.

OTC   Bronkaid mist asthma remedy

Manufacturer: Winthrop Laboratories
Ingredients: alcohol; ascorbic acid; epinephrine USP; hydrochloric acid and nitric acid buffers
Dosage Form: Oral inhalant: alcohol, 33%; ascorbic acid, 0.07%; epinephrine USP, 0.5%; hydrochloric acid and nitric acid buffers
Use: Temporary relief of acute paroxysms of bronchial asthma
Side Effects: Anxiety; chest pain; dizziness; headache; increase in blood pressure; insomnia; loss of appetite; nausea; nervousness; palpitations; sweating; tension; tremor; vomiting
Warnings: Persons with high blood pressure, diabetes, heart, or thyroid disease should use this product with caution. Consult your doctor or pharmacist if you have any questions concerning the use of this product.
Comments: Use this product only as directed. Side effects are rare when directions are followed. Relief of symptoms should occur within five to ten minutes. Do not use more than once every three to four hours except on the advice of your doctor. • After using this product, rinse or gargle with water or mouthwash to help avoid a "dry throat" feeling. • Do not use this product if it is discolored.

Bronkodyl bronchodilator (Breon Laboratories, Inc.), see Elixophyllin bronchodilator.

OTC   Bufferin analgesic

Manufacturer: Bristol-Myers Products
Ingredients: aspirin; aluminum glycinate; magnesium carbonate
Dosage Form: Tablet: aspirin, 324 mg (5 grains); aluminum glycinate, 48.6

mg (¾ grain); magnesium carbonate, 97.2 mg (1½ grains)

Use: Relief of pain of headache; temporary relief of minor arthritic pain, discomforts and fever of colds and "flu," menstrual cramps, muscle aches, toothache

Side Effects: Dizziness; mental confusion; nausea and vomiting; ringing in the ears; slight blood loss; sweating

Contraindications: This product may cause an increased bleeding tendency and should not be taken by persons with a history of bleeding, peptic ulcer, or stomach bleeding.

Warnings: Persons with kidney disease, asthma, hay fever, or other allergies should be extremely careful about using this product. The product may interfere with the treatment of gout. If you have any of these conditions, consult your doctor or pharmacist before using this medication. • Do not use this product if you are currently taking alcohol, methotrexate, oral anticoagulants, oral antidiabetics, probenecid, steroids, and/or sulfinpyrazone; if you are unsure of the type or contents of your medications, ask your doctor or pharmacist. • The dosage instructions listed on the package should be followed carefully; toxicity may occur in adults or children with repeated doses.

Comments: Magnesium interacts with tetracycline antibiotics. There may not be enough magnesium in this product to cause any problem, but if you are taking a tetracycline antibiotic in addition to this product, separate the dosages by at least two hours. • Pain-relief tablets, such as this product, that contain salts of magnesium or aluminum are known as buffered tablets. Such products dissolve faster than unbuffered products, but there is no evidence that they relieve pain faster or better than those products that do not contain buffers. Buffered tablets may be less likely to cause gastric upset in some people.

Butazolidin Alka anti-inflammatory (Geigy Pharmaceuticals), see Butazolidin anti-inflammatory.

R̸   **Butazolidin anti-inflammatory**

Manufacturer: Geigy Pharmaceuticals
Ingredient: phenylbutazone
Equivalent Products: Azolid, USV (P.R.) Development Corp.; phenylbutazone, various manufacturers
Dosage Form: Tablet: 100 mg (red)
Use: Reduction of pain, redness, and swelling due to arthritis or thrombophlebitis
Minor Side Effects: Diarrhea; nausea; rash; vomiting
Major Side Effects: Allergic reactions; blood in urine or stools; blurred vision; fatigue; hearing difficulty; heart disease; itching; jaundice; severe abdominal pain; sore throat; swelling; weight gain (more than two pounds per week); ulcer
Contraindications: This drug should not be taken by people who are allergic to it, or by those who have anemia or other blood problems, chronic stomach problems, high blood pressure, thyroid disorders, ulcers, or kidney, liver, or heart disease. The drug should not be taken by those who suffer from water retention or have experienced enlarged salivary glands while taking other drugs, especially anticoagulants. Consult your doctor immediately if this drug has been prescribed for you and you have any of these conditions. • This drug is not recommended for use by senile persons or by children under age 14.
Warnings: This drug should be used with special caution by people who are pregnant, nursing, or over age 40. • This drug can cause diabetes, thyroid

disease, and water retention to worsen; consult your doctor if you have any of these conditions and the drug is prescribed for you. • Use of this drug has been associated with leukemia, although there is no definite proof that the drug causes this disease. • This drug should not be used in conjunction with anticoagulants, cancer drugs, oral antidiabetics, or sulfonamides; if you are currently taking any drugs of these types, consult your doctor about their use. If you are unsure of the type or contents of your medications, ask your doctor or pharmacist. • Ophthalmologic adverse reactions and serious blood disorders have been reported to occur in patients using this drug; notify your doctor immediately if you suffer any visual disturbances (e.g., blurred vision), sore throat, fever, enlarged salivary glands, mouth sores, black stools, or weight gain. • While taking this drug, do not take aspirin or alcohol without first consulting your doctor.

Comments: This drug should never be used for trivial aches or pains. The drug should be used for a short time only, and in low doses. Follow your doctor's directions exactly and never exceed the recommended dosage. Blood checks should be done at least every two weeks, and you should request them even if your doctor does not order them. When first beginning treatment with this drug, a trial period of one week is recommended. If no relief is obtained in that time, the drug should be discontinued. • Take this drug with food or milk. • People who experience excessive stomachaches or pains when taking this drug might consider substituting Butazolidin Alka anti-inflammatory capsules; this product combines phenylbutazone with dried aluminum hydroxide gel and magnesium trisilicate to minimize gastric upset. Consult your doctor. • Another drug, oxyphenbutazone, has the same use, side effects, warnings, and comments as phenylbutazone. Oxyphenbutazone is available in trademarked forms as Tandearil (Geigy Pharmaceuticals) and Oxalid (USV (P.R.) Development Corp.) anti-inflammatories.

Butisol Sodium hypnotic (McNeil Laboratories), see Nembutal Sodium hypnotic.

R̻   Cafergot migraine remedy

Manufacturer: Sandoz Pharmaceuticals
Ingredients: caffeine; ergotamine tartrate
Equivalent Products: Cafermine, Spencer-Mead, Inc.; Cafertrate, Henry Schein, Inc.; Ergocaf, Robinson Laboratory, Inc.; Migrastat, Winston Pharmaceuticals, Inc.
Dosage Forms: Suppository: caffeine, 100 mg; ergotamine tartrate, 2 mg. Tablet: caffeine, 100 mg; ergotamine tartrate, 1 mg (pink)
Use: To abort or prevent migraine headache
Minor Side Effects: Drowsiness; itching; nausea; numbness; tingling in fingers and toes
Major Side Effects: Decreased or increased heart rate; localized edema; muscle pain in extremities; weakness in legs
Contraindications: This drug should not be used by people with blood vessel disease, heart disease, high blood pressure, liver or kidney disease, or infection. This drug should not be used during pregnancy. Consult your doctor immediately if this drug has been prescribed for you and you have any of these conditions. • This drug should not be used by people who are allergic to either of its ingredients. Consult your doctor immediately if this drug has been prescribed for you and you have such an allergy.
Warnings: To avoid toxicity, make sure that you stay within the dosage limits recommended.
Comments: Cafergot P-B tablets and suppositories have the same ingredients and dosages as Cafergot tablets and suppositories, plus the following:

Tablet: 0.125 mg l-alkaloids of belladonna and 30 mg sodium pentobarbital (bright green, coated). Suppository: 0.25 mg l-alkaloids of belladonna and 60 mg pentobarbital (sealed in blue aluminum foil). Other products are available which are similar to Cafergot, but they are not identical. Those products listed above which are identical may differ widely in price. Consult your doctor and pharmacist. • For best results, dosage should start at the first sign of a migraine attack. Learn to recognize the first symptoms of a migraine attack. If Cafergot dosing is delayed for several hours after the beginning of these symptoms, it may not work.

Cafergot P-B migraine remedy (Sandoz Pharmaceuticals), see Cafergot migraine remedy.

Cafermine migraine remedy (Spencer-Mead, Inc.), see Cafergot migraine remedy.

Cafertrate migraine remedy (Henry Schein, Inc.), see Cafergot migraine remedy.

OTC   Caladryl poison ivy remedy

Manufacturer: Parke-Davis
Ingredients: calamine; camphor; diphenhydramine hydrochloride; alcohol (lotion form only)
Dosage Forms: Cream: calamine; camphor, 0.1%; diphenhydramine hydrochloride, 1%. Lotion: alcohol, 2%; calamine; camphor, 0.1%; diphenhydramine hydrochloride, 1%
Use: Relief of itching due to insect bites; mild poison ivy or oak; mild sunburn; or other minor skin irritations
Side Effects: Allergic reactions (rash, itching, soreness); local irritation
Warnings: Do not apply this product to blistered, raw or oozing areas of the skin.
Comments: To prevent irritation and secondary infection, avoid scratching. • Before applying medication, soak the area in warm water or apply towels soaked in water for five to ten minutes. Dry the area gently by patting with a soft towel, then apply medication.

OTC   calamine lotion

Manufacturer: various manufacturers
Ingredients: zinc oxide; ferric oxide; glycerine in calcium hydroxide solution
Dosage Form: Suspension
Use: Relief of itching and pain of poison ivy and oak, insect bites, rashes, and other minor skin irritations
Side Effects: None when used topically. (May cause abdominal pains; nausea; numbness of extremities; or vomiting if swallowed.)
Comments: Shake the lotion thoroughly before each use. • As this product dries, a thin, pink-colored crust remains on the skin, which may be objectionable to some people. • If severe itching is a problem, purchase this product with 0.5 to 1% phenol (carbolic acid) added. (Or, ask your pharmacist to add the phenol to your calamine lotion.) The phenol will help relieve itching, but note that it may cause burning, rash, or skin irritation.

OTC   Campho-Phenique athlete's foot remedy and antiseptic

Manufacturer: Winthrop Laboratories
Ingredients: phenol; camphor
Dosage Forms: Liquid: phenol, 4.7%; camphor, 10.8%
Use: Treatment of athlete's foot; relief of pain of sores, cuts, burns, insect bites; aid in fighting infection from skin lesions and minor injuries
Side Effects: Allergy; local irritation
Warnings: Do not apply this product to mucous membranes, scraped skin, or to large areas of skin. • If your condition worsens, or if irritation occurs, stop using this product and consult your pharmacist.
Comments: Some lesions take months to heal, so it is important not to stop treatment too soon. • If foot lesions are consistently a problem, check the fit of your shoes. • Wash your hands thoroughly after applying this product. • When using the liquid form of this product, avoid contaminating the contents of the bottle by pouring some of the liquid into a separate container for each use.

Candex antifungal agent (Dome Division), see Mycostatin antifungal agent.

Capade antihistamine, anticholinergic, and adrenergic (Spencer-Mead, Inc.), see Ornade Spansule antihistamine, anticholinergic, and adrenergic.

Capital with Codeine analgesic (Carnrick Laboratories, Inc.), see Tylenol with Codeine analgesic.

OTC   Carter's Little Pills laxative

Manufacturer: Carter Products
Ingredient: bisacodyl
Dosage Form: Pill: bisacodyl, 5 mg
Use: Relief of constipation
Side Effects: Excess loss of fluids; faintness; griping (cramps); mucus in feces; rectal burning
Contraindications: Persons with high fever (100° F or more); black or tarry stools; nausea; vomiting; abdominal pain; or children under age three should not use this product unless directed by a doctor. • Do not use this product when constipation is caused by megacolon or other diseases of the intestines, or hypothyroidism.
Warnings: Excessive use (daily for a month or more) of this product may cause diarrhea, vomiting, and loss of certain blood electrolytes.
Comments: Do not take this product within one hour before or after taking an antacid and/or drinking milk. Severe abdominal cramping will result. • Evacuation may occur within 6 to 12 hours. Never self-medicate if constipation lasts longer than two weeks or if the medication does not produce a laxative effect within a week. • Limit use to seven days unless directed otherwise by a doctor since this product may cause laxative-dependence (addiction) if used for a longer time.

OTC   cascara sagrada laxative

Manufacturer: various manufacturers
Ingredient: active principles of cascara
Dosage Forms: Liquid; Tablet
Use: Relief of constipation; cathartic

Side Effects: Excess loss of fluid; griping (cramps); mucus in feces

Contraindications: Persons with high fever (100° F or more); black or tarry stools; nausea; vomiting; abdominal pain; or children under age three should not use this product unless directed by a doctor. • Do not use this product when constipation is caused by megacolon or other diseases of the intestine, or hypothyroidism.

Warnings: Excessive use (daily for a month or more) of this product may cause diarrhea, vomiting, and loss of certain blood electrolytes.

Comments: Evacuation may occur within six to eight hours. Never self-medicate with this product if constipation lasts longer than two weeks or if the medication does not produce a laxative effect within a week. • Limit use to seven days unless otherwise directed by a doctor since this product may cause laxative-dependence (addiction) if used for a longer period.

OTC   castor oil laxative

Manufacturer: various manufacturers
Ingredient: castor oil
Dosage Form: Liquid
Use: Relief of constipation; cathartic
Side Effects: Excess loss of fluid; griping (cramps); mucus in feces

Contraindications: Persons with high fever (100° F or more); black or tarry stools; nausea; vomiting; abdominal pain; or children under age three should not use this product unless directed by a doctor. • Do not use this product when constipation is caused by megacolon or other diseases of the intestine, or hypothyroidism.

Warnings: Excessive use (daily for a month or more) of this product may cause diarrhea, vomiting, and loss of certain blood electrolytes.

Comments: Generally, castor oil is not recommended for treatment of constipation; consult your pharmacist for recommendations on another product. • Evacuation may occur within 6 to 12 hours. Never self-medicate with this product if constipation lasts longer than two weeks or if the medication does not produce a laxative effect within a week. • Limit use to seven days unless directed otherwise by a doctor since this product may cause laxative-dependence (addiction) if used for a longer time. • Limit use to one dose per each infrequent bout of constipation.

℞   Catapres antihypertensive

Manufacturer: Boehringer Ingelheim Ltd.
Ingredient: clonidine hydrochloride
Dosage Form: Tablet: 0.1 mg (tan); 0.2 mg (orange); 0.3 mg (peach)
Use: Treatment of high blood pressure
Minor Side Effects: Constipation; dizziness; drowsiness; dry mouth; fatigue; headache; increased sensitivity to alcohol; insomnia; nasal congestion; nausea; rash; vomiting
Major Side Effects: Breathing difficulty; enlarged breasts (in both sexes); hair loss; impotence; jaundice; pain; urine retention; weight gain
Warnings: This drug is not recommended for use in women who are pregnant or who may become pregnant. • This drug should be used cautiously in children. • Tolerance to this drug may develop in some patients, necessitating a reevaluation of therapy. • Discontinuance of the use of this drug should be done slowly to avoid a rapid rise in blood pressure and certain other symptoms. Rare instances of stroke and death have been reported after abrupt stoppage of this drug. • Patients who engage in potentially dangerous activities, such as driving a motor vehicle or operating machinery should use this drug with caution, since it can cause drowsiness. • Patients receiving

this drug should take periodic eye examinations. Although there is no documented evidence on effect in humans, some research animals being given this drug have suffered retinal degradation. • This drug should be used with caution in persons with severe heart disease, stroke, or chronic kidney failure. Be sure your doctor knows if you have any of these conditions. • This drug should not be used with alcohol, barbiturates, or other sedatives. If you are currently taking any drugs of these types, consult your doctor about their use. If you are unsure of the type or content of the medications you are taking, ask your doctor or pharmacist.

Comments: This drug should be taken with food or milk. • Mild side effects from this drug (e.g., nasal congestion) are most noticeable during the first two weeks of therapy and become less bothersome after this period. • While taking this drug, do not take any nonprescription item for cough, cold, or sinus problems without first checking with your doctor. • Never stop taking this drug abruptly. Rather, you should decrease consumption over a period of two to four days. Do not discontinue or decrease the dose of this drug unless your doctor directs you to do so. • To avoid dizziness or light-headedness when you stand, contract and relax the muscles of your legs for a few moments before rising. Do this by pushing one foot against the floor while raising the other foot slightly, alternating feet so that you are "pumping" your legs in a pedaling motion. • Chew gum or suck on ice chips or a piece of hard candy to reduce mouth dryness.

Centet antibiotic (The Central Pharmacal Co.), see tetracycline hydrochloride antibiotic.

OTC   Cēpacol throat lozenges

Manufacturer: Merrell-National Laboratories
Ingredients: cetylpyridinium chloride; benzyl alcohol; aromatics
Dosage Form: Lozenge: cetylpyridinium chloride, 1:1500; benzyl alcohol, 0.3%; aromatics (yellow),
Use: Temporary relief of dryness and minor irritation of mouth and throat and resulting cough
Contraindications: Do not give this product to children under three years of age unless directed to do so by your doctor.
Warnings: A sore throat in a child under age six should never be treated without medical supervision. Consult your doctor. • If your sore throat is severe; is accompanied by headache, high fever, nausea, or vomiting; or lasts for more than two days, consult your doctor.
Comments: The antibacterial ingredient included represents an irrational use for this product if it is recommended to treat an infection-induced sore throat. Colds are caused by viruses, and the ingredients in these lozenges are not effective against viral infections. The value of this product lies in its temporary throat-soothing quality.

OTC   Cēpacol Troches anesthetic throat lozenges

Manufacturer: Merrell-National Laboratories
Ingredients: cetylpyridinium chloride; benzocaine; aromatics
Dosage Form: Lozenge: cetylpyridinium chloride, 1:1500; benzocaine, 10 mg; aromatics (green)
Use: Temporary relief of pain and discomfort due to minor sore throat, minor mouth irritations, stomatitis
Side Effects: Occasional nausea; vomiting
Contraindications: Do not give this product to children under three years of age unless directed to do so by your doctor.

Warnings: A sore throat in a child under age six should never be treated without medical supervision. Consult your doctor. • If your sore throat is severe; is accompanied by headache, high fever, nausea, or vomiting; or lasts for more than two days, consult your doctor.

Comments: The antibacterial ingredient included represents an irrational use for this product if it is recommended to treat a sore throat due to a cold. Colds are caused by viruses, and the ingredients in these lozenges are not effective against viral infections. The value of this product lies in its temporary pain-relieving qualities.

Cerespan smooth muscle relaxant (USV [P.R.] Development Corp.), see Pavabid Plateau Caps smooth muscle relaxant.

Cerylin expectorant and smooth muscle relaxant (Spencer-Mead, Inc.), see Quibron expectorant and smooth muscle relaxant.

OTC   Cetaphil Lotion skin cleanser

Manufacturer: Alcon Laboratories
Ingredients: cetyl alcohol; propylene glycol; sodium lauryl sulfate; stearyl alcohol; methylparaben; propylparaben; butylparaben
Dosage Form: Lotion (quantities of ingredients not specified)
Use: Cleansing agent for dermatitis, allergic eczema, and other soap-intolerant conditions
Side Effects: Allergy; burning; itching; rash; stinging. (If swallowed, nausea and vomiting may occur.)
Contraindications: This product should not be used by anyone who experiences an allergic reaction to it (e.g., itching or rash).
Warnings: Do not swallow this product. • Keep out of the reach of children.
Comments: This product contains no animal, mineral, or vegetable fats.

OTC   Cheracol cough remedy

Manufacturer: The Upjohn Company
Ingredients: codeine phosphate; guaifenesin; alcohol; wild cherry bark; white pine bark
Dosage Form: Liquid (content per 5 ml, or one teaspoon): codeine phosphate, 10 mg; guaifenesin, 100 mg; alcohol, 3%; wild cherry bark; white pine bark
Use: Temporary relief of cough due to colds or "flu"; also to convert a dry, nonproductive cough to a productive, phlegm-producing cough
Side Effects: Constipation; nausea; slight drying of respiratory passages; vomiting
Warnings: This product should be used with caution by persons who have asthma or other respiratory diseases. If you have such a condition, consult your doctor before taking this product. • Because this product contains codeine, it has the potential for abuse and must be used with caution. It usually should not be taken for more than seven to ten days. Tolerance may develop quickly, but do not increase the dose without consulting your doctor. • This product interacts with alcohol, guanethidine, monoamine oxidase inhibitors, sedative drugs, and tricyclic antidepressants. If you are currently taking any drugs of these types, check with your doctor before taking this product. If you are unsure of the type or contents of your medications, ask your doctor or pharmacist.
Comments: Do not use this product to treat chronic coughs, such as those from smoking or asthma. • Do not use this product to treat productive (hacking) coughs that produce phlegm. • If you require an expectorant, you need

more moisture in your environment. Drink eight to ten glasses of water daily. The use of a vaporizer or humidifier may also be beneficial. Consult your doctor. • Over-the-counter sale of this product may not be permitted in some states.

OTC   Cheracol D cough remedy

Manufacturer: The Upjohn Company
Ingredients: dextromethorphan hydrobromide; guaifenesin; alcohol
Dosage Form: Liquid (content per 5 ml, or one teaspoon): dextromethorphan hydrobromide, 10 mg; guaifenesin, 100 mg; alcohol, 3%
Use: Temporary relief of cough due to colds or "flu"; also to convert a dry, nonproductive cough to a productive, phlegm-producing cough
Side Effects: Drowsiness; nausea; vomiting
Warnings: This product interacts with monoamine oxidase inhibitors; if you are currently taking any drugs of this type, check with your doctor before taking this product. If you are unsure of the type or contents of your medications, ask your doctor or pharmacist.
Comments: Do not use this product to treat chronic coughs, such as those from smoking or asthma. • Do not use this product to treat productive (hacking) coughs that produce phlegm. • If you require an expectorant, you need more moisture in your environment. Drink eight to ten glasses of water daily. The use of a vaporizer or humidifier may also be beneficial. Consult your doctor.

Chloramead phenothiazine (Spencer-Mead, Inc.), see Thorazine phenothiazine.

OTC   Chloraseptic throat lozenges

Manufacturer: Norwich-Eaton Pharmaceuticals
Ingredients: phenol; sodium phenolate
Dosage Form: Lozenge: phenol and sodium phenolate to total 32.5 mg phenol
Use: Temporary relief of pain and discomfort due to minor sore throat, minor mouth irritations, stomatitis, and following oral surgery
Contraindications: Do not give this product to children under six years of age unless directed to do so by your doctor.
Warnings: A sore throat in a child under age six should never be treated without medical supervision. Consult your doctor. • If your sore throat is severe; is accompanied by headache, high fever, nausea, or vomiting; or lasts for more than two days, consult your doctor.
Comments: The antibacterial ingredients included represent an irrational use for this product if it is recommended to treat a sore throat due to a cold. Colds are caused by viruses, and the ingredients in these lozenges are not effective against viral infections. The value of this product lies in its temporary throat-soothing quality.

Chlordiazachel sedative and hypnotic (Rachelle Laboratories, Inc.), see Librium sedative and hypnotic.

Chlorofon-F analgesic (Rugby Laboratories), see Parafon Forte analgesic.

Chloroserpine diuretic and antihypertensive (Rugby Laboratories), see Diupres diuretic and antihypertensive.

Chlor-Pz phenothiazine (USV [P.R.] Development Corporation), see
Thorazine phenothiazine.

OTC Chlor-Trimeton decongestant cold and allergy remedy

Manufacturer: Schering Corporation
Ingredients: chlorpheniramine maleate; pseudoephedrine sulfate
Dosage Form: Tablet: chlorpheniramine maleate, 4 mg; pseudoephedrine
sulfate, 60 mg
Use: Temporary relief of nasal congestion due to colds, hay fever, and
sinusitis
Side Effects: Anxiety; blurred vision; chest pain; confusion; constipation;
diarrhea; difficult and painful urination; dizziness; headache; heartburn; increased blood pressure; insomnia; loss of appetite; nausea; nervousness;
palpitations; rash; reduced sweating; tension; tremor; vomiting; weakness
Contraindications: This product should not be used by persons who have
severe heart disease or severe high blood pressure. • This product should not
be given to newborn or premature infants.
Warnings: This product should be used with special caution by the elderly
or debilitated, and by persons who have asthma, diabetes, enlarged prostate,
glaucoma (certain types), heart disease, high blood pressure, kidney disease,
obstructed bladder, obstructed intestine, peptic ulcer, or thyroid disease. If
you have any of these conditions, consult your doctor before taking this product. • This product may cause drowsiness. Do not take it if you must drive,
operate heavy machinery, or perform other tasks requiring mental alertness.
To prevent oversedation, avoid the use of alcohol or other drugs that have
sedative properties. • This product interacts with alcohol, guanethidine,
monoamine oxidase inhibitors, sedative drugs, and tricyclic antidepressants.
If you are currently taking any drugs of these types, check with your doctor
before taking this product. If you are unsure of the type or contents of your
medications, ask your doctor or pharmacist. • Because this product reduces
sweating, avoid excessive work or exercise in hot weather.
Comments: Many other conditions (some serious) mimic the common cold.
If symptoms persist beyond one week or if they occur regularly without
regard to season, consult your doctor. • The effectiveness of this product
may diminish after being taken regularly for seven to ten days; consult your
pharmacist about substituting another product containing a different antihistamine if this product begins to lose its effectiveness for you. • Chew gum
or suck on ice chips or a piece of hard candy to reduce mouth dryness.

OTC   Chlor-Trimeton Expectorant cough remedy

Manufacturer: Schering Corporation
Ingredients: chlorpheniramine maleate; phenylephrine hydrochloride; ammonium chloride; sodium citrate; guaifenesin; alcohol
Dosage Form: Liquid (content per 5 ml, or one teaspoon): chlorpheniramine
maleate, 2 mg; phenylephrine hydrochloride, 10 mg; ammonium chloride, 100
mg; sodium citrate, 50 mg; guaifenesin, 50 mg; alcohol, 1% or less
Use: Temporary relief of cough, nasal congestion, and other symptoms of
colds or "flu"; also to convert a dry, nonproductive cough to a productive,
phlegm-producing cough
Side Effects: Anxiety; blurred vision; chest pain; confusion; constipation;
difficult and painful urination; dizziness; drowsiness; headache; increased
blood pressure; insomnia; loss of appetite; mild stimulation; nausea;
nervousness; palpitations; rash; reduced sweating; tension; tremor; vomiting
Contraindications: This product should not be used by persons who have
severe heart disease or severe high blood pressure. • This product should not

be given to newborn or premature infants.

Warnings: This product should be used with special caution by the elderly or debilitated, and by persons who have asthma, diabetes, enlarged prostate, glaucoma (certain types), heart disease, high blood pressure, kidney disease, obstructed bladder, obstructed intestine, peptic ulcer, or thyroid disease. If you have any of these conditions, consult your doctor before taking this product. • This product may cause drowsiness. Do not take it if you must drive, operate heavy machinery, or perform other tasks requiring mental alertness. To prevent oversedation, avoid the use of alcohol or other drugs that have sedative properties. • This product interacts with alcohol, guanethidine, monoamine oxidase inhibitors, sedative drugs, and tricyclic antidepressants. If you are currently taking any drugs of these types, check with your doctor before taking this product. If you are unsure of the type or contents of your medications, ask your doctor or pharmacist. • Because this product reduces sweating, avoid excessive work or exercise in hot weather.

Comments: Many other conditions (some serious) mimic the common cold. If symptoms persist beyond one week or if they occur regularly without regard to season, consult your doctor. • Do not use this product to treat chronic coughs, such as those from smoking or asthma. • Do not use this product to treat productive (hacking) coughs that produce phlegm. • If you require an expectorant, you need more moisture in your environment. Drink eight to ten glasses of water daily. The use of a vaporizer or humidifier may also be beneficial. Consult your doctor. • Chew gum or suck on ice chips or a piece of hard candy to reduce mouth dryness.

OTC Chlor-Trimeton Expectorant with Codeine cough remedy

Manufacturer: Schering Corporation

Ingredients: ammonium chloride; codeine phosphate; guaifenesin; phenylephrine hydrochloride; chlorpheniramine maleate; sodium citrate; alcohol

Dosage Form: Liquid (content per 5 ml, or one teaspoon): ammonium chloride, 100 mg; codeine phosphate, 10 mg; guaifenesin, 50 mg; phenylephrine hydrochloride, 10 mg; chlorpheniramine maleate, 2 mg; sodium citrate, 50 mg; alcohol, 5.25%

Use: Temporary relief of cough, nasal congestion, and other symptoms of colds or "flu"; also to convert a dry, nonproductive cough to a productive, phlegm-producing cough

Side Effects: Anxiety; blurred vision; chest pain; confusion; constipation; difficult and painful urination; dizziness; drowsiness; headache; increased blood pressure; insomnia; loss of appetite; mild stimulation; nausea; nervousness; palpitations; rash; reduced sweating; tension; tremor; vomiting

Contraindications: This product should not be used by persons who have severe heart disease or severe high blood pressure. • This product should not be given to newborn or premature infants.

Warnings: This product should be used with special caution by the elderly or debilitated, and by persons who have asthma or respiratory disease, diabetes, enlarged prostate, glaucoma (certain types), heart disease, high blood pressure, kidney disease, obstructed bladder, obstructed intestine, peptic ulcer, or thyroid disease. If you have any of these conditions, consult your doctor before taking this product. • This product may cause drowsiness. Do not take it if you must drive, operate heavy machinery, or perform other tasks requiring mental alertness. To prevent oversedation, avoid the use of alcohol or other drugs that have sedative properties. • This product interacts with alcohol, guanethidine, monoamine oxidase inhibitors, sedative drugs, and tricyclic antidepressants. If you are currently taking any drugs of these types, check with your doctor before taking this product. If you are unsure of the type or contents of your medications, ask your doctor or pharmacist. •

Because this product reduces sweating, avoid excessive work or exercise in hot weather. • Because this product contains codeine, it has the potential for abuse and must be used with caution. It usually should not be taken for more than seven to ten days. Tolerance may develop quickly, but do not increase the dose without consulting your doctor.

Comments: Many other conditions (some serious) mimic the common cold. If symptoms persist beyond one week or if they occur regularly without regard to season, consult your doctor. • Do not use this product to treat chronic coughs, such as those from smoking or asthma. • Do not use this product to treat productive (hacking) coughs that produce phlegm. • If you require an expectorant, you need more moisture in your environment. Drink eight to ten glasses of water daily. The use of a vaporizer or humidifier may also be beneficial. Consult your doctor. • Chew gum or suck on ice chips or a piece of hard candy to reduce mouth dryness. • Over-the-counter sale of this product may not be permitted in some states.

Chlorzide diuretic and antihypertensive (Foy Laboratories), see hydrochlorothiazide diuretic and antihypertensive.

Chlorzone Forte analgesic (Henry Schein, Inc.), see Parafon Forte analgesic.

OTC · **Chocks multivitamin (regular, Bugs Bunny, and Flintstones)**

Manufacturer: Miles Laboratories, Inc.
Ingredients: vitamin A; vitamin D; vitamin E; vitamin C; folic acid; thiamine; riboflavin; niacin; vitamin B_6; vitamin B_{12}
Dosage Form: Chewable tablet: vitamin A, 2500 IU; vitamin D, 400 IU; vitamin E, 15 IU; vitamin C, 60 mg; folic acid, 0.3 mg; thiamine, 1.05 mg; riboflavin, 1.2 mg; niacin, 13.5 mg; vitamin B_6, 1.05 mg; vitamin B_{12}, 4.5 mcg
Use: Dietary supplement
Warnings: This product contains ingredients that accumulate and are stored in the body. The recommended dose should not be exceeded for long periods (several weeks to months) except by doctor's orders.
Comments: If large doses are taken, this product may interfere with the results of urine tests. Inform your doctor and pharmacist you are taking this product. • Chewable tablets should never be referred to as "candy" or as "candy-flavored" vitamins. Your child may take you literally and swallow toxic amounts.

OTC · **Chocks Plus Iron multivitamin (regular, Bugs Bunny, and Flintstones)**

Manufacturer: Miles Laboratories, Inc.
Ingredients: vitamin A; vitamin D; vitamin E; vitamin C; folic acid; thiamine; riboflavin; niacin; vitamin B_6; vitamin B_{12}; iron
Dosage Form: Chewable tablet: vitamin A, 2500 IU; vitamin D, 400 IU; vitamin E, 15 IU; vitamin C, 60 mg; folic acid, 0.3 mg; thiamine, 1.05 mg; riboflavin, 1.2 mg; niacin, 13.5 mg; vitamin B_6, 1.05 mg; vitamin B_{12}, 4.5 mcg; iron (elemental), 15 mg
Use: Dietary supplement
Side Effects: Constipation; diarrhea; nausea; stomach pain
Contraindications: This product should not be used by persons who have active peptic ulcer or ulcerative colitis.
Warnings: The iron in this product interacts with oral tetracycline antibiotics and reduces the absorption of the antibiotics. If you are currently

taking tetracycline, consult your doctor or pharmacist before taking this product. If you are unsure of the type or contents of your medications, ask your doctor or pharmacist. • Alcoholics and persons who have chronic liver or pancreatic disease should use this product with special caution; such persons may have enhanced iron absorption and are therefore more likely than others to experience iron toxicity. • Accidental iron poisoning is common in children; be sure to keep this product safely out of their reach. • This product contains ingredients that accumulate and are stored in the body. The recommended dose should not be exceeded for long periods (several weeks to months) except by doctor's orders.

Comments: Because of its iron content, this product may cause constipation, diarrhea, nausea, or stomach pain. These symptoms usually disappear or become less severe after two to three days. Taking your dose with food or milk may help minimize these side effects. If they persist, ask your pharmacist to recommend another product. • Black, tarry stools are a normal consequence of iron therapy. If your stools are not black and tarry, this product may not be working for you. Ask your pharmacist to recommend another product. • If large doses are taken, this product may interfere with the results of urine tests. Inform your doctor and pharmacist you are taking this product. • Chewable tablets should never be referred to as "candy" or as "candy-flavored" vitamins. Your child may take you literally and swallow toxic amounts.

℞   **Choledyl bronchodilator**

Manufacturer: Parke-Davis
Ingredient: oxtriphylline
Dosage Form: Liquid (content per 5 ml, or one teaspoon): 100 mg. Tablet: 100 mg (red); 200 mg (yellow)
Use: Relief of acute bronchial asthma and reversible bronchospasm associated with bronchitis and emphysema
Minor Side Effects: Central nervous system stimulation; gastric distress
Major Side Effects: Convulsions; difficult breathing; palpitations
Warnings: This drug should be used cautiously by pregnant or nursing women. Women who may become pregnant should use this drug with caution. • This drug should not be used with other xanthine preparations, since adverse reactions, particularly central nervous system stimulation in children, may occur. Be sure your doctor knows if you are taking such preparations. Ask your doctor or pharmacist if you are unsure of the nature of your medications.
Comments: If you have mild gastrointestinal distress while taking this drug, take an over-the-counter product like Maalox or Gelusil antacid. This drug should be taken with food or milk. • Call your doctor if you have severe stomach pain, vomiting, or restlessness. • Tolerance to this drug occurs infrequently; it is useful for long-term therapy for bronchospasm. • Be sure to take your dosage at exactly the right time. • Do not crush the tablet form. • Drink at least eight to ten glasses of water each day. • Avoid drinking coffee, tea, cocoa, colas, or other beverages that contain caffeine while taking this drug. • Do not use over-the-counter items for asthma while taking this drug, unless your doctor has told you to do so.

Cin-Quin antiarrhythmic (Rowell Laboratories, Inc.), see quinidine sulfate antiarrhythmic.

Circanol vasodilator (Riker Laboratories, Inc.), see Hydergine vasodilator.

OTC   Clearasil Antibacterial Acne Lotion

Manufacturer: Vicks Toiletry Products Division
Ingredient: benzoyl peroxide
Dosage Form: Lotion: benzoyl peroxide, 5%
Use: Treatment of acne
Side Effects: Allergy; local irritation
Warnings: Do not get product in or near the eyes. • Persons with known sensitivity to benzoyl peroxide should not use this product.
Comments: If the condition worsens, stop using this product and call your pharmacist. • Wash area gently with warm water and pat dry before applying this acne preparation. • Avoid exposure to heat lamps, sunlamps, or direct sunlight when using this product. • This product may be especially active on fair-skinned people. • This product may damage certain fabrics including rayon.

OTC   Clearasil Medicated Cleanser acne preparation

Manufacturer: Vicks Toiletry Products Division
Ingredients: alcohol; allantoin; salicylic acid
Dosage Form: Solution: alcohol, 43%; allantoin, 0.1%; salicylic acid, 0.25%
Use: Treatment of acne
Side Effects: Allergy; local irritation
Warnings: Do not get product in or near the eyes.
Comments: If the condition worsens, stop using this product and call your pharmacist.

℞   Clinoril anti-inflammatory

Manufacturer: Merck Sharp & Dohme
Ingredient: sulindac
Dosage Form: Tablet: 150 mg; 200 mg (both yellow)
Use: Reduction of pain, redness, and swelling due to acute or chronic arthritis
Minor Side Effects: Abdominal pain; constipation; diarrhea; indigestion; gas; itching; loss of appetite; nausea; rash; vomiting
Major Side Effects: Depression; dizziness; edema and weight gain; gastrointestinal bleeding; headache; high blood pressure; nerve damage; nosebleed; numbness in fingers and toes; ringing in ears; visual disturbance
Contraindications: This drug should not be taken by people who are allergic to it or to aspirin or other nonsteroidal anti-inflammatory agents. Consult your doctor immediately if this drug has been prescribed for you and you have such an allergy.
Warnings: This drug should be used with caution in persons with peptic ulcer, certain blood diseases, gastrointestinal bleeding, history of gastrointestinal disease, blood clotting disorders, liver or kidney disease, or certain types of heart disease. Be sure your doctor knows if you have any of these conditions. • This drug should be used with caution by pregnant women, nursing mothers, and children. • Abnormal liver function tests may occur with the use of this drug. • Persons using this drug who experience eye problems should immediately bring these symptoms to their doctor's attention so that eye tests can be initiated. • This drug interacts with aspirin, anticoagulants, probenecid, or steroids. If you are currently taking any drugs of these types, consult your doctor about their use. If you are unsure about the type or contents of your medication, ask your doctor or pharmacist. • Do not stop taking this drug without informing your doctor.

358

Comments: This drug is a potent pain-killing drug and is not intended for general aches and pains. • Regular checkups by the doctor, including blood tests and eye examinations, are required of persons taking this drug. • This drug must be taken with food or milk. Never take this drug on an empty stomach or with aspirin, and never take more than directed.

Coastaldyne analgesic (Coastal Pharmaceuticals Co., Inc.), see Tylenol with Codeine analgesic.

Cocillin V-K antibiotic (Coastal Pharmaceutical Co., Inc.), see penicillin potassium phenoxymethyl antibiotic.

Cogentin antiparkinson drug (Merck Sharp & Dohme), see Artane antiparkinson drug.

OTC   Colace laxative

Manufacturer: Mead Johnson Nutritional Division
Ingredient: docusate sodium (dioctyl sodium sulfosuccinate)
Dosage Forms: Capsule: docusate sodium, 50 mg; 100 mg. Liquid: docusate sodium, 1%. Syrup (content per 5 ml): docusate sodium, 20 mg
Use: Relief of constipation and stool softener
Side Effects: Bitter taste; nausea; rash; throat irritation
Contraindications: Persons with high fever (100° F or more); black or tarry stools; nausea; vomiting; abdominal pain; or children under age three should not use this product unless directed by a doctor. • Do not use this product when constipation is caused by megacolon or other diseases of the intestine, or hypothyroidism.
Warnings: Excessive use (daily for a month or more) of this product may cause diarrhea, vomiting, and loss of certain blood electrolytes. • Pregnant women should not use this product except on the advice of a doctor.
Comments: Evacuation may occur within 72 hours. • This product is referred to as a stool softener and is recommended for prevention of constipation when the stool is hard and dry. Do not take another product containing mineral oil at the same time as you are taking this product. • Never self-medicate with this product if constipation lasts longer than two weeks or if the medication does not produce a laxative effect within a week. • Take the liquid form of this product in one-half glass of milk or fruit juice to help mask the taste. • Limit use to seven days unless directed otherwise by your doctor; this product may cause laxative-dependence (addiction) if used for a longer period.

ColBENEMID uricosuric (Merck Sharp & Dohme), see Benemid uricosuric.

Rx   colchicine gout remedy

Manufacturer: various manufacturers
Ingredient: colchicine
Equivalent Products: Colsalide, North American Pharmacal
Dosage Forms: Enteric-coated tablet; Tablet: various dosages and colors
Use: Relief of sudden (acute) pain from gout

Minor Side Effects: Abdominal pain; diarrhea; nausea; vomiting

Major Side Effects: Burning sensation in mouth, skin, stomach, and throat; convulsions; death; delirium; general vascular damage; kidney damage; loss of hair; muscle weakness; respiratory depression; severe bloody diarrhea; shock

Contraindications: This drug should not be taken by people who are allergic to it. Consult your doctor immediately if this drug has been prescribed for you and you have such an allergy.

Warnings: This drug should be used with extreme caution by elderly and debilitated persons, especially those with kidney, stomach, intestinal, or heart disease. • The dosage of this drug should be reduced if weakness, anorexia, nausea, vomiting, or diarrhea appears.

Comments: Although this drug is usually used to relieve attacks of gout pain, some doctors prescribe it as a preventive of gout pain. When taken as a preventive, one method is to take one tablet one to four times a week for moderately severe gout, or even one tablet once or twice a day for more severe cases. • This drug should be taken at the first sign of a gout attack. A delay of several hours will reduce its effectiveness. • One method for determining the correct dose of this drug is to take one tablet every one to two hours until pain is relieved, or until nausea, vomiting, or diarrhea develops. At this point, the medication dose should be decreased slightly. • If diarrhea becomes severe, paregoric may have to be taken to help relieve this symptom. If diarrhea persists for longer than one and one-half to two days, or if it is stained with blood, a doctor should be consulted.

Col-Decon adrenergic and antihistamine (Columbia Medical Co.), see Naldecon adrenergic and antihistamine.

OTC   **Collyrium Drops eyewash**

Manufacturer: Wyeth Laboratories

Ingredients: boric acid; sodium borate; thimerosal; antipyrine; sodium salicylate

Dosage Form: Liquid: boric acid; sodium borate; thimerosal; 0.002%; antipyrine, 0.4%; sodium salicylate, 0.056%

Use: Antiseptic eye wash

Side Effects: Mild irritation of the eye (rare). If swallowed, may cause abdominal cramping, nausea, and vomiting; large doses swallowed may cause flushing, whole-body rash, or liver or kidney disease.

Warnings: If the condition for which you are using this product persists, or if eye irritation occurs, consult your doctor promptly. • Keep this product out of the reach of children. • Carefully follow the usage instructions that are printed on the product label.

Comments: An eye cup is included with this product to use in washing the eyes; keep the eye cup clean and dry.

Colonil anticholinergic and antispasmodic (Mallinckrodt, Inc.), see Lomotil anticholinergic and antispasmodic.

Colsalide gout remedy (North American Pharmacal), see colchicine gout remedy.

Rx   **Combid Spansule anticholinergic and phenothiazine**

Manufacturer: Smith Kline & French Laboratories

Ingredients: isopropamide iodide; prochlorperazine maleate

Equivalent Products: Com-Pro-Span, Columbia Medical Co.; Prochlor-Iso, Henry Schein, Inc.

Dosage Form: Capsule: isopropamide iodide, 5 mg; prochlorperazine maleate, 10 mg (yellow/clear with multicolored pellets)

Use: Treatment of intestinal or stomach disorders, including peptic ulcer

Minor Side Effects: Blurred vision; change in urine color; constipation; diarrhea; difficult urination; drooling; drowsiness; dry mouth; headache; insomnia; increased sensitivity to light; jitteriness; loss of the sense of taste; menstrual irregularities; nasal congestion; nausea; nervousness; palpitations; rash; reduced sweating; restlessness; uncoordinated movements; vomiting

Major Side Effects: Difficult ejaculation; difficult swallowing; enlarged breasts (in both sexes); fluid retention; impotence; involuntary movements of the face, tongue, mouth, or jaw; jaundice; muscle stiffness; rise in blood pressure; tremors

Contraindications: This drug should not be used by people suffering drug-induced depression, or who have blood disease, liver disease, jaundice, glaucoma, enlarged prostate, obstructed intestine, obstructed bladder, or an allergy to the drug or any of its components. This drug may disguise symptoms of brain tumor or obstructed intestine, and should not be used by people in whom either condition is suspected. Consult your doctor immediately if this drug has been prescribed for you and you have, or might have, any of these conditions. • This drug should not be used by children under the age of 12.

Warnings: This drug should be used cautiously by pregnant or nursing women, the elderly, and people who have a past history of jaundice, liver disease, blood disease, or allergy to other drugs. Be sure your doctor knows if any of these conditions apply to you. • This drug interacts with amantadine, haloperidol, antacids, other phenothiazines, other anticholinergics, alcohol, and depressants; if you are currently taking any drugs of these types, consult your doctor about their use. If you are unsure of the type or contents of your medications, ask your doctor or pharmacist. • This drug may cause drowsiness; avoid tasks that require alertness. To prevent oversedation, avoid the use of alcohol or other drugs that have sedative properties. • While taking this drug, do not take any nonprescription item for cough, cold, or sinus problems without first checking with your doctor. • This drug has sustained action; never take it more frequently than your doctor prescribes. A serious overdose could result. • Because this drug reduces sweating, avoid excessive work or exercise in hot weather. • Call your doctor if you notice a rash, flushing, or pain in the eye. • This drug may influence the results of thyroid function tests; remind your doctor that you are taking the drug if you are scheduled for a thyroid test.

Comments: The effects of therapy with this drug may not be apparent for at least two weeks. • This drug does not cure ulcers but may help them improve. • This drug is best taken one-half to one hour before meals. • Chew gum or suck on ice chips or a piece of hard candy to reduce mouth dryness. • To avoid dizziness or light-headedness when you stand, contract and relax the muscles of your legs for a few moments before rising. Do this by pushing one foot against the floor while raising the other foot slightly, alternating feet so that you are "pumping" your legs in a pedaling motion.

℞   **Compazine phenothiazine**

Manufacturer: Smith Kline & French Laboratories
Ingredient: prochlorperazine
Dosage Form: Liquid concentrate (per 1 ml): 10 mg. Suppository: 2.5 mg; 5 mg; 25 mg. Time-release capsule: 10 mg; 15 mg; 30 mg; 75 mg (all are

black/clear with yellow and white beads). Tablet: 5 mg; 10 mg; 25 mg (all yellow)

Use: Control of severe nausea and vomiting; relief of certain kinds of anxiety, tension, agitation, psychiatric disorders

Minor Side Effects: Blurred vision; change in urine color; constipation; diarrhea; drooling; drowsiness; dry mouth; jitteriness; menstrual irregularities; nasal congestion; nausea; rash; reduced sweating; restlessness; uncoordinated movements; vomiting

Major Side Effects: Difficulty in swallowing; enlarged or painful breasts (in both sexes); fluid retention; impotence; involuntary movements of the face, mouth, tongue, or jaw; jaundice; muscle stiffness; rise in blood pressure; sore throat; tremors

Contraindications: This drug should not be taken by people who have blood diseases or by those who are suffering drug-induced depression. Consult your doctor immediately if this drug has been prescribed for you and you have such a condition. • This drug should not be given to people who are comatose or to children undergoing surgery. • People who have previously had an allergic reaction to any phenothiazine should not take this drug.

Warnings: This drug should be used cautiously by pregnant women. • This drug may cause drowsiness; avoid tasks that require alertness. To prevent oversedation, avoid the use of alcohol or other drugs that have sedative properties. • This drug interacts with oral antacids or anticholinergics; if you are currently taking any drugs of these types, consult your doctor about their use. If you are unsure of the type or contents of your medications, ask your doctor or pharmacist. • When taking this drug, do not take any nonprescription item for cough, cold, or sinus problems without first checking with your doctor. • This drug may cause motor restlessness, uncoordinated movements, and muscle spasms. If so, it should be discontinued or the dosage should be adjusted. Contact your doctor immediately if you notice any such symptoms. • The antivomiting action of this drug may mask symptoms of severe disease or toxicity due to overdose of other drugs. • People with acute illnesses should take this drug only under close supervision. Their dosage may need adjustment. • This drug has sustained action. Never take it more frequently than your doctor prescribes. A serious overdose may result.

Comments: The effects of this drug may not be apparent for at least two weeks. • Chew gum or suck on ice chips or a piece of hard candy to reduce mouth dryness. • To avoid dizziness or light-headedness when you stand, contract and relax the muscles of your legs for a few moments before rising. Do this by pushing one foot against the floor while raising the other foot slightly, alternating feet so that you are "pumping" your legs in a pedaling motion. • This drug reduces sweating; therefore, avoid excessive work or exercise in hot weather. • The liquid concentrate form of this drug should be added to 60 ml (2 fluid ounces) or more of water, milk, juice, coffee, tea, or a carbonated beverage, or to pulpy foods (applesauce, etc.) immediately prior to administration.

OTC   Compound W wart remover

Manufacturer: Whitehall Laboratories

Ingredients: acetone; alcohol; camphor; ether; glacial acetic acid; menthol; salicylic acid

Dosage Form: Liquid: acetone; alcohol; camphor, 1.5%; ether, 57%; glacial acetic acid, 9%; menthol, 2%; salicylic acid, 14%

Use: Removes common warts

Side Effects: Allergy; local irritation

Contraindications: Do not use this product if you have diabetes or poor circulation.

Warnings: Use externally only. Do not apply wart remover to mucous membranes. • Keep away from eyes. • This product is flammable; do not use around an open flame. • This product is extremely corrosive. Follow directions carefully and exactly. Protect surrounding skin with petroleum jelly before use.

Comments: Overuse causes death of surrounding skin. • Do not use this product on moles, birthmarks, or on areas that do not have the typical appearance of a common wart. • This product creates a film over the area as it is applied. Do not be alarmed and do not remove the film. • Do not use this product for more than a week. • If the condition worsens, stop using wart remover and call your pharmacist. • Keep the bottle tightly closed between uses.

OTC   Compoz Tablets sleeping aid

Manufacturer: Jeffrey Martin, Inc.
Ingredient: pyrilamine maleate
Dosage Form: Tablet: pyrilamine maleate, 10 mg
Use: To induce drowsiness and assist in falling asleep
Side Effects: Blurred vision; confusion; constipation; difficult urination; dizziness; drowsiness; dry mouth and respiratory passages; headache; insomnia; low blood pressure; nausea; nervousness; palpitations; rash; restlessness; vomiting. Children may react with primary symptoms of excitement (convulsions; flushed skin; nervousness; tremors; twitching of muscles; uncoordinated movements).

Contraindications: This product should not be given to children under 12 years of age. • Do not take this product if you are pregnant or nursing.

Warnings: This product must be used with extreme caution by persons who have asthma, glaucoma, or enlarged prostate. If you have any of these conditions, do not take this product without first consulting your doctor. • This product may interact with other drugs; if you are currently taking any other prescription or over-the-counter medication, do not take this product without first consulting your doctor or pharmacist. • Tolerance to this drug may develop; do not increase the recommended dosage of this drug unless your doctor directs you to do so. • This drug may cause drowsiness; avoid driving, operating heavy machinery, or performing other tasks requiring mental alertness. To prevent oversedation, avoid the use of alcohol or other sedative drugs.

Comments: Insomnia may be a symptom of a serious illness; consult a doctor if sleeplessness lasts for more than two weeks.

Com-Pro-Span anticholinergic and phenothiazine (Columbia Medical Co.), see Combid Spansule anticholinergic and phenothiazine.

OTC   Comtrex cold remedy

Manufacturer: Bristol-Myers Products
Ingredients: acetaminophen; phenylpropanolamine hydrochloride; chlorpheniramine maleate; dextromethorphan hydrobromide; alcohol (liquid form only)
Dosage Forms: Capsule and tablet: acetaminophen, 325 mg; phenylpropanolamine hydrochloride, 12.5 mg; chlorpheniramine maleate, 1 mg; dextromethorphan hydrobromide, 10 mg. Liquid (content per 30 ml, or one fluid ounce): acetaminophen, 650 mg; phenylpropanolamine hydrochloride, 25 mg; chlorpheniramine maleate, 2 mg; dextromethorphan hydrobromide, 20 mg; alcohol, 20%
Use: Relief of major cold symptoms
Side Effects: Anxiety; blurred vision; chest pain; confusion; constipation;

difficult and painful urination; dizziness; headache; increased blood pressure; insomnia; loss of appetite; nausea; nervousness; palpitations; rash; reduced sweating; tension; tremor; vomiting

Contraindications: This product should not be used by persons who have severe heart disease or severe high blood pressure. • This product should not be given to newborn or premature infants.

Warnings: This product should be used with special caution by the elderly or debilitated, and by persons who have asthma, diabetes, enlarged prostate, glaucoma (certain types), heart disease, high blood pressure, kidney disease, obstructed bladder, obstructed intestine, peptic ulcer, or thyroid disease. If you have any of these conditions, consult your doctor before taking this product. • This product may cause drowsiness. Do not take it if you must drive, operate heavy machinery, or perform other tasks requiring mental alertness. To prevent oversedation, avoid the use of alcohol or other drugs that have sedative properties. • This product interacts with alcohol, guanethidine, monoamine oxidase inhibitors, sedative drugs, and tricyclic antidepressants. If you are currently taking any drugs of these types, check with your doctor before taking this product. If you are unsure of the type or contents of your medications, ask your doctor or pharmacist. • Because this product reduces sweating, avoid excessive work or exercise in hot weather. • When taken in overdose, acetaminophen is more toxic than aspirin. Follow dosage instructions carefully.

Comments: Many other conditions (some serious) mimic the common cold. If symptoms persist beyond one week or if they occur regularly without regard to season, consult your doctor. • The effectiveness of this product may diminish after being taken regularly for seven to ten days; consult your pharmacist about substituting another product containing a different antihistamine if this product begins to lose its effectiveness for you. • Chew gum or suck on ice chips or a piece of hard candy to reduce mouth dryness.

OTC Conceptrol contraceptive cream

Manufacturer: Ortho Pharmaceutical Corporation
Ingredient: nonoxynol 9
Dosage Form: Vaginal cream: nonoxynol 9, 5%
Use: Intravaginal contraception
Side Effects: Local irritation to user or partner
Contraindications: This product should not be used if either partner is allergic to nonoxynol.
Comments: Be sure to insert a new dose of contraceptive cream for each intercourse. • Do not douche for at least six hours after intercourse. • Used alone, this product is not as effective as when used with a diaphragm.

Congens No. 1 estrogen hormone (Blaine Co., Inc.), see Premarin estrogen hormone.

OTC Congespirin children's cold and allergy remedy

Manufacturer: Bristol-Myers Products
Ingredients: aspirin; phenylephrine hydrochloride
Dosage Form: Chewable tablet: aspirin, 81 mg (1¼ grains); phenylephrine hydrochloride, 1.25 mg
Use: Temporary relief of nasal congestion, fever, sneezing, aches and pains of colds or "flu"
Side Effects: Dizziness; mental confusion; mild to moderate stimulation; nausea and vomiting; ringing in the ears; slight blood loss; sweating
Contraindications: This product should not be used by persons who have significant drug or food allergies, aspirin sensitivity, asthma, blood-clotting

disease, gout, or vitamin-K deficiency.

Warnings: This product should be used with special caution by persons who have diabetes, heart disease, high blood pressure, or thyroid disease. If your child has any of these conditions, consult your doctor before administering this product. • This product interacts with alcohol, ammonium chloride, guanethidine, methotrexate, monoamine oxidase inhibitors, oral anticoagulants, oral antidiabetics, probenecid, sedative drugs, steroids, sulfinpyrazone, tricyclic antidepressants, and vitamin C. If your child is currently taking any drugs of these types, check with your doctor before administering this product. If you are unsure of the type or contents of your child's medications, ask your doctor or pharmacist.

Comments: Many other conditions (some serious) mimic the common cold. If symptoms persist beyond one week or if they occur regularly without regard to season, consult your doctor. • The effectiveness of this product may diminish after being taken regularly for seven to ten days; consult your pharmacist about substituting another product containing a different antihistamine if this product begins to lose its effectiveness for your child. • Have your child chew gum or suck on ice chips to reduce mouth dryness.

OTC　　　　　Contac cold and allergy remedy

Manufacturer: Menley & James Laboratories

Ingredients: atropine sulfate; belladonna alkaloids; phenylpropanolamine hydrochloride; chlorpheniramine maleate; scopolamine hydrobromide; sulfate

Dosage Form: Time-release capsule: atropine sulfate, 0.0375 mg; belladonna alkaloids, 0.2 mg; phenylpropanolamine hydrochloride, 50 mg; chlorpheniramine maleate, 4 mg; scopolamine hydrobromide, 0.0219 mg; sulfate, 0.19 mg.

Use: Relief of symptoms of colds

Side Effects: Anxiety; blurred vision; chest pain; confusion; constipation; difficult and painful urination; dizziness; headache; increased blood pressure; insomnia; loss of appetite; nausea; nervousness; palpitations; rash; reduced sweating; tension; tremor; vomiting

Contraindications: Unless directed otherwise by a doctor, this product should not be used by the elderly or debilitated, nor by persons who have asthma, enlarged prostate, eye disease, glaucoma (certain types), heart disease, high blood pressure, kidney disease, liver disease, myasthenia gravis, obstructed bladder, obstructed intestine, peptic ulcer, or thyroid disease. This product should not be given to children or infants.

Warnings: This product should be used with special caution by persons who have diabetes. If you have this condition, consult your doctor before taking this product. • This product may cause drowsiness. Do not take it if you must drive, operate heavy machinery, or perform other tasks requiring mental alertness. To prevent oversedation, avoid the use of alcohol or other drugs that have sedative properties. • This product interacts with alcohol, amantadine, guanethidine, haloperidol, monoamine oxidase inhibitors, sedative drugs, and tricyclic antidepressants. If you are currently taking any drugs of these types, check with your doctor before taking this product. If you are unsure of the type or contents of your medications, ask your doctor or pharmacist. • Because this product reduces sweating, avoid excessive work or exercise in hot weather. • This product has sustained action; never increase the recommended dose or take it more frequently than directed.

Comments: Many other conditions (some serious) mimic the common cold. If symptoms persist beyond one week or if they occur regularly without regard to season, consult your doctor. • The effectiveness of this product may diminish after being taken regularly for seven to ten days; consult your pharmacist about substituting another product containing a different anti-histamine if this product begins to lose its effectiveness for you. • Chew gum or suck on ice chips or a piece of hard candy to reduce mouth dryness.

OTC Contac Jr. children's cold and allergy remedy

Manufacturer: Menley & James Laboratories
Ingredients: phenylpropanolamine hydrochloride; acetaminophen; dextromethorphan hydrobromide; alcohol
Dosage Form: Liquid (content per 5 cc, or one teaspoon): phenylpropanolamine hydrochloride, 9.375 mg; acetaminophen, 162.5 mg; dextromethorphan hydrobromide, 5 mg; alcohol, 10%
Use: Relief of congestion, coughing, body aches, and fever due to colds
Side Effects: Mild to moderate stimulation, nausea, vomiting drowsiness, dry mouth
Warnings: This product should be used with special caution by persons who have diabetes, high blood pressure, or thyroid disease. If your child has any of these conditions, consult your doctor before administering this product. • This product interacts with alcohol, ammonium chloride, guanethidine, monoamine oxidase inhibitors, sedative drugs, and tricyclic antidepressants. If your child is currently taking any drugs of these types, check with your doctor before administering this product. If you are unsure of the type or contents of your child's medications, ask your doctor or pharmacist. • When taken in overdose, acetaminophen is more toxic than aspirin. Follow dosage instructions carefully.
Comments: Many other conditions (some serious) mimic the common cold. If symptoms persist beyond one week or if they occur regularly without regard to season, consult your doctor. Have your child chew gum or suck on ice chips or a piece of hard candy to reduce mouth dryness.

Contraceptives (oral), see oral contraceptives.

Coprobate sedative and hypnotic (Coastal Pharmaceutical Co., Inc.), see meprobamate sedative and hypnotic.

℞ Cordran steroid hormone

Manufacturer: Dista Products Company
Ingredient: flurandrenolide
Dosage Forms: Cream: 0.025%; 0.05%. Lotion: 0.05%. Ointment: 0.025%; 0.05%. Tape (content per square cm): 4 mcg
Use: Relief of pruritus and inflammations of the skin such as eczema and poison ivy
Minor Side Effects: Burning sensation; dryness; irritation; itching; rash
Major Side Effect: Secondary infection
Contraindications: This drug should not be used by people who are allergic to it. Consult your doctor immediately if this drug has been prescribed for you and you have such an allergy.
Warnings: If irritation develops, discontinue use of this drug and notify your doctor. This drug should be used with caution if an extensive area is involved or if an occlusive dressing is being used, since there will be increased absorption of the drug into the bloodstream. This is particularly true concerning the use of this drug in children and infants. • This drug should be used cautiously by pregnant women. Be sure your doctor knows if you are pregnant. • This product is not to be used on or in the eyes.
Comments: If the affected area of the skin is extremely dry or is scaling,

the skin may be moistened before applying this drug by soaking in water or by applying water with a clean cloth. The ointment form is probably better for dry skin. • Do not use this drug with an occlusive wrap unless instructed to do so by your doctor. If it is necessary for you to use this drug under a wrap, follow your doctor's instructions exactly; do not leave the wrap in place longer than specified. • The tape form of this drug is used in place of an occlusive wrap bandage. If the tape fails to stick to the skin, rub the area lightly with rubbing alcohol before applying the tape.

OTC   Coricidin cold and allergy remedy

Manufacturer: Schering Corporation
Ingredients: chlorpheniramine maleate; aspirin
Dosage Form: Tablet: chlorpheniramine maleate, 2 mg; aspirin, 325 mg (5 grains)
Use: Temporary relief of cold and allergy symptoms
Side Effects: Anxiety; blurred vision; chest pain; confusion; constipation; difficult and painful urination; dizziness; headache; increased blood pressure; insomnia; loss of appetite; nausea; nervousness; palpitations; rash; ringing in the ears; slight blood loss; reduced sweating; tension; tremor; vomiting
Contraindications: This product should not be used by persons who have significant drug and food allergies, aspirin sensitivity, asthma, blood-clotting disease, enlarged prostate, glaucoma, gout, peptic ulcer, or vitamin-K deficiency. • This product should not be given to newborn or premature infants, nor to children under six years of age.
Warnings: This product may cause drowsiness. Do not take it if you must drive, operate heavy machinery, or perform other tasks requiring mental alertness. To prevent oversedation, avoid the use of alcohol or other drugs that have sedative properties. • This product interacts with alcohol, ammonium chloride, guanethidine, methotrexate, monoamine oxidase inhibitors, oral anticoagulants, oral antidiabetics, probenecid, sedative drugs, steroids, sulfinpyrazone, tricyclic antidepressants, and vitamin C. If you are currently taking any drugs of these types, check with your doctor before taking this product. If you are unsure of the type or contents of your medications, ask your doctor or pharmacist. • Because this product reduces sweating, avoid excessive work or exercise in hot weather.
Comments: Many other conditions (some serious) mimic the common cold. If symptoms persist beyond one week or if they occur regularly without regard to season, consult your doctor. • The effectiveness of this product may diminish after being taken regularly for seven to ten days; consult your pharmacist about substituting another product containing a different antihistamine if this product begins to lose its effectiveness for you. • Chew gum or suck on ice chips or a piece of hard candy to reduce mouth dryness.

OTC   Coricidin cough remedy

Manufacturer: Schering Corporation
Ingredients: dextromethorphan hydrobromide; phenylpropanolamine hydrochloride; guaifenesin; alcohol
Dosage Form: Liquid (content per 5 ml, or one teaspoon): dextromethorphan hydrobromide, 10 mg; phenylpropanolamine hydrochloride, 12.5 mg; guaifenesin, 100 mg; alcohol, less than 0.5%
Use: Temporary relief of cough and nasal congestion due to colds or "flu"; also to convert a dry, nonproductive cough to a productive, phlegm-producing cough

Side Effects: Drowsiness; nausea; vomiting

Warnings: This product should be used with special caution by children under two years of age, and by persons who have diabetes, heart disease, high blood pressure, or thyroid disease. If you have any of these conditions, consult your doctor before taking this product. • This product interacts with guanethidine and monoamine oxidase inhibitors. If you are currently taking any drugs of these types, check with your doctor before taking this product. If you are unsure of the type or contents of your medications, ask your doctor or pharmacist.

Comments: Do not use this product to treat chronic coughs, such as those from smoking or asthma. • Do not use this product to treat productive (hacking) coughs that produce phlegm. • If you require an expectorant, you need more moisture in your environment. Drink eight to ten glasses of water daily. The use of a vaporizer or humidifier may also be beneficial. Consult your doctor.

OTC   Coricidin 'D' decongestant cold and allergy remedy

Manufacturer: Schering Corporation

Ingredients: chlorpheniramine maleate; phenylpropanolamine hydrochloride; aspirin

Dosage Form: Tablet: chlorpheniramine maleate, 2 mg; phenylpropanolamine hydrochloride, 12.5 mg; aspirin, 325 mg (5 grains)

Use: Temporary relief of congestion, cold, allergy, and sinus symptoms

Side Effects: Anxiety; blurred vision; chest pain; confusion; constipation; difficult and painful urination; dizziness; headache; increased blood pressure; insomnia; loss of appetite; nausea; nervousness; palpitations; rash; ringing in the ears; slight blood loss; reduced sweating; tension; tremor; vomiting

Contraindications: This product should not be used by persons who have significant drug and food allergies, aspirin sensitivity, asthma, blood-clotting disease, diabetes, enlarged prostate, glaucoma, gout, heart disease, high blood pressure, peptic ulcer, thyroid disease, or vitamin-K deficiency. • This product should not be given to newborn or premature infants, nor to children under six years of age.

Warnings: This product should be used with special caution by the elderly or debilitated, and by persons who have kidney disease, obstructed bladder, or obstructed intestine. If you have any of these conditions, consult your doctor before taking this product. • This product may cause drowsiness. Do not take it if you must drive, operate heavy machinery, or perform other tasks requiring mental alertness. To prevent oversedation, avoid the use of alcohol or other drugs that have sedative properties. • This product interacts with alcohol, ammonium chloride, guanethidine, methotrexate, monoamine oxidase inhibitors, oral anticoagulants, oral antidiabetics, probenecid, sedative drugs, steroids, sulfinpyrazone, tricyclic antidepressants, and vitamin C. If you are currently taking any drugs of these types, check with your doctor before taking this product. If you are unsure of the type or contents of your medications, ask your doctor or pharmacist. • Because this product reduces sweating, avoid excessive work or exercise in hot weather.

Comments: Many other conditions (some serious) mimic the common cold. If symptoms persist beyond one week or if they occur regularly without regard to season, consult your doctor. • The effectiveness of this product may diminish after being taken regularly for seven to ten days; consult your pharmacist about substituting another product containing a different antihistamine if this product begins to lose its effectiveness for you. • Chew gum or suck on ice chips or a piece of hard candy to reduce mouth dryness.

OTC   Coricidin Demilets children's cold and allergy remedy

Manufacturer: Schering Corporation
Ingredients: chlorpheniramine maleate; aspirin; phenylephrine hydrochloride
Dosage Form: Chewable tablet: chlorpheniramine maleate, 0.5 mg; aspirin, 80 mg (1¼ grains); phenylephrine hydrochloride, 2.5 mg
Use: Temporary relief of symptoms of colds, or hay fever and other upper respiratory allergies
Side Effects: Blurred vision; confusion; constipation; convulsions; difficult urination; dizziness; drowsiness; dry mouth and respiratory passages; flushed skin; headache; increased blood pressure; insomnia; low blood pressure; nausea; nervousness; palpitations; rash; restlessness; ringing in the ears; tremor; twitching of muscles; uncoordinated movements; vomiting
Contraindications: This product should not be used by persons who have aspirin sensitivity, asthma, blood-clotting disease, gout, significant drug or food allergies, or vitamin-K deficiency. • This product should not be given to newborn or premature infants.
Warnings: This product should be used with special caution by persons who have diabetes, heart disease, high blood pressure, or thyroid disease. If your child has any of these conditions, consult your doctor before administering this product. • This product interacts with alcohol, ammonium chloride, guanethidine, methotrexate, monoamine oxidase inhibitors, oral anticoagulants, oral antidiabetics, probenecid, sedative drugs, steroids, sulfinpyrazone, tricyclic antidepressants, and vitamin C. If your child is currently taking any drugs of these types, check with your doctor before administering this product. If you are unsure of the type or contents of your child's medications, ask your doctor or pharmacist.
Comments: Many other conditions (some serious) mimic the common cold. If symptoms persist beyond one week or if they occur regularly without regard to season, consult your doctor. • The effectiveness of this product may diminish after being taken regularly for seven to ten days; consult your pharmacist about substituting another product containing a different antihistamine if this product begins to lose its effectiveness for your child. • Have your child chew gum or suck on ice chips or a piece of hard candy to reduce mouth dryness.

OTC   Coricidin nasal decongestant

Manufacturer: Schering Corporation
Ingredient: phenylephrine hydrochloride
Dosage Form: Nasal spray: phenylephrine hydrochloride, 0.5%
Use: Temporary relief of nasal congestion due to colds, sinusitis, hay fever, or other upper respiratory allergies
Side Effects: Blurred vision; burning, dryness of nasal mucosa; increased nasal congestion or discharge; sneezing, and/or stinging; dizziness; drowsiness; headache; insomnia; nervousness; palpitations; slight increase in blood pressure; stimulation
Contraindications: This product should not be used by persons who have glaucoma (certain types).
Warnings: This product should be used with special caution by persons who have diabetes, advanced hardening of the arteries, heart disease, high blood pressure, or thyroid disease. If you have any of these conditions, consult your doctor before taking this product. • This product interacts with guanethidine, monoamine oxidase inhibitors, and thyroid preparations. If you are currently taking any drugs of these types, check with your doctor before taking this product. If you are unsure of the type or contents of your medica-

tions, ask your doctor or pharmacist. • To avoid side effects such as burning, sneezing, or stinging, and a "rebound" increase in nasal congestion and discharge, do not exceed the recommended dosage and do not use this product for more than three or four continuous days. • This product should not be used by more than one person; sharing the dispenser may spread infection.

Corphed adrenergic and antihistamine (Bell Pharmacal Corp.), see Actifed adrenergic and antihistamine.

OTC   Correctol laxative

Manufacturer: Plough, Inc.
Ingredients: docusate sodium (dioctyl sodium sulfosuccinate); yellow phenolphthalein
Dosage Form: Tablet: docusate sodium, 100 mg; yellow phenolphthalein, 65 mg
Use: Relief of constipation and stool softener
Side Effects: Excess loss of fluid; griping (cramps); mucus in feces; pink to purple rash with blistering
Contraindications: Persons with high fever (100° F or more); black or tarry stools; nausea; vomiting; abdominal pain; or children under age three should not use this product unless directed by a doctor. • Do not use this product when constipation is caused by megacolon or other diseases of the intestine, or hypothyroidism. • Persons with a sensitivity to phenolphthalein should not use this product.
Warnings: Excessive use (daily for a month or more) of this product may cause diarrhea, vomiting, and loss of certain blood electrolytes. • Pregnant women should not use this product except on the advice of a doctor.
Comments: This product may discolor the urine and feces. • Evacuation may occur within 6 to 12 hours. Never self-medicate if constipation lasts longer than two weeks or if the medication does not produce a laxative effect within a week. • Limit use to seven days unless directed otherwise by a doctor since this product may cause laxative-dependence (addiction) if used for a longer time. • An ingredient in this product is referred to as a stool softener. This product is recommended for prevention of constipation when the stool is hard and dry. Do not take another product containing mineral oil at the same time as you are taking this product.

OTC   Cortaid topical steroid product

Manufacturer: The Upjohn Company
Ingredient: hydrocortisone acetate
Dosage Forms: Cream, lotion, and ointment: hydrocortisone acetate, 0.5%
Use: Temporary relief of skin inflammation, irritation, itching and rashes associated with such conditions as dermatitis, eczema, or poison ivy
Side Effects: Burning sensation; dryness; irritation; itching; rash; secondary infections
Contraindications: Do not use this product in the presence of diseases that severely impair blood circulation or in the presence of a bacterial or viral infection.
Warnings: Use this product externally only. • Avoid contact with eyes. Do not use for prolonged periods of time. If the condition persists, call your doctor. • Consult a physician for use on children under two years of age.
Comments: If the affected area is extremely dry or is scaling, the skin may be moistened before applying the medication by soaking in water or by applying water with a clean cloth. The ointment form of this product is preferred for dry skin. • Hydrocortisone-containing products, until recently, required a

prescription for purchase. They are now sold over-the-counter in strengths of up to 0.5%.

Cortan steroid hormone (Halsey Drug Co., Inc.), see prednisone steroid hormone.

Cortin steroid hormone and anti-infective (C & M Pharmacal, Inc.), see Vioform-Hydrocortisone steroid hormone and anti-infective.

R̽ Cortisporin ophthalmic suspension

Manufacturer: Burroughs Wellcome Co.
Ingredients: polymyxin B sulfate; neomycin sulfate; hydrocortisone; thimerosal
Dosage Form: Drop(content per ml): polymyxin B sulfate, 10,000 units; neomycin sulfate, 5 mg; hydrocortisone, 10 mg; thimerosal, 0.001%
Use: Short-term treatment of bacterial infections of the eye
Minor Side Effects: Burning; stinging
Major Side Effects: Perception of a "halo" effect around lights; worsening of the condition
Contraindications: This product should not be used for fungal or viral infections of the eye or for eye infections with pus. Nor should this product be used for conditions involving the back part of the eye. • This drug should not be used by people who are allergic to any of its ingredients. Consult your doctor immediately if this drug has been prescribed for you and you have such an allergy.
Warnings: Frequent eye examinations are advisable while this drug is being used, particularly if it is necessary to use the drug for an extended period of time. • Prolonged use of this drug may result in glaucoma, secondary infection, and eye damage. Contact your doctor immediately if you notice any visual disturbances (dimming or blurring of vision, reduced night vision, halos around lights), eye pain, or headache.
Comments: As with all eyedrops, this drug may cause minor, temporary clouding or blurring of vision when first applied. • Discard any unused portion of this drug. • Consult your doctor if symptoms reappear. • This product should be shaken well before using. • Be careful about the contamination of medications used for the eyes. Wash your hands before administering eyedrops. Do not touch the dropper to the eye. Do not wash or wipe the dropper before replacing it in the bottle. Close the bottle tightly to keep out moisture.

R̽ Cortisporin otic solution/suspension

Manufacturer: Burroughs Wellcome Company
Ingredients: hydrocortisone; neomycin sulfate; polymyxin B sulfate
Equivalent Product: Otobione suspension, Schering Corporation
Dosage Forms: Solution (per 1 ml): hydrocortisone, 10 mg; neomycin sulfate, 5 mg; polymyxin B sulfate, 10,000 units. Suspension (per 1 ml): hydrocortisone, 10 mg; neomycin sulfate, 5 mg; polymyxin B sulfate, 10,000 units
Use: Treatment of superficial bacterial infections of the outer ear
Minor Side Effects: Burning sensation; hives; itching
Contraindications: This drug should not be used to treat viral infections. • This drug should not be taken by people who are allergic to it. Notify your doctor if your skin becomes red and swollen, scaly, or itchy; allergic reactions to neomycin are common.
Warnings: This drug should not be used for more than ten days. • This drug should be used cautiously if there is a possibility that the patient has a punctured eardrum.

Comments: To administer eardrops, tilt your head to one side with the affected ear turned upward. Grasp the earlobe and pull it upward and back to straighten the ear canal. (If administering eardrops to a child, gently pull the earlobe downward and back.) Fill the dropper and place the prescribed number of drops in the ear. Be careful not to touch the dropper to the ear canal, as the dropper can easily become contaminated this way. Keep the ear tilted upward for five to ten seconds, then gently insert a small piece of cotton into the ear to prevent the drops from escaping. • Do not wash or wipe the dropper after use. Close the bottle tightly to keep out moisture. • Discard any remaining medicine after treatment has been completed so that you will not be tempted to use the medication for a subsequent ear problem without consulting a doctor. • If you wish to warm the drops before administration, roll the bottle back and forth between your hands. Do not place the bottle in boiling water; the medication will lose potency if heated above body temperature.

OTC   Coryban-D cough remedy

Manufacturer: Pfipharmecs Division
Ingredients: dextromethorphan hydrobromide; guaifenesin; phenylephrine hydrochloride; acetaminophen; alcohol
Dosage Form: Liquid (content per 5 ml, or one teaspoon): dextromethorphan hydrobromide, 7.5 mg; guaifenesin, 50 mg; phenylephrine hydrochloride, 5 mg; acetaminophen, 120 mg; alcohol, 7.5%
Use: Temporary relief of cough, nasal congestion, fever, aches, and pains due to colds or "flu"; also to convert a dry, nonproductive cough to a productive, phlegm-producing cough
Side-Effects: Drowsiness; mild stimulation; nausea; vomiting
Contraindications: This product should not be given to children under six years of age.
Warnings: This product should be used with special caution by persons who have diabetes, heart disease, high blood pressure, or thyroid disease. If you have any of these conditions, consult your doctor before taking this product. • This product interacts with guanethidine and monamine oxidase inhibitors. If you are currently taking any drugs of these types, check with your doctor before taking this product. If you are unsure of the type or contents of your medications, ask your doctor or pharmacist. • When taken in overdose, acetaminophen is more toxic than aspirin. Follow dosage instructions carefully.
Comments: Do not use this product to treat chronic coughs, such as those from smoking or asthma. • Do not use this product to treat productive (hacking) coughs that produce phlegm. • If you require an expectorant, you need more moisture in your environment. Drink eight to ten glasses of water daily. The use of a vaporizer or humidifier may also be beneficial. Consult your doctor.

OTC   Coryban-D decongestant cold remedy

Manufacturer: Pfipharmecs Division
Ingredients: caffeine; chlorpheniramine maleate; phenylpropanolamine hydrochloride
Dosage Form: Capsule: caffeine, 30 mg; chlorpheniramine maleate, 2 mg; phenylpropanolamine hydrochloride, 25 mg
Use: Temporary relief of nasal/sinus congestion and other symptoms of colds
Side Effects: Anxiety; blurred vision; chest pain; confusion; constipation; difficult and painful urination; dizziness; drowsiness; headache; increased blood pressure; insomnia; loss of appetite; nausea; nervousness; palpita-

tions; rash; reduced sweating; tension; tremor; vomiting

Contraindications: This product should not be used by persons who have severe heart disease or severe high blood pressure. • This product should not be given to newborn or premature infants.

Warnings: This product should be used with special caution by the elderly or debilitated, and by persons who have asthma, diabetes, enlarged prostate, glaucoma (certain types), heart disease, high blood pressure, kidney disease, obstructed bladder, obstructed intestine, peptic ulcer, or thyroid disease. If you have any of these conditions, consult your doctor before taking this product. • This product may cause drowsiness. Do not take it if you must drive, operate heavy machinery, or perform other tasks requiring mental alertness. To prevent oversedation, avoid the use of alcohol or other drugs that have sedative properties. • This product interacts with alcohol, guanethidine, monoamine oxidase inhibitors, sedative drugs, and tricyclic antidepressants. If you are currently taking any drugs of these types, check with your doctor before taking this product. If you are unsure of the type or contents of your medications, ask your doctor or pharmacist. • Because this product reduces sweating, avoid excessive work or exercise in hot weather.

Comments: Many other conditions (some serious) mimic the common cold. If symptoms persist beyond one week or if they occur regularly without regard to season, consult your doctor. • The effectiveness of this product may diminish after being taken regularly for seven to ten days; consult your pharmacist about substituting another product containing a different antihistamine if this product begins to lose its effectiveness for you. • Chew gum or suck on ice chips or a piece of hard candy to reduce mouth dryness.

OTC   Co-Salt salt substitute

Manufacturer: Norcliff Thayer Inc.

Ingredients: potassium chloride; ammonium chloride; choline bitartrate; silica; lactose

Dosage Form: Crystalline powder (quantities of ingredients not specified)

Use: As a substitute for table salt by persons on low-sodium diets

Contraindications: Persons who have kidney disease or oliguria (small urinary output) should not use this product.

Warnings: Remember that sodium is an essential daily nutrient—the body needs a certain amount each day. If generalized symptoms of sodium depletion occur, such as muscle cramping, nausea, and weakness, the use of table salt should be reinstituted.

Comments: Use this product the same way you would use table salt on food or in cooking. • Because this product is rich in potassium, some doctors and pharmacists recommend its use when taking diuretics or other drugs that cause a potassium loss from the body. • Neocurtasal (Winthrop Laboratories) is another commonly used salt substitute.

OTC   CoTylenol children's cold remedy

Manufacturer: McNeil Consumer Products Company

Ingredients: pseudoephedrine hydrochloride; chlorpheniramine maleate; acetaminophen; alcohol

Dosage Form: Liquid (content per 5 ml, or one teaspoon): pseudoephedrine hydrochloride, 7.5 mg; chlorpheniramine maleate, 0.5 mg; acetaminophen, 120 mg; alcohol, 7%

Use: Temporary relief of nasal congestion, fever, aches, pains, and general discomfort due to colds

Side Effects: Anxiety; blurred vision; chest pain; confusion; constipation; difficult and painful urination; dizziness; drowsiness; headache; increased blood pressure; insomnia; loss of appetite; nausea; nervousness; palpitations; rash; sweating; tension; tremor; vomiting

Contraindications: This product should not be used by persons who have severe heart disease or severe high blood pressure. • This product should not be given to newborn or premature infants.

Warnings: This product should be used with special caution by persons who have asthma, diabetes, enlarged prostate, glaucoma (certain types), heart disease, high blood pressure, kidney disease, obstructed bladder, obstructed intestine, peptic ulcer, or thyroid disease. If your child has any of these conditions, consult your doctor before administering this product. • This product interacts with alcohol, guanethidine, monoamine oxidase inhibitors, sedative drugs, and tricyclic antidepressants. If your child is currently taking any drugs of these types, check with your doctor before administering this product. If you are unsure of the type or contents of your child's medications, ask your doctor or pharmacist. • When taken in overdose, acetaminophen is more toxic than aspirin. Follow dosage instructions carefully.

Comments: Many other conditions (some serious) mimic the common cold. If symptoms persist beyond one week or if they occur regularly without regard to season, consult your doctor. • The effectiveness of this product may diminish after being taken regularly for seven to ten days; consult your pharmacist about substituting another product containing a different antihistamine if this product begins to lose its effectiveness for your child. • Have your child suck on ice chips or a piece of hard candy to reduce mouth dryness.

OTC   **CoTylenol cold remedy**

Manufacturer: McNeil Consumer Products Company

Ingredients: acetaminophen; chlorpheniramine maleate; pseudoephedrine hydrochloride

Dosage Form: Tablet: acetaminophen, 325 mg; chlorpheniramine maleate, 2 mg; pseudoephedrine hydrochloride, 30 mg

Use: Temporary relief of nasal congestion, fever, aches, pains, and general discomfort due to colds

Side Effects: Anxiety; blurred vision; chest pain; confusion; constipation; difficult and painful urination; dizziness; drowsiness; headache; increased blood pressure; insomnia; loss of appetite; nausea; nervousness; palpitations; rash; reduced sweating; tension; tremor; vomiting

Contraindications: This product should not be used by persons who have severe heart disease or severe high blood pressure. • This product should not be given to newborn or premature infants.

Warnings: This product should be used with special caution by the elderly or debilitated, and by persons who have asthma, diabetes, enlarged prostate, glaucoma (certain types), heart disease, high blood pressure, kidney disease, obstructed bladder, obstructed intestine, peptic ulcer, or thyroid disease. If you have any of these conditions, consult your doctor before taking this product. • This product may cause drowsiness. Do not take it if you must drive, operate heavy machinery, or perform other tasks requiring mental alertness. To prevent oversedation, avoid the use of alcohol or other drugs that have sedative properties. • This product interacts with alcohol, guanethidine, monoamine oxidase inhibitors, sedative drugs, and tricyclic antidepressants. If you are currently taking any drugs of these types, check with your doctor before taking this product. If you are unsure of the type or contents of your medications, ask your doctor or pharmacist. • Because this product reduces sweating, avoid excessive work or exercise in hot weather. • When used in overdose, acetaminophen is more toxic than aspirin. Follow dosage instructions carefully.

Comments: Many other conditions (some serious) mimic the common cold. If symptoms persist beyond one week or if they occur regularly without regard to season, consult your doctor. • The effectiveness of this product may diminish after being taken regularly for seven to ten days; consult your pharmacist about substituting another product containing a different antihistamine if this product begins to lose its effectiveness for you. • Chew gum or suck on ice chips or a piece of hard candy to reduce mouth dryness.

OTC   CoTylenol liquid cold formula

Manufacturer: McNeil Consumer Products Company
Ingredients: acetaminophen; chlorpheniramine maleate; pseudoephedrine hydrochloride; dextromethorphan hydrobromide; alcohol
Dosage Form: Liquid (content per 30 ml): acetaminophen, 650 mg; chlorpheniramine maleate, 4 mg; pseudoephedrine hydrochloride, 60 mg; dextromethorphan hydrobromide, 20 mg; alcohol, 7.5%
Use: Temporary relief of nasal congestion, fever, aches, pains, coughing, and general discomfort due to colds
Side Effects: Anxiety; blurred vision; chest pain; confusion; constipation; difficult and painful urination; dizziness; drowsiness; headache; increased blood pressure; insomnia; loss of appetite; nausea; nervousness; palpitations; rash; reduced sweating; tension; tremor; vomiting
Contraindications: This product should not be used by persons who have severe heart disease or severe high blood pressure. • This product should not be given to newborn or premature infants.
Warnings: This product should be used with special caution by the elderly or debilitated, and by persons who have asthma, diabetes, enlarged prostate, glaucoma (certain types), heart disease, high blood pressure, kidney disease, obstructed bladder, obstructed intestine, peptic ulcer, or thyroid disease. If you have any of these conditions, consult your doctor before taking this product. • This product may cause drowsiness. Do not take it if you must drive, operate heavy machinery, or perform other tasks requiring mental alertness. To prevent oversedation, avoid the use of alcohol or other drugs that have sedative properties. • This product interacts with alcohol, guanethidine, monoamine oxidase inhibitors, sedative drugs, and tricyclic antidepressants. If you are currently taking any drugs of these types, check with your doctor before taking this product. If you are unsure of the type or contents of your medications, ask your doctor or pharmacist. • Because this product reduces sweating, avoid excessive work or exercise in hot weather. • When used in overdose, acetaminophen is more toxic than aspirin.
Comments: Many other conditions (some serious) mimic the common cold. If symptoms persist beyond one week, or if they occur regularly without regard to season, consult your doctor. • The effectiveness of this product may diminish after being taken regularly for seven to ten days; consult your pharmacist about substituting another product containing a different antihistamine if this product begins to lose its effectiveness for you. • Chew gum or suck on ice chips or a piece of hard candy to reduce mouth dryness.

℞   Coumadin anticoagulant

Manufacturer: Endo Laboratories, Inc.
Ingredient: sodium warfarin
Equivalent Product: Panwarfin, Abbott Laboratories
Dosage Form: Tablet: 2 mg (lavender); 2.5 mg (orange); 5 mg (peach); 7.5 mg (yellow); 10 mg (white)
Use: Prevention of blood clot formation in conditions such as heart disease and pulmonary embolism

Minor Side Effects: Change in urine color; diarrhea; nausea

Major Side Effects: Black stools; bleeding; fever; rash; red urine

Contraindications: This drug should not be taken if any condition or circumstance exists in which bleeding is likely to be worsened by taking the drug (such as ulcers or certain surgeries). Be sure that you have given your doctor a complete medical history. • This drug should not be taken by people who are allergic to it, or by pregnant women. Consult your doctor immediately if this drug has been prescribed for you and you have either condition.

Warnings: This drug should be used cautiously by people who have any condition where bleeding is an added risk, including those suffering malnutrition, or who have liver disease, kidney disease, intestinal infection, wounds or injuries, high blood pressure, blood disease (certain types), diabetes, menstrual difficulties, indwelling catheters, and congestive heart failure. The drug should be used cautiously by nursing mothers. Be sure your doctor knows if you have any of these conditions. • This drug interacts with alcohol, allopurinol, anabolic steroids, antipyrine, barbiturates, chloral hydrate, chloramphenicol, cholestyramine, clofibrate, dextrothyroxine, diazoxide, disulfiram, ethacrynic acid, ethchlorvynol, glucagon, glutethimide, griseofulvin, indomethacin, mefenamic acid, neomycin, oral antidiabetics, oral contraceptives, oxyphenbutazone, phenylbutazone, phenytoin, quinidine, rifampin, salicylates, steroids, thyroid, triclofos, and antidepressants. If you are currently taking any drugs of these types, consult your doctor about their use. If you are unsure of the type or contents of your medications, ask your doctor or pharmacist. • Do not start or stop taking any other medication, including aspirin, without checking with your doctor. • Regular blood coagulation tests are essential while you are taking this drug. Many factors—including diet, environment, exercise, and other medications—may affect your response to this drug, so blood tests will need to be repeated often. If clots fail to form over cuts and bruises, or if purple or brown spots appear under bruised skin, call your doctor immediately. • Do not increase your dose or take this drug more frequently than your doctor prescribes. • While taking this drug, avoid drinking alcoholic beverages. • A change in urine color may or may not be serious; if you notice a change, contact your doctor or pharmacist. • Be sure all of your health care professionals know you are taking this drug.

OTC   Covangesic cold and allergy remedy

Manufacturer: Mallinckrodt, Inc.

Ingredients: phenylpropanolamine hydrochloride; phenylephrine hydrochloride; pyrilamine maleate; chlorpheniramine maleate; acetaminophen; alcohol (liquid form only)

Dosage Forms: Liquid (content per 5 ml, or one teaspoon): phenylpropanolamine hydrochloride, 6.25 mg; phenylephrine hydrochloride, 3.75 mg; pyrilamine maleate, 6.25 mg; chlorpheniramine maleate, 1 mg; acetaminophen, 120 mg; alcohol, 7.5%. Tablet: phenylpropanolamine hydrochloride, 12.5 mg; phenylephrine hydrochloride, 7.5 mg; pyrilamine maleate, 12.5 mg; chlorpheniramine maleate, 2 mg; acetaminophen, 275 mg

Use: Temporary relief of nasal congestion, fever, aches, pains, and general discomfort due to colds or upper respiratory allergies

Side Effects: Anxiety; blurred vision; chest pain; confusion; constipation; difficult and painful urination; dizziness; drowsiness; headache; increased blood pressure; insomnia; loss of appetite; nausea; nervousness; palpitations; rash; reduced sweating; tension; tremor; vomiting

Contraindications: This product should not be used by persons who have severe heart disease or severe high blood pressure. • This product should not be given to newborn or premature infants.

Warnings: This product should be used with special caution by the elderly or debilitated, and by persons who have asthma, diabetes, enlarged prostate, glaucoma (certain types), heart disease, high blood pressure, kidney disease, obstructed bladder, obstructed intestine, peptic ulcer, or thyroid disease. If you have any of these conditions, consult your doctor before taking this product. • This product may cause drowsiness. Do not take it if you must drive, operate heavy machinery, or perform other tasks requiring mental alertness. To prevent oversedation, avoid the use of alcohol or other drugs that have sedative properties. • This product interacts with alcohol, guanethidine, monoamine oxidase inhibitors, sedative drugs, and tricyclic antidepressants. If you are currently taking any drugs of these types, check with your doctor before taking this product. If you are unsure of the type or contents of your medications, ask your doctor or pharmacist. • Because this product reduces sweating, avoid excessive work or exercise in hot weather. • When taken in overdose, acetaminophen is more toxic than aspirin. Follow dosage instructions carefully.

Comments: Many other conditions (some serious) mimic the common cold. If symptoms persist beyond one week, or if they occur regularly without regard to season, consult your doctor. • The effectiveness of this product may diminish after being taken regularly for seven to ten days; consult your pharmacist about substituting another product containing a different antihistamine if this product begins to lose its effectiveness for you. • Chew gum or suck on ice chips or a piece of hard candy to reduce mouth dryness.

OTC   Cruex athlete's foot remedy

Manufacturer: Pharmacraft Division
Ingredients: calcium undecylenate; zinc undecylenate; p-chloro-m-xylenol (Ingredients vary with dosage form; see below.)
Dosage Forms: Cream: zinc undecylenate, 20%; p-chloro-m-xylenol, 3%. Powder (regular and aerosol): calcium undecylenate, 10%
Use: Relief and prevention of athlete's foot and jock itch
Side Effects: Allergy; local irritation
Warnings: Do not apply this product to mucous membranes, scraped skin, or to large areas of skin. • If your condition worsens, or if irritation occurs, stop using this product and consult your pharmacist. • When using the aerosol form of this product, be careful not to inhale any of the powder.
Comments: Some lesions take months to heal, so it is important not to stop treatment too soon. • If foot lesions are consistently a problem, check the fit of your shoes. • Wash your hands thoroughly after applying this product. The cream form of this product is preferable to the powders for effectiveness; the best action of the powders may be in drying the infected area. • The aerosol powder may be more expensive than the other forms of this product; check prices before paying for convenience you do not need.

Cyclanfor vasodilator (Forest Laboratories, Inc.), see Cyclospasmol vasodilator.

Cyclopar antibiotic (Parke-Davis), see tetracycline hydrochloride antibiotic.

R   Cyclospasmol vasodilator

Manufacturer: Ives Laboratories, Inc.
Ingredient: cyclandelate
Equivalent Products: cyclandelate, various manufacturers; Cyclanfor, Forest Laboratories, Inc.; Cydel, W. E. Hauck, Inc.

Dosage Forms: Capsule: 200 mg (blue); 400 mg (blue/red). Tablet: 100 mg (orange)

Use: Dilation of blood vessels

Minor Side Effects: Flushing; headache; stomach distress

Major Side Effects: Palpitations; weakness

Contraindications: This drug should not be used by people allergic to it or by those who are pregnant. Consult your doctor immediately if this drug has been prescribed for you and you have either condition.

Warnings: This drug may cause prolonged bleeding time; people with active bleeding or a bleeding tendency should be monitored carefully while taking this drug. • This drug should be used cautiously by people with glaucoma, severe hardening of the arteries, or heart disease. Be sure your doctor knows if you have any of these conditions.

Comments: Although this drug dilates blood vessels, a government panel of experts has determined that the drug is only "possibly" effective in the treatment of hardening of the arteries, leg cramps, and in the prevention of stroke. • While taking this drug, do not take any nonprescription item for cough, cold, or sinus problems without first checking with your doctor. • Take this drug with food or an antacid to avoid stomach distress. • Mild side effects are most noticeable during the first two weeks of therapy and become less bothersome after this period.

Cydel vasodilator (W. E. Hauck, Inc.), see Cyclospasmol vasodilator.

Cyprodine antihistamine (Spencer-Mead, Inc.), see Periactin antihistamine.

OTC   Dalkon kit contraceptive

Manufacturer: A. H. Robins Company

Ingredients: benzethonium chloride; nonoxynol 9

Dosage Form: Vaginal foam: benzethonium chloride; nonoxynol 9, 8%

Use: Intravaginal contraception

Side Effects: Local irritation to user or partner

Contraindications: This product should not be used if either partner has an allergy to either component.

Comments: Be sure to insert a new dose of contraceptive foam for each intercourse. • Do not douche for at least six hours after intercourse. • Used alone, this product is not as effective as when it is combined with a diaphragm.

R   Dalmane hypnotic

Manufacturer: Roche Products Inc.

Ingredient: flurazepam hydrochloride

Dosage Form: Capsule: 15 mg (orange/ivory); 30 mg (red/ivory)

Use: Sleeping aid

Minor Side Effects: Confusion; constipation; depression; difficult urination; dizziness; drowsiness; dry mouth; fatigue; headache; nausea; rash; slurred speech; uncoordinated movements

Major Side Effects: Blurred vision; decreased sexual drive; double vision; jaundice; low blood pressure; stimulation; tremors

Contraindications: This drug should not be taken by people who are allergic to it. Consult your doctor immediately if this drug has been prescribed for you and you have such an allergy.

Warnings: This drug should not be taken with alcohol and other sedative drugs or central nervous system depressants. If you are currently taking any drugs of these types, consult your doctor about their use. If you are unsure of the type or contents of your medications, ask your doctor or pharmacist. • Patients involved in occupations or activities requiring complete mental alertness, such as driving a vehicle or operating machinery, should use this drug with extreme caution. • This drug should almost always be avoided during pregnancy, particularly during the first trimester. • This drug is not currently recommended for use by persons under the age of 15. • This drug should be used with caution by the elderly and debilitated patients. • This drug should be cautiously used in severely depressed persons and in those in whom there is seen evidence of latent depression, particularly if suicidal tendencies are evident. If so, protective measures may be necessary. • Periodic blood counts and liver function tests should be performed if this drug is used repeatedly. This drug should be used cautiously by people with impaired liver or kidney function. • This drug has the potential for abuse and must be used with caution. Tolerance may develop quickly; do not increase the dose of the drug without first consulting your doctor. • This is a safe drug when used alone. When it is combined with other sedative drugs or alcohol, serious adverse reactions may develop. • This drug should not be stopped suddenly.

Comments: This drug currently is the most widely used drug for inducing sleep. It is effective, but eliminating the cause of the insomnia is also important. Phenobarbital is also an effective sleep-inducer, and it is cheaper. Consult your doctor. • This drug should be taken 30 to 60 minutes before retiring, and other sedatives and alcohol should be avoided to prevent oversedation.

℞ Darvocet-N analgesic

Manufacturer: Eli Lilly and Company

Ingredients: propoxyphene napsylate; acetaminophen

Dosage Form: Tablet: Darvocet-N 50: propoxyphene napsylate, 50 mg; acetaminophen, 325 mg (orange). Darvocet-N 100: propoxyphene napsylate, 100 mg; acetaminophen, 650 mg (orange)

Use: Relief of mild to moderate pain

Minor Side Effects: Abdominal pain; blurred vision; constipation; dizziness; drowsiness; headache; light-headedness; nausea; rash; sedation; vomiting; weakness

Major Side Effect: Liver dysfunction

Contraindications: This drug should not be used by persons allergic to either of its ingredients. Consult your doctor immediately if this drug has been prescribed for you and you have such an allergy.

Warnings: This drug should not be prescribed for patients who are suicidal or who are addiction-prone. • This drug should be used with extreme caution by patients taking tranquilizers or antidepressant drugs, as well as by patients who use alcohol in excess. If you are currently taking any drugs of these types, consult your doctor about their use. If you are unsure of the type or contents of your medications, ask your doctor or pharmacist. • The recommended dosage of this drug should not be exceeded. • Alcohol intake should be limited while taking this drug. • This drug, when taken in higher-than-recommended doses over long periods, can produce drug dependency, both physical and psychological, and tolerance. • This drug can cause drowsiness; avoid tasks that require alertness. • This drug should be used with extreme caution in patients with peptic ulcer or blood coagulation problems. Be sure your doctor knows if you have such conditions. • This drug should be used cautiously during pregnancy and by nursing mothers. • This drug is not recommended for use in children.

Comments: Aspirin or acetaminophen should be tried before therapy with this drug is undertaken. If aspirin or acetaminophen does not relieve pain, this drug may be effective. • You may want to ask your doctor to prescribe an inexpensive brand of propoxyphene hydrochloride instead of the napsylate form, since it will be less expensive and the napsylate form is converted to hydrochloride once it is in the stomach. • This drug has the potential for abuse and must be used with caution. Tolerance may develop quickly; do not increase the dose of the drug without consulting your doctor.

℞ Darvon analgesic

Manufacturer: Eli Lilly and Company
Ingredient: propoxyphene hydrochloride
Equivalent Products: Dolene, Lederle Laboratories; Doraphen, H. R. Cenci Laboratories, Inc.; Margesic Improved, North American Pharmacal, Inc.; Paragesic-65, Parmed Pharmaceuticals, Inc.; Progesic-65, Ulmer Pharmacal Company; propoxyphene hydrochloride, various manufacturers; Proxagesic, Tutag Pharmaceuticals, Inc.; Proxene, Bowman Pharmaceuticals; SK-65, Smith Kline & French Laboratories
Dosage Form: Capsule: 32 mg; 65 mg (both pink)
Use: Relief of mild pain
Minor Side Effects: Abdominal pain; blurred vision; constipation; dizziness; drowsiness; headache; light-headedness; nausea; rash; sedation; vomiting; weakness
Major Side Effects: Liver dysfunction
Contraindications: This drug should not be used by people allergic to it or by those who are pregnant. Consult your doctor immediately if this drug has been prescribed for you and you have either condition.
Warnings: This drug should be used cautiously by children and people with ulcers. • This drug may cause drowsiness; avoid tasks that require alertness. To prevent oversedation, avoid the use of alcohol or other central nervous system depressants or drugs that have sedative qualities. • This drug should not be used in conjunction with orphenadrine; if you are currently taking orphenadrine, consult your doctor. If you are unsure about the content of your medications, ask your doctor or pharmacist. • This drug has the potential for abuse and must be used with caution. Tolerance may develop quickly; do not increase the dose of this drug without first consulting your doctor.
Comments: An aspirin or acetaminophen product should be tried before this drug. If aspirin or acetaminophen does not relieve pain, this drug may be effective.

℞ Darvon Compound-65 analgesic

Manufacturer: Eli Lilly and Company
Ingredients: aspirin; caffeine; phenacetin; propoxyphene hydrochloride
Equivalent Products: Bexophene, Mallard Incorporated; Dolene Compound 65, Lederle Laboratories; Elder 65 Compound, Paul B. Elder Company; ICN 65 Compound, ICN Pharmaceuticals, Inc.; Margesic Compound No. 65, North American Pharmacal, Inc.; Pargesic Compound 65, Parmed Pharmaceuticals Inc.; Poxy Compound-65, Sutliff & Case Co., Inc.; Progesic Compound-65, Ulmer Pharmacal Company; Proxagesic Compound-65, Tutag Pharmaceuticals, Inc.; Repro Compound 65, Reid-Provident Laboratories, Inc.; Scrip-Dyne Compound, Scrip-Physician Supply Co.; SK-65 Compound, Smith Kline & French Laboratories
Dosage Form: Capsule: aspirin, 227 mg; caffeine, 32.4 mg; phenacetin, 162

mg; propoxyphene hydrochloride, 65 mg (crimson/light gray)

Use: Relief of mild pain

Minor Side Effects: Abdominal pain; blurred vision; constipation; dizziness; drowsiness; headache; light-headedness; nausea; rash; ringing in the ears; sedation; vomiting; weakness

Major Side Effects: Kidney disease; liver dysfunction

Contraindications: This drug should not be used by people allergic to any of its ingredients or by those who are pregnant. • This drug may cause allergic reactions and should not, therefore, be taken by people who have asthma, severe hay fever, or other significant allergies. Be sure your doctor knows if you have such a condition.

Warnings: This drug may cause drowsiness; avoid tasks that require alertness. To prevent oversedation, avoid the use of alcohol or other central nervous system depressants or drugs that have sedative qualities. • This drug should not be used in conjunction with alcohol, ammonium chloride, methotrexate, oral anticoagulants, oral antidiabetics, orphenadrine, probenecid, steroids, sulfinpyrazone, or vitamin C; if you are currently taking any drugs of these types, consult your doctor about their use. If you are unsure of the type or contents of your medications, ask your doctor or pharmacist. • This drug has the potential for abuse and must be used with caution. Tolerance may develop quickly; do not increase the dose of this drug without first consulting your doctor. • If your ears feel unusual, or you hear buzzing or ringing, or if your stomach hurts, your dosage may need adjustment. Call your doctor.

Comments: An aspirin or acetaminophen product should be tried before this drug. If aspirin or acetaminophen does not relieve pain, this drug may be effective.

Deapril-ST vasodilator (Mead Johnson Pharmaceutical Division), see Hydergine vasodilator.

OTC   Debrox eardrops

Manufacturer: Marion Laboratories, Inc.

Ingredients: anhydrous glycerol; carbamide peroxide

Dosage Form: Drop: anhydrous glycerol; carbamide peroxide, 6.5%

Use: Earwax removal

Side Effects: allergic reactions (rash, itching, soreness); local irritation

Contraindications: Do not use product if your eardrum is punctured.

Warnings: Stop using eardrops if a rash or redness occurs.

Comments: Do not rinse dropper or touch it to the ear. To do so may contaminate the dropper and consequently the solution. • To warm eardrops to body temperature, hold bottle in your hands or rotate it between your palms before use. • If you do not feel better in two days, call your doctor.

OTC   Deep-Down external analgesic

Manufacturer: The J. B. Williams Company, Inc.

Ingredients: alcohol; camphor; menthol; methyl nicotinate; methyl salicylate

Dosage Form: Ointment: alcohol, 5%; camphor, 0.5%; menthol, 5%; methyl nicotinate, 0.7%; methyl salicylate, 15%

Use: Temporary relief of pain in muscles and other areas

Side Effects: Allergic reactions (rash, itching, soreness); local irritation

Warnings: Use this product externally only. • Do not use on broken or irritated skin or on large areas of the body; avoid contact with eyes. • When using this product avoid exposure to direct sunlight, heat lamp, or sunlamp. •

Before using this product on children under 12 years of age, consult your doctor. • If the condition persists, call your doctor.

Comments: This greaseless ointment smells good and may be attractive to a child. It should be stored safely out of the reach of children. • Be sure to rub this product well into the skin.

Delapav smooth muscle relaxant (Dunhall Pharmaceuticals, Inc.), see Pavabid Plateau Caps smooth muscle relaxant.

Delaxin muscle relaxant (Ferndale Laboratories, Inc.), see Robaxin muscle relaxant.

Delco-Retic diuretic and antihypertensive (Delco Chemical Co., Inc.), see hydrochlorothiazide diuretic and antihypertensive.

OTC   Delfen contraceptive

Manufacturer: Ortho Pharmaceutical Corporation
Ingredient: nonoxynol 9
Dosage Forms: Vaginal cream: nonoxynol 9, 5%. Vaginal foam: nonoxynol 9, 12.5%
Use: Intravaginal contraception
Side Effects: Local irritation to user or partner
Contraindications: This product should not be used if either partner has an allergy to nonoxynol 9.
Comments: Be sure to insert a new dose of this contraceptive for each intercourse. • Do not douche for at least six hours after intercourse. • Used alone, this product is not as effective as when it is combined with a diaphragm.

Delta-E antibiotic (Trimen Laboratories, Inc.), see erythromycin antibiotic.

Deltamycin antibiotic (Trimen Laboratories, Inc.), see tetracycline hydrochloride antibiotic.

Deltapen-VK antibiotic (Trimen Laboratories, Inc.), see penicillin potassium phenoxymethyl antibiotic.

Deltasone steroid hormone (The Upjohn Company), see prednisone steroid hormone.

R   Demerol analgesic

Manufacturer: Winthrop Laboratories
Ingredient: meperidine hydrochloride
Equivalent Products: meperidine hydrochloride, various manufacturers; Pethadol, Halsey Drug Co., Inc.
Dosage Forms: Liquid (content per 5 ml): 50 mg. Tablet: 50 mg, 100 mg (both white)
Use: Relief of severe pain
Minor Side Effects: Constipation; drowsiness; dry mouth; euphoria; flushing; light-headedness; nausea; palpitations; rash; sweating; uncoordinated movements; urine retention; vomiting
Major Side Effects: Breathing difficulties; faintness; rapid heartbeat; tremors

Contraindications: This drug should not be taken by persons who are allergic to it or by those who are using or have recently used monoamine oxidase inhibitors. Consult your doctor or pharmacist if you are unsure.

Warnings: This drug should be used with extreme caution by the elderly and pregnant or nursing women. • This drug should be used cautiously by people who have asthma and other respiratory problems; epilepsy; head injuries; diseases of the liver, kidney, prostate, or thyroid; or an acute abdominal condition. Be sure your doctor knows if you have any of these conditions. • This drug should be used with caution by people who are taking central nervous system depressants. Be sure your doctor is aware of every medication you use. • This drug has the potential for abuse and must be used with caution. Tolerance may develop quickly; do not increase the dose of the drug without first consulting your doctor. • This drug may cause drowsiness; avoid tasks that require alertness. To prevent oversedation, avoid the use of alcohol or other drugs that have sedative properties. • This drug may cause a drop in blood pressure and should be used cautiously by people with heart disease. • This drug should not be used in conjunction with alcohol, monoamine oxidase inhibitors, phenothiazines, and antidepressants; if you are currently taking any drugs of these types, consult your doctor about their use. If you are unsure of the type or contents of your medications, ask your doctor or pharmacist. • Because it contains a narcotic, this drug should not be used for more than seven to ten days.

Comments: To avoid dizziness or light-headedness when you stand, contract and relax the muscles of your legs for a few moments before rising. Do this by pushing one foot against the floor while raising the other foot slightly, alternating feet so that you are "pumping" your legs in a pedaling motion. • The liquid form of this drug should be taken in one-half glass of water to avoid numbing the inside of the mouth. This drug is also available in two other forms: Demerol APAP analgesic from Breon Laboratories, Inc. (meperidine hydrochloride, aspirin, phenacetin, caffeine, and acetaminophen) and A.P.C. with Demerol from Winthrop Laboratories (meperidine hydrochloride, aspirin, phenacetin, and caffeine).

Demerol APAP analgesic (Breon Laboratories, Inc.), see Demerol analgesic.

Demi-Regroton diuretic and antihypertensive (USV [P.R.] Development Corp.), see Regroton diuretic and antihypertensive.

OTC   Dermolate anal-itch ointment

Manufacturer: Schering Corporation
Ingredients: hydrocortisone
Dosage Form: Ointment: hydrocortisone, 0.5%
Use: Temporary relief of burning, minor pain, skin inflammation, and itching around the rectum associated with hemorrhoids
Side Effects: Burning sensation; dryness; irritation; itching; rash; secondary infections
Contraindications: Do not use this product in the presence of diseases that severely impair blood circulation or in the presence of a bacterial or viral infection.
Warnings: Use this product externally only. • Avoid contact with eyes. • Do not use for prolonged periods of time or if hemorrhoids are bleeding. If the condition persists, contact your doctor. • Consult a physician for use on children under two years of age.
Comments: If the affected area is extremely dry or is scaling, the skin may be moistened before applying the medication by soaking in water or by apply-

ing water with a clean cloth. • Hydrocortisone-containing products, until recently, required a prescription for their purchase. They are now sold OTC in strengths of up to 0.5%. • This product comes packaged in an over-size box which is deceiving. There is no applicator for the ointment.

OTC — Dermolate topical steroid

Manufacturer: Schering Corporation
Ingredients: Cream: hydrocortisone. Spray: alcohol; hydrocortisone
Dosage Forms: Cream: hydrocortisone, 0.5%. Spray: alcohol, 24%; hydrocortisone, 0.5%
Use: Temporary relief of skin inflammation, irritation, itching, and rashes associated with conditions such as dermatitis, eczema, or poison ivy
Side Effects: Burning sensation; dryness; irritation; itching; rash; secondary infections
Contraindications: Do not use this product in the presence of diseases that severely impair blood circulation or in the presence of a bacterial or viral infection.
Warnings: Use this product externally only. • Avoid contact with eyes. • Do not use for prolonged periods of time. If the condition persists, contact your doctor. • Consult a physician for use on children under two years of age.
Comments: If the affected area is extremely dry or is scaling, the skin may be moistened before applying the medication by soaking in water or by applying water with a clean cloth. • Hydrocortisone-containing products, until recently, required a prescription for their purchase. They are now sold OTC in strengths of up to 0.5%.

Desamycin antibiotic (Pharmics, Inc.), see tetracycline hydrochloride antibiotic.

OTC — Desenex athlete's foot remedy

Manufacturer: Pharmacraft Division
Ingredients: undecylenic acid; zinc undecylenate; isopropyl alcohol (Ingredients vary with dosage form; see below.)
Dosage Forms: Ointment: undecylenic acid, 5%; zinc undecylenate, 20%. Powder (regular and aerosol): undecylenic acid, 2%; zinc undecylenate, 20%. Soap: undecylenic acid, 2%. Solution: undecylenic acid, 10%; isopropyl alcohol, 47%.
Use: Treatment of athlete's foot and ringworm of the body exclusive of the nails and scalp
Side Effects: Allergy; local irritation
Warnings: Diabetics and persons with impaired circulation should not use this product without first consulting a physician. • Do not apply this product to mucous membranes, scraped skin, or to large areas of skin. • If your condition worsens, or if irritation occurs, stop using this product and consult your pharmacist. When using the aerosol form of this product, be careful not to inhale any of the powder.
Comments: Some lesions take months to heal, so it is important not to stop treatment too soon. • If foot lesions are consistently a problem, check the fit of your shoes. • Wash your hands thoroughly after applying this product. • The ointment and solution forms of this product are preferable to the powders and soap for effectiveness; the best action of the powders may be in drying the infected area. Use the soap frequently for best results, unless directed otherwise by your doctor. • The aerosol powder may be more expensive than the other forms of this product; check prices before paying for convenience you do not need.

OTC   Desitin Ointment rash remedy

Manufacturer: Leeming Division
Ingredients: cod liver oil; lanolin; petrolatum; talc; zinc oxide
Dosage Form: Ointment (quantities of ingredients not specified)
Use: Treatment of diaper rash; minor skin irritations; superficial wounds and burns
Side Effects: Local irritation

OTC   Desitin rash remedy

Manufacturer: Leeming Division
Ingredients: talc; fragrance
Dosage Form: Powder (quantities of ingredients not specified)
Use: For keeping baby skin dry; soothing diaper rash, prickly heat, and chafing
Side Effects: Allergy; local irritation
Comments: While using this product, be careful not to inhale any of the powder.

OTC   DeWitt's Pills analgesic

Manufacturer: DeWitt International Corporation
Ingredients: buchu; caffeine; methylene blue; potassium nitrate; salicylamide; uva ursi
Dosage Form: Tablet (quantities of ingredients not specified)
Use: Temporary relief of pain of backache and joints
Side Effects: Nausea; slight stimulation; temporary warm feeling
Comments: The caffeine component of this product may cause a slight stimulation; there is no scientific evidence that it has any pain-relieving effect. • This product may color the urine blue. This is not dangerous. • Salicylamide (the only active ingredient in this product) has a shorter duration of action and is less effective than aspirin for the relief of pain. • This product may be safe individuals who are allergic to aspirin.

Dexedrine anorectic (Smith Kline & French Laboratories), see **Biphetamine anorectic.**

Rx   Diabinese oral antidiabetic

Manufacturer: Pfizer Laboratories Division
Ingredient: chlorpropamide
Dosage Form: Tablet: 100 mg; 250 mg (both blue)
Use: Treatment of diabetes mellitus
Minor Side Effects: Diarrhea; dizziness; fatigue; headache; loss of appetite; nausea; rash; vomiting; weakness
Major Side Effects: Jaundice; low blood sugar level; sore throat
Contraindications: This drug should not be used by people with juvenile or growth-onset diabetes (see Comments); severe or unstable "brittle" diabetes; diabetes complicated by ketosis and acidosis, major surgery, severe infection, or severe trauma; or severe liver, thyroid, or kidney disease. Be sure your doctor knows if you have any of these conditions. • This drug should not be used by pregnant women or women of childbearing age.
Warnings: This drug should be used cautiously in conjunction with alcohol, antibacterial sulfonamides, barbiturates, dicumarol, guanethidine, monoamine oxidase inhibitors, phenylbutazone, probenecid, or salicylates. If you are currently taking any drugs of these types, consult your doctor about

their use. If you are unsure of the type or contents of your medications, ask your doctor or pharmacist. • Use of this drug in combination with certain other drugs may bring about hypoglycemia. When starting this drug, the patient's urine should be tested for sugar and acetone at least three times daily and the results reviewed by the physician at least once a week. Frequent laboratory tests of liver function should also be seriously considered. (See Comments regarding visits with the doctor.) • This drug should not be used as a substitute for diet regulation, weight control, exercise control, proper hygiene, or prompt care of infection. • Alcohol and decreased food, coupled with this drug, may lead to hypoglycemia, ketosis, coma, and death. Certain diuretics, on the other hand, when taken with this drug, have been shown to suppress insulin secretion, and, therefore, will contribute to hyperglycemia. • The severity of the diabetes, the nature of any complications, and the availability of lab facilities determine if therapy with this drug can be continued or should be discontinued while insulin is being used. • It takes from three to five days for complete elimination of this drug from the body. Thus, accidental ingestion of the drug by children necessitates that the children be kept under close observation for this period, even if recovery seems to have occurred. • Persons taking this drug should still be instructed in the use of insulin. Hyperglycemic reactions may occur during the initial period of therapy with this drug, particularly during any transition from insulin to this oral drug. Hypoglycemia, if it occurs, may be long-lasting.

Comments: Oral antidiabetic drugs, such as this drug, are not effective in the treatment of diabetes in children under age 12. • Studies have shown that a balanced diet and exercise program may be just as effective as this drug. However, drugs of this type allow diabetics more leeway in their lifestyle. Nonetheless, persons taking this drug should carefully watch their diet and exercise program. • During the first six weeks of therapy with this drug, visit your doctor at least once a week. • While taking this drug, check your urine for sugar and ketone at least three times a day. • A patient taking this drug will have to be switched to insulin therapy if complications (e.g., ketoacidosis, severe trauma, severe infection, diarrhea, nausea, or vomiting) or the need for major surgery develop. • This drug should be taken at the same time each day. • Ask your doctor how to recognize the first signs of low blood sugar. • Do not take alcohol while taking this drug. Avoid any other drugs, including nonprescription cold remedies and aspirin, unless your doctor tells you to take them. • You may sunburn easily while taking this product. Avoid exposure to the sun as much as possible. • You may retain fluid while taking this drug. Be careful to watch for swollen feet or hands or a rapid weight gain, each of which could be indicative of fluid retention.

Diacin vitamin supplement (Lemmon Company), see nicotinic acid vitamin supplement.

Dialex antianginal (Trimen Laboratories, Inc.), see Nitro-Bid Plateau Caps antianginal.

OTC   Dialose laxative

Manufacturer: Stuart Pharmaceuticals
Ingredients: carboxymethylcellulose sodium; docusate sodium (dioctyl sodium sulfosuccinate)
Dosage Form: Capsule: carboxymethylcellulose sodium, 400 mg; docusate sodium, 100 mg
Use: Relief of constipation
Side Effects: Excess loss of fluid; griping (cramps); mucus in feces

Contraindications: Persons with high fever (100 °F or more); black or tarry stools; nausea; vomiting; abdominal pain; or children under age three should not use this product unless directed by a doctor. • Do not use this product when constipation is caused by megacolon or other diseases of the intestine, or hypothyroidism. • Persons with intestinal ulcers should not use this product.

Warnings: Excessive use (daily for a month or more) of this product may cause diarrhea, vomiting, and loss of certain blood electrolytes. • Pregnant women should not use this product except on the advice of a doctor.

Comments: Evacuation may not occur for 12 to 72 hours. If you are taking other drugs, do not take this product until you have checked with your doctor or pharmacist. • An ingredient in this product is referred to as a stool softener. This product is recommended for prevention of constipation when the stool is hard and dry. Do not take another product containing mineral oil at the same time as you are taking this product. • Never self-medicate with this product if constipation lasts longer than two weeks or if the medication does not produce a laxative effect within a week. • Limit use to seven days unless directed otherwise by your doctor; this product may cause laxative-dependence (addiction) if used for a longer time.

OTC — Dialose Plus laxative

Manufacturer: Stuart Pharmaceuticals
Ingredients: carboxymethylcellulose sodium; casanthranol; docusate sodium (dioctyl sodium sulfosuccinate)
Dosage Form: Capsule: carboxymethylcellulose sodium, 400 mg; casanthranol, 30 mg; docusate sodium, 100 mg
Use: Relief of constipation and stool softener
Side Effects: Excess loss of fluid; griping (cramps); mucus in feces
Contraindications: Persons with high fever (100° F or more); black or tarry stools; nausea; vomiting; abdominal pain; or children under age three should not use this product unless directed by a doctor. • Do not use this product when constipation is caused by megacolon or other diseases of the intestine, or hypothyroidism. • Persons with intestinal ulcers should not use this product.

Warnings: Excessive use (daily for a month or more) of this product may cause diarrhea, vomiting, and loss of certain blood electrolytes. • Pregnant women should not use this product except on the advice of a doctor.

Comments: This product may discolor the urine. • Evacuation may occur within 6 to 12 hours, or it may not occur for up to 72 hours. • Never self-medicate if constipation lasts longer than two weeks or if the medication does not produce a laxative effect within a week. • Limit use to seven days unless directed otherwise by a doctor since this product may cause laxative-dependence (addiction) if used for a longer time. • If you are taking other drugs, do not take this product until you have checked with your doctor or pharmacist. • An ingredient in this product is referred to as a stool softener. This product is recommended for prevention of constipation when the stool is hard and dry. Do not take another product containing mineral oil at the same time as you are taking this product.

Rx — Diamox diuretic

Manufacturer: Lederle Laboratories
Ingredient: acetazolamide
Equivalent Products: acetazolamide, various manufacturers; Rozolamide, Robinson Laboratory, Inc.
Dosage Forms: Sustained-release capsule: 500 mg (orange). Tablet: 125

mg; 250 mg (both white); 500 mg (orange)

Use: Treatment of certain types of glaucoma; fluid retention; epilepsy

Minor Side Effects: Constipation; diarrhea; drowsiness; loss of appetite; nausea; tingling in the fingers and toes; vomiting

Major Side Effects: Blood in the urine; convulsions; darkened skin; jaundice; visual disturbances

Contraindications: This drug should not be taken by people who have severe diseases of the kidney, liver, or adrenal glands; glaucoma (certain types); or low blood levels of sodium or potassium. Consult your doctor immediately if this drug has been prescribed for you and you have any of these conditions.

Warnings: This drug should be used cautiously by pregnant women. • This drug may cause certain lung diseases (e.g., emphysema) to worsen and should not be used in conjunction with amphetamine, methenamine, or quinidine sulfate; if you are currently taking any of these drugs, consult your doctor about their use. If you are unsure about the content of your medications, ask your doctor or pharmacist. • Do not increase the dose of this drug without consulting your doctor. • This drug may cause drowsiness; avoid tasks that require alertness. To prevent oversedation, avoid the use of alcohol or other drugs that have sedative properties. • People allergic to sulfa drugs may likewise be allergic to this drug. • People taking this product and digitalis should watch carefully for symptoms of increased toxicity (e.g., nausea, blurred vision, palpitations). • Contact your doctor if you develop a fever, rash, or sore throat while taking this drug.

Comments: This drug can cause potassium loss. To help avoid potassium loss, take this drug with a glass of fresh or frozen orange juice, or eat a banana each day. The use of Co-Salt salt substitute also helps prevent potassium loss.

OTC   Diaparene Baby Powder rash remedy

Manufacturer: Glenbrook Laboratories

Ingredients: cornstarch; fragrance; magnesium carbonate; methylbenzethonium chloride, 1:1800

Dosage Form: Powder (quantities of ingredients not specified)

Use: Keeping baby skin dry; soothing diaper rash, prickly heat, and chafing

Side Effects: Local irritation

Comments: While using this product, be careful not to inhale any of the powder.

OTC   Diaparene Peri-Anal Cream rash remedy

Manufacturer: Glenbrook Laboratories

Ingredients: cod liver oil; methylbenzethonium chloride, 1:1000; water repellent base

Dosage Form: Cream (quantities of ingredients not specified)

Use: Relief of diaper rash

Side Effects: Allergy; local irritation

Diaqua diuretic and antihypertensive (W. E. Hauck, Inc.), see hydrochlorothiazide diuretic and antihypertensive.

Diazachel sedative and hypnotic (North American Pharmacal, Inc.), see Librium sedative and hypnotic.

Di-Azo analgesic (Kay Pharmacal Company, Inc.), see Pyridium analgesic.

388

Dibent antispasmodic (W. E. Hauck, Inc.), see Bentyl antispasmodic.

OTC   Di-Gel antacid and antiflatulent

Manufacturer: Plough, Inc.

Ingredients: aluminum hydroxide; aluminum hydroxide-magnesium carbonate codried gel; magnesium hydroxide; simethicone

Dosage Forms: Liquid (content per teaspoon): aluminum hydroxide, 282 mg; magnesium hydroxide, 87 mg; simethicone, 25 mg. Tablet: aluminum hydroxide-magnesium carbonate codried gel, 282 mg; magnesium hydroxide, 85 mg; simethicone, 25 mg

Use: Relief of acid indigestion, heartburn, sour stomach, and accompanying painful gas symptoms

Side Effects: Abdominal discomfort; constipation; diarrhea; dizziness; mouth irritation; nausea; rash; vomiting

Contraindications: Persons with kidney disease or those on a salt-free diet should not use this product. In persons with kidney disease repeated daily use may cause nausea, vomiting, depressed reflexes, and breathing difficulties.

Warnings: Long-term (several weeks) use of this product may lead to intestinal obstruction and dehydration. • Phosphate depletion may occur leading to weakness, loss of appetite, and eventually bone pain. You can prevent this by drinking at least one glass of milk a day.

Comments: Self-treatment of severe or repeated attacks of heartburn, indigestion, or upset stomach is not recommended. If you do self-treat, limit therapy to two weeks, then call your doctor if symptoms persist. • Never self-medicate with this product if your symptoms occur regularly (two to three times or more a month); if they are particularly worse than normal; if you feel a "tightness" in your chest, have chest pains, or are sweating; or if you are short of breath. Consult your doctor. • To prevent constipation, drink at least eight glasses of water a day. If constipation persists, consult your doctor or pharmacist. • This product works best when taken one hour after meals or at bedtime, unless otherwise directed by your doctor or pharmacist. • The liquid form of this product is superior to the tablet form and should be used unless you have been specifically directed to use the tablet. • Do not take this product within two hours of a dose of a tetracycline antibiotic. Also, if you are taking iron, a vitamin-mineral product, chlorpromazine, phenytoin, digoxin, quinidine, or warfarin, remind your doctor or pharmacist that you are taking this product. • Simethicone is included to relieve bloating and gas formation by enhancing belching or flatus formation. If you do not suffer from these symptoms, use a product without simethicone to save money.

R_X   **Dilantin anticonvulsant**

Manufacturer: Parke-Davis

Ingredient: phenytoin sodium (diphenylhydantoin)

Equivalent Products: Di-Phen, various manufacturers; Diphenylan Sodium, The Lannett Company, Inc.; Ditan, Mallard Incorporated; phenytoin sodium, various manufacturers

Dosage Forms: Capsule: 30 mg (white with pink stripe); 100 mg (white with orange stripe). Flavored tablet: 50 mg (yellow). Liquid (content per 5 ml): 30 mg; 125 mg

Use: Control of epilepsy and other convulsive disorders

Minor Side Effects: Change in urine color; constipation; drowsiness; headache; nausea; rash; vomiting

Major Side Effects: Confusion; dizziness; gum enlargement; nervousness; slurred speech; uncoordinated movements.

Contraindications: This drug should not be taken by people who are allergic to it. Consult your doctor immediately if this drug has been prescribed for you and you have such an allergy.

Warnings: This drug should be used cautiously by people who have heart disease, impaired liver function, or a slow rate of metabolism; and by pregnant women. Be sure your doctor knows if you have any of these conditions. • Diabetics who need to take this drug should check their urine sugar more frequently than usual. • This drug should not be used to treat seizures due to hypoglycemia. Careful diagnosis is essential before this drug is prescribed. • Because the metabolism of this drug may be significantly altered by the use of other drugs, great care must be taken when this drug is used concomitantly with other drugs. Be sure that your doctor is aware of every medication that you take. This drug interacts with barbiturates, chloramphenicol, corticosteroids, disulfiram, isoniazid, oral anticoagulants, propranolol, thyroid hormones, and tricyclic antidepressants; if you are currently taking any drugs of these types, consult your doctor about their use. If you are unsure of the type or contents of your medications, ask your doctor or pharmacist. • The results of certain lab tests may be altered if the patient has been taking this drug. If you need any tests, remind your doctor that you are taking this drug. • Depending on the type of disorder being treated, this drug may be used in combination with other anticonvulsants. • This drug may cause low blood pressure, lymph node enlargement, and rash. Consult your doctor if you feel faint or light-headed, notice that your glands are swollen, or develop a rash. • This drug may cause a bone disease. • Do not use this drug to treat headaches unless your doctor specifically recommends it. • Therapy with this drug may cause the gums to enlarge enough to cover the teeth. Gum enlargement can be minimized, at least partially, by good dental care—frequent brushing and massaging the gums with the rubber tip of a good toothbrush. • This drug may cause drowsiness; avoid tasks that require alertness. To prevent oversedation, avoid the use of alcohol or other drugs that have sedative properties. • Do not stop taking this drug suddenly; you may start to convulse. • If you take phenobarbital in addition to this drug, you may be able to take them together in a single product, Dilantin with Phenobarbital anticonvulsant. Consult your doctor.

Dilantin with Phenobarbital anticonvulsant (Parke-Davis), see Dilantin anticonvulsant.

Dilart smooth muscle relaxant (Trimen Laboratories, Inc.), see Pavabid Plateau Caps smooth muscle relaxant.

OTC   **Dimacol cough remedy**

Manufacturer: A. H. Robins Company

Ingredients: guaifenesin; pseudoephedrine hydrochloride; dextromethorphan hydrobromide; alcohol (liquid form only)

Dosage Forms: Capsule: guaifenesin, 100 mg; pseudoephedrine hydrochloride, 30 mg; dextromethorphan hydrobromide, 15 mg. Liquid (content per 5 ml, or one teaspoon): guaifenesin, 100 mg; pseudoephedrine hydrochloride, 30 mg; dextromethorphan hydrobromide, 15 mg; alcohol, 4.75%

Use: Temporary relief of cough and nasal congestion due to colds or "flu"; also to convert a dry, nonproductive cough to a productive, phlegm-producing cough

Side Effects: Drowsiness; mild stimulation; nausea; vomiting

Warnings: This product should be used with special caution by children under two years of age, and by persons who have diabetes, heart disease, high blood pressure, or thyroid disease. If you have any of these conditions, consult your doctor before taking this product. • This product interacts with guanethidine and monoamine oxidase inhibitors. If you are currently taking any drugs of these types, check with your doctor before taking this product. If you are unsure of the type or contents of your medications, ask your doctor or pharmacist.

Comments: Do not use this product to treat chronic coughs, such as from smoking or asthma. • Do not use this product to treat productive (hacking) coughs that produce phlegm. • If you require an expectorant, you need more moisture in your environment. Drink eight to ten glasses of water daily. The use of a vaporizer or humidifier may also be beneficial. Consult your doctor.

OTC   Dimetane allergy remedy

Manufacturer: A.H. Robins Company

Ingredients: brompheniramine maleate

Dosage Forms: Liquid (content per 5 ml, or one teaspoon): brompheniramine maleate, 2 mg. Tablet: brompheniramine maleate, 4 mg (peach), 8 mg (Persian rose), or 12 mg (peach)

Use: Temporary relief of symptoms of hay fever and upper respiratory allergy; treatment of mild inflammatory skin conditions requiring antihistamines

Side Effects: Blurred vision; confusion; constipation; diarrhea; difficult urination; dizziness; drowsiness; dry mouth; headache; insomnia; nasal congestion; nausea; nervousness; palpitations; rash; rash from exposure to sunlight; reduced sweating; restlessness; severe abdominal cramping; sore throat; vomiting

Contraindications: This product should not be used by people who are allergic to it or by those who have asthma. • This product should not be taken by newborn infants or nursing mothers.

Warnings: The elderly should use this product with special caution; they are more likely to suffer side effects to the medication than are other people. • Children taking this product may become restless and excited; administer the drug cautiously. • While taking this product, do not take any other nonprescription item for cough, cold, or sinus problems without first consulting your doctor. • This product may cause drowsiness. Do not take it if you must drive, operate heavy machinery, or perform other tasks requiring mental alertness. To prevent oversedation, avoid the use of alcohol or other drugs that have sedative properties. • Because this product reduces sweating, avoid excessive work or exercise in hot weather.

Comments: Chew gum or suck on ice chips or a piece of hard candy to reduce mouth dryness. • The effectiveness of this product may diminish after being taken regularly for seven to ten days. Consult your doctor or pharmacist about substituting another product containing a different antihistamine if this occurs.

Rx   Dimetane DC expectorant

Manufacturer: A. H. Robins Company

Ingredients: brompheniramine maleate; codeine phosphate; guaifenesin; phenylephrine hydrochloride; phenylpropanolamine hydrochloride

Equivalent Products: Midatane DC, Vangard Laboratories; Normatane DC, North American Pharmacal, Inc.; Puretane DC, Purepac Pharmaceutical Co.; Spentane DC, Spencer-Mead, Inc.

Dosage Form: Liquid (content per 5 ml): brompheniramine maleate, 2 mg; codeine phosphate, 10 mg; guaifenesin, 100 mg; phenylephrine hydrochloride, 5 mg; phenylpropanolamine hydrochloride, 5 mg

Use: Relief of coughing and other symptoms of allergy and the common cold

Minor Side Effects: Blurred vision; confusion; constipation; diarrhea; difficult urination; dizziness; drowsiness; dry mouth; headache; heartburn; insomnia; loss of appetite; nasal congestion; nausea; palpitations; rash; reduced sweating; restlessness; vomiting; weakness

Major Side Effects: Chest pain; high blood pressure; low blood pressure; severe abdominal pain; sore throat

Contraindications: This drug should not be used to treat asthma or other symptoms of the lower respiratory tract. • This drug should not be given to infants, or taken by nursing mothers. • This drug should not be taken by people who are allergic to any of its components or by people who are using monoamine oxidase inhibitors (ask your pharmacist if you are unsure). Consult your doctor immediately if this drug has been prescribed for you and you have any of these conditions.

Warnings: This drug should be used cautiously by people who have asthma, glaucoma, ulcer, enlarged prostate, obstructed bladder, obstructed intestine, high blood pressure, heart or vessel disease, or thyroid disease; and by those who are pregnant. Be sure your doctor knows if you have any of these conditions. • This drug must be used cautiously by the elderly, who are more likely than others to experience side effects, especially sedation, from the drug. • Use this drug cautiously with children; overdosage may cause excitation leading to convulsions and death. • This drug should not be used in conjunction with antidepressants, guanethidine, monoamine oxidase inhibitors, or phenothiazines; if you are currently taking any drugs of these types, consult your doctor about their use. If you are unsure of the type or contents of your medications, ask your doctor or pharmacist. • While taking this drug, do not take any nonprescription item for cough, cold, or sinus problems without first checking with your doctor. • This drug may cause drowsiness; avoid tasks that require alertness. To prevent oversedation, avoid the use of alcohol or other drugs that have sedative properties. • Because this product contains codeine, it has the potential for abuse and must be used with caution. It usually should not be taken for more than ten days. Tolerance may develop quickly, but do not increase the dosage without consulting your doctor. • Because this drug reduces sweating, avoid excessive work or exercise in hot weather.

Comments: If you need an expectorant, you need more moisture in your environment. Drink nine to ten glasses of water each day. The use of a vaporizer or humidifier may also be beneficial. Consult your doctor. • Chew gum or suck on ice chips or a piece of hard candy to reduce mouth dryness.

Rₓ   **Dimetane expectorant**

Manufacturer: A. H. Robins Company

Ingredients: brompheniramine maleate; guaifenesin; phenylephrine hydrochloride; phenylpropanolamine hydrochloride

Equivalent Products: Midatane, Vangard Laboratories; Normatane, North American Pharmacal, Inc.; Puretane, Purepac Pharmaceutical Co.; Spentane, Spencer-Mead, Inc.

Dosage Form: Liquid (content per 5 ml): brompheniramine maleate, 2 mg; guaifenesin, 100 mg; phenylephrine hydrochloride, 5 mg; phenylpropanolamine hydrochloride, 5 mg

Use: Relief of symptoms of allergy and the common cold

Minor Side Effects: Blurred vision; confusion; constipation; diarrhea; difficult urination; dizziness; drowsiness; dry mouth; headache; heartburn; insomnia; loss of appetite; nasal congestion; nausea; palpitations; rash; reduced sweating; restlessness; vomiting; weakness

Major Side Effects: Chest pain; high blood pressure; low blood pressure;

severe abdominal pain; sore throat

Contraindications: This drug should not be used to treat asthma or other symptoms of the lower respiratory tract. • This drug should not be given to infants, or taken by nursing mothers. • This drug should not be taken by people who are allergic to any of its components or by people who are using monoamine oxidase inhibitors (ask your pharmacist if you are unsure). Consult your doctor immediately if this drug has been prescribed for you and you have any of these conditions.

Warnings: This drug should be used cautiously by people who have asthma, glaucoma, ulcer, enlarged prostate, obstructed bladder, obstructed intestine, high blood pressure, heart or vessel disease, or thyroid disease; and by those who are pregnant. Be sure your doctor knows if you have any of these conditions. • This drug must be used cautiously by the elderly, who are more likely than others to experience side effects, especially sedation, from the drug. • Use this drug cautiously with children; overdosage may cause excitation leading to convulsions and death. • This drug should not be used in conjunction with guanethidine or monoamine oxidase inhibitors; if you are currently taking any drugs of these types, consult your doctor about their use. If you are unsure of the type or contents of your medications, ask your doctor or pharmacist. • While taking this drug, do not take any nonprescription item for cough, cold, or sinus problems without first checking with your doctor. • This drug may cause drowsiness; avoid tasks that require alertness. To prevent oversedation, avoid the use of alcohol or other drugs that have sedative properties. • Because this drug reduces sweating, avoid excessive work or exercise in hot weather.

Comments: If you need an expectorant, you need more moisture in your environment. Drink nine to ten glasses of water each day. The use of a vaporizer or humidifier may also be beneficial. Consult your doctor. • Chew gum or suck on ice chips or a piece of hard candy to reduce mouth dryness.

R̽   **Dimetapp antihistamine**

Manufacturer: A. H. Robins Company

Ingredients: brompheniramine maleate; phenylephrine hydrochloride; phenylpropanolamine hydrochloride

Equivalent Products: Brocon, Forest Laboratories, Inc.; Bromatapp, Henry Schein, Inc.; Bromepaph, Columbia Medical Co.; Bromophen, Rugby Laboratories; Eldatapp, Paul B. Elder Co.; Histatapp, Upsher-Smith Laboratories, Inc.; Midatap, Vangard Laboratories; Normatane, North American Pharmacal, Inc.

Dosage Forms: Liquid (content per 5 ml): brompheniramine maleate, 4 mg; phenylephrine hydrochloride, 5 mg; phenylpropanolamine hydrochloride, 5 mg. Sustained-release tablet: brompheniramine maleate, 12 mg; phenylephrine hydrochloride, 15 mg; phenylpropanolamine hydrochloride, 15 mg (blue)

Use: Relief of hay fever symptoms and respiratory congestion

Minor Side Effects: Blurred vision; confusion; constipation; diarrhea; difficult urination; dizziness; drowsiness; dry mouth; headache; heartburn; insomnia; loss of appetite; nasal congestion; nausea; palpitations; rash; reduced sweating; restlessness; vomiting; weakness

Major Side Effects: Chest pain; high blood pressure; low blood pressure; severe abdominal pain; sore throat

Contraindications: This drug should not be used to treat asthma or other symptoms of the lower respiratory tract. • This drug should not be taken by people allergic to it or to other antihistamines similar in chemical structure. • This drug should not be taken by pregnant women or by people who are using monoamine oxidase inhibitors (ask your pharmacist if you are unsure). • The tablet form of this drug should not be taken by children under 12 years of age.

Warnings: This drug should be used cautiously by people who have heart disease, vessel disease, or high blood pressure. Be sure your doctor knows if you have any of these conditions. • Use this drug cautiously with children; overdosage may cause excitation leading to convulsions and death. • This drug should not be used in conjunction with guanethidine or monoamine oxidase inhibitors; if you are currently taking any drugs of these types, consult your doctor about their use. If you are unsure of the type or contents of your medications, ask your doctor or pharmacist. • While taking this drug, do not take any nonprescription item for cough, cold, or sinus problems without first checking with your doctor. • This drug may cause drowsiness; avoid tasks that require alertness. To prevent oversedation, avoid the use of alcohol or other drugs that have sedative properties. • Because this drug reduces sweating, avoid excessive work or exercise in hot weather. • The tablet form of this drug has sustained action; never increase your dose or take it more frequently than your doctor prescribes. A serious overdose could result.

Comments: The tablet form of this drug must be swallowed whole. • Chew gum or suck on ice chips or a piece of hard candy to reduce mouth dryness.

OTC Diothane hemorrhoidal preparation

Manufacturer: Merrell-National Laboratories

Ingredients: diperodon; 8-quinolinol benzoate; propylene glycol; sorbitan sequioleate

Dosage Form: Ointment: diperodon, 1%; 8-quinolinol benzoate, 0.1%; propylene glycol; sorbitan sequioleate

Use: Relief of pain, burning, and itching of hemorrhoids

Warnings: Sensitization (continued itching and redness) may occur with long-term and repeated use.

Comments: Hemorrhoidal (pile) preparations relieve itching, reduce pain and inflammation, and check bleeding, but do not heal, dry up, or give lasting relief from hemorrhoids. • Certain ingredients in this product may cause an allergic reaction; do not use for longer than seven days at a time unless your doctor has advised you otherwise. • Never self-medicate for hemorrhoids if pain is continuous or throbbing, if bleeding or itching is excessive, or if you feel a large pressure within the rectum.

Dipav smooth muscle relaxant (Lemmon Company), see Pavabid Plateau Caps smooth muscle relaxant.

Di-Phen anticonvulsant (various manufacturers), see Dilantin anticonvulsant.

Diphenatol anticholinergic and antispasmodic (Rugby Laboratories), see Lomotil anticholinergic and antispasmodic.

Diphenylan Sodium anticonvulsant (The Lannett Company, Inc.), see Dilantin anticonvulsant.

Disophrol Chronotab allergy and congestion remedy (Schering Corporation), see Drixoral allergy and congestion remedy.

Di-Spaz antispasmodic (North American Pharmacal, Inc.), see Bentyl antispasmodic.

Ditan anticonvulsant (Mallard Incorporated), see Dilantin anticonvulsant.

Diucen-H diuretic and antihypertensive (Central Pharmacal Company), see hydrochlorothiazide diuretic and antihypertensive.

℞   Diupres diuretic and antihypertensive

Manufacturer: Merck Sharp & Dohme
Ingredients: chlorothiazide; reserpine
Equivalent Products: Chloroserpine, Rugby Laboratories; Ro-Cloro-Serp-500, Robinson Laboratory, Inc.; Thiaserp, Spencer-Mead, Inc.
Dosage Form: Tablet: chlorothiazide, 250 mg, 500 mg; reserpine, 0.125 mg (both pink)
Use: Treatment of high blood pressure
Minor Side Effects: Cramps; diarrhea; dizziness; headache; itch; loss of appetite; nasal congestion; nausea; palpitations; rash; restlessness; tingling in the fingers and toes; vomiting
Major Side Effects: Blurred vision; chest pain; depression; elevated blood sugar; elevated uric acid; glaucoma; muscle spasm; nightmares; sore throat; weakness
Contraindications: This drug should not be taken by people who are allergic to it or to sulfa drugs. The drug should not be taken by those who have ulcers, ulcerative colitis, anuria (inability to urinate), depression; and by people receiving electroshock therapy. Consult your doctor immediately if this drug has been prescribed for you and you have any of these conditions.
Warnings: This drug should be used cautiously by pregnant women and people who have asthma or allergies, kidney or liver disease, or diabetes. Be sure your doctor knows if you have any of these conditions. • Nursing women who must take this drug should stop nursing. • This drug interacts with amphetamine, colestipol hydrochloride, decongestants, digitalis, levodopa, lithium carbonate, monoamine oxidase inhibitors, oral antidiabetics, and steroids; if you are currently taking any drugs of these types, consult your doctor about their use. If you are unsure of the type or contents of your medications, ask your doctor or pharmacist. • This drug must be used cautiously with digitalis and quinidine; be sure your doctor knows if you are taking either of these drugs. Watch for symptoms of increased toxicity (e.g., nausea, blurred vision, palpitations) and notify your doctor if they occur. • Notify your doctor if this drug makes you feel unusually depressed. • While taking this drug, do not take any nonprescription item for cough, cold, or sinus problems without first checking with your doctor. • This drug may cause drowsiness; avoid tasks that require alertness. To prevent oversedation, avoid the use of alcohol or other drugs that have sedative properties. • To help avoid potassium loss while using this product, take your dose with a glass of fresh or frozen orange juice and eat a banana each day. The use of a salt substitute also helps prevent potassium loss. • This drug may influence the results of thyroid function tests; if you are scheduled to have such a test, remind your doctor that you are taking this drug. • This drug may cause gout, ulcers, ulcerative colitis, gallstones, asthma, or high blood levels of calcium. The drug may cause the onset of diabetes that has been latent. • One of the components of this product, reserpine, causes cancer in rats. It has not been shown to cause cancer in people.
Comments: This product combines two antihypertensive ingredients in a single tablet. A doctor probably should not prescribe this or other "fixed dose" combination products as the first choice in the treatment of high blood pressure. The patient should receive each of the ingredients individually. If response is adequate to the fixed doses contained in this product, it may then be substituted. The advantage of a combination product such as this one is based on increased convenience to the patient. • Take this product at

the same time each day. • Take your dose with food or milk. • The effects of therapy with this drug may not be apparent for at least two weeks. • Mild side effects (e.g., nasal congestion) are most noticeable during the first two weeks of drug therapy and become less bothersome after this period. • This drug causes frequent urination. Expect this effect; it should not alarm you. • To avoid dizziness or light-headedness when you stand, contract and relax the muscles of your legs for a few moments before rising. Do this by pushing one foot against the floor while raising the other foot slightly, alternating feet so that you are "pumping" your legs in a pedaling motion.

OTC   Diurex diuretic

Manufacturer: Alva-Amco Pharmacal Companies, Inc.
Ingredients: buchu extract; methylene blue; powdered extract of juniper; caffeine; potassium salicylate
Dosage Form: Tablet (quantities of ingredients not specified)
Use: To help relieve water retention
Contraindications: This product should not be used to relieve water retention due to disease conditions such as heart or kidney disease.
Comments: This product is not recommended for purchase or use; it has no diuretic activity that you couldn't get from drinking a cup of coffee. • This product may color your urine blue; this effect is harmless and temporary and should not alarm you.

Rx   Diuril diuretic and antihypertensive

Manufacturer: Merck Sharp & Dohme
Ingredient: chlorothiazide sodium
Equivalent Products: chlorothiazide, various manufacturers; Ro-Chlorozide, Robinson Laboratory, Inc.
Dosage Forms: Liquid (content per 5 ml): 250 mg. Tablet: 250 mg; 500 mg (both white)
Use: Treatment of high blood pressure; removal of fluid from tissues
Minor Side Effects: Cramps, diarrhea; dizziness; headache; loss of appetite; nausea; rash; restlessness; tingling in the fingers and toes; vomiting
Major Side Effects: Blurred vision; elevated blood sugar; elevated uric acid; muscle spasm; sore throat; weakness
Contraindications: This drug should not be used by people who are allergic to it or to sulfa drugs, or by people who are suffering a lack of urination. Consult your doctor immediately if this drug has been prescribed for you and you have any of these conditions.
Warnings: This drug should be used cautiously by people who have diabetes, kidney or liver disease, a history of allergy or asthma, or by those who are pregnant or nursing. Be sure your doctor knows if you have any of these conditions. • This drug may affect the potency of, or the patient's need for, other blood pressure drugs, antidiabetics, and some surgical muscle relaxants; dosage adjustment may be necessary. • This drug interacts with colestipol hydrochloride, digitalis, lithium, and steroids. If you are currently taking any drugs of these types, consult your doctor about their use. If you are unsure of the type or contents of your medications, ask your doctor or pharmacist. • This drug may affect thyroid and laboratory tests; be sure your doctor knows that you are taking this drug if you are having any tests done. • This drug may cause gout or high blood levels of calcium. The drug may cause the onset of diabetes that has been latent. • This drug can cause potassium loss. To help avoid this, take this product with a glass of fresh or frozen orange juice, or eat a banana every day. The use of a salt substitute also helps prevent potassium loss. • While taking this product, limit your consumption of

alcoholic beverages in order to prevent dizziness or light-headedness. • If you are taking digitalis in addition to this drug, watch carefully for symptoms of increased digitalis toxicity (e.g., nausea, blurred vision, palpitations) and notify your doctor immediately if they occur. • If you have high blood pressure, do not take any nonprescription item for cough, cold, or sinus problems without first checking with your doctor.

Comments: Try to plan your dosage schedule to avoid taking this drug at bedtime. • To avoid dizziness or light-headedness when you stand, contract and relax the muscles of your legs for a few moments before rising. Do this by pushing one foot against the floor while raising the other foot slightly, alternating feet so that you are "pumping" your legs in a pedaling motion. • This product causes frequent urination.

Diu-Scrip diuretic and antihypertensive (Scrip-Physician Supply Co.), see hydrochlorothiazide diuretic and antihypertensive.

Dizmiss antinauseant (Bowman Pharmaceuticals), see Antivert antinauseant.

OTC   Doan's Pills analgesic

Manufacturer: Purex Corporation
Ingredients: caffeine; magnesium salicylate
Dosage Form: Pill: caffeine, 32 mg; magnesium salicylate, 325 mg
Use: Temporary relief from pain of backache
Side Effects: Minor nausea
Contraindications: This product may cause an increased bleeding tendency and should not be taken by persons with a history of bleeding, peptic ulcer, or stomach bleeding.
Warnings: Persons with asthma, hay fever, or other allergies should be extremely careful about using this product. This product may interfere with the treatment of gout. If you have any of these conditions, consult your doctor or pharmacist before using this medication. • Do not use this product if you are currently taking alcohol, methotrexate, oral anticoagulants, oral antidiabetics, probenecid, steroids, or sulfinpyrazone; if you are unsure of the type or contents of your medications, ask your doctor or pharmacist. • The dosage instructions listed on the package should be followed carefully; toxicity may occur in adults or children with repeated doses. Salicylates are involved in more poisonings in children under age five than any other group of drugs.
Comments: The caffeine component of this product may cause a slight stimulation. You can get the same effect by taking an aspirin tablet with a cup of coffee, and it is cheaper.

OTC   Dr. Scholl's Corn/Callus Salve corn and callus remedy

Manufacturer: Scholl, Inc.
Ingredients: eucalyptus oil; lanolin; mineral oil; petrolatum; salicylic acid
Dosage Form: Ointment (quantities of ingredients not specified)
Use: For removal of corns and calluses
Contraindications: Do not use this product if you have diabetes or poor circulation.
Comments: This product is extremely corrosive. Follow the package directions carefully and exactly. Protect surrounding skin with petroleum jelly before use. • It is important not to stop treatment too soon. Some lesions take months to heal. Also, remember to check the fit of your shoes. • If the condition worsens, stop using this remedy and call your pharmacist. • After applying this product, wash your hands thoroughly.

OTC   **Dr. Scholl's "2" Drop Corn-Callus Remover**
corn and callus remedy

Manufacturer: Scholl, Inc.

Ingredients: alcohol; camphor; ether; salicylic acid

Dosage Form: Liquid (content per ounce): alcohol, 15%; camphor; ether, 9.62 gm; salicylic acid

Use: For removal of corns and calluses

Side Effects: Allergy; local irritation

Contraindications: Do not use this product if you have diabetes or poor circulation.

Warnings: Overuse of this product causes death of surrounding skin.

Comments: This product is extremely corrosive. Follow package directions carefully and exactly. Protect surrounding skin with petroleum jelly before use. • This product is flammable; do not use around an open flame. • This product creates a film over the area as it is applied. Do not be alarmed and do not remove the film. • It is important not to stop treatment too soon. Some lesions take months to heal. Also, remember to check the fit of your shoes. • If the condition worsens, stop using this product and call your pharmacist. • Keep the bottle tightly capped between uses.

Dolene analgesic (Lederle Laboratories), see Darvon analgesic.

Dolene Compound 65 analgesic (Lederle Laboratories), see Darvon Compound-65 analgesic.

Domeform-HC steroid hormone and anti-infective (Dome Division), see Vioform-Hydrocortisone steroid hormone and anti-infective.

OTC   **Donnagel diarrhea remedy**

Manufacturer: A. H. Robins Company

Ingredients: alcohol; atropine sulfate; hyoscine hydrobromide; hyoscyamine sulfate; kaolin; pectin; sodium benzoate

Dosage Form: Suspension (content per ounce): alcohol, 3.8%; atropine sulfate, 0.0194 mg; hyoscine hydrobromide, 0.0065 mg; hyoscyamine sulfate, 0.1037 mg; kaolin, 6 g; pectin, 142.8 mg; sodium benzoate, 60 mg

Use: Treatment of common diarrhea

Side Effects: Blurred vision; coughing and sore throat; difficult urination; drowsiness; dry mouth; fever; headache; nervousness; palpitations; warm skin; weakness

Contraindications: Persons with glaucoma, myasthenia gravis, and certain types of heart, liver, or kidney disease should not use this product.

Warnings: This product should not be used without first consulting a doctor by a person who is under age three or over age 60, has a history of asthma, heart disease, peptic ulcer, or is pregnant.

Comments: Diarrhea should stop in two to three days. If it persists longer, recurs frequently or in presence of high fever, call your doctor and be sure to tell him of any drugs you are taking. Be sure to drink at least eight glasses of water each day. • If you are taking other drugs, do not take this product until you have checked with your doctor or pharmacist. • This product may cause dryness of the mouth. To reduce this feeling, chew gum or suck on ice chips or a piece of hard candy. Since this product reduces sweating, avoid excessive work or exercise in hot weather.

OTC   **Donnagel-PG diarrhea remedy**

Manufacturer: A. H. Robins Company

Ingredients: alcohol; atropine sulfate; hyoscine hydrobromide; hyoscyamine sulfate; kaolin; pectin; powdered opium; sodium benzoate

Dosage Form: Suspension (content per ounce): alcohol, 5%; atropine sulfate, 0.018 mg; hyoscine hydrobromide, 0.0065 mg; hyoscyamine sulfate, 0.105 mg; kaolin, 6 g; pectin, 142.8 mg; powdered opium, 24 mg; sodium benzoate, 60 mg

Use: Treatment of common diarrhea

Side Effects: Blurred vision; coughing and sore throat; difficult urination; dizziness; drowsiness; dry mouth; faintness; fever; flushing of face; headache; loss of appetite; mental confusion; nervousness; palpitations; sedation; skin rash; warm skin; weakness

Contraindications: Persons with glaucoma, myasthenia gravis, and certain types of heart, liver, or kidney disease should not use this product.

Warnings: This product should not be used without first consulting a doctor by a person who is under age three or over age 60, has a history of asthma, heart disease, peptic ulcer, or is pregnant. • Persons with heart, liver, lung, or thyroid disease should use this product with caution. Consult your doctor or pharmacist if you have any questions concerning the use of this product.

Comments: Over-the-counter sale of this product may not be permitted in some states. • Diarrhea should stop in two to three days. If it persists longer, recurs frequently or in the presence of high fever, call your doctor and be sure to tell him of any drugs you are taking. Be sure to drink at least eight glasses of water each day. • This product contains a narcotic, but when used as directed, you need not worry about addiction to it. • If you are taking other drugs, do not take this product until you have first checked with your doctor or pharmacist. • Avoid excessive use of alcohol, tranquilizers, or any drug that sedates the nervous system if you are taking large and repeated doses of this product. • This product may cause dryness of the mouth. To reduce this feeling, chew gum or suck on ice chips or a piece of hard candy. Since this product reduces sweating, avoid excessive work or exercise in hot weather.

℞ Donnatal sedative and anticholinergic

Manufacturer: A. H. Robins Company

Ingredients: atropine sulfate; hyoscine hydrobromide; hyoscyamine sulfate; phenobarbital

Equivalent Products: Hyosophen, Rugby Laboratories; Sedralex, Kay Pharmacal Co., Inc.; Setamine, Tutag Pharmaceuticals, Inc.; Spalix, Reid-Provident Laboratories, Inc.; Spasmolin, Spencer-Mead, Inc.

Dosage Forms: Capsule (green/white); Tablet (white): atropine sulfate, 0.0194 mg; hyoscine hydrobromide, 0.0065 mg; hyoscyamine sulfate, 0.1037 mg; phenobarbital, 16 mg. Liquid (content per 5 ml): same as capsule and tablet. Sustained-action tablet: atropine sulfate, 0.0582 mg; hyoscine hydrobromide, 0.0195 mg; hyoscyamine sulfate, 0.3111 mg; phenobarbital, 48.6 mg (green)

Use: Treatment of bed-wetting; motion sickness; premenstrual tension; stomach and intestinal disorders; urinary frequency

Minor Side Effects: Blurred vision; constipation; difficult urination; nausea; nervousness; palpitations; reduced sweating; vomiting; increased sensitivity to light

Major Side Effects: Breathing difficulty; cold clammy skin; impotence; rash

Contraindications: This drug should not be taken by people who have glaucoma (certain types), enlarged prostate, obstructed bladder, or liver or kidney disease; or by those who are allergic to this drug. Consult your doctor immediately if the drug has been prescribed for you and you have any of these conditions.

Warnings: This drug should not be used in conjunction with amantadine, haloperidol, antacids, phenothiazines, alcohol, griseofulvin, tranquilizers, oral anticoagulants, steroids, sulfonamides, tetracycline, tricyclic antidepressants, or phenytoin; if you are currently taking any drugs of these types, consult your doctor about their use. If you are unsure of the type or contents of your medications, ask your doctor or pharmacist. • While taking this drug, do not take any nonprescription item for cough, cold, or sinus problems without first checking with your doctor. • This drug may cause drowsiness; avoid tasks that require alertness. To prevent oversedation, avoid taking alcohol or other drugs that have sedative properties.

Comments: This drug is best taken one-half to one hour before meals. • This drug does not cure ulcers but may help them improve. • Although this product contains phenobarbital, it has not been shown to have a high potential for abuse. • If you are taking an anticoagulant drug in addition to this product, remind your doctor. • If this drug is prescribed for you in its capsule form, ask your doctor to prescribe tablets instead—the tablets are less expensive.

Doraphen analgesic (H. R. Cenci Laboratories, Inc.), see Darvon analgesic.

OTC   Dorbane laxative

Manufacturer: Riker Laboratories, Inc.
Ingredient: danthron
Dosage Form: Tablet: danthron, 75 mg
Use: Relief of constipation
Side Effects: Excess loss of fluid; griping (cramps); mucus in feces
Contraindications: Persons with high fever (100° F or more); black or tarry stools; nausea; vomiting; abdominal pain; or children under age three should not use this product unless directed by a doctor. • Do not use this product when constipation is caused by megacolon or other diseases of the intestine, or hypothyroidism.
Warnings: Excessive use (daily for a month or more) of this product may cause diarrhea, vomiting, and loss of certain blood electrolytes.
Comments: This product may discolor the urine. • Evacuation may occur within 6 to 12 hours. Never self-medicate if constipation lasts longer than two weeks or if the medication does not produce a laxative effect within a week. • Limit use to seven days unless directed otherwise by a doctor since this product may cause laxative-dependence (addiction) if used for a longer time.

OTC   Dorbantyl laxative, Dorbantyl Forte laxative

Manufacturer: Riker Laboratories, Inc.
Ingredients: danthron; docusate sodium (dioctyl sodium sulfosuccinate)
Dosage Forms: Dorbantyl capsule: danthron, 25 mg; docusate sodium, 50 mg. Dorbantyl Forte capsule: danthron, 50 mg; docusate sodium, 100 mg
Use: Relief of constipation and stool softener
Side Effects: Excess loss of fluid; griping (cramps); mucus in feces
Contraindications: Persons with high fever (100° F or more); black or tarry stools; nausea; vomiting; abdominal pain; or children under age three should not use these products unless directed by a doctor. • Do not use these products when constipation is caused by megacolon or other diseases of the intestine, or hypothyroidism.
Warnings: Excessive use (daily for a month or more) of these products may cause diarrhea, vomiting, and loss of certain blood electrolytes. • Pregnant women should not use these products except on the advice of a doctor.

400

Comments: These products may discolor the urine. • Evacuation may occur within 6 to 12 hours. Never self-medicate if constipation lasts longer than two weeks or if the medication does not produce a laxative effect within a week. • Limit use to seven days unless directed otherwise by a doctor since these products may cause laxative-dependence (addiction) if used for a longer time. • An ingredient in these products is referred to as a stool softener. These products are recommended for prevention of constipation when the stool is hard and dry. Do not take another product containing mineral oil at the same time as you are taking these products.

OTC Doxidan laxative

Manufacturer: Hoechst-Roussel Pharmaceuticals, Inc.
Ingredients: danthron; docusate calcium (dioctyl calcium sulfosuccinate)
Dosage Form: Capsule: danthron, 50 mg; docusate calcium, 60 mg
Use: Relief of chronic constipation and stool softener
Side Effects: Excess loss of fluid; griping (cramps); mucus in feces; nausea; rash
Contraindications: Persons with high fever (100° F or more); black or tarry stools; nausea; vomiting; abdominal pain; or children under age six should not use this product unless directed by a doctor. • Do not use this product when constipation is caused by megacolon or other diseases of the intestine, or hypothyroidism.
Warnings: Excessive use (daily for a month or more) of this product may cause diarrhea, vomiting, and loss of certain blood electrolytes. • Pregnant women should not use this product except on the advice of a doctor.
Comments: This product may discolor the urine. • Evacuation may occur within 6 to 12 hours. Never self-medicate if constipation lasts longer than two weeks or if the medication does not produce a laxative effect within a week. • Limit use to seven days unless directed otherwise by a doctor since this product may cause laxative-dependence (addiction) if used for a longer time. • An ingredient in this product is referred to as a stool softener. This product is recommended for prevention of constipation when the stool is hard and dry. Do not take another product containing mineral oil at the same time as you are taking this product.

Doxychel antibiotic (Rachelle Laboratories, Inc.), see Vibramycin antibiotic.

Doxy-II antibiotic (USV [P.R.] Development Corp.), see Vibramycin antibiotic.

Dralzine antihypertensive (Lemmon Pharmacal Company), see Apresoline antihypertensive.

OTC Dramamine antinauseant

Manufacturer: Searle Pharmaceuticals Inc.
Ingredient: dimenhydrinate
Dosage Forms: Liquid (content per 15 ml): dimenhydrinate, 15 mg. Tablet: dimenhydrinate, 50 mg
Use: Antinauseant for prevention or treatment of motion sickness
Side Effects: Blurred vision; drowsiness; dry mouth
Contraindications: Persons with asthma or enlargement of the prostate gland should not use this product.
Warnings: Persons with glaucoma should use this product with caution. Consult your doctor or pharmacist if you have any questions concerning the

use of this drug. • This product should be used with caution. Large doses (10 to 15 tablets) are reported to cause euphoria and can cause severe toxicity to the brain and heart and may even cause death. • Do not take this product without telling your doctor. If you are taking an aminoglycoside antibiotic (e.g., streptomycin, gentamycin, neomycin, kanamycin) do not take this product without first checking with your doctor.

Comments: Vomiting is one of the body's defense mechanisms to rid itself of toxic or poisonous substances. Do not self-medicate with this product if vomiting has occurred for two or more days. Call your doctor. • Nausea and vomiting in women, especially early in the day, are early symptoms of pregnancy. Never take this product, or any other drug, until pregnancy has been ruled out. • If your vomitus has blood in it, or if you have headache or abdominal pain, call your doctor. • This product is recommended only for nausea or vomiting caused by motion sickness. It is less effective for other disorders. • For best results, take this product one hour before departure. • Avoid the excessive use of alcohol, tranquilizers, or any drug that sedates the nervous system.

OTC　　　　　**Dramamine Junior antinauseant**

Manufacturer: Searle Pharmaceuticals Inc.
Ingredients: dimenhydrinate; ethyl alcohol; sucrose; glucose; methylparaben
Dosage Form: Liquid syrup (content per 4 ml, teaspoonful): dimenhydrinate, 12.5 mg (quantities of other ingredients not specified)
Use: Antinauseant for prevention or treatment of motion sickness
Side Effects: Blurred vision; drowsiness; dry mouth
Contraindications: Persons with asthma or enlargement of the prostate gland should not use this product.
Warnings: Persons with glaucoma should use this product with caution. Consult your doctor or pharmacist if you have any questions concerning the use of this drug. • This product should be used with caution. Large doses, especially in children, have been known to cause euphoria and can cause severe toxicity to the brain and heart and may even cause death. • Do not take this product without telling your doctor. If you are taking an aminoglycoside antibiotic (e.g., streptomycin, gentamycin, neomycin, kanamycin) do not take this product without first checking with your doctor.
Comments: Vomiting is one of the body's defense mechanisms to rid itself of toxic or poisonous substances. Do not self-medicate with this product if vomiting has occurred for two or more days. Call your doctor. • Nausea and vomiting in women, especially early in the day, are early symptoms of pregnancy. Never take this product, or any other drug, until pregnancy has been ruled out. • If your vomitus has blood in it, or if you have a headache or abdominal pain, call your doctor. • This product is recommended only for nausea or vomiting caused by motion sickness. It is less effective for other disorders. • For best results, take this product one hour before departure. • Avoid the excessive use of alcohol, tranquilizers, or any drug that sedates the nervous system.

Dri-Phed adrenergic and antihistamine (Stayner Corp.), see Actifed adrenergic and antihistamine.

Dri-Phed-C expectorant (Stayner Corp.), see Actifed-C expectorant.

OTC　　　　　**Dristan cold and allergy remedy**

Manufacturer: Whitehall Laboratories

Ingredients: phenylephrine hydrochloride; chlorpheniramine maleate; aspirin; caffeine

Dosage Form: Tablet: phenylephrine hydrochloride, 5 mg; chlorpheniramine maleate, 2 mg; aspirin, 325 mg (5 grains); caffeine, 16.2 mg

Use: Temporary relief of nasal congestion, fever, aches, pains, and general discomfort due to colds or upper respiratory allergies

Side Effects: Anxiety; blurred vision; chest pain; confusion; constipation; difficult and painful urination; dizziness; drowsiness; headache; increased blood pressure; insomnia; loss of appetite; nausea; nervousness; palpitations; rash; reduced sweating; ringing in the ears; slight blood loss; tension; tremor; vomiting

Contraindications: This product should not be used by persons who have aspirin sensitivity, asthma, blood-clotting disease, gout, severe heart disease, severe high blood pressure, significant drug or food allergies, or vitamin-K deficiency. • This product should not be given to newborn or premature infants.

Warnings: This product should be used with special caution by the elderly or debilitated, and by persons who have diabetes, enlarged prostate, glaucoma (certain types), heart disease, high blood pressure, kidney disease, obstructed bladder, obstructed intestine, peptic ulcer, or thyroid disease. If you have any of these conditions, consult your doctor before taking this product. • This product may cause drowsiness. Do not take it if you must drive, operate heavy machinery, or perform other tasks requiring mental alertness. To prevent oversedation, avoid the use of alcohol or other drugs that have sedative properties. • This product interacts with alcohol, ammonium chloride, guanethidine, methotrexate, monoamine oxidase inhibitors, oral anticoagulants, oral antidiabetics, probenecid, sedative drugs, steroids, sulfinpyrazone, tricyclic antidepressants, and vitamin C. If you are currently taking any drugs of these types, check with your doctor before taking this product. If you are unsure of the type or contents of your medications, ask your doctor or pharmacist. • Because this product reduces sweating, avoid excessive work or exercise in hot weather.

Comments: Many other conditions (some serious) mimic the common cold. If symptoms persist beyond one week or if they occur regularly without regard to season, consult your doctor. • The effectiveness of this product may diminish after being taken regularly for seven to ten days; consult your pharmacist about substituting another product containing a different antihistamine if this product begins to lose its effectiveness for you. • Chew gum or suck on ice chips or a piece of hard candy to reduce mouth dryness.

Dristan Long-Lasting Nasal Mist decongestant (Whitehall Laboratories), see Dristan nasal decongestant.

OTC   Dristan nasal decongestant

Manufacturer: Whitehall Laboratories

Ingredients: propylhexedrine; methyl salicylate; methol; eucalyptol

Dosage Form: Inhaler: propylhexedrine, 250 mg (quantities of other ingredients not specified)

Use: Temporary relief of nasal congestion due to colds, sinusitis, hay fever, or other upper respiratory allergies

Side Effects: Blurred vision; burning, dryness of nasal mucosa; increased nasal congestion or discharge; sneezing, and/or stinging; dizziness; drowsiness; headache; insomnia; nervousness; palpitations; slight increase in blood pressure; stimulation

Contraindications: This product should not be used by persons who have glaucoma (certain types).

Warnings: This product should be used with special caution by persons who have diabetes, advanced hardening of the arteries, heart disease, high blood pressure, or thyroid disease. If you have any of these conditions, consult your doctor before taking this product. • This product interacts with monoamine oxidase inhibitors, thyroid preparations, and tricyclic antidepressants. If you are currently taking any drugs of these types, check with your doctor before taking this product. If you are unsure of the type or contents of your medications, ask your doctor or pharmacist. • To avoid side effects such as burning, sneezing, or stinging, and a "rebound" increase in nasal congestion and discharge, do not exceed the recommended dosage and do not use this product for more than three or four continuous days. • This product should not be used by more than one person; sharing the dispenser may spread infection.

Comments: Whitehall Laboratories also produces Dristan Long-Lasting Nasal Mist decongestant (nasal spray). This product contains xylometazoline hydrochloride and has a duration of action of approximately 12 hours. Because of this product's dosing schedule, it is less likely to cause "rebound" congestion during use than nasal decongestants that do not contain this ingredient.

OTC   Dristan nasal decongestant

Manufacturer: Whitehall Laboratories

Ingredients: phenylephrine hydrochloride; pheniramine maleate; benzalkonium chloride; thimerosal

Dosage Form: Nasal spray: phenylephrine hydrochloride, 0.5%; pheniramine maleate, 0.2%; benzalkonium chloride, 1:5000; thimerosal, 0.002%

Use: Temporary relief of nasal congestion due to colds, sinusitis, hay fever, or other upper respiratory allergies

Side Effects: Blurred vision; burning, dryness of nasal mucosa; increased nasal congestion or discharge; sneezing, and/or stinging; dizziness; drowsiness; headache; insomnia; nervousness; palpitations; slight increase in blood pressure; stimulation

Contraindications: This product should not be used by persons who have glaucoma (certain types).

Warnings: This product should be used with special caution by persons who have diabetes, advanced hardening of the arteries, heart disease, high blood pressure, or thyroid disease. If you have any of these conditions, consult your doctor before taking this product. • This product interacts with guanethidine, monoamine oxidase inhibitors, thyroid preparations, and tricyclic antidepressants. If you are currently taking any drugs of these types, check with your doctor before taking this product. If you are unsure of the type or contents of your medications, ask your doctor or pharmacist. • To avoid side effects such as burning, sneezing, or stinging, and a "rebound" increase in nasal congestion and discharge, do not exceed the recommended dosage and do not use this product for more than three or four continuous days. • This product should not be used by more than one person; sharing the dispenser may spread infection.

Comments: Whitehall Laboratories also produces Dristan Long-Lasting Nasal Mist decongestant (nasal spray). This product contains xylometazoline hydrochloride and has a duration of action of approximately 12 hours. Because of this product's dosing schedule, it is less likely to cause "rebound" congestion during use than nasal decongestants that do not contain this ingredient.

OTC   Dristan timed-release cold and allergy remedy

Manufacturer: Whitehall Laboratories

Ingredients: chlorpheniramine maleate; phenylephrine hydrochloride

Dosage Form: Timed-release capsule: chlorpheniramine maleate, 4 mg; phenylephrine hydrochloride, 20 mg

Use: Relief of nasal congestion and other symptoms of colds and upper respiratory allergies

Side Effects: Anxiety; blurred vision; chest pain; confusion; constipation; difficult and painful urination; dizziness; drowsiness; headache; increased blood pressure; insomnia; loss of appetite; nausea; nervousness; palpitations; rash; reduced sweating; tension; tremor; vomiting

Contraindications: This product should not be used by persons who have severe heart disease or severe high blood pressure. • This product should not be given to newborn or premature infants.

Warnings: This product should be used with special caution by the elderly or debilitated, and by persons who have asthma, diabetes, enlarged prostate, glaucoma (certain types), heart disease, high blood pressure, kidney disease, obstructed bladder, obstructed intestine, peptic ulcer, or thyroid disease. If you have any of these conditions, consult your doctor before taking this product. • This product may cause drowsiness. Do not take it if you must drive, operate heavy machinery, or perform other tasks requiring mental alertness. To prevent oversedation, avoid the use of alcohol or other drugs that have sedative properties. • This product interacts with alcohol, guanethidine, monoamine oxidase inhibitors, sedative drugs, and tricyclic antidepressants. If you are currently taking any drugs of these types, check with your doctor before taking this product. If you are unsure of the type or contents of your medications, ask your doctor or pharmacist. • Because this product reduces sweating, avoid excessive work or exercise in hot weather. • This product has sustained action; never increase the recommended dose or take it more frequently than directed. A serious overdose could result.

Comments: Many other conditions (some serious) mimic the common cold. If symptoms persist beyond one week or if they occur regularly without regard to season, consult your doctor. • The effectiveness of this product may diminish after being taken regularly for seven to ten days; consult your pharmacist about substituting another product containing a different antihistamine if this product begins to lose its effectiveness for you. • Chew gum or suck on ice chips or a piece of hard candy to reduce mouth dryness.

℞   **Drixoral allergy and congestion remedy**

Manufacturer: Schering Corporation

Ingredients: dexbrompheniramine maleate; pseudoephedrine sulfate

Equivalent Products: Disophrol Chronotab, Schering Corporation; Duo-Hist, Henry Schein, Inc.; Histodrix T.D., Spencer-Mead, Inc.

Dosage Form: Sustained-action tablet: dexbrompheniramine maleate, 6 mg; pseudoephedrine sulfate, 120 mg (green)

Use: Relief of hay fever symptoms; respiratory and middle ear congestion

Minor Side Effects: Blurred vision; confusion; constipation; diarrhea; difficult urination; dizziness; drowsiness; dry mouth; headache; heartburn; insomnia; loss of appetite; nasal congestion; nausea; palpitations; rash; reduced sweating; restlessness; vomiting; weakness

Major Side Effects: Chest pain; high or low blood pressure; severe abdominal pain; sore throat

Contraindications: This drug should not be taken by people who have severe heart disease or severe high blood pressure, children under the age of 12, or pregnant or nursing women. Consult your doctor immediately if this drug has been prescribed for you and you fit into any of these categories.

Warnings: This drug should be used cautiously by people who have high blood pressure, heart or thyroid disease, glaucoma, enlarged prostate, or diabetes. Be sure your doctor knows if you have any of these conditions. • This drug may cause drowsiness. Avoid tasks that require alertness, and to prevent oversedation avoid the use of alcohol and other drugs that have sedative properties. • This drug interacts with guanethidine and monoamine oxidase inhibitors; if you are currently taking any drugs of these types, consult your doctor about their use. If you are unsure of the type or contents of your medications, ask your doctor or pharmacist. • While taking this drug, do not take any nonprescription item for cough, cold, or sinus problems without first checking with your doctor. • This drug has sustained action; never take it more frequently than your doctor prescribes. A serious overdose may result.

Comments: Chew gum or suck on ice chips or a piece of hard candy to reduce mouth dryness. • Because this drug reduces sweating, avoid excessive work or exercise in hot weather. • This product must be swallowed whole.

OTC   Dulcolax laxative

Manufacturer: Boehringer Ingelheim Ltd.
Ingredient: bisacodyl
Dosage Forms: Suppository: bisacodyl, 10 mg. Tablet: bisacodyl, 5 mg
Use: Relief of constipation
Side Effects: Allergic reactions (including bronchial asthma); excess loss of fluid; faintness; griping (cramps); mucus in feces
Contraindications: Persons with high fever (100° F or more); black or tarry stools; nausea; vomiting; abdominal pain; or children under age three should not use this product unless directed by a doctor. • Do not use this product when constipation is caused by megacolon or other diseases of the intestine, or hypothyroidism.
Warnings: Excessive use (daily for a month or more) of this product may cause diarrhea, vomiting, and loss of certain blood electrolytes.
Comments: Do not take this product with milk or antacids. Severe abdominal cramping will result. • The suppository may cause a burning sensation within the rectum. • Evacuation may occur within 6 to 12 hours. Never self-medicate if constipation lasts longer than two weeks or if the medication does not produce a laxative effect within a week. • Limit use to seven days unless directed otherwise by a doctor since this product may cause laxative-dependence (addiction) if used for a longer time.

Duo-Hist allergy and congestion remedy (Henry Shein, Inc.), see Drixoral allergy and congestion remedy.

Duratet antibiotic (Meyer Laboratories, Inc.), see tetracycline hydrochloride antibiotic.

OTC   Duration nasal decongestant

Manufacturer: Plough, Inc.
Ingredients: oxymetazoline hydrochloride; phenylmercuric acetate
Dosage Forms: Drop; Nasal spray: oxymetazoline hydrochloride, 0.05%; phenylmercuric acetate, 0.002%
Use: Temporary relief of nasal congestion due to colds, sinusitis, hay fever, or other upper respiratory allergies
Side Effects: Blurred vision; burning, dryness of nasal mucosa; increased nasal congestion or discharge; sneezing, and/or stinging; dizziness; drowsiness; headache; insomnia; nervousness; palpitations; slight increase in blood pressure; stimulation

Contraindications: This product should not be used by persons who have glaucoma (certain types).

Warnings: This product should be used with special caution by persons who have diabetes, advanced hardening of the arteries, heart disease, high blood pressure, or thyroid disease. If you have any of these conditions, consult your doctor before taking this product. • This product interacts with monoamine oxidase inhibitors, thyroid preparations, and tricyclic antidepressants. If you are currently taking any drugs of these types, check with your doctor before taking this product. If you are unsure of the type or contents of your medications, ask your doctor or pharmacist. • To avoid side effects such as burning, sneezing, or stinging, and a "rebound" increase in nasal congestion and discharge, do not exceed the recommended dosage and do not use this product for more than three or four continuous days. • This product should not be used by more than one person; sharing the dispenser may spread infection.

Comments: This product has a duration of action of approximately 12 hours. Because it needs to be administered only twice per day, this product is less likely to cause "rebound" congestion than nasal products containing different ingredients. • The spray form of this product, although slightly more expensive than the drops, is preferred for adult use. The spray penetrates far back into the nose, covering the nasal area more completely, and is more convenient to use. The drops are preferable for administration to children.

℞   **Dyazide diuretic and antihypertensive**

Manufacturer: Smith Kline & French Laboratories

Ingredients: hydrochlorothiazide; triamterene

Dosage Form: Capsule: hydrochlorothiazide, 25 mg; triamterene, 50 mg (maroon/white)

Use: Treatment of high blood pressure; removal of fluid from the tissues

Minor Side Effects: Constipation; diarrhea; drowsiness; dry mouth; fatigue; headache; nausea; rash; restlessness; vomiting; weakness

Major Side Effects: Elevated blood sugar; elevated uric acid; muscle cramps or spasms; sore throat

Contraindications: This drug should not be used for persons with severe liver or kidney disease, hyperkalemia (high blood levels of potassium), or anuria (inability to urinate). Be sure your doctor knows if you have any of these conditions. This drug should not be used routinely during pregnancy in otherwise healthy women, since mother and fetus are being exposed unnecessarily to possible hazards. • This drug should not be used by persons allergic to it or to sulfa drugs. Consult your doctor immediately if this drug has been prescribed for you and you have such an allergy.

Warnings: Patients should not be placed on dietary potassium supplements or potassium salts when taking this drug unless they develop low blood levels of potassium or their dietary intake of potassium is insufficient. Abnormal elevation of serum potassium is probably the most severe disturbance with this drug. Hyperkalemia is more likely to occur in patients who are severely ill, with relatively small urine outputs, or in elderly or diabetic patients with kidney problems. • This drug should be used cautiously in pregnant women, nursing mothers, and children. Low potassium blood levels (hypokalemia) may occur when using this drug. • Use of this drug may produce an elevated blood urea nitrogen level, creatinine level, or both. Should one or both of these problems arise, this drug should be discontinued. • This drug can produce hepatic coma in patients with severe liver disease. Be sure your doctor knows if you have such disease. • Periodic blood studies of patients taking this drug are recommended. • This drug should be used cautiously in patients with diabetes, anemia, blood disease, or gout. Be sure your doctor knows if you have such conditions. • This drug interacts with colestipol hydrochloride, digitalis, lithium carbonate, oral antidiabetics, potassium salts, steroids, or spironolactone. If you are currently taking any drugs of these types, consult your doctor about their use. If you are unsure of the type or contents of your medications, ask your doctor or pharmacist. • This drug should be used cautiously in patients undergoing surgery.

Comments: This drug causes frequent urination. Expect this effect; it should not alarm you. • This drug does not cause potassium loss, and potassium supplements are usually not necessary. • Although the price of this drug is relatively high compared to some other drugs used to treat high blood pressure, the price is justified because it does not cause potassium loss. • Do not take potassium supplements while taking this drug, unless directed to do so by your doctor. • While taking this drug (as with many drugs that lower blood pressure), you should limit your consumption of alcoholic beverages in order to prevent dizziness or light-headedness. To avoid dizziness or light-headedness when you stand, contract and relax the muscles of your legs for a few moments before rising. Do this by pushing one foot against the floor while raising the other foot slightly, alternating feet so that you are "pumping" your legs in a pedaling motion. • If you are allergic to a sulfa drug, you may likewise be allergic to this drug. Be sure to inform your doctor if you have a sulfa-drug allergy. • When taking this drug, do not take any nonprescription item for cough, cold, or sinus problems without first checking with your doctor. • A doctor should probably not prescribe this drug or other "fixed dose" products as the first choice in the treatment of high blood pressure. The patient should receive each of the individual ingredients singly, and if the response is adequate to the fixed doses contained in Dyazide, it can be substituted. The advantage of a combination product such as this drug is increased convenience to the patient. • There are other "generic brands" of triamterene with hydrochlorothiazide. Consult your pharmacist concerning their equivalence to Dyazide diuretic and antihypertensive.

Eardro otic solution (Jenkins Laboratories, Inc.), see Auralgan otic solution.

OTC   **Ecotrin analgesic**

Manufacturer: Menley & James Laboratories
Ingredient: aspirin
Dosage Form: Enteric-coated tablet: aspirin, 325 mg (5 grains)
Use: Temporary relief of minor aches and pains of arthritis and rheumatism; protection against gastric upset sometimes caused by regular, uncoated aspirin
Side Effects: Dizziness; mental confusion; nausea and vomiting; ringing in the ears; slight blood loss; sweating
Contraindications: This product may cause an increased bleeding tendency and should not be taken by persons with a history of bleeding, peptic ulcer, or stomach bleeding.
Warnings: Persons with asthma, hay fever, or other allergies should be extremely careful about using this product. The product may interfere with the treatment of gout. If you have any of these conditions, consult your doctor or pharmacist before using this medication. • Do not use this product if you are currently taking alcohol, methotrexate, oral anticoagulants, oral antidiabetics, probenecid, steroids, and/or sulfinpyrazone; if you are unsure of the type or contents of your medications, ask your doctor or pharmacist. • The dosage instructions listed on the package should be followed carefully; toxicity may occur in adults or children with repeated doses.
Comments: Enteric-coated tablets such as this product are formulated

with a coating so that they dissolve in the intestine rather than in the stomach, thus preventing stomach upset. Enteric-coated products do not have a rapid onset for use in relief of headache, but they may be useful for treatment at bedtime of prolonged aches and pains such as arthritis and rheumatism. • Do not take this product with antacids or milk. The tablets must be swallowed whole.

E. E. S. antibiotic (Abbott Laboratories), see erythromycin antibiotic.

Rx   **Elavil antidepressant**

Manufacturer: Merck Sharp & Dohme
Ingredient: amitriptyline hydrochloride
Equivalent Products: Amitril, Parke-Davis; amitriptyline hydrochloride, various manufacturers; Endep, Roche Products, Inc.
Dosage Form: Tablet: 10 mg (blue); 25 mg (yellow); 50 mg (beige); 75 mg (orange); 100 mg (mauve); 150 mg (blue)
Use: Relief of depression
Minor Side Effects: Diarrhea; difficult urination; dizziness; drowsiness; dry mouth; fatigue; hair loss; headache; increased sensitivity to light; loss of appetite; nausea; numbness in fingers or toes; palpitations; rash; reduced sweating; uncoordinated movements; vomiting; weakness
Major Side Effects: Enlarged or painful breasts (in both sexes); fatigue; heart attack; high or low blood pressure; imbalance; impotence; jaundice; mood changes; mouth sores; nervousness; ringing in the ears; sleep disorders; sore throat; stroke; tremors; weight loss or gain (in children)
Contraindications: This drug should not be taken by people who are allergic to it, those who have recently had a heart attack, or those who are taking monoamine oxidase inhibitors (ask your pharmacist if you are unsure). Consult your doctor immediately if this drug has been prescribed for you and you fit into any of these categories.
Warnings: This drug is not recommended for use by children under age 12. • This drug should be used cautiously by people who have glaucoma (certain types), heart disease (certain types), epilepsy, liver disease, or hyperthyroidism; and by pregnant women. Be sure your doctor knows if you have any of these conditions. • This drug should be used cautiously by patients who are potentially suicidal, those who are receiving electroshock therapy, or those who are about to undergo surgery. • Close medical supervision is required when this drug is taken with guanethidine or Placidyl hypnotic. • This drug may cause changes in blood sugar levels. • This drug interacts with alcohol, amphetamine, barbiturates, clonidine, epinephrine, oral anticoagulants, phenylephrine, and depressants; if you are currently taking any drugs of these types, consult your doctor about their use. If you are unsure of the type or contents of your medications, ask your doctor or pharmacist. • This drug may cause drowsiness; avoid tasks that require alertness. To prevent oversedation, avoid the use of alcohol or other drugs that have sedative properties. • While taking this drug, do not take any nonprescription item for cough, cold, or sinus problems without first checking with your doctor. Be sure your doctor is aware of every medication you use, and do not stop or start any other drug without your doctor's approval.
Comments: The effects of therapy with this drug may not be apparent for two weeks. • Chew gum or suck on ice chips or a piece of hard candy to reduce mouth dryness. • Because this drug reduces sweating, avoid excessive work or exercise in hot weather. • Avoid long exposure to the sun while taking this drug. • To avoid dizziness or light-headedness when you stand, contract and relax the muscles of your legs for a few moments before

rising. Do this by pushing one foot against the floor while raising the other foot slightly, alternating feet so that you are "pumping" your legs in a pedaling motion. • Many people receive as much benefit from taking a single dose of this drug at bedtime as from taking multiple doses throughout the day. Talk to your doctor about this.

Eldatapp antihistamine (Paul B. Elder Co.), see Dimetapp antihistamine.

Eldefed adrenergic and antihistamine (Elder Pharmaceuticals), see Actifed adrenergic and antihistamine.

Elder 65 Compound analgesic (Paul B. Elder Company), see Darvon Compound-65 analgesic.

Eldezine antinauseant, (Paul B. Elder Co.), see Antivert antinauseant.

R̥   **Elixophyllin bronchodilator**

Manufacturer: Cooper Laboratories, Inc.
Ingredient: theophylline
Equivalent Products: Bronkodyl, Breon Laboratories, Inc.; Lanophyllin, The Lannett Company, Inc.; Somophyllin-T, Fisons Corporation; Theocap, Meyer Laboratories, Inc.; theophylline, various manufacturers
Dosage Forms: Capsule: 100 mg (off-white, soft gelatin); 200 mg (red, soft gelatin). Elixir (content per 15 ml): 80 mg. Sustained-release capsule: 125 mg (white); 250 mg (clear)
Use: Symptomatic relief of bronchial asthma, bronchospasm, emphysema, and other lung diseases
Minor Side Effects: Gastrointestinal disturbances (stomach pain, nausea, vomiting); nervousness
Major Side Effects: Convulsions; difficult breathing; palpitations
Contraindications: This drug should not be taken by people who are allergic to it. Consult your doctor immediately if this drug has been prescribed for you and you have such an allergy.
Warnings: This drug should be used cautiously by people who have peptic ulcer, heart disease, high blood pressure, or thyroid disease; or by those who are pregnant. Be sure your doctor knows if you have any of these conditions. • This drug should not be used in conjunction with disulfiram, ephedrine, lithium carbonate, oral antidiabetics, propranolol, or other xanthines; if you are currently taking any drugs of these types, consult your doctor about their use. If you are unsure of the type or contents of your medications, ask your doctor or pharmacist. • While taking this drug, do not use any nonprescription item for asthma without first checking with your doctor. Avoid drinking coffee, tea, cola drinks, cocoa, or other beverages that contain caffeine. • Call your doctor if you have severe stomach pain, vomiting, or restlessness, because this drug may aggravate an ulcer. • The elixir form of this drug is 40-proof alcohol; use caution when taking it with other drugs with which alcohol interacts, or switch to a similar product that does not contain alcohol.
Comments: While taking this drug, drink at least eight glasses of water daily. • Be sure to take your dose at exactly the right time. • Take this drug with food or milk. • If taking this drug causes you minor gastrointestinal distress, use a nonprescription antacid product, such as Maalox or Gelusil, for relief. • You may save money by buying the elixir in quarts or gallons.

OTC   **Emetrol antinauseant**

Manufacturer: William H. Rorer, Inc.

Ingredients: dextrose; levulose; orthophosphoric acid
Dosage Form: Liquid (quantities of ingredients not specified)
Use: Relieves nausea and vomiting due to epidemic vomiting as intestinal flu, etc.; psychogenic factors and regurgitation in infants; morning sickness; motion sickness; drug therapy or inhalation of anesthesia
Side Effects: Larger than recommended doses may cause abdominal cramping and diarrhea.
Warnings: Persons with diabetes or gout should use this product with caution. Consult your doctor or pharmacist if you have any questions concerning the use of this drug.
Comments: Vomiting is one of the body's defense mechanisms to rid itself of toxic or poisonous substances. Do not self-medicate with this product if vomiting has occurred for two or more days. Call your doctor. • If your vomitus has blood in it, or if you have headache or abdominal pain, call your doctor. • Do not take this product with water and do not drink any fluids for at least 15 minutes after taking.

OTC Emko contraceptive

Manufacturer: Schering Corporation
Ingredients: benzethonium chloride; dichlorodifluoromethane; dichloro-tetrafluoroethane; glyceryl monostearate; nonoxynol 9; poloxamer 188; polyethylene glycol 600; stearic acid; substituted adamantane; triethanolamine
Dosage Form: Vaginal foam: benzethonium chloride, 0.2%; (quantities of other ingredients not specified)
Use: Intravaginal contraception
Side Effects: Local irritation to user or partner
Contraindications: This product should not be used if either partner has an allergy to either component.
Comments: Be sure to insert a new dose of this contraceptive for each intercourse. • Do not douche for at least six hours after intercourse. • Used alone, this product is not as effective as when it is combined with a diaphragm. This product is not effective until at least ten minutes after insertion of the product. • Do not insert this product longer than one hour before intercourse.

OTC Empirin Compound analgesic

Manufacturer: Burroughs Wellcome Co.
Ingredient: aspirin
Dosage Form: Tablet: aspirin, 325 mg (5 grains)
Use: Relief of pain of headache, toothache, sprains, muscular aches, nerve inflammation, menstruation; relief of discomforts and fever of colds; temporary relief of minor aches and pains of arthritis and rheumatism
Side Effects: Dizziness; mental confusion; nausea and vomiting; ringing in the ears; slight blood loss; sweating
Contraindications: This product may cause an increased bleeding tendency and should not be taken by persons with a history of bleeding, peptic ulcer, or stomach bleeding.
Warnings: Persons with asthma, hay fever, or other allergies should be extremely careful about using this product. The product may interfere with the treatment of gout. If you have any of these conditions, consult your doctor or pharmacist before using this medication. • Do not use this product if you are currently taking alcohol, methotrexate, oral anticoagulants, oral antidiabetics, probenecid, steroids, and/or sulfinpyrazone; if you are unsure of the type or contents of your medications, ask your doctor or pharmacist. • The dosage instructions listed on the package should be followed carefully; tox-

icity may occur in adults or children with repeated doses.

Comments: This product has recently been reformulated. The current product looks like the former, but no longer contains phenacetin or caffeine; aspirin is now its only ingredient. "Compound" does not mean multiple active ingredients. You will save money by purchasing generic aspirin instead.

℞   **Empirin Compound with Codeine analgesic**

Manufacturer: Burroughs Wellcome Co.

Ingredients: aspirin; caffeine; codeine phosphate; phenacetin

Dosage Form: Tablet: aspirin, 227 mg; codeine phosphate (see Comments)

Use: Relief of moderate to severe pain

Minor Side Effects: Confusion; constipation; dizziness; drowsiness; dry mouth; flushing; light-headedness; nausea; palpitations; rash; ringing in ears; slight blood loss; sweating; urine retention; vomiting

Major Side Effects: Breathing difficulties; jaundice; low blood sugar; rapid heartbeat; tremors

Contraindications: This drug should not be used by people who are allergic to any of its ingredients. Consult your doctor immediately if this drug has been prescribed for you and you have such an allergy.

Warnings: This drug has the capability of causing drug dependence. Use with extreme caution. • This drug may cause drowsiness; avoid activities requiring alertness, including driving a motor vehicle or operating machinery. To prevent oversedation, avoid the use of other sedative drugs or alcohol. • This drug should be used cautiously in pregnant women and in persons with head injury, diseases of the abdomen, allergies, thyroid disease, or prostate problems. Be sure your doctor knows if you have any of these conditions. • This drug should be used cautiously by elderly or debilitated persons. • This drug interacts with alcohol, ammonium chloride, vitamin C, methotrexate, oral anticoagulants, probenecid, steroids, and sulfinpyrazone. If you are currently taking any drugs of these types, consult your doctor about their use. If you are unsure of the type or contents of your medications, ask your doctor or pharmacist.

Comments: For this and other preparations containing codeine, the number which follows the drug name always refers to the amount of codeine present. Hence, #1 has 1/8 grain codeine; #2 has 1/4 grain; #3 has 1/2 grain; and #4 contains 1 grain. These numbers are standard for amounts of codeine. • Products containing narcotics (e.g., codeine) are usually not used for more than seven to ten days. • If you are also taking an anticoagulant ("blood thinner"), remind your doctor. • This drug has the potential for abuse and must be used with caution. Tolerance may develop quickly; do not increase the dose of this drug without first consulting your doctor. • Although no exact equivalent to this product is available, similar products are, and they may save you money. Discuss them with your doctor. • Take this drug with food or milk. • If your ears feel strange, if you hear buzzing or ringing, or if your stomach hurts, your dosage may need adjustment. Call your doctor.

Empracet with Codeine analgesic (Burroughs Wellcome Co.), see Tylenol with Codeine analgesic.

E-Mycin antibiotic (The Upjohn Company), see erythromycin antibiotic.

OTC   **Encare Oval contraceptive**

Manufacturer: Ortho Pharmaceutical Corporation

Ingredient: nonoxynol 9
Dosage Form: Vaginal suppository: nonoxynol 9, 2.27%
Use: Intravaginal contraception
Side Effects: Local irritation to user or partner
Contraindications: This product should not be used if either partner has an allergy to nonoxynol.
Comments: Be sure to insert a new dose of this contraceptive for each intercourse. • Do not douche for at least six hours after intercourse. • Used alone, this product is not as effective as when it is combined with a diaphragm. Do not try intercourse for at least ten minutes after insertion of this product.

Endep antidepressant (Roche Products, Inc.), see Elavil antidepressant.

R̲   **Enduron diuretic and antihypertensive**

Manufacturer: Abbott Laboratories
Ingredient: methyclothiazide
Equivalent Product: Aquatensen, Wallace Laboratories
Dosage Form: Tablet: 2.5 mg (orange); 5 mg (salmon)
Use: Treatment of high blood pressure; removal of fluid from the tissues
Minor Side Effects: Cramps; diarrhea; dizziness; headache; nausea; rash; restlessness; tingling in the fingers and toes; vomiting
Major Side Effects: Blurred vision; muscle spasms; sore throat; weakness
Contraindications: This drug should not be taken by people who have severe kidney disease, or who are allergic to this drug or sulfa drugs. Consult your doctor immediately if this drug has been prescribed for you and you have such a condition or such an allergy.
Warnings: This drug should be used cautiously by pregnant women and by people who have asthma or allergies, kidney or liver disease, or diabetes. Be sure your doctor knows if you have any of these conditions. • Nursing women who must take this drug should stop nursing. • This drug interacts with colestipol hydrochloride, digitalis, lithium carbonate, oral antidiabetics, and steroids; if you are currently taking any drugs of these types, consult your doctor about their use. If you are unsure of the type or contents of your medications, ask your doctor or pharmacist. • This drug may affect the potency of, or the patient's need for, other blood pressure drugs and antidiabetics; dosage adjustment may be necessary. • This drug must be used cautiously with digitalis; be sure your doctor knows if you are taking digitalis in addition to this drug. Watch for symptoms of increased toxicity (e.g., nausea, blurred vision, palpitations) and notify your doctor if they occur. • If you have high blood pressure, do not take any nonprescription item for cough, cold, or sinus problems without first checking with your doctor. • While taking this product (as with many drugs that lower blood pressure), you should limit your consumption of alcoholic beverages in order to prevent dizziness or light-headedness. • This drug may influence the results of thyroid function tests; if you are scheduled to have such a test, remind your doctor that you are taking this drug. • This drug may cause gout, high blood levels of calcium, or the onset of diabetes that has been latent; periodic measurement of blood levels of sugar, calcium, uric acid, and potassium are advisable while you are using this drug.
Comments: Try to plan your dosage schedule to avoid taking this drug at bedtime. • This drug causes frequent urination. Expect this effect; it should not alarm you. • To avoid dizziness or light-headedness when you stand, con-

tract and relax the muscles of your legs for a few moments before rising. Do this by pushing one foot against the floor while raising the other foot slightly, alternating feet so that you are "pumping" your legs in a pedaling motion. • To help avoid potassium loss while using this product, take your dose with a glass of fresh or frozen orange juice and eat a banana each day. The use of Co-Salt salt substitute also helps prevent potassium loss.

Enoxa anticholinergic and antispasmodic (Tutag Pharmaceuticals, Inc.), see Lomotil anticholinergic and antispasmodic.

OTC　　　　　Enzactin athlete's foot remedy

Manufacturer: Ayerst Laboratories
Ingredient: triacetin
Dosage Form: Cream (content per gram): 250 mg
Use: Treatment of athlete's foot
Side Effects: Allergy; local irritation
Warnings: Do not apply this product to mucous membranes, scraped skin, or to large areas of skin. • If your condition worsens, or if irritation occurs, stop using this product and consult your pharmacist.
Comments: Some lesions take months to heal, so it is important not to stop treatment too soon. • If foot lesions are consistently a problem, check the fit of your shoes. • Wash your hands thoroughly after applying this product. • This product may damage certain fabrics, including rayon.

OTC　　　　　Epi-Clear acne preparation

Manufacturer: E. R. Squibb & Sons, Inc.
Ingredients: alcohol; benzoyl peroxide; sulfur
Dosage Form: Lotion: alcohol, 10%; benzoyl peroxide, 10%; sulfur, 10%
Use: Treatment of acne
Side Effects: Allergy; local irritation
Warnings: Do not get in or near the eyes.
Comments: If the condition worsens, stop using this product and call your pharmacist. • Wash hands gently in warm water and pat dry before applying lotion. • Avoid exposure to heat lamps, sunlamps, or direct sunlight when using this product.

OTC　　　　　Epi-Clear Scrub Cleanser acne preparation

Manufacturer: E. R. Squibb & Sons, Inc.
Ingredient: aluminum oxide
Dosage Form: Cleanser, coarse: aluminum oxide, 65%; medium: aluminum oxide, 52%; fine: aluminum oxide, 38%
Use: Treatment of acne
Side Effects: Allergy; local irritation
Warnings: Do not get product in or near the eyes.
Comments: If the condition worsens, stop using this product and call your pharmacist. • Wash area gently with warm water and pat dry before using this product. • Avoid exposure to heat lamps, sunlamps, or direct sunlight when using this product.

OTC　　　　　Epi-Clear Soap for Oily Skin acne preparation

Manufacturer: E. R. Squibb & Sons, Inc.
Ingredients: hydrocarbon hydrotropes; sulfated surfactants
Dosage Form: Cleanser: hydrocarbon hydrotropes; sulfated surfactants, 6.3%
Use: Treatment of acne
Side Effects: Allergy; local irritation

414

Warnings: Do not get product in or near the eyes.

Comments: If the condition worsens, stop using this product and call your pharmacist.

R_x   **Equagesic analgesic**

Manufacturer: Wyeth Laboratories

Ingredients: aspirin, ethoheptazine citrate, meprobamate

Equivalent Product: Meprogesic, Premo Pharmaceutical Laboratories, Inc.

Dosage Form: Tablet: aspirin, 250 mg; ethoheptazine citrate, 75 mg; meprobamate, 150 mg (yellow/white/red layered)

Use: Relief of tension headache, or pain in muscles or joints accompanied by tension and/or anxiety

Minor Side Effects: Diarrhea; dizziness; drowsiness; fatigue; light-headedness; nausea; rash; ringing in the ears; vomiting

Major Side Effects: Fainting; fever; palpitations; sore throat

Contraindications: This drug should not be used by people who have an allergy or intolerance to aspirin or to the product's other components. Consult your doctor immediately if this drug has been prescribed for you and you have such an allergy. • This drug should not be used by children under the age of 12.

Warnings: This drug should be used cautiously by pregnant or nursing women. • This drug interacts with central nervous system depressants, ammonium chloride, anticoagulants, methotrexate, oral antidiabetics, probenecid, steroids, sulfinpyrazone, and vitamin C; if you are currently taking any drugs of these types, consult your doctor about their use. If you are unsure of the type or contents of your medications, ask your doctor or pharmacist. • This drug may cause drowsiness; avoid tasks that require alertness. To prevent oversedation, avoid the use of alcohol or other drugs that have sedative properties. • This drug has the potential for abuse and must be used with caution. Tolerance develops quickly; do not take the drug more frequently than prescribed or increase the dose without first consulting your doctor. • If you are taking an anticoagulant ("blood thinner") in addition to this drug, remind your doctor. • Notify your doctor if your ears feel strange, if you hear buzzing or ringing, if your stomach hurts, or if you get a rash, sore throat or fever. Your dosage may need adjustment, or you may have an allergy to one of the drug's ingredients.

Comments: Take this drug with food or milk.

Equanil sedative and hypnotic (Wyeth Laboratories), see meprobamate sedative and hypnotic.

Ergocaf migraine remedy (Robinson Laboratory, Inc.), see Cafergot migraine remedy.

Erypar antibiotic (Parke-Davis), see erythromycin antibiotic.

Erythrocin, antibiotic (Abbott Laboratories), see erythromycin antibiotic.

R_x   **erythromycin antibiotic**

Manufacturer: various manufacturers

Ingredient: erythromycin

Equivalent Products: Bristamycin, Bristol Laboratories; Delta-E, Trimen Laboratories, Inc.; E. E. S., Abbott Laboratories; E-Mycin, The Upjohn Company; Erypar, Parke-Davis; Erythrocin, Abbott Laboratories; Ethril, E. R. Squibb & Sons, Inc.; Ilosone, Dista Products Company; Ilotycin, Dista Products Company; Pediamycin, Ross Laboratories; Pfizer-E, Pfipharmecs Division; Robimycin, A. H. Robins Company; Romycin, W. E. Hauck, Inc.; RP-Mycin, Reid-Provident Laboratories, Inc.; SK-Erythromycin, Smith Kline & French Laboratories; Wintrocin, Winston Pharmaceuticals, Inc.; Wyamycin, Wyeth Laboratories

Dosage Forms: Capsule; Chewable tablet; Drops; Liquid; Tablet (various dosages and various colors)

Use: Treatment of a wide variety of bacterial infections

Minor Side Effects: Abdominal cramps; diarrhea; fatigue; fever; nausea; vomiting

Major Side Effects: "Black tongue;" cough; irritation of the mouth; rash; rectal and vaginal itching; severe diarrhea; superinfection

Contraindications: This drug should not be taken by people who are allergic to it. Consult your doctor immediately if this drug has been prescribed for you and you have such an allergy.

Warnings: This drug should be used cautiously by people who have liver disease and by pregnant or nursing women. • This drug may affect the potency of theophylline; if you are currently taking theophylline, consult your doctor about its use. If you are unsure about the contents of your medications, ask your doctor or pharmacist.

Comments: Take this drug on an empty stomach (one hour before or two hours after a meal). • This drug should be taken for at least ten full days, even if symptoms disappear within that time. • The liquid forms of this drug should be stored in the refrigerator.

Esidrix diuretic and antihypertensive (CIBA Pharmaceutical Company), see hydrochlorothiazide diuretic and antihypertensive.

Eskabarb sedative and hypnotic (Smith Kline & French Laboratories), see phenobarbital sedative and hypnotic.

℞   **Eskatrol adrenergic and phenothiazine**

Manufacturer: Smith Kline & French Laboratories

Ingredients: dextroamphetamine sulfate; prochlorperazine

Dosage Form: Sustained-release capsule: dextroamphetamine sulfate, 15 mg; prochlorperazine, 7.5 mg (white/clear with multicolored pellets)

Use: Short-term treatment of obesity

Minor Side Effects: Blurred vision; change in urine color; constipation; diarrhea; dizziness; drooling; drowsiness; dry mouth; headache; insomnia; jitteriness; menstrual irregularities; nasal congestion; nausea; palpitations; rash; reduced sweating; restlessness; uncoordinated movements; unpleasant taste in the mouth

Major Side Effects: Difficulty in swallowing; enlarged or painful breasts (in both sexes); euphoria; fluid retention; impotence; involuntary movements of the face, mouth, tongue, or jaw; jaundice; muscle stiffness; rapid heartbeat; rise in blood pressure; sore throat; tremors

Contraindications: This drug should not be used by people with advanced arteriosclerosis, symptomatic cardiovascular disease, moderate to severe high blood pressure, hyperthyroidism, or known hypersensitivity or idiosyncrasy to the sympathomimetic amines. Be sure your doctor knows if you have any of these conditions. • This drug should not be used by people with history of drug abuse, phenothiazine-induced jaundice or blood disorders, or in the presence of bone-marrow depression. • This drug should not be taken during or within 14 days following the administration of monoamine oxidase inhibitors, since high blood pressure may result. If you are currently taking any drugs of this type, consult your doctor about their use. If you are unsure of the type or contents of your medications, ask your doctor or pharmacist. • This drug should not be used by nursing mothers. • Because of the anti-vomiting action of this drug, it should not be used where nausea and vomiting are believed to be manifestations of intestinal obstruction or brain tumor.

Warnings: This drug can mask extreme fatigue, which can impair the ability to perform potentially hazardous tasks, so use this drug cautiously if you must drive or operate machinery, or perform other tasks that require alertness. • This drug has a high potential for abuse and psychological dependence. Should psychological dependence to this drug occur, use should be discontinued, under your doctor's guidance. • This drug should be used with caution by pregnant women and is not recommended for use as an anorectic agent in children under 12 years of age. • This drug should be used with extreme care in persons with mild high blood pressure and in persons taking insulin for treatment of diabetes mellitus. Be sure your doctor knows if you have either of these conditions. • The smallest quantity feasible of this drug should be prescribed or dispensed at one time in order to minimize the possibility of overdose. • Use of this drug may intensify and prolong the action of central nervous system depressants, including alcohol. This drug also interacts with acetazolamide, anticholinergics, guanethidine, levodopa, monoamine oxidase inhibitors, oral antacids, and sodium bicarbonate. If you are currently taking any drugs of these types, consult your doctor about their use. If you are unsure about the type or contents of your medications, ask your doctor or pharmacist.

Comments: To be effective, this drug must be accompanied by a low-calorie diet. • The effects of this drug on appetite control wear off; do not take this drug for more than three weeks at a time. One way to get full benefit from this drug is to take it for three weeks, stop for three weeks, then resume drug therapy. Consult your doctor about this regimen. • This drug has sustained action; do not take it more frequently than your doctor prescribes. A serious overdose may result. • To avoid sleeplessness, do not take this drug later than 3:00 P.M. • While taking this drug, do not take any nonprescription item for cough, cold, or sinus problems without first checking with your doctor. • This drug may mask symptoms of fatigue and pose serious danger; do not take this drug as a stimulant to keep awake. • This drug may cause drowsiness; to prevent oversedation, avoid the use of other sedative drugs or alcohol. • This drug reduces sweating; avoid excessive work or exercise in hot weather. • As with any other drug that has antivomiting activity, symptoms of severe disease or toxicity due to overdose of other drugs may be masked by this drug. • Do not increase the dose of this drug without first consulting your doctor.

Estroate estrogen hormone (Kay Pharmacal Company, Inc.), see Premarin estrogen hormone.

Estrocon estrogen hormone (Mallard Incorporated), see Premarin estrogen hormone.

E.T.H. Compound adrenergic, sedative, and smooth muscle relaxant (Stayner Corporation), see Marax adrenergic, sedative, and smooth muscle relaxant.

Ethril antibiotic (E. R. Squibb & Sons, Inc.), see erythromycin antibiotic.

Etrafon phenothiazine and antidepressant (Schering Corporation), see Triavil phenothiazine and antidepressant.

OTC   **Excedrin analgesic**

Manufacturer: Bristol-Myers Products
Ingredients: aspirin; acetaminophen; salicylamide; caffeine
Dosage Form: Tablet: aspirin, 194.4 mg (3 grains); acetaminophen, 97.2 mg (1½ grains); salicylamide, 129.6 mg (2 grains); caffeine, 64.8 mg (1 grain)
Use: Relief of pain of headache, toothache, sprains, muscular aches, nerve inflammation, menstruation; relief of discomforts and fever of colds; temporary relief of minor aches and pains of arthritis and rheumatism
Side Effects: Dizziness; mental confusion; mild to moderate stimulation; nausea and vomiting; ringing in the ears; slight blood loss; sweating
Contraindications: This product may cause an increased bleeding tendency and should not be taken by persons with a history of bleeding, peptic ulcer, or stomach bleeding.
Warnings: Persons with asthma, hay fever, or other allergies should be extremely careful about using this product. The product may interfere with the treatment of gout. If you have any of these conditions, consult your doctor or pharmacist before using this medication. • Do not use this product if you are currently taking alcohol, methotrexate, oral anticoagulants, oral antidiabetics, probenecid, steroids, and/or sulfinpyrazone; if you are unsure of the type or contents of your medications, ask your doctor or pharmacist. • When taken in overdose, this product is more toxic than plain aspirin. The dosage instructions listed on the package should be followed carefully; toxicity may occur in adults or children with repeated doses.
Comments: You can save money by taking plain aspirin or acetaminophen instead of this product; there is no evidence that combinations of ingredients are more effective than similar doses of a single-ingredient product. The caffeine in this product may have a slight stimulant effect but has no pain-relieving value.

OTC   **Excedrin P.M. analgesic**

Manufacturer: Bristol-Myers Products
Ingredients: acetaminophen; pyrilamine maleate
Dosage Form: Tablet: acetaminophen, 500 mg; pyrilamine maleate, 25 mg
Use: Relief of pain of headache, bursitis, colds of "flu," sinusitis, muscle aches, menstruation; temporary relief of toothache and minor arthritic pain; sleep aid
Side Effects: When taken in overdose: blood disorders; blurred vision; chest pain; confusion; constipation; difficult and painful urination; loss of appetite; nausea; palpitations; rash; reduced sweating; vomiting
Contraindications: This product should not be used by persons who have severe heart disease or severe high blood pressure. • This product should not be given to newborn or premature infants.
Warnings: This product should be used with special caution by the elderly or debilitated, and by persons who have asthma, diabetes, enlarged prostate, glaucoma (certain types), heart disease, high blood pressure, kidney disease, obstructed bladder, obstructed intestine, or peptic ulcer. If you have any of these conditions, consult your doctor before taking this product. • This product interacts with alcohol, guanethidine, monoamine oxidase inhibitors, sedative drugs, and tricyclic antidepressants. If you are currently taking any drugs of these types, check with your doctor before taking this product. If you are unsure of the type or contents of your medications, ask your doctor or pharmacist. • Because this product reduces sweating, avoid excessive work or exercise in hot weather. • When taken in overdose, this product is more toxic than aspirin. The dosage instructions listed on the package should be

418

followed carefully; toxicity may occur in adults or children with repeated doses. • This product may cause drowsiness. Do not take it if you must drive, operate heavy machinery, or perform other tasks requiring mental alertness. To prevent oversedation, avoid the use of alcohol or other drugs that have sedative properties.

Comments: Chew gum or suck on ice chips or a piece of hard candy to reduce mouth dryness.

OTC   Ex-Lax laxative

Manufacturer: Ex-Lax Pharmaceutical Co., Inc.
Ingredient: yellow phenolphthalein
Dosage Form: Chocolate tablet; Unflavored pill: yellow phenolphthalein, 90 mg
Use: Relief of constipation
Side Effects: Excess loss of fluid; griping (cramps); mucus in feces; pink to purple rash with blistering
Contraindications: Persons with high fever (100° F or more); black or tarry stools; nausea; vomiting; abdominal pain; or children under age three should not use this product unless directed by a doctor. • Do not use this product when constipation is caused by megacolon or other diseases of the intestine, or hypothyroidism. • Persons with a sensitivity to phenolphthalein should not use this product.
Warnings: Excessive use (daily for a month or more) of this product may cause diarrhea, vomiting, and loss of certain blood electrolytes.
Comments: This product may discolor the urine and feces. • Evacuation may occur within 6 to 12 hours. Never self-medicate if constipation lasts longer than two weeks or if the medication does not produce a laxative effect within a week. • Limit use to seven days unless directed otherwise by a doctor since this product may cause laxative-dependence (addiction) if used for a longer time.

Exsel seborrheic shampoo (Herbert Laboratories), see Selsun seborrheic shampoo.

Rx   Fastin anorectic

Manufacturer: Beecham Laboratories
Ingredient: phentermine hydrochloride
Equivalent Products: Adipex-P, Lemmon Company; Anoxine, Winston Pharmaceuticals, Inc.; phentermine hydrochloride, various manufacturers
Dosage Form: Capsule: 30 mg (blue/white)
Use: Short-term treatment of obesity
Minor Side Effects: Diarrhea; dizziness; dry mouth; headache; insomnia; nausea; palpitations; restlessness; unpleasant taste in the mouth; vomiting
Major Side Effects: Chest pain; high blood pressure; overstimulation of nerves
Contraindications: This drug should not be used by people who have certain types of heart disease, severe high blood pressure, thyroid disease, glaucoma, or by those who are allergic to it, those in an agitated state, or those who are taking monoamine oxidase inhibitors. Consult your doctor immediately if this drug has been prescribed for you and you have any of these conditions.
Warnings: This drug has the potential for abuse and must be used with caution. Tolerance to this drug may develop quickly; do not increase the dose without first consulting your doctor. • This drug should be used cautiously by pregnant women and by people with mild high blood pressure or diabetes. Be

sure your doctor knows if you have any of these conditions. • This drug is not recommended for use by children. • This drug interacts with acetazolamide, guanethidine, phenothiazines, sodium bicarbonate, and antidepressants; if you are currently taking any drugs of these types, consult your doctor about their use. If you are unsure of the type or contents of your medications, ask your doctor or pharmacist. • While taking this drug, do not take any non-prescription item for cough, cold, or sinus problems without first checking with your doctor. • This drug may mask symptoms of fatigue and impair the ability to perform tasks that require alertness. Do not take this drug as a stimulant to keep awake.

Comments: The effects of this drug on appetite control wear off; do not take this drug for more than three weeks at a time. One way to get full benefit from this drug is to take it for three weeks, stop for another three weeks, and then resume drug therapy. Consult your doctor about this regimen. • To be effective, therapy with this drug must be accompanied by a low-calorie diet. • To avoid sleeplessness, do not take this drug later than 3:00 P.M. • Ionamin anorectic (Pennwalt Pharmaceutical Division) is not a generic equivalent of this drug, but in the body they become identical substances.

OTC   Feen-A-Mint laxative

Manufacturer: Plough, Inc.
Ingredients: docusate sodium (dioctyl sodium sulfosuccinate); yellow phenolphthalein
Dosage Forms: Chewable tablet: docusate sodium, 100 mg; yellow phenolphthalein, 64.8 mg. Chewing gum: docusate sodium, 100 mg; yellow phenolphthalein, 97.2 mg
Use: Stool softener; relief of constipation
Side Effects: Excess loss of fluid; griping (cramps); mucus in feces; pink to purple rash with blistering
Contraindications: Persons with high fever (100° F or more); black or tarry stools; nausea; vomiting; abdominal pain; or children under age three should not use this product unless directed to do so by a doctor. • Do not use this product when constipation is caused by megacolon or other diseases of the intestine, or hypothyroidism. • Persons with a sensitivity to phenolphthalein should not use this product.
Warnings: Excessive use (daily for a month or more) of this product may cause diarrhea, vomiting, and loss of certain blood electrolytes. • Pregnant women should not use this product except on the advice of a doctor.
Comments: This product may discolor the urine and feces. • Evacuation may occur within 6 to 12 hours. Never self-medicate if constipation lasts longer than two weeks or if the medication does not produce a laxative effect within a week. • Limit use to seven days unless directed otherwise by a doctor since this product may cause laxative-dependence (addiction) if used for a longer time. • This product is recommended for prevention of constipation when the stool is hard and dry. Do not take another product containing mineral oil at the same time as you are taking this product.

OTC   Femiron iron supplement

Manufacturer: The J. B. Williams Company, Inc.
Ingredient: iron
Dosage Form: Tablet: iron (from ferrous fumarate), 20 mg
Use: Dietary supplement
Side Effects: Constipation; diarrhea; nausea; stomach pain
Contraindications: This product should not be used by persons who have active peptic ulcer or ulcerative colitis.

Warnings: Alcoholics and persons who have chronic liver or pancreatic disease should use this product with special caution; such persons may have enhanced iron absorption and are therefore more likely than others to experience iron toxicity. • This product interacts with oral tetracycline antibiotics and reduces the absorption of the antibiotics. If you are currently taking tetracycline, consult your doctor or pharmacist before taking this product. If you are unsure of the type or contents of your medications, ask your doctor or pharmacist. • Accidental iron poisoning is common in children; be sure to keep this product safely out of their reach.

Comments: This product may cause constipation, diarrhea, nausea, or stomach pain. These symptoms usually disappear or become less severe after two to three days. Taking your dose with food or milk may help minimize these side effects. If they persist, ask your pharmacist to recommend another product. • Black, tarry stools are a normal consequence of iron therapy. If your stools are not black and tarry, this product may not be working for you. Ask your pharmacist to recommend another product.

OTC   Femiron multivitamin and iron supplement

Manufacturer: The J. B. Williams Company, Inc.

Ingredients: iron; vitamin A; vitamin D; thiamine (vitamin B$_1$); riboflavin (vitamin B$_2$); niacinamide; ascorbic acid (vitamin C); pyridoxine (vitamin B$_6$); cyanocobalamin (vitamin B$_{12}$); calcium pantothenate; folic acid; tocopherol acetate (vitamin E)

Dosage Form: Tablet: iron (from ferrous fumarate), 20 mg; vitamin A, 5000 IU; vitamin D, 400 IU; thiamine, 1.5 mg; riboflavin, 1.7 mg; niacinamide, 20 mg; ascorbic acid, 60 mg; pyridoxine, 2 mg; cyanocobalamin, 6 mcg; calcium pantothenate, 10 mg; folic acid, 0.4 mg; tocopherol acetate, 15 IU

Use: Dietary supplement

Side Effects: Constipation; diarrhea; nausea; stomach pain

Contraindications: This product should not be used by persons who have active peptic ulcer or ulcerative colitis.

Warnings: The iron in this product interacts with oral tetracycline antibiotics and reduces the absorption of the antibiotics. If you are currently taking tetracycline, consult your doctor or pharmacist before taking this product. If you are unsure of the type or contents of your medications, ask your doctor or pharmacist. • Alcoholics and persons who have chronic liver or pancreatic disease should use this product with special caution; such persons may have enhanced iron absorption and are therefore more likely than others to experience iron toxicity. • Accidental iron poisoning is common in children; be sure to keep this product safely out of their reach. • This product contains ingredients that accumulate and are stored in the body. The recommended dose should not be exceeded for long periods (several weeks to months) except by doctor's orders.

Comments: Because of its iron content, this product may cause constipation, diarrhea, nausea, or stomach pain. These symptoms usually disappear or become less severe after two to three days. Taking your dose with food or milk may help minimize these side effects. If they persist, ask your pharmacist to recommend another product. • Black, tarry stools are a normal consequence of iron therapy. If your stools are not black and tarry, this product may not be working for you. Ask your pharmacist to recommend another product. • If large doses are taken, this product may interfere with the results of urine tests. Inform your doctor and pharmacist you are taking this product.

Fenbutal analgesic and sedative (Tutag Pharmaceuticals, Inc.), see Fiorinal analgesic and sedative.

Fenylhist antihistamine (Mallard Incorporated), see Benadryl antihistamine.

OTC   Feosol iron supplement

Manufacturer: Menley & James Laboratories
Ingredients: iron; alcohol (liquid form only)
Dosage Forms: Liquid (content per 5 ml, or one teaspoon): ferrous sulfate, 220 mg (yielding 44 mg of elemental iron); alcohol, 5%. Spansule capsule: dried ferrous sulfate, 167 mg (equivalent to ferrous sulfate, 250 mg, and yielding 50 mg of elemental iron). Tablet: dried ferrous sulfate, 200 mg (equivalent to ferrous sulfate, 325 mg, and yielding 65 mg of elemental iron)
Use: Dietary supplement
Side Effects: Constipation; diarrhea; nausea; stomach pain
Contraindications: This product should not be used by persons who have active peptic ulcer or ulcerative colitis.
Warnings: Alcoholics and persons who have chronic liver or pancreatic disease should use this product with special caution; such persons may have enhanced iron absorption and are therefore more likely than others to experience iron toxicity. • This product interacts with oral tetracycline antibiotics and reduces the absorption of the antibiotics. If you are currently taking tetracycline, consult your doctor or pharmacist before taking this product. If you are unsure of the type or contents of your medications, ask your doctor or pharmacist. • Accidental iron poisoning is common in children; be sure to keep this product safely out of their reach.
Comments: This product may cause constipation, diarrhea, nausea, or stomach pain. These symptoms usually disappear or become less severe after two to three days. Taking your dose with food or milk may help minimize these side effects. The capsule form of this product is less likely to induce stomach upset. If side effects persist, ask your pharmacist to recommend another product. • Black, tarry stools are a normal consequence of iron therapy. If your stools are not black and tarry, this product may not be working for you. Ask your pharmacist to recommend another product.

OTC   Fergon iron supplement

Manufacturer: Breon Laboratories Inc.
Ingredient: iron (ferrous gluconate)
Dosage Forms: Capsule: ferrous gluconate, 435 mg (yielding 50 mg of elemental iron). Liquid (content per 5 ml, or one teaspoon): ferrous gluconate, 300 mg. Tablet: ferrous gluconate, 320 mg
Use: Dietary supplement
Side Effects: Constipation; diarrhea; nausea; stomach pain
Contraindications: This product should not be used by persons who have active peptic ulcer or ulcerative colitis.
Warnings: Alcoholics and persons who have chronic liver or pancreatic disease should use this product with special caution; such persons may have enhanced iron absorption and are therefore more likely than others to experience iron toxicity. • This product interacts with oral tetracycline antibiotics and reduces the absorption of the antibiotics. If you are currently taking tetracycline, consult your doctor or pharmacist before taking this product. If you are unsure of the type or contents of your medications, ask your doctor or pharmacist. • Accidental iron poisoning is common in children; be sure to keep this product safely out of their reach.
Comments: This product may cause constipation, diarrhea, nausea, or stomach pain. These symptoms usually disappear or become less severe after two to three days. Taking your dose with food or milk may help minimize

these side effects. If they persist, ask your pharmacist to recommend another product. • Black, tarry stools are a normal consequence of iron therapy. If your stools are not black and tarry, this product may not be working for you. Ask your pharmacist to recommend another product.

OTC   Fer-In-Sol iron supplement

Manufacturer: Mead Johnson Nutritional Division
Ingredient: iron
Dosage Forms: Capsule: dried ferrous sulfate, 190 mg (yielding 60 mg of elemental iron). Drop (content per 0.6 ml): ferrous sulfate, 75 mg (yielding 15 mg of elemental iron). Liquid (content per 5 ml, or one teaspoon): ferrous sulfate, 90 mg (yielding 18 mg of elemental iron)
Use: Dietary supplement
Side Effects: Constipation; diarrhea; nausea; stomach pain
Contraindications: This product should not be used by persons who have active peptic ulcer or ulcerative colitis.
Warnings: Alcoholics and persons who have chronic liver or pancreatic disease should use this product with special caution; such persons may have enhanced iron absorption and are therefore more likely than others to experience iron toxicity. • This product interacts with oral tetracycline antibiotics and reduces the absorption of the antibiotics. If you are currently taking tetracycline, consult your doctor or pharmacist before taking this product. If you are unsure of the type or contents of your medications, ask your doctor or pharmacist. • Accidental iron poisoning is common in children; be sure to keep this product safely out of their reach.
Comments: This product may cause constipation, diarrhea, nausea, or stomach pain. These symptoms usually disappear or become less severe after two to three days. Taking your dose with food or milk may help minimize these side effects. If they persist, ask your pharmacist to recommend another product. • Black, tarry stools are a normal consequence of iron therapy. If your stools are not black and tarry, this product may not be working for you. Ask your pharmacist to recommend another product.

Fernisone steroid hormone (Ferndale Laboratories, Inc.), see prednisone steroid hormone.

Rx   Fiorinal analgesic and sedative

Manufacturer: Sandoz Pharmaceuticals
Ingredients: aspirin, butalbital, caffeine, phenacetin
Equivalent Products: Fenbutal, Tutag Pharmaceuticals, Inc.; Forbutal, Vangard Laboratories; I-PAC, Spencer-Mead, Inc.; Isollyl, Rugby Laboratories; Lanorinal, The Lannett Company, Inc.; Marnal, North American Pharmacal, Inc.; Ten-Shun, Bowman Pharmaceuticals, Inc.
Dosage Forms: Capsule (bright green/light green); Tablet (white): aspirin, 200 mg; butalbital, 50 mg; caffeine, 40 mg; phenacetin, 130 mg
Use: Relief of pain associated with tension
Minor Side Effects: Constipation; dizziness; drowsiness; nausea; rash; ringing in the ears; vomiting
Major Side Effects: Breathing difficulty; cold, clammy skin; kidney diseases
Contraindications: This drug should not be taken by people who have porphyria or by those who are allergic to it. Consult your doctor immediately if this drug has been prescribed for you and you have either condition.
Warnings: This drug should be used cautiously by people who have ulcers, coagulation problems, or kidney disease; and by those who are pregnant or

nursing. Be sure your doctor knows if you have any of these conditions. • Because of the butalbital (barbiturate) content, this drug may be habit-forming; do not take this drug unless absolutely necessary. This drug has the potential for abuse and must be used with caution. Tolerance may develop quickly; do not increase the dose without first consulting your doctor. • This drug may cause drowsiness; avoid tasks that require alertness. To prevent oversedation, avoid the use of alcohol or other drugs that have sedative properties. • The safety and effectiveness of this drug when used by children under the age of 12 has not been established. • This drug interacts with alcohol, ammonium chloride, anticoagulants, methotrexate, oral antidiabetics, probenecid, steroids, sulfinpyrazone, vitamin C, central nervous system depressants, griseofulvin, phenytoin, sulfonamides, tetracyclines, and antidepressants; if you are currently taking any drugs of these types, consult your doctor about their use. If you are unsure of the type or contents of your medications, ask your doctor or pharmacist. • If your ears feel strange, if you hear buzzing or ringing, or if your stomach hurts, your dosage may need adjustment. Call your doctor.

Comments: Take this drug with food or milk.

R̞ₓ   **Fiorinal with Codeine analgesic and sedative**

Manufacturer: Sandoz Pharmaceuticals
Ingredients: aspirin; butalbital; caffeine; codeine phosphate; phenacetin
Dosage Form: Capsule #1 (red/yellow), #2 (grey/yellow), #3 (blue/yellow): aspirin, 200 mg; butalbital, 50 mg; caffeine, 40 mg; codeine phosphate (see "Comments"); phenacetin, 130 mg
Use: Relief of pain associated with tension
Minor Side Effects: Blurred vision; confusion; constipation; dizziness; drowsiness; itching; nausea; ringing in the ears; skin rash; slight blood loss; sweating; vomiting
Contraindications: This drug should not be taken by people who are allergic to any of its ingredients. Consult your doctor immediately if this drug has been prescribed for you and you have such an allergy.
Warnings: The use of this drug may be habit-forming, due to the presence of codeine and butalbital. This drug has the potential for abuse and must be used with caution. Tolerance to this drug may develop quickly; do not increase the dose of this drug without consulting your doctor.
Comments: For this and other preparations containing codeine, the number that follows the drug name always refers to the amount of codeine present. Hence, #1 has 1/8 grain (7.5 mg) codeine; #2 has 1/4 grain (15 mg); #3 has 1/2 grain (30 mg). These numbers are standard for amounts of codeine contained in any codeine product. • Many headaches are believed to be caused by nervousness or tension or prolonged contraction of the head and neck muscles. This drug is reported to relieve these conditions to help control headache. • Take this drug with food or milk. • If your ears feel strange, if you hear ringing or buzzing, or if your stomach hurts, your dosage may need adjustment. Call your doctor. • Since this drug may cause drowsiness, do not drive a motor vehicle or operate machinery.

OTC   **Fizrin Powder analgesic and antacid**

Manufacturer: Glenbrook Laboratories
Ingredients: aspirin; citric acid; sodium bicarbonate; sodium carbonate
Dosage Form: Packet of powder: aspirin, 325 mg; citric acid, 1449 mg; sodium bicarbonate, 1825 mg; sodium carbonate, 400 mg
Use: For relief from acid indigestion, heartburn or sour stomach; headache or minor aches and pains

Side Effects: Bloating; constipation; dizziness; gas; gastric fullness; mental confusion; nausea and vomiting; ringing in the ears; slight blood loss; sweating

Contraindications: Persons with heart or kidney disease, blood clotting diseases, vitamin-K deficiency, gout, asthma, allergies, aspirin sensitivity, or those on a salt-free diet should not use this product.

Warnings: Long-term use (several weeks) may lead to increased calcium in the blood, abnormal kidney function, and metabolic alkalosis (nausea, vomiting, mental confusion, loss of appetite).

Comments: This product first must be dissolved in water. Wait until all gas bubbles are dissolved before swallowing. • Self-treatment of severe or repeated attacks of heartburn, indigestion, or upset stomach is not recommended. If you do self-treat, limit therapy to two weeks, then call your doctor if symptoms persist. Never self-medicate with this product if your symptoms occur regularly (two to three times or more a month); if they are particularly worse than normal; if you feel a "tightness" in your chest, have chest pains, or are sweating; or if you are short of breath. Consult your doctor. • This product is safe and effective when used on an occasional basis only. Repeated administrations for longer than one or two weeks may cause "rebound acidity," an increase in gastric acid production. If this happens, your symptoms get worse. • This product works best when taken one hour after meals or at bedtime, unless otherwise directed by your doctor or pharmacist. • Do not take this product within two hours of a dose of a tetracycline antibiotic. Also, if you are taking iron, a vitamin-mineral product, chlorpromazine, phenytoin, digoxin, quinidine, or warfarin, remind your doctor or pharmacist that you are taking this product. • If you are taking ammonium chloride, vitamin C, methotrexate, oral anticoagulants, oral antidiabetics, probenecid, steroids, or sulfinpyrazone, check with your doctor or pharmacist before taking this product.

℞ Flagyl anti-infective

Manufacturer: Searle & Co.
Ingredient: metronidazole
Dosage Form: Tablet: 250 mg (white)
Use: Treatment of certain genitourinary tract infections and amebiasis

Minor Side Effects: Abdominal cramps; change in urine color; constipation; diarrhea; dizziness; dry mouth; flushing; headache; itching; loss of appetite; metallic taste in mouth; mouth sores; nasal congestion; nausea; rash; superinfection with yeast in mouth or vagina; vomiting

Contraindications: This drug should not be used by people with a history of blood disease or with active physical disease of the central nervous system. Be sure your doctor knows if you have such a condition. • This drug should not be taken by pregnant women during the first trimester. • This drug should not be taken by people who are allergic to it. Consult your doctor immediately if this drug has been prescribed for you and you have such an allergy.

Warnings: This drug should be used with caution by pregnant women and nursing mothers. • This drug should not be taken with anticoagulants or alcoholic beverages. If you are currently taking anticoagulants or alcoholic beverages, consult your doctor about their use. If you are unsure about the type or contents of your medications, ask your doctor or pharmacist. • Total and differential blood tests are recommended before and during therapy with this drug. • Known or previously unrecognized vaginal fungal infections may present more prominent signs during therapy with this drug. • Mild blood disease has been reported during administration of this drug.

Comments: This drug has been shown to produce cancers in mice and rats. • This drug should be taken for seven days. Four to six weeks should elapse before a repeat course of treatment. • If this drug is being used to treat a sex-

ually transmitted disease, your sexual partner may also need to be treated. •
This drug may cause darkening of the urine. Do not be alarmed.

OTC   Fleet Enema laxative

Manufacturer: C. B. Fleet Co., Inc.
Ingredients: sodium biphosphate; sodium phosphate
Dosage Forms: Adult enema: sodium biphosphate, 19 g; sodium phosphate, 7 g. Pediatric enema: half the adult content
Use: For relief of constipation
Contraindications: Persons with heart or kidney disease or those on a salt-
free diet should not use this product. • Persons with high fever (100° F or
more); black or tarry stools; nausea; vomiting; abdominal pain; or children
under age three should not use this product unless directed by a doctor. • Do
not use this product when constipation is caused by megacolon or other diseases of the intestine, or hypothyroidism.
Warnings: Excessive use (daily for a month or more) of this product may
cause diarrhea, vomiting, and loss of certain blood electrolytes.
Comments: Evacuation may occur within several hours. • A glass (eight
ounces) of water should be taken with each dose. • Limit use to seven days
unless directed otherwise by your doctor; this product may cause laxative-
dependence (addiction) if used for longer periods. • Never self-medicate with
this product if constipation lasts longer than two weeks or if the medication
does not produce a laxative effect within a week.

OTC   Fletcher's Castoria laxative

Manufacturer: Glenbrook Laboratories
Ingredient: senna
Dosage Form: Liquid: senna, 6.5%
Use: Relief of constipation
Side Effects: Excess loss of fluid; griping (cramps); mucus in feces
Contraindications: Persons with high fever (100° F or more); black or tarry
stools; nausea; vomiting; abdominal pain; or children under age three should
not use this product unless directed by a doctor. • Do not use this product
when constipation is caused by megacolon or other diseases of the intestine,
or hypothyroidism.
Warnings: Excessive use (daily for a month or more) of this product may
cause diarrhea, vomiting, and loss of certain blood electrolytes.
Comments: This product may discolor the urine. • Evacuation may occur
within 6 to 12 hours. Never self-medicate if constipation lasts longer than two
weeks of if the medication does not produce a laxative effect within a week. •
Limit use to seven days unless directed otherwise by a doctor since this product may cause laxative-dependence (addiction) if used for a longer time.

℞   Flexeril analgesic and muscle relaxant

Manufacturer: Merck Sharp & Dohme
Ingredient: cyclobenzaprine hydrochloride
Dosage Form: Tablet: 10 mg (butterscotch yellow)
Use: Relief of muscle spasm
Minor Side Effects: Blurred vision; decreased urination; dizziness; drowsi-
ness; dry mouth; dyspepsia; fatigue; insomnia; nausea; nervousness; numb-
ness in fingers and toes; sweating; unpleasant taste in the mouth; weakness
Major Side Effects: Confusion; depression; disturbed concentration; hal-
lucinations; headache; increased heart rate; itching; rash; swelling of the face
and tongue; tremors

Contraindications: This drug should not be taken by people who are allergic to it. Consult your doctor immediately if this drug has been prescribed for you and you have such an allergy.

Warnings: This drug interacts with monoamine oxidase inhibitors (or within 14 days after their discontinuation); alcohol, barbiturates, and other central nervous system depressants; anticholinergics; and some antihypertensives. If you are currently taking any drugs of these types, consult your doctor about their use. If you are unsure of the type or contents of your medications, ask your doctor or pharmacist. • This drug should be used with extreme caution by people who have urinary retention, narrow-angle glaucoma, congestive heart failure, arrhythmias, increased intraocular pressure, or thyroid disease. Be sure your doctor knows if you have any of these conditions. • Children below the age of 15 and pregnant women should use this drug with caution. • This drug is not recommended for use by nursing mothers. • This drug may cause drowsiness; avoid tasks that require alertness. • Use of this drug for periods longer than two to three weeks is not recommended.

Comments: This drug is not useful to reduce muscle spasm associated with diseases of the central nervous system or spine, such as cerebral palsy. • This drug should not be taken as a substitute for rest, physical therapy, or other measures recommended by your doctor to treat your condition. • While taking this drug, do not take any nonprescription item for cough, cold, or sinus problems without first checking with your doctor. • Since this drug may cause dryness of the mouth, chew gum or suck on ice chips or a piece of hard candy to reduce this feeling.

Fluonid steroid hormone (Herbert Laboratories), see Synalar steroid hormone.

F.M.-200, F.M.-400 sedative and hypnotic (Amfre-Grant, Inc.), see meprobamate sedative and hypnotic.

OTC   **Foille burn remedy**

Manufacturer: Carbisulphoil Co.

Ingredients: benzocaine; benzyl alcohol; 8-hydroxyquinoline and sulfur in a bland vegetable oil base

Dosage Forms: Aerosol; Liquid; Ointment: benzocaine, 2%; benzyl alcohol, 4%; 8-hydroxyquinoline and sulfur in a bland vegetable oil base

Use: First aid product for treatment of sunburn and burns

Side Effects: Allergy; local irritation

Warnings: Do not use this product on broken skin. • This product should not be used on large areas of the body since enough of the medication can be absorbed to be toxic.

Comments: Remember that ointments that are put on serious (second- or third-degree) burns will have to be taken off before definitive treatment can be given. Consult your doctor or pharmacist if you have any questions concerning the use of this product.

Forbaxin muscle relaxant (Forest Laboratories, Inc.), see Robaxin muscle relaxant.

Forbutal analgesic and sedative (Vangard Laboratories), see Fiorinal analgesic and sedative.

Formtone-HC steroid hormone and anti-infective (Dermik Laboratories, Inc.), see Vioform-Hydrocortisone steroid hormone and anti-infective.

OTC   Formula 44 Cough Control Discs cough remedy

Manufacturer: Vicks Health Care Division
Ingredients: dextromethorphan; benzocaine; menthol; anethole; peppermint oil
Dosage Form: Lozenge: dextromethorphan equivalent to dextromethorphan hydrobromide, 5 mg; benzocaine, 1.25 mg; menthol, anethole, peppermint oil, 0.35%
Use: Temporary relief of cough and throat irritation due to colds or "flu"
Side Effects: Itching, occasional nausea, vomiting
Contraindications: Do not give this product to children under four years of age.
Warnings: If your cough persists, or is accompanied by high fever, consult your doctor promptly. • A sore throat in a child under age six should never be treated without medical supervision. Consult your doctor. • This product interacts with monoamine oxidase inhibitors; if you are currently taking any drugs of this type, check with your doctor before taking this product. If you are unsure of the type or contents of your medications, ask your doctor or pharmacist.

OTC   Formula 44-D cough remedy

Manufacturer: Vicks Health Care Division
Ingredients: dextromethorphan hydrobromide; phenylpropanolamine hydrochloride; guaifenesin; alcohol
Dosage Form: Liquid (content per 5 ml, or one teaspoon): dextromethorphan hydrobromide, 10 mg; phenylpropanolamine hydrochloride, 12.5 mg; guaifenesin, 50 mg; alcohol, 10%
Use: Temporary relief of cough and nasal congestion due to colds or "flu"; also to convert a dry, nonproductive cough to a productive, phlegm-producing cough
Side Effects: Drowsiness; mild stimulation; nausea; vomiting
Warnings: This product should be used with special caution by children under two years of age, and by persons who have diabetes, heart disease, high blood pressure, or thyroid disease. If you have any of these conditions, consult your doctor before taking this product. • This product interacts with guanethidine and monoamine oxidase inhibitors. If you are currently taking any drugs of these types, check with your doctor before taking this product. If you are unsure of the type or contents of your medications, ask your doctor or pharmacist.
Comments: Do not use this product to treat chronic coughs, such as those from smoking or asthma. • Do not use this product to treat productive (hacking) coughs that produce phlegm. • If you require an expectorant, you need more moisture in your environment. Drink eight to ten glasses of water daily. The use of a vaporizer or humidifier may also be beneficial. Consult your doctor.

OTC   Fostex acne preparation

Manufacturer: Westwood Pharmaceuticals Inc.
Ingredients: salicylic acid; sulfur
Dosage Forms: Cream; Liquid; Soap: salicylic acid, 2%; sulfur, 2%
Use: Treatment of acne
Side Effects: Allergy; local irritation
Warnings: Do not get product in or near the eyes.
Comments: If the condition worsens, stop using this product and call your pharmacist.

OTC   **Fostril acne preparation**

Manufacturer: Westwood Pharmaceuticals Inc.
Ingredients: laureth-4; sulfur; talc; zinc oxide
Dosage Form: Liquid: laureth-4, 6%; sulfur, 2%; talc; zinc oxide
Use: Treatment of acne
Side Effects: Allergy; local irritation
Warnings: Do not get product in or near the eyes.
Comments: If the condition worsens, stop using this product and call your pharmacist.

OTC   **4-Way cold remedy**

Manufacturer: Bristol-Myers Products
Ingredients: aspirin; phenylpropanolamine hydrochloride; chlorpheniramine maleate
Dosage Form: Tablet: aspirin, 324 mg (5 grains); phenylpropanolamine hydrochloride, 12.5 mg; chlorpheniramine maleate, 2 mg
Use: Temporary relief of nasal congestion, fever, aches, pains, and general discomfort due to colds
Side Effects: Anxiety; blurred vision; chest pain; confusion; constipation; difficult and painful urination; dizziness; drowsiness; headache; increased blood pressure; insomnia; loss of appetite; nausea; nervousness; palpitations; rash; reduced sweating; ringing in the ears; slight blood loss; tension; tremor; vomiting
Contraindications: This product should not be used by persons who have aspirin sensitivity, asthma, blood-clotting disease, gout, significant drug or food allergies, or vitamin-K deficiency. • This product should not be given to newborn or premature infants.
Warnings: This product should be used with special caution by the elderly or debilitated, and by persons who have diabetes, enlarged prostate, glaucoma (certain types), heart disease, high blood pressure, kidney disease, obstructed bladder, obstructed intestine, peptic ulcer, or thyroid disease. If you have any of these conditions, consult your doctor before taking this product. • This product may cause drowsiness. Do not take it if you must drive, operate heavy machinery, or perform other tasks requiring mental alertness. To prevent oversedation, avoid the use of alcohol or other drugs that have sedative properties. • This product interacts with alcohol, ammonium chloride, guanethidine, methotrexate, monoamine oxidase inhibitors, oral anticoagulants, oral antidiabetics, probenecid, sedative drugs, steroids, sulfinpyrazone, tricyclic antidepressants, and vitamin C. If you are currently taking any drugs of these types, check with your doctor before taking this product. If you are unsure of the type or contents of your medications, ask your doctor or pharmacist. • Because this product reduces sweating, avoid excessive work or exercise in hot weather.
Comments: Many other conditions (some serious) mimic the common cold. If symptoms persist beyond one week or if they occur regularly without regard to season, consult your doctor. • The effectiveness of this product may diminish after being taken regularly for seven to ten days; consult your pharmacist about substituting another product containing a different antihistamine if this product begins to lose its effectiveness for you. • Chew gum or suck on ice chips or a piece of hard candy to reduce mouth dryness.

OTC   **Freezone Corn and Callus Remover**

Manufacturer: Whitehall Laboratories
Ingredients: collodion; alcohol; ether; Oregon balsam fir; hypophospho-

rous acid; salicylic acid; zinc chloride

Dosage Form: Liquid: collodion; alcohol, 20.5%; ether, 64.8%; Oregon balsam fir; hypophosphorous acid; salicylic acid, 13.6%; zinc chloride, 2.18%

Use: Removal of corns and calluses

Side Effects: Allergy; local irritation

Contraindications: Do not use this product if you have diabetes or poor circulation.

Warnings: Overuse of this product causes death of surrounding skin. • Do not apply if corn or callus is infected.

Comments: This product is extremely corrosive. Follow the directions on the package carefully and exactly. Protect surrounding skin with petroleum jelly before use. When applying between the toes hold them apart until product is dry. • This product is flammable; do not use around an open flame. • This product creates a film over the area as it is applied. Do not be alarmed and do not remove the film. • It is important not to stop treatment too soon. Some lesions take months to heal. Also, remember to check the fit of your shoes. • If the condition worsens, stop using this product and call your pharmacist. • After applying this product, wash your hands thoroughly. • Keep the bottle tightly capped between uses.

Rₓ Fulvicin-U/F antifungal

Manufacturer: Schering Corporation

Ingredient: griseofulvin

Equivalent Products: griseofulvin (various manufacturers); Grifulvin V, Ortho Pharmaceutical Corporation; Grisactin, Ayerst Laboratories; grisOwen, Owen Laboratories

Dosage Form: Tablet: 250 mg; 500 mg (both white)

Use: Treatment of certain fungal (ringworm) infections of the skin, hair, and nails

Minor Side Effects: Abdominal pain; diarrhea; dizziness; fatigue; headache; impaired performance of routine activities; insomnia; nausea; numbness and tingling in hands and feet; vomiting

Major Side Effects: Blood and kidney disorders; edema; itching; mental confusion; rash

Contraindications: This drug should not be taken by people with porphyria or liver failure. Consult your doctor immediately if this drug has been prescribed for you and you have either of these conditions. • This drug should not be used by people who are allergic to it. Consult your doctor immediately if this drug has been prescribed for you and you have such an allergy.

Warnings: This drug should not be used for the prevention of fungal infections. • Pregnant women should use this drug with caution. • This drug should be taken only under close medical supervision. This drug may cause allergic reactions in people who are allergic to penicillin. • People using this drug should avoid exposure to intense natural or artificial sunlight, since a photosensitivity reaction has been observed. • This drug should not be used in conjunction with warfarin-type anticoagulants or barbiturates. If you are currently taking any drugs of these types, consult your doctor about their use. If you are unsure of the type of your medications, ask your doctor or pharmacist.

Comments: This drug is not effective for bacterial infections. Nor should it be used for minor or trivial fungal infections that will respond to topical agents alone. • The absorption of this drug may be enhanced if taken with a high-fat diet, including butter or milk. • Prior to the use of this drug, there should be a clear identification made of the type of fungus responsible for the infection. • This drug may need to be taken for several months to achieve its full benefit. • Do not skip doses, even though the beneficial effects are not readily noticed. Since fungal infections are readily transmitted from one person to another, strict sanitary measures should be observed.

Gamene pediculocide and scabicide (Barnes-Hind Pharmaceuticals, Inc.), see Kwell pediculocide and scabicide.

℞   Gantanol antibacterial

Manufacturer: Roche Products Inc.
Ingredient: sulfamethoxazole
Dosage Forms: Liquid (content per 5 ml, or one teaspoon): 500 mg. Tablet: 500 mg (green); 1 g (light orange)
Use: Treatment of a variety of bacterial infections, especially of the urinary tract
Minor Side Effects: Abdominal pain; depression; diarrhea; headache; nausea; vomiting
Major Side Effects: Blood disorders; fluid retention; hallucinations; itching; jaundice; rash; ringing in the ears; sore throat
Contraindications: This drug should not be used by pregnant women at term, or by nursing mothers, or given to infants less than two months old. This drug should not be used by people allergic to it. Consult your doctor immediately if this drug has been prescribed for you and you fit either description or have such an allergy. • This drug should not be used for treatment of strep throat.
Warnings: This drug should be used with caution during pregnancy. • This drug should be used with caution in persons with kidney disease, liver disease, blood disease, bronchial asthma, severe hay fever, or other allergies. Be sure your doctor knows if you have any of these conditions. • Complete blood counts and frequent urinalysis should be done in persons receiving this drug. Report any symptoms of fever or sore throat to your doctor at once; these are early signs of blood disorders. • Adequate fluid intake must be maintained when taking this drug in order to prevent crystalluria and stone formation. • This drug may cause you to be especially sensitive to the sun. Avoid exposure to the sun as much as possible while taking this medication. • This drug should not be taken with barbiturates, methenamine hippurate, methenamine mandelate, methotrexate, oral antidiabetics, oxacillin, para-aminobenzoic acid, or phenytoin. If you are currently taking any drugs of these types, consult your doctor about their use. If you are unsure of the type or contents of your medications, ask your doctor or pharmacist.
Comments: This drug should be taken with at least a full glass of water. Drink at least nine glasses of water each day. • This drug should be taken for at least ten full days, even if symptoms have disappeared within that time.

℞   Gantrisin antibacterial

Manufacturer: Roche Products, Inc.
Ingredient: sulfisoxazole
Equivalent Products: Rosoxol, Robinson Laboratory, Inc.; SK-Soxazole, Smith Kline & French Laboratories; Sulfalar, Parke-Davis; sulfisoxazole, various manufacturers
Dosage Forms: Liquid (content per 5 ml): 0.5 Gm; 1 Gm (long-acting form). Tablet: 500 mg (white)
Use: Treatment of a variety of bacterial infections, especially of the urinary tract
Minor Side Effects: Abdominal pain; depression; diarrhea; headache; nausea; vomiting
Major Side Effects: Fluid retention; hallucinations; itching; jaundice; rash; ringing in the ears; sore throat

Contraindications: This drug should not be taken by people who are allergic to it, or by those who are pregnant or nursing. Consult your doctor immediately if this drug has been prescribed for you and you have any of these conditions. • In most cases, this drug should not be given to infants under two months of age. • This drug should not be used to treat strep throat.

Warnings: This drug may cause allergic reactions and should, therefore, be used cautiously by people who have asthma, severe hay fever, or other significant allergies. People who have liver or kidney disease should also use this drug with caution. Be sure your doctor knows if you have any of these conditions. • This drug can cause blood diseases; notify your doctor immediately if you experience fever, sore throat, or skin discoloration, as these can be early signs of blood disorders. • This drug should not be used in conjunction with barbiturates, local anesthetics, methenamine hippurate, methenamine mandelate, methotrexate, oral antidiabetics, oxacillin, para-aminobenzoic acid, or phenytoin; if you are currently taking any drugs of these types, consult your doctor about their use. If you are unsure of the type or contents of your medications, ask your doctor or pharmacist. • This drug may cause you to be especially sensitive to the sun, so avoid exposure to the sun as much as possible and use an effective sunscreen that does not contain para-aminobenzoic acid (PABA).

Comments: This drug should be taken for at least ten full days, even if symptoms disappear within that time. • Take this drug with at least a full glass of water. Drink at least nine glasses of water each day. • This drug is also available as an ophthalmic suspension and as a vaginal cream.

OTC   Gaviscon antacid

Manufacturer: Marion Laboratories, Inc.

Ingredients: aluminum hydroxide; magnesium trisilicate

Dosage Forms: Liquid (content per tablespoon): aluminum hydroxide, 160 mg; magnesium trisilicate, 40 mg. Tablet: aluminum hydroxide, 80 mg; magnesium trisilicate, 20 mg

Use: For relief from acid indigestion, heartburn, and/or sour stomach

Side Effects: Constipation or diarrhea

Contraindications: Persons with kidney disease or those on a salt-free diet should not use this product. In persons with kidney disease, repeated (daily) use of this product may cause nausea, vomiting, depressed reflexes, and breathing difficulties.

Warnings: Long-term (several weeks) use of this product may lead to intestinal obstruction and dehydration. • Phosphate depletion may occur leading to weakness, loss of appetite, and eventually bone pain. This may be prevented by drinking at least one glass of milk a day.

Comments: This product has been reformulated, but its advertising has not reflected the change in ingredients.• Self-treatment of severe or repeated attacks of heartburn, indigestion, or upset stomach is not recommended. If you do self-treat, limit therapy to two weeks, then call your doctor if symptoms persist. Never self-medicate with this product if your symptoms occur regularly (two to three times or more a month); if they are particularly worse than normal; if you feel "tightness" in your chest, have chest pains, or are sweating; or if you are short of breath. Consult your doctor. • To prevent constipation, drink at least eight glasses of water a day. If constipation persists, consult your doctor or pharmacist. • This product is safe and effective when used on an occasional basis only. Repeated administrations for longer than one to two weeks may cause "rebound acidity" where gastric acid production is actually increased. If this happens, your symptoms get worse. • This product works best when taken one hour after meals or at bedtime, unless otherwise directed by your doctor or pharmacist. • The liquid form of this product is superior to the tablet form and should be used unless you have been specifically directed to use the tablet. • Do not take this product within two hours of a dose of a tetracycline antibiotic. Also, if you are taking iron, a vitamin-mineral product, chlorpromazine, phenytoin, digoxin, quinidine, or warfarin, remind your doctor or pharmacist that you are taking this product.

OTC   Gelusil antacid

Manufacturer: Parke-Davis
Ingredients: aluminum hydroxide; magnesium hydroxide; simethicone
Dosage Forms: Liquid (content per teaspoon); Tablet: aluminum hydroxide, 200 mg; magnesium hydroxide, 200 mg; simethicone, 25 mg
Use: Relief from acid indigestion, heartburn, sour stomach and/or hyper-acidity associated with such conditions as peptic ulcer and hiatal hernia
Side Effects: Abdominal discomfort; constipation; diarrhea; dizziness; mouth irritation; nausea; rash; vomiting
Contraindications: Persons with kidney disease should not use this product. In persons with kidney disease, repeated daily use of this product may cause nausea, vomiting, depressed reflexes, and breathing difficulties.
Warnings: Long-term (several weeks) use of this product may lead to intestinal obstruction and dehydration. • Phosphate depletion may occur leading to weakness, loss of appetite, and eventually bone pain. This may be prevented by drinking at least one glass of milk a day.
Comments: Self-treatment of severe or repeated attacks of heartburn, indigestion, or upset stomach is not recommended. If you do self-treat, limit therapy to two weeks, then call your doctor if your symptoms persist. Never self-medicate with this product if your symptoms occur regularly (two to three times or more a month); if they are particularly worse than normal; if you feel a "tightness" in your chest, have chest pains, or are sweating; or if you are short of breath. Consult your doctor. • To prevent constipation, drink at least eight glasses of water a day. If constipation persists, consult your doctor or pharmacist. • This product works best when taken one hour after meals or at bedtime, unless otherwise directed by your doctor or pharmacist. • The liquid form of this product is superior to the tablet form and should be used unless you have been specifically directed to use the tablet. • Do not take this product within two hours of a dose of a tetracycline antibiotic. Also, if you are taking iron, a vitamin-mineral product, chlorpromazine, phenytoin, digoxin, quinidine, or warfarin, remind your doctor or pharmacist that you are taking this product. • Simethicone is included to relieve bloating and gas formation by enhancing belching or flatus formation. If you do not suffer from these symptoms, use a product without simethicone to save money.

OTC   Gelusil II antacid

Manufacturer: Parke-Davis
Ingredients: aluminum hydroxide; magnesium hydroxide; simethicone
Dosage Form: Liquid (content per teaspoon); Tablet: aluminum hydroxide, 400 mg; magnesium hydroxide, 400 mg; simethicone, 30 mg
Use: Relief from acid indigestion, heartburn, sour stomach and/or hyper-acidity associated with such conditions as peptic ulcer and hiatal hernia
Side Effects: Abdominal discomfort; constipation; diarrhea; dizziness; mouth irritation; nausea; rash; vomiting
Contraindications: Persons with kidney disease should not take this product. In persons with kidney disease, repeated daily use of this product may cause nausea, vomiting, depressed reflexes, and breathing difficulties.
Warnings: Long-term (several weeks) use of this product may lead to intes-

tinal obstruction and dehydration. • Phosphate depletion may occur leading to weakness, loss of appetite, and eventually bone pain. This may be prevented by drinking at least one glass of milk a day.

Comments: Self-treatment of severe or repeated attacks of heartburn, indigestion, or upset stomach is not recommended. If you do self-treat, limit therapy to two weeks, then call your doctor if your symptoms persist. Never self-medicate with this product if your symptoms occur regularly (two to three times or more a month); if they are particularly worse than normal; if you feel a "tightness" in your chest, have chest pains, or are sweating; or if you are short of breath. Consult your doctor. • To prevent constipation, drink at least eight glasses of water a day. If constipation persists, consult your doctor or pharmacist. • This product works best when taken one hour after meals or at bedtime, unless otherwise directed by your doctor or pharmacist. • The liquid form of this product is superior to the tablet form and should be used unless you have been specifically directed to use the tablet. • Do not take this product within two hours of a dose of a tetracycline antibiotic. Also, if you are taking iron, a vitamin-mineral product, chlorpromazine, phenytoin, digoxin, quinidine, or warfarin, remind your doctor or pharmacist that you are taking this product. • Simethicone is included to relieve bloating and gas formation by enhancing belching or flatus formation. If you do not suffer from these symptoms, use a product without simethicone to save money.

Genecillin-VK-400 antibiotic (General Pharmaceutical Prods. Inc.), see penicillin potassium phenoxymethyl antibiotic.

OTC   Gentz Wipes hemorrhoidal preparation

Manufacturer: Philips Roxane Laboratories, Inc.
Ingredients: aluminum chlorhydroxy allantoinate; cetylpyridinium chloride; fragrance; hamamelis water; pramoxine hydrochloride; propylene glycol
Dosage Form: Medicated pad: aluminum chlorhydroxy allantoinate, 0.2%; cetylpyridinium chloride, 0.5%; fragrance; hamamelis water, 50%; pramoxine hydrochloride, 1%; propylene glycol, 0.1%
Use: Relief of pain, burning, and itching of hemorrhoids
Warnings: Sensitization (continued itching and redness) may occur with long-term and repeated use.
Comments: Hemorrhoidal (pile) preparations relieve itching, reduce pain and inflammation, and check bleeding, but do not heal, dry up, or give lasting relief from the hemorrhoids. • Certain ingredients in this product may cause an allergic reaction; do not use for longer than seven days at a time unless your doctor has advised you otherwise. • Never self-medicate for hemorrhoids if pain is continuous or throbbing, if bleeding or itching is excessive, or if you feel a large pressure within the rectum.

Gerigine vasodilator (Rugby Laboratories), see Hydergine vasodilator.

OTC   Geritol Junior multivitamin

Manufacturer: The J. B. Williams Company, Inc.
Ingredients: vitamin A palmitate; vitamin D; thiamine (vitamin B₁); riboflavin (vitamin B₂); niacinamide; pyridoxine hydrochloride (vitamin B₆); cyanocobalamin (vitamin B₁₂); panthenol; iron ammonium citrate
Dosage Form: Liquid (content per 5 ml, or one teaspoon): vitamin A palmitate, 8000 IU; vitamin D, 400 IU; thiamine, 5 mg; riboflavin, 5 mg; niacinamide, 100 mg; pyridoxine hydrochloride, 1 mg; cyanocobalamin, 3 mcg;

panthenol, 4 mg; iron ammonium citrate, 100 mg

Use: Dietary supplement

Side Effects: Constipation; diarrhea; nausea; stomach pain

Contraindications: This product should not be used by persons who have active peptic ulcer or ulcerative colitis.

Warnings: The iron in this product interacts with oral tetracycline antibiotics and reduces the absorption of the antibiotics. If you are currently taking tetracycline, consult your doctor or pharmacist before taking this product. If you are unsure of the type or contents of your medications, ask your doctor or pharmacist. • Alcoholics and persons who have chronic liver or pancreatic disease should use this product with special caution; such persons may have enhanced iron absorption and are therefore more likely than others to experience iron toxicity. • Accidental iron poisoning is common in children; be sure to keep this product safely out of their reach. • This product contains ingredients that accumulate and are stored in the body. The recommended dose should not be exceeded for long periods (several weeks to months) except by doctor's orders.

Comments: Because of its iron content, this product may cause constipation, diarrhea, nausea, or stomach pain. These symptoms usually disappear or become less severe after two to three days. Taking your dose with food or milk may help minimize these side effects. If they persist, ask your pharmacist to recommend another product. • Black, tarry stools are a normal consequence of iron therapy. If your stools are not black and tarry, this product may not be working for you. Ask your pharmacist to recommend another product. • This product will taste better chilled, although refrigeration is not required for its stability. • The form of iron in this product is not absorbed into the bloodstream as well as that in other products. If you are taking this product expressly for its iron content, ask your pharmacist to recommend a different supplement product.

OTC   Geritol Junior multivitamin

Manufacturer: The J. B. Williams Company, Inc.

Ingredients: vitamin A; vitamin D; ascorbic acid (vitamin C); thiamine (vitamin B_1); riboflavin (vitamin B_2); niacinamide; pyridoxine hydrochloride (vitamin B_6); cyanocobalamin (vitamin B_{12}); calcium pantothenate; iron sulfate

Dosage Form: Tablet: vitamin A, 5000 IU; vitamin D, 100 IU; ascorbic acid, 30 mg; thiamine, 2.5 mg; riboflavin, 2.5 mg; niacinamide, 20 mg; pyridoxine hydrochloride, 1 mg; cyanocobalamin, 2.5 mcg; calcium pantothenate, 2 mg; iron sulfate, 25 mg

Use: Dietary supplement

Side Effects: Constipation; diarrhea; nausea; stomach pain

Contraindications: This product should not be used by persons who have active peptic ulcer or ulcerative colitis.

Warnings: The iron in this product interacts with oral tetracycline antibiotics and reduces the absorption of the antibiotics. If you are currently taking tetracycline, consult your doctor or pharmacist before taking this product. If you are unsure of the type or contents of your medications, ask your doctor or pharmacist. • Alcoholics and persons who have chronic liver or pancreatic disease should use this product with special caution; such persons may have enhanced iron absorption and are therefore more likely than others to experience iron toxicity. • Accidental iron poisoning is common in children; be sure to keep this product safely out of their reach. • This product contains ingredients that accumulate and are stored in the body. The recommended dose should not be exceeded for long periods (several weeks to months) except by doctor's orders.

Comments: Because of its iron content, this product may cause constipation, diarrhea, nausea, or stomach pain. These symptoms usually disappear or become less severe after two to three days. Taking your dose with food or milk may help minimize these side effects. If they persist, ask your pharmacist to recommend another product. • Black, tarry stools are a normal consequence of iron therapy. If your stools are not black and tarry, this product may not be working for you. Ask your pharmacist to recommend another product. • If large doses are taken, this product may interfere with the results of urine tests. Inform your doctor and pharmacist you are taking this product.

OTC   Geritol multivitamin

Manufacturer: The J. B. Williams Company, Inc.

Ingredients: iron; thiamine (vitamin B_1); riboflavin (vitamin B_2); niacinamide; panthenol; pyridoxine (vitamin B_6); cyanocobalamin (vitamin B_{12}); methionine; choline bitartrate

Dosage Form: Liquid (content per fluid ounce): iron (from ferric ammonium citrate), 100 mg; thiamine, 5 mg; riboflavin, 5 mg; niacinamide, 100 mg; panthenol, 4 mg; pyridoxine, 1 mg; cyanocobalamin, 1.5 mcg; methionine, 50 mg; choline bitartrate, 100 mg

Use: Dietary supplement

Side Effects: Constipation; diarrhea; nausea; stomach pain

Contraindications: This product should not be used by persons who have active peptic ulcer or ulcerative colitis.

Warnings: The iron in this product interacts with oral tetracycline antibiotics and reduces the absorption of the antibiotics. If you are currently taking tetracycline, consult your doctor or pharmacist before taking this product. If you are unsure of the type or contents of your medications, ask your doctor or pharmacist. • Alcoholics and persons who have chronic liver or pancreatic disease should use this product with special caution; such persons may have enhanced iron absorption and are therefore more likely than others to experience iron toxicity. • Accidental iron poisoning is common in children; be sure to keep this product safely out of their reach.

Comments: Because of its iron content, this product may cause constipation, diarrhea, nausea, or stomach pain. These symptoms usually disappear or become less severe after two to three days. Taking your dose with food or milk may help minimize these side effects. If they persist, ask your pharmacist to recommend another product. • Black, tarry stools are a normal consequence of iron therapy. If your stools are not black and tarry, this product may not be working for you. Ask your pharmacist to recommend another product. • The need for dietary supplements of methionine and choline bitartrate has not been demonstrated. This product will taste better chilled, although refrigeration is not required for its stability. • The form of iron in this product is not absorbed into the bloodstream as well as that in other products. If you are taking this product expressly for its iron content, ask your pharmacist to recommend a different supplement product.

OTC   Geritol multivitamin

Manufacturer: The J. B. Williams Company, Inc.

Ingredients: iron; thiamine (vitamin B_1); riboflavin (vitamin B_2); vitamin C; niacinamide; calcium pantothenate; pyridoxine (vitamin B_6); cyanocobalamin (vitamin B_{12})

Dosage Form: Tablet: iron (as ferrous sulfate), 50 mg; thiamine, 5 mg; riboflavin, 5 mg; vitamin C (as sodium ascorbate), 75 mg; niacinamide, 30 mg; calcium pantothenate, 2 mg; pyridoxine, 0.5 mg; cyanocobalamin, 3 mcg

Use: Dietary supplement

Side Effects: Constipation; diarrhea; nausea; stomach pain

Contraindications: This product should not be used by persons who have active peptic ulcer or ulcerative colitis.

Warnings: The iron in this product interacts with oral tetracycline antibiotics and reduces the absorption of the antibiotics. If you are currently taking tetracycline, consult your doctor or pharmacist before taking this product. If you are unsure of the type or contents of your medications, ask your doctor or pharmacist. • Alcoholics and persons who have chronic liver or pancreatic disease should use this product with special caution; such persons may have enhanced iron absorption and are therefore more likely than others to experience iron toxicity. • Accidental iron poisoning is common in children; be sure to keep this product safely out of their reach.

Comments: Because of its iron content, this product may cause constipation, diarrhea, nausea, or stomach pain. These symptoms usually disappear or become less severe after two to three days. Taking your dose with food or milk may help minimize these side effects. If they persist, ask your pharmacist to recommend another product. • Black, tarry stools are a normal consequence of iron therapy. If your stools are not black and tarry, this product may not be working for you. Ask your pharmacist to recommend another product. • If large doses are taken, this product may interfere with the results of urine tests. Inform your doctor and pharmacist you are taking this product.

OTC   glycerin suppositories

Manufacturer: various manufacturers

Ingredients: glycerin; monohydrated sodium carbonate; stearic acid

Dosage Form: Suppository (adult- or child-length) (quantities of ingredients not specified)

Use: Relief of simple constipation, especially in children

Side Effects: Diarrhea

Contraindications: This product should not be used by persons who have abdominal pain, black or tarry stools, high fever (100° F or more), nausea, or vomiting. • This product should not be used by children under three years of age unless otherwise directed by a doctor. • This product should not be used if constipation is caused by megacolon or other diseases of the intestine, or by hypothyroidism.

Warnings: If constipation lasts longer than two weeks or if the medication does not produce a laxative effect within a week, discontinue use of this product and consult your doctor. • Limit use of this product to seven continuous days unless otherwise directed by a doctor; if used for a longer period of time, this product may cause laxative-dependence (addiction).

Comments: Bowel evacuation may occur within 6 to 12 hours.

Glyceryl-T expectorant and smooth muscle relaxant (Rugby Laboratories), see Quibron expectorant and smooth muscle relaxant.

OTC   Gly-Oxide canker sore and fever blister remedy

Manufacturer: Marion Laboratories, Inc.

Ingredients: anhydrous glycerol; carbamide peroxide; flavors

Dosage Form: Liquid: anhydrous glycerol; carbamide peroxide, 10%; flavors

Use: Local treatment of minor oral inflammations such as canker sores and fever blisters

Comments: If you have an oral ulcer which does not heal within three weeks, see your dentist. • This product costs more than most of the more common preparations intended for treating mouth sores. However, the extra cost is justified.

Gly-Trate Meta-Kaps antianginal (Sutliff & Case Co., Inc.), see Nitro-Bid Plateau Caps antianginal.

G-Mycin antibiotic (Coast Laboratories, Inc.), see tetracycline hydrochloride antibiotic.

G-Recillin antibiotic (Reid-Provident Laboratories), see penicillin G antibiotic.

Grifulvin V antifungal (Ortho Pharmaceutical Corporation), see Fulvicin-U/F antifungal.

Grisactin antifungal (Ayerst Laboratories), see Fulvicin-U/F antifungal.

grisOwen antifungal (Owen Laboratories), see Fulvicin-U/F antifungal.

Gyne-Lotrimin antifungal agent (Schering Corporation), see Lotrimin antifungal agent.

Habdryl antihistamine (Bowman Pharmaceuticals), see Benadryl antihistamine.

℞   Haldol antipsychotic agent

Manufacturer: McNeil Laboratories
Ingredient: haloperidol
Dosage Forms: Liquid concentrate (content per ml): 2 mg. Tablet: 0.5 mg (white); 1 mg (yellow); 2 mg (pink); 5 mg (green); 10 mg (aqua)
Use: Treatment of certain psychotic disorders; certain symptoms of Gilles de la Tourette's syndrome in children and infants; severe behavior problems in children; short-term treatment of hyperactive children
Minor Side Effects: Blurred vision; change in urine color; constipation; diarrhea; dizziness; drooling; drowsiness; dry mouth; jitteriness; menstrual irregularities; nasal congestion; rash; reduced sweating; restlessness; uncoordinated movements; vomiting
Major Side Effects: Difficulty in swallowing; enlarged or painful breasts (in both sexes); fluid retention; impotence; involuntary movements of the face, mouth, tongue, or jaw; jaundice; muscle stiffness; rise in blood pressure; sore throat; tremors
Contraindications: This drug should not be taken by people who are severely depressed, comatose, have central nervous system depression due to alcohol or other centrally acting depressants, or have Parkinson's disease. Be sure your doctor knows if you have any of these conditions. • This drug should not be taken by people who are allergic to it. Consult your doctor immediately if this drug has been prescribed for you and you have such an allergy.
Warnings: This drug should be used with caution by pregnant women. • Infants should not be nursed during drug treatment. • This drug should not be taken in combination with lithium. • Bronchopneumonia may result from usage of this drug. • This drug may impair mental and/or physical abilities required for performance of hazardous tasks such as operating machinery or driving a motor vehicle. • This drug should not be taken with alcohol. • This drug should be taken cautiously by patients with severe cardiovascular disorders, those receiving anticoagulant or anticonvulsant therapy, those with known allergies, or with thyrotoxicosis. Be sure your doctor knows if you

have any of these conditions or if you are taking any of these drug types, or any of the following: alcohol, oral antacids, anticholinergics, depressants. If you are unsure about the type or contents of your medications, ask your doctor or pharmacist.

Comments: The effects of this drug therapy may not be apparent for at least two weeks. • This drug has a persistent action; never take it more frequently than your doctor prescribes. A serious overdose may result. • While taking this drug, do not take any nonprescription item for cough, cold, or sinus problems without first checking with your doctor. This drug may cause dryness of the mouth. To reduce this feeling, chew gum or suck on ice chips or a piece of hard candy. • This drug reduces sweating; avoid excessive work or exercise in hot weather. • To avoid dizziness or light-headedness when you stand, contract and relax the muscles of your legs for a few moments before rising. Do this by pushing one foot against the floor while raising the other foot slightly, alternating feet so that you are "pumping" your legs in a pedaling motion. • As with any other drug that has antivomiting activity, symptoms of severe disease or toxicity due to overdose of other drugs may be masked by this drug.

OTC   Haley's M-O laxative

Manufacturer: Winthrop Laboratories
Ingredients: magnesium hydroxide; mineral oil
Dosage Form: Emulsion: magnesium hydroxide, 75%; mineral oil, 25%
Use: Relief of constipation
Contraindications: Persons with high fever (100° F or more); black or tarry stools; nausea; vomiting; abdominal pain; or children under age six should not use this product unless directed by a doctor. • Do not use this product when constipation is caused by megacolon or other diseases of the intestine, or hypothyroidism.
Warnings: Excessive use (daily for a month or more) of this product may cause diarrhea, vomiting, and loss of certain blood electrolytes. • Repeated (daily) use of this product may cause nausea, vomiting, depressed reflexes, and breathing difficulties in persons with kidney disease. • A type of pneumonia may occur after prolonged (more than two months) and repeated (daily) use.
Comments: Mineral oil may interfere with the absorption of vitamins A and D, calcium, and phosphate. • This product is best taken at bedtime; it should not be taken at mealtime. • If this product leaks through the rectum, the dose should be reduced until this symptom disappears. • Do not take a stool softener at the same time you are taking this product. • Evacuation may occur within several hours. A glass (eight ounces) of water should be taken with each dose. • Never self-medicate with this product if constipation lasts longer than two weeks or if the medication does not produce a laxative effect within a week. • Limit use to seven days unless directed otherwise by a doctor since this product may cause laxative-dependence (addiction) if used for a longer time.

OTC   Hazel-Balm hemorrhoidal preparation

Manufacturer: Arnar-Stone Laboratories, Inc.
Ingredients: benzethonium chloride; hamamelis water; water soluble lanolin derivative
Dosage Form: Aerosol: benzethonium chloride, 0.1%; hamamelis water, 79.9%; water soluble lanolin derivative, 20%
Use: Relief of pain, burning, and itching of hemorrhoids
Warnings: Sensitization (continued itching and redness) may occur with long-term and repeated use.

Comments: Hemorrhoidal (pile) preparations relieve itching, reduce pain and inflammation, and check bleeding, but do not heal, dry up, or give lasting relief from the hemorrhoids. • Certain ingredients in this product may cause an allergic reaction; do not use for longer than seven days at a time unless your doctor has advised you otherwise. • Never self-medicate for hemorrhoids if pain is continuous or throbbing, if bleeding or itching is excessive, or if you feel a large pressure within the rectum.

HCV steroid hormone and anti-infective (Saron Pharmacal Corp.), see Vioform-Hydrocortisone steroid hormone and anti-infective.

OTC **Head & Shoulders Cream,
Head & Shoulders Shampoo dandruff treatment**

Manufacturer: Procter & Gamble
Ingredients: cocamide MEA; ethanolamine; hydroxypropyl methylcellulose; magnesium aluminum silicate; TEA-lauryl sulfate; triethanolamine; zinc pyrithione
Dosage Forms: Shampoo, lotion: zinc pyrithione, 2% (quantities of other ingredients not specified). Cream: zinc pyrithione, 2% (quantities of other ingredients not specified)
Use: Controls dandruff and seborrheic dermatitis of the scalp
Side Effects: Burning of the skin; discoloration of hair; dryness or oiliness of hair or scalp; eye irritation
Warnings: Do not use this product if the skin is broken.
Comments: Although this shampoo has not been reported to cause serious toxicity, if you swallow any, call your doctor or pharmacist right away. • Leave the shampoo on the scalp for a few minutes before rinsing.

Heb-Cort steroid hormone and anti-infective (Barnes-Hind Pharmaceuticals, Inc.), see Vioform-Hydrocortisone steroid hormone and anti-infective.

OTC **Heet external analgesic**

Manufacturer: Whitehall Laboratories
Ingredients: alcohol; camphor; methyl salicylate; oleoresin capsicum
Dosage Form: Lotion: alcohol, 70%; camphor, 3.6%; methyl salicylate, 15%; oleoresin capsicum (as Capsaicin), 0.025%
Use: Used externally for temporary relief of pain in muscles and other areas
Side Effects: Allergic reactions (rash, itching, soreness); local irritation; local numbness
Warnings: If you have diabetes or impaired circulation, use this product only upon the advice of a physician. • Use this product externally only. • Do not use on broken or irritated skin or on large areas of the body; avoid contact with eyes. • When using this product, avoid exposure to direct sunlight, heat lamp, or sunlamp. • Before using this product on children under 12 years of age, consult your doctor. • If the condition persists, call your doctor.
Comments: This lotion smells good and may be attractive to a child. It should be stored safely out of the reach of children. • Do not rub this product into the skin.

Henotal sedative and hypnotic (Bowman Pharmaceuticals), see phenobarbital sedative and hypnotic.

Hexaderm I.Q. steroid hormone and anti-infective (Amfre-Grant, Inc.), see Vioform-Hydrocortisone steroid hormone and anti-infective.

Hexyphen antiparkinson drug (Robinson Laboratory, Inc.), see Artane antiparkinson drug.

Hiserpia antihypertensive (Bowman Pharmaceuticals), see reserpine antihypertensive.

Histatapp antihistamine (Upsher-Smith Laboratories, Inc.), see Dimetapp antihistamine.

Histodrix T.D. allergy and congestion remedy (Spencer-Mead, Inc.), see Drixoral allergy and congestion remedy.

OTC   Hold cough suppressant lozenges

Manufacturer: Beecham Products
Ingredients: benzocaine; dextromethorphan hydrobromide
Dosage Form: Lozenge: benzocaine; dextromethorphan hydrobromide, 7.5 mg
Use: Temporary suppression of coughs
Side Effects: Occasional nausea; vomiting
Contraindications: Do not give this product to children under six years of age.
Warnings: If your cough persists, or is accompanied by high fever, consult your doctor promptly. • A sore throat in a child under age six should never be treated without medical supervision. Consult your doctor. • This product interacts with monoamine oxidase inhibitors; if you are currently taking any drugs of this type, check with your doctor before taking this product. If you are unsure of the type or contents of your medications, ask your doctor or pharmacist.

OTC   Hold liquid cough suppressant and decongestant

Manufacturer: Beecham Products
Ingredients: dextromethorphan hydrobromide; phenylpropanolamine hydrochloride; alcohol
Dosage Form: Liquid (content per two teaspoonfuls): dextromethorphan hydrobromide, 20 mg; phenylpropanolamine hydrochloride, 25 mg; alcohol, 9.5%
Use: Temporary relief of cough and nasal congestion due to colds or "flu"
Side Effects: Drowsiness; mild stimulation; nausea; vomiting
Warnings: This product should be used with special caution by children under two years of age, and by persons who have diabetes, heart disease, high blood pressure, or thyroid disease. If you have any of these conditions, consult your doctor before taking this product. • This product interacts with guanethidine and monoamine oxidase inhibitors. If you are currently taking any drugs of these types, check with your doctor before taking this product. If you are unsure of the type or contents of your medications, ask your doctor or pharmacist.
Comments: Do not use this product to treat chronic coughs, such as from smoking or asthma. • Do not use this product to treat productive (hacking) coughs that produce phlegm.

HRC-Proclan VC with Codeine expectorant (H. R. Cenci Laboratories, Inc.), see Phenergan VC with Codeine expectorant.

HRC-Proclan with Codeine expectorant (H. R. Cenci Laboratories, Inc.), see Phenergan with Codeine expectorant.

Rx   **Hydergine vasodilator**

Manufacturer: Sandoz Pharmaceuticals
Ingredients: dihydroergocornine mesylate; dihydroergocristine mesylate; dihydroergocryptine mesylate
Equivalent Products: Circanol, Riker Laboratories, Inc.; Deapril-ST, Mead Johnson Pharmaceutical Division; Gerigine, Rugby Laboratories; Spengine, Spencer-Mead, Inc.; Tri-Ergone, Columbia Medical Co.; Trigot, E. R. Squibb & Sons, Inc.
Dosage Forms: Sublingual tablet: dihydroergocornine mesylate, 0.333 mg; 0.167 mg; dihydroergocristine mesylate, 0.333 mg, 0.167 mg; dihydroergocryptine mesylate, 0.333 mg, 0.167 mg (both white). Tablet: 0.333 mg (each ingredient) (white)
Use: To reduce symptoms associated with senility
Minor Side Effects: Irritation under the tongue (sublingual form only); nausea; vomiting
Contraindications: This drug should not be taken by people who are allergic to it. Consult your doctor immediately if this drug has been prescribed for you and you have such an allergy.
Warnings: Although this drug may increase the flow of blood to the brain, objective improvement of symptoms of senility is difficult to document. Because it is difficult to determine the cause of symptoms associated with senility, careful diagnosis is advised before this drug is prescribed.
Comments: Effects of this therapy may not be apparent for three to four weeks. • The sublingual form of this drug must be placed under the tongue and allowed to dissolve completely. Try not to swallow for as long as possible. Do not drink any liquids for ten minutes after placing the tablet under the tongue. • The oral tablet form of this drug must be swallowed.

Hydro-Chlor diuretic and antihypertensive (North American Pharmacal, Inc.), see hydrochlorothiazide diuretic and antihypertensive.

Rx   **hydrochlorothiazide diuretic and antihypertensive**

Manufacturer: various manufacturers
Ingredient: hydrochlorothiazide
Equivalent Products: Chlorzide, Foy Laboratories; Delco-Retic, Delco Chemical Co., inc.; Diaqua, W.E. Hauck, Inc.; Diucen-H, Central Pharmacal Company; Diu-Scrip, Scrip-Physician Supply Co.; Esidrix, CIBA Pharmaceutical Company; Hydro-Chlor, North American Pharmacal, Inc.; HydroDIURIL, Merck Sharp & Dohme; Hydromal, Mallard Incorporated; Hydro-Z-50, Mayrand, Inc.; Jen-Diril, Jenkins Laboratories, Inc.; Lexor, Lemmon Company; Loqua, Columbia Medical Co.; Oretic, Abbot Laboratories; Tri-Zide, Tri-County Pharmaceuticals; X-Aqua, General Pharmaceutical Prods., Inc.; Zide, Tutag Pharmaceuticals, Inc.
Dosage Form: Tablet: various dosages and various colors
Use: Treatment of high blood pressure; removal of fluid from body tissues
Minor Side Effects: Cramps; diarrhea; dizziness; headache; loss of appetite; nausea; rash; restlessness; tingling in the fingers and toes; vomiting
Major Side Effects: Blurred vision; elevated blood sugar; elevated uric acid; muscle spasms; sore throat; weakness
Contraindications: This drug should not be taken by people who have demonstrated an allergy to this or sulfa drugs and by those who are suffering a lack of urination. Consult your doctor immediately if this drug has been prescribed for you and you have any of these conditions.

Warnings: This drug should be used cautiously by people who have kidney or liver disease, a history of allergy or asthma, and by those who are pregnant. Be sure your doctor knows if you have any of these conditions. • Nursing women who must take this drug should stop nursing. • This drug interacts with colestipol hydrochloride, lithium carbonate, oral antidiabetics, and steroids; if you are currently taking any drugs of these types, consult your doctor about their use. If you are unsure of the type or contents of your medications, ask your doctor or pharmacist. • This drug may affect the potency of, or the patient's need for, other blood pressure drugs and antidiabetics; dosage adjustment may be necessary. • If you are taking digitalis in addition to this drug, watch carefully for symptoms of increased toxicity (e.g., nausea, blurred vision, palpitations) and notify your doctor if they occur. • This drug may cause gout, high levels of calcium in the blood, and the onset of diabetes that has been latent. While taking this drug, periodic measurements of blood levels of sugar, calcium, uric acid, and potassium are advisable. This drug can affect the results of laboratory and thyroid tests and your responsiveness to surgical muscle relaxants. Be sure your doctor knows that you are taking this drug. • While taking this drug (as with many drugs that lower blood pressure), you should limit your consumption of alcoholic beverages in order to prevent dizziness or light-headedness. • If you have high blood pressure, do not take any nonprescription item for cough, cold, or sinus problems without first checking with your doctor.

Comments: Try to plan your dosage schedule to avoid taking this drug at bedtime. • To avoid dizziness or light-headedness when you stand, contract and relax the muscles of your legs for a few moments before rising. Do this by pushing one foot against the floor while raising the other foot slightly, alternating feet so that you are "pumping" your legs in a pedaling motion. • This drug causes frequent urination. Expect this effect; it should not alarm you. • To help avoid potassium loss while using this drug, take your dose with a glass of fresh or frozen orange juice and eat a banana each day. The use of Co-Salt salt substitute also helps prevent potassium loss.

HydroDIURIL diuretic and antihypertensive (Merck Sharp & Dohme), see hydrochlorothiazide diuretic and antihypertensive.

OTC   hydrogen peroxide

Manufacturer: various manufacturers
Ingredient: hydrogen peroxide
Dosage Form: Liquid: hydrogen peroxide, 3%
Use: To clean wounds and prevent infection by killing germs; also used as a mouthwash
Side Effects: None when used topically. (May cause mild nausea and a feeling of fullness or bloating if swallowed)
Contraindications: Do not use hydrogen peroxide to bleach hair.
Warnings: Do not use this product on abscesses. • Do not apply bandages to the wound until the hydrogen peroxide has stopped bubbling.
Comments: Store this product in the refrigerator once the container has been opened. Keep the container tightly capped. • The bubbling action of this product indicates that oxygen is being released, removing debris from wounds. If this product does not bubble when placed on an open wound, it is no longer effective and should be replaced. • This product has no activity on unbroken skin.

Hydromal diuretic and antihypertensive (Mallard Incorporated), see hydrochlorothiazide diuretic and antihypertensive.

Hydrophed adrenergic, sedative, and smooth muscle relaxant (Rugby Laboratories), see Marax adrenergic, sedative, and smooth muscle relaxant.

R_x   **Hydropres diuretic and antihypertensive**

Manufacturer: Merck Sharp & Dohme
Ingredients: hydrochlorothiazide; reserpine
Equivalent Products: Aquaserp, Spencer-Mead, Inc.; Hydroserp, various manufacturers; Hydroserpine, various manufacturers; Hydrotensin, Mayrand, Inc.; Loquapres, Columbia Medical Co.; Thia-Serp, Robinson Laboratories, Inc.
Dosage Form: Tablet: hydrochlorothiazide, 25 mg, 50 mg; reserpine, 0.125 mg (both green)
Use: Treatment of high blood pressure
Minor Side Effects: Cramping; diarrhea; dizziness; headache; itching; loss of appetite; nasal congestion; nausea; palpitations; rash; restlessness; tingling in the fingers and toes; vomiting
Major Side Effects: Blurred vision; chest pain; depression; drowsiness; elevated blood sugar; elevated uric acid; muscle spasms; nightmares; sore throat; weakness
Contraindications: This drug should not be taken by people who are allergic to it or to sulfa drugs, those who are suffering a lack of urination, those who have peptic ulcers or colitis, those who are in a state of depression, and those who are about to undergo electroshock therapy. Consult your doctor immediately if this drug has been prescribed for you and you have any of these conditions.
Warnings: This drug should be used cautiously by people who have liver or kidney diseases, bronchial asthma, gallstones, diabetes, and gout; and by pregnant or nursing women. Be sure your doctor knows if you have any of these conditions. A doctor should probably not prescribe a combination product like this as the first choice in the treatment of high blood pressure. The patient should receive each of the individual ingredients singly, and if response is adequate to the fixed components contained in this product, it can then be substituted. The advantage of a "fixed dose" combination product is based on increased convenience to the patient. • This product interacts with amphetamine, colestipol hydrochloride, decongestants, digitalis, levodopa, lithium carbonate, monoamine oxidase inhibitors, oral antidiabetics, quinidine, and steroids; if you are currently taking any drugs of these types, consult your doctor about their use. If you are unsure of the type or contents of your medications, ask your doctor or pharmacist. • This drug may add to the effect of other antihypertensive drugs. If you are taking more than one drug to control your blood pressure, your dosages may need adjustment. Consult your doctor. • This drug may cause or worsen bronchial asthma, liver and kidney diseases, allergy, and depression. • Persons taking this drug should have blood tests to monitor levels of sodium, potassium, and calcium. • This drug can cause potassium loss. • This drug may affect thyroid tests, anesthesia, and responsiveness to surgical muscle relaxants. Be sure that your doctor knows that you are taking this drug. • While taking this drug, do not take any nonprescription item for cough, cold, or sinus problems without first consulting your doctor. • This drug may cause drowsiness; avoid tasks that require alertness. • To prevent oversedation and/or light-headedness, avoid the use of alcohol and other sedative drugs while taking this product. • Persons taking this product and digitalis should watch carefully for symptoms of increased digitalis toxicity (e.g., nausea, blurred vision, palpitations). • Reserpine causes cancer in rats. It has not been shown to cause cancer in humans.

444

Comments: Take this drug with food or milk at the same time each day. •
The effects of this drug may not be apparent for at least two weeks. Mild side
effects (e.g., nasal congestion) are most noticeable during the first two weeks
of therapy and become less bothersome after this period. • To avoid dizziness or light-headedness when you stand, contract and relax the muscles
of your legs for a few moments before rising. Do this by pushing one foot
against the floor while raising the other foot slightly, alternating feet so that
you are "pumping" your legs in a pedaling motion. • To help avoid potassium
loss, take this drug with a glass of fresh or frozen orange juice, or eat a
banana each day. The use of Co-Salt salt substitute helps prevent potassium
loss.

**Hydroquin steroid hormone and anti-infective (Robinson
Laboratory, Inc.),** see Vioform-Hydrocortisone steroid hormone
and anti-infective.

Hydroserp diuretic and antihypertensive (various manufacturers),
see Hydropres diuretic and antihypertensive.

Hydroserpine diuretic and antihypertensive (various manufacturers),
see Hydropres diuretic and antihypertensive.

Hydrotensin diuretic and antihypertensive (Mayrand, Inc.), see
Hydropres diuretic and antihypertensive.

Hydro-Z-50 diuretic and antihypertensive (Mayrand, Inc.), see
hydrochlorothiazide diuretic and antihypertensive.

R̽   Hygroton diuretic and antihypertensive

Manufacturer: USV Laboratories Inc.
Ingredient: chlorthalidone
Dosage Form: Tablet: 25 mg (peach); 50 mg (aqua); 100 mg (white)
Use: Treatment of high blood pressure and removal of fluid from body
tissues
Minor Side Effects: Constipation; cramping; diarrhea; headache; itching;
loss of appetite; nausea; numbness or tingling in fingers and toes; rash
Major Side Effects: Dizziness; elevated blood sugar; impotence; muscle
spasms; restlessness; sore throat; weakness
Contraindications: This drug should not be taken by persons suffering
from anuria (inability to urinate). This drug should not be taken by people who
are allergic to it or to sulfa drugs. Consult your doctor immediately if this
drug has been prescribed for you and you have anuria or such an allergy.
Warnings: This drug should be used with caution in persons with kidney
disease, liver disease, allergies, or asthma. Be sure your doctor knows if you
have any of these conditions. • This drug should be used with caution, since
it may cause low blood levels of potassium, gout, and diabetes. • Use of this
drug may affect thyroid tests. • Use of this drug requires the periodic taking
of lab tests. • This drug may add to the actions of other blood pressure drugs.
This drug interacts with colestipol hydrochloride, digitalis, lithium carbonate,
oral antidiabetics, steroids, and tubocurarine. If you are currently taking any
drugs of these types, consult your doctor about their use. If you are unsure of
the type or contents of your medications, ask your doctor or pharmacist. •
This drug should be used cautiously in pregnant women and by nursing
mothers.
Comments: This drug causes frequent urination. Expect this effect; it
should not alarm you. • This drug can cause potassium loss. To help avoid

potassium loss, take this drug with a glass of fresh or frozen orange juice. You may also eat a banana each day. The use of a salt substitute helps prevent potassium loss. • Try not to take this drug at bedtime. • While taking this drug, as with many drugs that lower blood pressure, you should limit your consumption of alcoholic beverages in order to prevent dizziness or light-headedness. • To avoid dizziness or light-headedness when you stand, contract and relax the muscles of your legs for a few moments before rising. Do this by pushing one foot against the floor while raising the other foot slightly, alternating feet so that you are "pumping" your legs in a pedaling motion. • Persons taking this drug and digitalis should watch carefully for signs of increased toxicity (e.g., nausea, blurred vision, palpitations), and notify their doctors immediately if symptoms occur. • If you are allergic to a sulfa drug, you may likewise be allergic to this drug. • If you have high blood pressure, do not take any nonprescription item for cough, cold, or sinus problems without first checking with your doctor.

Hyosophen sedative and anticholinergic (Rugby Laboratories), see Donnatal sedative and anticholinergic.

Hysone steroid hormone and anti-infective (Mallard Incorporated), see Vioform-Hydrocortisone steroid hormone and anti-infective.

ICN 65 Compound analgesic (ICN Pharmaceuticals, Inc.), see Darvon Compound-65 analgesic.

Ilosone antibiotic (Dista Products Company), see erythromycin antibiotic.

Ilotycin antibiotic (Dista Products Company), see erythromycin antibiotic.

Imavate antidepressant (A. H. Robins Company), see Tofranil antidepressant.

R_X   **Inderal beta blocker**

Manufacturer: Ayerst Laboratories
Ingredient: propranolol hydrochloride
Dosage Form: Tablet: 10 mg (peach); 20 mg (blue); 40 mg (green); 80 mg (yellow)
Use: Treatment of angina pectoris, certain heart arrhythmias, high blood pressure; prevention of migraine headaches
Minor Side Effects: Abdominal cramps; constipation; diarrhea; insomnia; nausea; vomiting
Major Side Effects: Dizziness; low blood pressure; rash; shortness of breath; sore throat; tingling in fingers or toes; visual disturbances
Contraindications: This drug should not be used by persons with bronchial asthma, severe hay fever, or certain types of heart disease. Be sure your doctor knows if you have any of these conditions. • This drug should not be used with monoamine oxidase inhibitors, or during the two-week withdrawal period from such drugs. If you are currently taking any drugs of this type, consult your doctor about their use. If you are unsure of the type or contents of your medications, ask your doctor or pharmacist.
Warnings: This drug should be used with caution in persons with certain respiratory problems, diabetes, certain heart problems, liver and kidney diseases, or thyroid disease. Be sure your doctor knows if you have any of these conditions. • This drug should be used cautiously by pregnant women and by

women of childbearing age. • This drug should be used with care during anesthesia and in patients undergoing major surgery. This drug should be withdrawn 48 hours prior to surgery. • This drug should be used cautiously when reserpine is taken.

Comments: This drug is a potent medication, and it should not be stopped abruptly. Deaths from heart attacks have occurred when the medication was stopped suddenly. • Your doctor may want you to take your pulse every day while you take this medication. Consult your doctor. • This drug may cause drowsiness; avoid tasks that require alertness. • Be sure to take your medication doses at the same time each day. • While taking this drug, do not take any nonprescription item for cough, cold, or sinus problems without first checking with your doctor. • The action of this drug is similar to Lopressor beta blocker.

℞ Indocin anti-inflammatory

Manufacturer: Merck Sharp & Dohme
Ingredient: indomethacin
Dosage Form: Capsule: 25 mg; 50 mg (both are blue/white)
Use: Reduction of pain, redness, and swelling due to arthritis
Minor Side Effects: Constipation; diarrhea; dizziness; drowsiness; headache; nausea; rash; ringing in ears; vomiting
Major Side Effects: Blood in stools, urine, or mouth; blurred vision; fatigue; fluid retention; high blood pressure; itching; jaundice; paleness; severe abdominal pain; sore throat; weight gain
Contraindications: This drug should not be used by people who are allergic to it. Consult your doctor immediately if this drug has been prescribed for you and you have such an allergy. • This drug should not be used by persons with nasal polyps associated with a severe allergic reaction to aspirin or other nonsteroidal anti-inflammatory drugs. If you have this condition or such a history and this drug has been prescribed for you, consult your doctor immediately.
Warnings: The lowest dose possible of this drug should be prescribed. Increased dosage tends to increase adverse effects. • Careful instructions to, and observations of, the individual patient are essential to the prevention of serious adverse reactions. • This drug should be used with extreme caution in the elderly, in children 14 years old and under, in pregnant women, in nursing mothers, in epileptics, and in persons with infections, Parkinson's disease, ulcers, bleeding diseases, or psychiatric illness. Be sure your doctor knows if you have any of these conditions. • This drug has been known to cause corneal deposits and retinal disturbances after long-term therapy. Report any visual disturbances to your doctor immediately. Thorough, periodic eye examinations are desirable in persons undergoing long-term therapy with this drug. • This drug may mask the usual signs and symptoms of infection. • This drug can inhibit coagulation of blood, thus prolonging bleeding time; persons with coagulation defects, and those taking anticoagulant drugs must use this drug with caution. • This drug interacts with aspirin, oral anticoagulants, probenecid, steroids, and furosemide. If you are currently taking any drugs of these types, consult your doctor about their use. If you are unsure about the type or contents of your medications, ask your doctor or pharmacist. • This drug may cause drowsiness; avoid tasks requiring alertness, such as driving a motor vehicle. • If any severe adverse reactions to this drug occur, notify your doctor immediately.
Comments: This drug is a potent pain killer and is not intended for general aches and pains. • Regular checkups by the doctor, including blood tests, are required of persons taking this drug. • This drug must be taken with food or

milk, immediately after meals, or with antacids. Never take this drug on an empty stomach or with aspirin or alcohol. • If you are taking an anticoagulant ("blood thinner"), remind your doctor. • This drug may cause discoloration of the urine or feces. If you notice a change in color, call your doctor. • It may take a month before you feel the full effect of this drug.

OTC   Infra-Rub external analgesic

Manufacturer: Whitehall Laboratories
Ingredients: glycol monosalicylate; histamine dihydrochloride; lanolin; methyl nicotinate; capsicum oleoresin
Dosage Form: Cream: histamine dihydrochloride, 0.1%; oleoresin capsicum, 0.4%
Use: Used externally for temporary relief of pain in muscles and other areas
Side Effects: Allergic reactions (rash, itching, soreness); local irritation
Warnings: If you have diabetes or impaired circulation, use this product only upon the advice of a physician. • Use this product externally only. • Do not use on broken or irritated skin or on large areas of the body; avoid contact with eyes. • When using this product avoid exposure to direct sunlight, heat lamp, or sunlamp. • Before using this product on children under 12 years of age, consult your doctor. • If the condition persists, call your doctor.
Comments: Be sure to rub this product well into skin.

Rx   insulin antidiabetic

Manufacturer: various manufacturers
Equivalent Products: This drug is usually prescribed by strength rather than by trade name.
Dosage Forms: This drug is available only as an injectable. Various types of insulin provide different times of onset and duration of action. The types of insulin and their times of onset and duration are as follows:

	Onset (hr.)	Duration (hr.)
regular insulin	1/2	6
insulin zinc suspension, prompt	1/2	14
isophane insulin (NPH)	1	24
insulin zinc suspension	1	24
globin zinc insulin	2	24
protamine zinc insulin (PZI)	6	36
insulin zinc suspension, extended	6	36

Use: Treatment of diabetes mellitus
Minor Side Effects: Low blood sugar level
Major Side Effects: No major side effects when used as directed
Warnings: This drug should only be used under the direction of a doctor, and a prescribed diet should be followed precisely. • Do not substitute one type of this drug for another. Stick to your prescribed type. • When using this drug, be on guard for signs of low blood sugar. Your doctor will instruct you on what to watch for. • This drug interacts with guanethidine, monoamine oxidase inhibitors, propranolol, steroids, tetracycline, and thyroid hormone. If you are currently taking any drugs of these types, consult your doctor about their use. If you are unsure of the type or contents of your medications, ask your doctor or pharmacist.
Comments: This drug is stored in the refrigerator in the pharmacy, but once the bottle has been opened, most forms (except U-500 strength) may be kept at room temperature for the normal life of the vial. • This drug comes in various strengths, currently U-40, U-100, and U-500. Eventually, U-40 will be taken off the market, and insulin strength will be less confusing. Until then, be sure to buy the right strength of the drug and the right syringes. • Purchase dis-

posable syringes if possible and remember to dispose of them properly. Once you have started using a particular brand of disposable insulin syringe and needle, do not switch brands without first talking with your doctor. A dosage error may occur. • Special injection kits are available for blind diabetics. Ask your doctor for help in obtaining them. • Doses of this drug may be prepared in advance. Ask your pharmacist for advice. • Most insulin products are composed of a mixture of both pork and beef insulins. However, products are available that contain all beef insulin or all pork insulin. Never switch from one form to another unless your doctor tells you to do so. • Thoroughly blend insulin before withdrawing a dose in the syringe. • While taking this drug, do not take any nonprescription item for cough, cold, or sinus problems without first checking with your doctor. • Injection sites for this drug should be rotated using various parts of the body. It is important that this be done. Be sure to follow your doctor's instructions carefully.

OTC Intercept Contraceptive Inserts

Manufacturer: Ortho Pharmaceutical Corporation
Ingredient: nonoxynol-9
Dosage Form: Vaginal insert: 100 mg
Use: Prevention of pregnancy
Side Effects: Allergy; local irritation (user or partner)
Comments: This product can be inserted with or without the special applicator. • To ensure that the medication is fully dispersed, wait at least ten minutes after inserting this product before having intercourse. • Insert a new dose of contraceptive for each intercourse. • Do not douche for six to eight hours after intercourse. • This product is not as effective used alone as when it is combined with a diaphragm.

OTC iodine tincture

Manufacturer: various manufacturers
Ingredients: alcohol; iodine; sodium iodide
Dosage Form: Liquid: iodine, 2%; sodium iodide, 2.5%; alcohol, at least 50%
Use: To disinfect minor burns, cuts, and scrapes
Side Effects: Blistering; burning; itching; weeping; stinging. (If large doses are swallowed, may cause abdominal cramping, nausea, diarrhea and vomiting; delirium; fever; shock; thirst or metallic taste in the mouth; and death.)
Warnings: Do not swallow this product. • Keep this product out of the reach of children. • Do not get this product in the eyes or use on mucous membranes.
Comments: Do not use any iodine product stronger than a 2-percent solution. The stronger solutions have no additional benefits, but are more toxic.

Iodocort steroid hormone and anti-infective (Ulmer Pharmacal Company), see Vioform-Hydrocortisone steroid hormone and anti-infective.

Ionamin anorectic (Pennwalt Pharmaceutical Division), see Fastin anorectic.

OTC Ionax Foam acne preparation

Manufacturer: Owen Laboratories
Ingredients: benzalkonium chloride; owenethers (polyoxyethylene ethers), soapless surfactant

Dosage Form: Aerosol spray: benzalkonium chloride, 0.2% (quantities of other ingredients not specified)
Use: Treatment of acne
Side Effects: Allergy; local irritation
Warnings: Do not get product in or near the eyes.
Comments: If the condition worsens, stop using this product and call your pharmacist. • Wash area gently with warm water and pat dry before applying this product. • Avoid exposure to heat lamps, sunlamps, or direct sunlight when using this preparation. • Spray is lemon scented.

OTC   Ionax Scrub acne preparation

Manufacturer: Owen Laboratories
Ingredients: alcohol; benzalkonium chloride in a special base; owenethers (polyoxyethylene ethers); polyethylene granules
Dosage Form: Abradant cleanser: alcohol, 10% (quantities of other ingredients not specified)
Use: Treatment of acne
Side Effects: Allergy; local irritation
Warnings: Do not get product in or near the eyes.
Comments: If the condition worsens, stop using this product and call your pharmacist. • Wash area gently with warm water and pat dry before applying this product. • Avoid exposure to heat lamps, sunlamps, or direct sunlight when using this preparation. • Cleanser is lime scented. • This product is to be used instead of soap. Apply to wet face and massage in skin for one to two minutes.

Iosel 250 seborrheic shampoo (Owen Drug Company), see Selsun seborrheic shampoo.

I-PAC analgesic and sedative (Spencer-Mead, Inc.), see Fiorinal analgesic and sedative.

OTC   ipecac syrup

Manufacturer: various manufacturers
Ingredient: ipecac
Dosage Form: Liquid
Use: To induce vomiting (emesis) following poisoning
Side Effects: Abdominal cramping; nausea; vomiting. Rarely, heart damage and impaired muscular movements occur.
Warnings: Before administering ipecac syrup, call your doctor, pharmacist, or Poison Control Center for instructions. • Do not try to induce vomiting if the victim is unconscious; this could result in choking and death. • Do not use the fluid extract form of ipecac. It is 14 times stronger than ipecac syrup and may cause severe toxicity.
Comments: Give one or two glasses of water to a child and two or three glasses of water to an adult before or immediately after giving ipecac syrup. One teaspoon of ipecac syrup usually is given to a child; one tablespoonful usually is given to an adult. • Vomiting should occur in about 15 minutes. If it does not, the dose can be repeated once, 15 to 30 minutes after the first dose. • Ipecac syrup must be readily available in case of an emergency; purchase a bottle now and keep it handy.

Isollyl analgesic and sedative (Rugby Laboratories), see Fiorinal analgesic and sedative.

Rx   isoniazid antitubercular

Manufacturer: various manufacturers
Ingredient: isonicotinic acid hydrazide (INH)
Equivalent Products: Laniazid, The Lannett Company, Inc.; Niconyl, Parke-Davis; Nydrazid, E. R. Squibb & Sons; Panazid, Panray Division
Dosage Form: Tablet: 50 mg; 100 mg; 300 mg (various colors)
Use: Treatment and prevention of tuberculosis
Minor Side Effects: Abdominal pain; nausea; vomiting
Major Side Effects: Blood disorders; darkening of the urine; chills; fatal hepatitis; fever; hyperglycemia; jaundice; liver damage; malaise; memory impairment; numbness and tingling of fingers and toes; pellagra; skin eruptions; toxic psychosis; vitamin-B_6 deficiency; weakness
Contraindications: This drug should not be taken by people who have had previous liver damage resulting from isoniazid therapy. This drug should not be taken by people who have had severe adverse reactions to it, such as drug fever, chills, arthritis. Make sure your doctor knows if you have had such reactions. • This drug should not be taken by people who have acute liver disease from any cause. Be sure your doctor knows if you have this condition.
Warnings: Persons undergoing therapy with this drug should have their eyes examined before and during its use. • This drug should be used with caution by pregnant women and nursing mothers. • The use of this drug should be discontinued at the first sign of hypersensitivity to it. • This drug should be used cautiously by people with kidney disease. Be sure your doctor is aware of your having this condition. • This drug should not be taken with aluminum-containing antacids, phenytoin, or aminosalicylic acid (PAS). If you are currently taking drugs of these types, consult your doctor about their use. If you are unsure about the type or contents of your medications, ask your doctor or pharmacist. • This drug should not be taken with daily ingestion of alcohol. • Vitamin B_6 (pyridoxine) should be taken each day while taking this drug to help reduce the incidence of side effects.
Comments: This drug is also referred to as INH. • This drug must be taken for long periods (months to years) to assure that the tuberculosis organism is completely eradicated. Do not discontinue therapy, except on the advice of your doctor. • Doses of this drug should not be skipped. This drug should be taken on an empty stomach, at least one hour before or two hours after meals. • Consult your doctor if any of the major side effects listed are observed. • This drug has been reported to induce lung tumors in a number of strains of mice.

Rx   Isopto Carpine ophthalmic solution

Manufacturer: Alcon Labs, Inc.
Ingredient: pilocarpine hydrochloride
Equivalent Products: Adsorbocarpine, Burton, Parsons & Company, Inc.; Almocarpine, Ayerst Laboratories; Mi-Pilo, Barnes-Hines Pharmaceuticals, Inc.; Mistura P, Lederle Laboratories; Pilocar, Smith, Miller & Patch; pilocarpine hydrochloride, various manufacturers; Pilomiotin, Smith, Miller & Patch; P.V. Carpine Liquifilm, Allergan Pharmaceuticals
Dosage Forms: Drops: 0.25%, 0.5%, 1%, 1.5%, 2%, 3%, 4%, 5%, 6%, 8%, 10%. Ocular therapeutic system (see Comments): 20 mcg, 40 mcg
Use: Treatment of glaucoma
Minor Side Effects: Blurred vision; brow-ache; loss of night vision
Contraindications: This drug should not be used by people who are allergic to pilocarpine. Consult your doctor immediately if this drug has been prescribed for you and you have such an allergy.
Warnings: Be careful about the contamination of solutions used for the

eyes. Wash your hands before administering eyedrops. Do not touch the dropper to your eye. Do not wash or wipe the dropper before replacing it in the bottle. Close the bottle tightly to keep out moisture.

Comments: To administer eyedrops, lie or sit down and tilt your head back. Carefully pull your lower eyelid down to form a pouch. Hold the dropper close to, but not touching, the eyelid, and place the prescribed number of drops into the pouch. Do not place the drops directly on the eyeball; you probably will blink and lose the medication. Close your eye and keep it shut for a few moments. • This drug may sting when first administered; this sensation usually goes away quickly. • Like other eyedrops, this drug may cause some clouding or blurring of vision. This side effect will go away quickly. • The ocular therapeutic system mentioned is an oval ring of plastic that contains pilocarpine. This ring is placed in the eye, and the drug is released gradually over a period of seven days. Use of these rings has made possible the control of glaucoma for some patients. If you are having trouble controlling glaucoma, ask your doctor about the possibility of using one of these devices.

OTC   Isopto-Frin eyedrops

Manufacturer: Alcon Laboratories
Ingredients: benzethonium chloride; hydroxypropyl methylcellulose; phenylephrine hydrochloride; sodium biphosphate; sodium citrate; sodium phosphate
Dosage Form: Drop: hydroxypropyl methylcellulose, 0.5%; phenylephrine hydrochloride, 0.12% (quantities of other ingredients not specified)
Use: Relief from minor eye irritation
Side Effects: Allergic reactions (rash, itching, soreness); local irritation; momentary blurred vision
Contraindications: Do not use this product if you have glaucoma.
Warnings: Do not use this product for more than two days without checking with your doctor.
Comments: Do not touch the dropper or bottle top to the eye or other tissue because contamination of the solution may result. • The use of more than one eye product at a time may cause severe irritation to the eye. Consult your pharmacist before doing so.

OTC   Isopto Plain artificial tears

Manufacturer: Alcon Laboratories
Ingredients: benzalkonium chloride; hydroxypropyl methylcellulose
Dosage Form: Drop: benzalkonium chloride, 0.01%; hydroxypropyl methylcellulose, 0.5%
Use: Lubricates dry eyes
Side Effects: Momentary blurred vision
Comments: Do not touch the dropper or bottle top to the eye or other tissue because contamination of the solution may result. • The use of more than one eye product at a time may cause severe irritation to the eye. Consult your pharmacist before doing so.

℞   Isordil antianginal

Manufacturer: Ives Laboratories, Inc.
Ingredient: isosorbide dinitrate
Equivalent Products: isosorbide dinitrate, various manufacturers; Isotrate Timecelles, W. E. Hauck, Inc.; Sorate, Trimen Laboratories; Sorbide, Mayrand, Inc.; Sorbitrate, Stuart Pharmaceuticals; Vasotrate, Reid-Provident Laboratories, Inc.

Dosage Forms: Chewable tablet: 10 mg (yellow). Sublingual tablet: 2.5 mg (yellow); 5 mg (pink). Sustained-action capsule: 40 mg (blue/clear with beads). Sustained-action tablet (green). Tablet: 5 mg (pink); 10 mg (white); 20 mg (green); 30 mg (blue)

Use: Prevention (tablet and capsule) and relief (chewable and sublingual tablet) of chest pain due to heart disease

Minor Side Effects: Dizziness; flushing; headache; nausea; vomiting

Major Side Effects: Low blood pressure; palpitations; rash; weakness

Contraindications: This drug should not be taken by people allergic to it. Consult your doctor immediately if this drug has been prescribed for you and you have such an allergy.

Warnings: Alcoholic beverages should be avoided or used with caution, as they may enhance the severity of this drug's side effects. • This drug interacts with nitroglycerin; if you are currently using nitroglycerin, consult your doctor about its use. • Before using this drug to relieve chest pain, be certain pain arises from the heart and is not due to a muscle spasm or to indigestion. • If your chest pain is not relieved by use of this drug, if pain arises from a different location or differs in severity, consult your doctor immediately.

Comments: Although the sublingual and chewable tablets are effective in relieving chest pain, there is some question about the effectiveness of the other forms in preventing pain. Carefully discuss the possible benefits of this drug with your doctor before purchasing it. • With continued use, you may develop a tolerance to this drug; many adverse side effects disappear after two to three weeks of drug use, but you may also become less responsive to the drug's beneficial effects. • The chewable tablets must be chewed to release the medication they contain. • The sustained-action forms must be swallowed whole. • To take a sublingual tablet properly, place the tablet under your tongue, close your mouth, and hold the saliva in your mouth and under your tongue as long as you can before swallowing it. If you have a bitter taste in your mouth after five minutes, the drug has not been completely absorbed. Wait five more minutes before drinking water. • To avoid dizziness or light-headedness when you stand, contract and relax the muscles of your legs for a few moments before rising. Do this by pushing one foot against the floor while raising the other foot slightly, alternating feet.

Isotrate Timecelles antianginal (W. E. Hauck, Inc.), see Isordil antianginal.

OTC   Ivy Dry Cream poison ivy remedy

Manufacturer: Ivy Corp.

Ingredients: benzocaine; camphor; isopropyl alcohol; menthol; methylparaben; propylparaben; tannic acid

Dosage Form: Cream: alcohol, 7.5%; tannic acid, 8% (quantities of other ingredients not specified)

Use: Relief of itching due to poison ivy and poison oak

Side Effects: Allergic reactions (rash, itching, soreness); local irritation

Comments: To prevent irritation and secondary infection, avoid scratching. • Before applying medication, soak the area in warm water or apply towels soaked in water for five to ten minutes. Dry area gently; apply medication.

Janimine antidepressant (Abbott Laboratories), see Tofranil antidepressant.

Jen-Diril diuretic and antihypertensive (Jenkins Laboratories, Inc.), see hydrochlorothiazide diuretic and antihypertensive.

J-Gan-VC expectorant (J. Pharmacal Co.), see Phenergan VC expectorant.

OTC   Johnson & Johnson Medicated Powder rash remedy

Manufacturer: Johnson & Johnson Products, Incorporated
Ingredients: fragrance; menthol; talc; zinc oxide
Dosage Form: Powder (quantities of ingredients not specified)
Use: For keeping baby skin dry; soothing diaper rash, prickly heat, and chafing
Side Effects: Allergy; local irritation
Comments: While using this product, be careful not to inhale any of the powder.

OTC   Johnson's Baby Cream rash remedy

Manufacturer: Johnson & Johnson Products, Incorporated
Ingredients: ceresin; glyceryl stearate; lanolin; mineral oil; paraffin; sodium borate; white beeswax
Dosage Form: Cream (quantities of ingredients not specified)
Use: Relief of baby diaper rash
Side Effects: Allergy; local irritation

OTC   Johnson's Baby Powder rash remedy

Manufacturer: Johnson & Johnson Products, Incorporated
Ingredients: fragrance; talc
Dosage Form: Powder (quantities of ingredients not specified)
Use: For keeping baby skin dry; soothing diaper rash, prickly heat, and chafing
Comments: While using this product, be careful not to inhale any of the powder.

Kaochlor-Eff potassium chloride replacement (Warren-Teed Laboratories), see potassium chloride replacement.

Kaochlor potassium chloride replacement (Warren-Teed Laboratories), see potassium chloride replacement.

Kaon-Cl potassium chloride replacement (Warren-Teed Laboratories), see potassium chloride replacement.

OTC Kaopectate, Kaopectate Concentrate diarrhea remedies

Manufacturer: The Upjohn Company
Ingredients: kaolin; pectin
Dosage Forms: Liquid (content per ounce): kaolin, 90 grains; pectin, 2 grains. Concentrate (content per ounce): kaolin, 135 grains; pectin, 3 grains
Use: For treatment of common diarrhea
Side Effects: Constipation after long-term use (seven days to two months)
Contraindications: This product or any other product for diarrhea should not be used to self-medicate without first consulting a doctor if the person is under age three or over age 60, has a history of asthma, heart disease, peptic ulcer, or is pregnant.
Comments: Diarrhea should stop in two to three days. If it persists longer, recurs frequently or in presence of high fever, call your doctor and be sure to tell him of any drugs you are taking. • Be sure to drink at least eight glasses

454

of water each day. • If you are taking other drugs, do not take this product until you have first checked with your doctor or pharmacist.

Kavrin smooth muscle relaxant (Hyrex Pharmaceuticals), see Pavabid Plateau Caps smooth muscle relaxant.

Kay Ciel potassium chloride replacement (Berlex Laboratories, Inc.), see potassium chloride replacement.

KEFF potassium chloride replacement (Lemmon Company), see potassium chloride replacement.

R̥   Keflex antibiotic

Manufacturer: Eli Lilly and Company
Ingredient: cephalexin
Dosage Forms: Capsule: 250 mg (white/dark green); 500 mg (light green/dark green). Drop (content per ml): 100 mg. Liquid (content per 5 ml, or one teaspoon): 125 mg; 250 mg. Tablet: 1 gm (green)
Use: Treatment of bacterial infections
Minor Side Effects: Abdominal pain; diarrhea; dizziness; fatigue; headache; itching; nausea; vomiting
Major Side Effects: "Black tongue"; cough; irritation of the mouth; rash; rectal and vaginal itching; severe diarrhea; superinfection
Contraindications: This drug should not be used by people who are allergic to it or other antibiotics in the cephalosporin group. Consult your doctor immediately if this drug has been prescribed for you and you have such an allergy.
Warnings: This drug should be used with extreme caution in persons with hypersensitivity to penicillin. Be sure your doctor knows if you have such hypersensitivity. • This drug should be used cautiously in patients with a history of any allergy. Be sure your doctor knows about any allergies that you have. • This drug should be used with caution during pregnancy. • Prolonged use of this drug may result in secondary infection. • This drug should be administered with caution to persons with kidney disease. Under such conditions, careful clinical observation and laboratory studies should be made because safe dosage may be lower than that usually recommended.
Comments: Although the medical and pharmaceutical literature contains many different opinions, general consensus is that about 10 percent of all persons who are allergic to penicillin will also be allergic to an antibiotic like this drug. This drug is frequently prescribed for many infections for which penicillin is adequate. For example, penicillin is the usual drug of choice for treatment of a strep throat, even though Keflex antibiotic may be prescribed. Ask your doctor if you really need this drug, or if you could take penicillin, which is less expensive. • This drug should be taken for at least ten full days, even if symptoms have disappeared within that time. • Diabetics using Clinitest urine-testing product may get a false high sugar reading. Change to Clinistix urine-testing product or Tes-Tape urine-testing product to avoid this problem. • Take this drug on an empty stomach (one hour before or two hours after a meal). The liquid form of this drug should be stored in the refrigerator.

Kemadrin antiparkinson drug (Burroughs Wellcome), see Artane antiparkinson drug.

Kenacort steroid hormone (E. R. Squibb & Sons), see Aristocort steroid hormone.

Kenalog steroid hormone

℞

Manufacturer: E. R. Squibb & Sons, Inc.

Ingredient: triamcinolone acetonide

Equivalent Products: Aristocort, Lederle Laboratories; triamcinolone acetonide, various manufacturers

Dosage Forms: Cream (content per gram): 0.25 mg; 1 mg; 5 mg. Lotion (content per ml): 0.25 mg; 1 mg. Ointment (content per gram): 0.25 mg; 1 mg; 5 mg. Spray (content per gram): 0.147 mg

Use: Relief of skin inflammation associated with conditions such as eczema or poison ivy

Minor Side Effects: Burning sensation; dryness; irritation of affected area; itching; rash

Major Side Effects: Secondary infection

Contraindications: This drug should not be taken by people who are allergic to it. Consult your doctor immediately if this drug is prescribed for you and you have such an allergy.

Warnings: If irritation develops when using this drug, immediately discontinue its use and notify your doctor. • If extensive areas are treated or if an occlusive bandage is used, there will be increased systemic absorption of this drug and suitable precautions should be taken, particularly in children and infants. • This drug is not for use in the eyes. • When the spray form of this drug is used about the face, the eyes should be covered and inhalation of the spray should be avoided. • This drug should be used cautiously with pregnant women.

Comments: The spray form of this drug produces a cooling sensation, which may be uncomfortable for some persons. • If the affected area is extremely dry or is scaling, the skin may be moistened before applying the product by soaking in water or by applying water with a clean cloth. The ointment form is probably the better product for dry skin. • Do not use the drug with an occlusive wrap of transparent plastic film unless directed to do so by your doctor. • If it is necessary for you to use this drug under a wrap, follow your doctor's instructions exactly; do not leave the wrap in place longer than specified. • Aristogel gel and Aristoderm lotion, manufactured by Lederle Laboratories, are—for all practical purposes—the same as this drug.

Kestrin estrogen hormone (Hyrex Pharmaceuticals), see Premarin estrogen hormone.

KLOR-CON potassium chloride replacement (Upsher-Smith Laboratories, Inc.), see potassium chloride replacement.

Kloride potassium chloride replacement (Amfre-Grant, Inc.), see potassium chloride replacement.

K-Lor potassium chloride replacement (Abbott Laboratories), see potassium chloride replacement.

KLOR potassium chloride replacement (Upsher-Smith Laboratories, Inc.), see potassium chloride replacement.

Klorvess potassium chloride replacement (Dorsey Laboratories), see potassium chloride replacement.

K-Lyte/Cl potassium chloride replacement (Mead Johnson Pharmaceutical Division), see potassium chloride replacement.

K-Lyte DS potassium replacement (Mead Johnson Pharmaceutical Division), see K-Lyte potassium replacement.

℞   K-Lyte potassium replacement

Manufacturer: Mead Johnson Pharmaceutical Division
Ingredients: potassium bicarbonate; potassium citrate
Dosage Form: Effervescent tablet: 25 mEq (lime or orange flavored)
Use: Prevention or treatment of potassium deficiency
Minor Side Effects: Abdominal discomfort; diarrhea; nausea; vomiting
Major Side Effects: Confusion; numbness or tingling in the arms or legs
Contraindications: This drug should not be taken by people with severe kidney disease, Addison's disease, or high blood potassium. Consult your doctor immediately if this drug has been prescribed for you and you have any of these conditions.
Warnings: Supplements of potassium should be administered with caution, since the amount of potassium deficiency may be difficult to determine accurately. • Potassium intoxication rarely occurs in patients with normal kidney function. • This drug should be given cautiously to digitalized patients and such patients should be monitored by ECG for heart problems.
Comments: Patients should carefully dissolve each dose completely in the stated amount of water. Do not take this tablet whole. • Potassium supplements usually have a low rate of patient compliance. If a potassium product is prescribed, be sure to take the medication as directed and do not stop taking it without first consulting your doctor. • This drug should be taken with meals. • Consult your doctor about using salt substitutes instead of this drug; they are similar, less expensive, and more convenient. Another product, K-Lyte DS, is identical to K-Lyte, except it is twice the strength.

OTC   Kolantyl antacid

Manufacturer: Merrell-National Laboratories
Ingredients: aluminum hydroxide; magnesium oxide
Dosage Forms: Gel (content per teaspoon): aluminum hydroxide, 150 mg; magnesium hydroxide, 150 mg. Tablet: aluminum hydroxide, 300 mg; magnesium oxide, 185 mg. Wafer: aluminum hydroxide, 180 mg; magnesium hydroxide, 170 mg
Use: Relief from acid indigestion, heartburn, sour stomach and/or hyperacidity associated with such conditions as peptic ulcer and hiatal hernia
Side Effects: Abdominal discomfort; constipation; diarrhea; dizziness; mouth irritation; nausea; rash; vomiting
Contraindications: Persons with kidney disease should not use this product. In persons with kidney disease, repeated daily use of this product may cause nausea, vomiting, depressed reflexes, and breathing difficulties.
Warnings: Long-term (several weeks) use of this product may lead to intestinal obstruction and dehydration. • Phosphate depletion may occur leading to weakness, loss of appetite, and eventually bone pain. This may be prevented by drinking at least one glass of milk a day.
Comments: Self-treatment of severe or repeated attacks of heartburn, indigestion, or upset stomach is not recommended. If you do self-treat, limit therapy to two weeks, then call your doctor if your symptoms persist. Never self-medicate with this product if your symptoms occur regularly (two to three times or more a month); if they are particularly worse than normal; if you feel a "tightness" in your chest, have chest pains, or are sweating; or if you

are short of breath. Consult your doctor. • To prevent constipation, drink at least eight glasses of water a day. If constipation persists, consult your doctor or pharmacist. • This product works best when taken one hour after meals or at bedtime, unless otherwise directed by your doctor or pharmacist. • The liquid form of this product is superior to the tablet form and should be used unless you have been specifically directed to use the tablet. Do not take this product within two hours of a dose of a tetracycline antibiotic. Also, if you are taking iron, a vitamin-mineral product, chlorpromazine, phenytoin, digoxin, quinidine, or warfarin, remind your doctor or pharmacist that you are taking this product.

OTC   Komed acne preparation

Manufacturer: Barnes-Hind Pharmaceuticals, Inc.
Ingredients: camphor; colloidal alumina; isopropyl alcohol; menthol; resorcinol; salicylic acid; sodium thiosulfate
Dosage Form: Lotion: isopropyl alcohol, 22%; resorcinol, 2%; salicyclic acid, 2%; sodium thiosulfate, 8% (quantities of other ingredients not specified)
Use: Treatment of acne
Side Effects: Allergy; local irritation
Warnings: Do not get product in or near the eyes.
Comments: This preparation may stain the skin. • If the condition worsens, stop using this product and call your pharmacist.

Korostatin antifungal agent (Holland-Rantos Company, Inc.), see Mycostatin antifungal agent.

K-Pava smooth muscle relaxant (Kay Pharmacal Company, Inc.), see Pavabid Plateau Caps smooth muscle relaxant.

K-Pen antibiotic (Kay Pharmacal Company, Inc.), see penicillin G antibiotic.

K-Phen with Codeine expectorant (Kay Pharmacal Company, Inc.), see Phenergan with Codeine expectorant.

K-10 potassium chloride replacement (H. R. Cenci Laboratories, Inc.), see potassium chloride replacement.

Rx   Kwell pediculocide and scabicide

Manufacturer: Reed & Carnrick
Ingredient: gamma benzene hexachloride (lindane)
Equivalent Product: Gamene, Barnes-Hind Pharmaceuticals, Inc.
Dosage Forms: Cream; Lotion; Shampoo (all 1% lindane)
Use: Elimination of crab lice, head lice, and their nits, and scabies
Minor Side Effects: Rash; skin irritation if product is improperly used
Major Side Effects: See "Warnings"
Contraindications: This drug should not be used by people who are allergic to it. Consult your doctor immediately if this drug has been prescribed for you and you have such an allergy.
Warnings: Side effects to this drug are rare if the directions for use are followed. However, convulsions and even death can result if the drug is swallowed or overused. If swallowed, do not take mineral oil; call your doctor or pharmacist immediately. • Do not use this drug with other skin products. • Special caution must be used in treating children, infants, and pregnant women with this drug.

Comments: Complete directions for the use of this drug are supplied by the manufacturers. Ask your pharmacist for these directions if he does not supply them. • Lice are easily transmitted from one person to another. All family members should be carefully examined. Personal items (clothing, towels) need only be machine-washed on the "hot" temperature cycle and dried. No unusual cleaning measures are required. Combs, brushes, and other such washable items may be cleaned with the shampoo form of this drug.

OTC   Lactinex diarrhea remedy

Manufacturer: Hynson, Westcott & Dunning
Ingredients: lactobacillus acidophilus; lactobacillus bulgaricus
Dosage Forms: Granules; Tablet (quantities of ingredients not specified)
Use: For treatment of common diarrhea and acute fever blisters and canker sores
Contraindications: This product or any other product for diarrhea should not be used to self-medicate without first consulting a doctor if the person is under age three or over age 60, has a history of asthma, heart disease, peptic ulcer, or is pregnant.
Comments: Diarrhea should stop in two to three days. If it persists longer, recurs frequently or in presence of high fever, call your doctor and be sure to tell him of any drugs you are taking. • Be sure to drink at least eight glasses of water each day. • The granules should be added to cereal, food, or milk before taking. • This product contains live bacteria that work to re-establish the normal bacteria in the intestine. While this diarrhea remedy is highly recommended by many doctors and pharmacists, several glasses of milk each day may work just as well. • Store this product in the refrigerator.

OTC   Lanacane hemorrhoidal preparation

Manufacturer: Combe Incorporated
Ingredients: benzocaine; chlorothymol; resorcinol; water washable base
Dosage Form: Cream: benzocaine, 5%; chlorothymol; resorcinol, 2%; water washable base
Use: Relief from rectal and vaginal itching and other irritated skin conditions
Warnings: Sensitization (continued itching and redness) may occur with long-term and repeated use.
Comments: Hemorrhoidal (pile) preparations relieve itching, reduce pain and inflammation, and check bleeding, but do not heal, dry up, or give lasting relief from hemorrhoids. • Certain ingredients in this product may cause an allergic reaction; do not use for longer than seven days at a time unless your doctor has advised you otherwise. • Never self-medicate for hemorrhoids if pain is continuous or throbbing, if bleeding or itching is excessive, or if you feel a large pressure within the rectum.

Laniazid antitubercular (The Lannett Company, Inc.), see isoniazid antitubercular.

Lanophyllin bronchodilator (The Lannett Company, Inc.), see Elixophyllin bronchodilator.

Lanophyllin-GG expectorant and smooth muscle relaxant (The Lannett Company, Inc.), see Quibron expectorant and smooth muscle relaxant.

Lanorinal analgesic and sedative (The Lannett Company, Inc.), see Fiorinal analgesic and sedative.

R_x   Lanoxin heart drug

Manufacturer: Burroughs Wellcome Co.

Ingredient: digoxin

Equivalent Products: digoxin, various manufacturers (see "Comments")

Dosage Forms: Elixir, pediatric (content per 1 cc): 0.05 mg. Tablet: 0.125 mg (yellow); 0.25 mg (white); 0.5 mg (green)

Use: To strengthen heartbeat and improve heart rhythm

Minor Side Effects: Diarrhea; nausea; vomiting

Major Side Effects: Loss of appetite; palpitations; visual disturbances (such as blurred or yellow vision)

Contraindications: People who have demonstrated a toxic reaction to any digitalis preparation, and people who are allergic to this drug should not take it; consult your doctor immediately if this drug has been prescribed for you and you have either of these conditions.

Warnings: This drug should be used cautiously by people who have kidney disease, potassium depletion, or calcium accumulation. Be sure your doctor knows if you have any of these conditions. • This drug should be used cautiously in infants. • Some people develop toxic reactions to this drug. If you suffer any side effects that are prolonged or especially bothersome, contact your doctor. • The elderly may have more side effects from this drug than younger people, and they should have regular checkups while taking it. • This drug interacts with aminoglycosides, antibiotics, amphotericin B, cholestyramine, colestipol hydrochloride, diuretics, phenylbutazone, propantheline, and propranolol; if you are currently taking any drugs of these types, consult your doctor about their use. If you are unsure of the type or contents of your medications, ask your doctor or pharmacist. • While taking this drug, do not take any nonprescription item for cough, cold, or sinus problems without first checking with your doctor. • This drug should never be used for weight loss.

Comments: The pharmacologic activity of the different brands of this drug varies widely due to how well the tablets dissolve in the stomach and bowels. Because of this variation it is important not to change brands of the drug without consulting your doctor. • Dosages of this drug must be carefully adjusted to the needs and responses of the individual patient. Your doctor may find it necessary to adjust your dosage of this drug frequently. • Your doctor may want you to take your pulse daily while you are using this drug. • Take this drug at the same time every day.

Lapav Graduals smooth muscle relaxant (Amfre-Grant, Inc.), see Pavabid Plateau Caps smooth muscle relaxant.

Larotid antibiotic (Roche Products, Inc.), see amoxicillin antibiotic.

R_x   Lasix diuretic and antihypertensive

Manufacturer: Hoechst-Roussel Pharmaceuticals Inc.

Ingredient: furosemide

Dosage Forms: Liquid (content per ml): 10 mg. Tablet: 20 mg; 40 mg; 80 mg (all are white)

Use: Treatment of high blood pressure; removal of fluid from body tissues

Minor Side Effects: Blurred vision; constipation; cramping; diarrhea; dizziness; nausea; rash; tingling in the fingers and toes; vomiting

Major Side Effects: Anemia; anorexia; jaundice; pancreatitis; ringing in the ears

Contraindications: This drug should not be used by pregnant women or by persons with anuria (no urine). This drug should not be used by people who are allergic to it. Consult your doctor immediately if this drug has been prescribed for you and you fit either description or have such an allergy.

Warnings: Use of this drug may cause gout, diabetes, hearing loss, and loss of potassium, calcium, water, and salt. • Persons hypersensitive to sulfa drugs may also be hypersensitive to this drug. If this drug has been prescribed for you and you are allergic to sulfa drugs, consult your doctor immediately. • Persons taking this drug should have periodic blood and urine tests. • This drug should be used cautiously in persons with cirrhosis of the liver or other liver problems, or with kidney disease. This drug should be used cautiously in children, pregnant women, and nursing mothers. • This drug should be used with caution in conjunction with other high blood pressure drugs. • Use of this drug may activate the appearance of systemic lupus erythematosus. Whenever adverse reactions to this drug are moderate to severe, this drug should be reduced or discontinued. Consult your doctor promptly if side effects occur. • This drug interacts with aspirin, curare, cephalosporins, clofibrate, digitalis, lithium carbonate, steroids, or cephaloridine. If you are currently taking any drugs of these types, consult your doctor about their use. If you are unsure of the type or contents of your medications, ask your doctor or pharmacist.

Comments: This drug causes more frequent urination. Expect this effect; it should not alarm you. • This drug has potent activity. If another drug to decrease blood pressure is also prescribed, your doctor may decide to decrease the dose of one of the drugs to avoid an excessive drop in blood pressure. • This drug can cause potassium loss. To help avoid such loss, take this drug with a glass of fresh or frozen orange juice. You may also eat a banana each day. The use of a salt substitute helps prevent potassium loss. • To avoid dizziness or light-headedness when you stand, contract and relax the muscles of your legs for a few moments before rising. Do this by pushing one foot against the floor while raising the other foot slightly, alternating feet so that you are "pumping" your legs in a pedaling motion. • Persons taking this product and digitalis should watch carefully for symptoms of increased toxicity (e.g., nausea, blurred vision, palpitations), and notify their doctors immediately if symptoms occur. • A generic furosemide product is available but it has not been approved by the FDA. It is not generically equivalent to this drug. • If you have high blood pressure, do not take any nonprescription item for cough, cold, or sinus problems without first checking with your doctor.

Ledercillin VK antibiotic (Lederle Laboratories), see penicillin potassium phenoxymethyl antibiotic.

Levoid thyroid hormone (Nutrition Control Products), see Synthroid thyroid hormone.

Levothroid thyroid hormone (Armour Pharmaceutical Company), see Synthroid thyroid hormone.

Lexor diuretic and antihypertensive (Lemmon Company), see hydrochlorothiazide diuretic and antihypertensive.

OTC   **Li-Ban Spray lice-control spray**

Manufacturer: Pfipharmecs Division
Ingredients: (5-Benzyl-3-furyl) methyl 2.2-dimethyl-3-(2-methylpropenyl) cyclopropanecarboxylate; related compounds; aromatic petroleum hydrocarbons
Dosage Form: Aerosol spray: (5-Benzyl-3-furyl) methyl 2.2-dimethyl-3-

(2-methylpropenyl) cyclopropanecarboxylate, 0.500%; related compounds, 0.068%; aromatic petroleum hydrocarbons, 0.664%

Use: To kill lice and louse eggs on clothing, bedding, furniture, and other inanimate objects

Side Effects: Allergy; burning; itching; rash; sneezing; stinging (if sprayed on skin or inhaled)

Warnings: This product should not be used on humans or animals; do not spray on skin and avoid inhaling the spray.

Comments: This product should be used only for items that cannot be laundered or dry cleaned. • Allow all treated articles to dry thoroughly before use.

R_x   ## Librax sedative and anticholinergic

Manufacturer: Roche Products, Inc.
Ingredients: chlordiazepoxide hydrochloride; clidinium bromide
Equivalent Product: Lidinium, Spencer-Mead, Inc.
Dosage Form: Capsule: chlordiazepoxide hydrochloride, 5 mg; clidinium bromide, 2.5 mg (green)
Use: In conjunction with other drugs, treatment of peptic ulcer or irritable bowel syndrome
Minor Side Effects: Blurred vision; confusion; constipation; depression; difficult urination; dizziness; drowsiness; dry mouth; fatigue; headache; increased sensitivity to light; insomnia; loss of the sense of taste; nausea; nervousness; palpitations; rash; reduced sweating; slurred speech; uncoordinated movements; vomiting
Major Side Effects: Double vision; impotence; jaundice; low blood pressure; tremors
Contraindications: This drug should not be taken by people who have glaucoma, enlarged prostate, or obstructed bladder. Consult your doctor immediately if this drug has been prescribed for you and you have any of these conditions.
Warnings: This drug should be used cautiously by people who have severe heart disease, liver or kidney disease; or by those who are pregnant or nursing. Be sure your doctor knows if you have any of these conditions. • This drug should not be used in conjunction with amantadine, haloperidol, other central nervous system depressants, phenothiazines, alcohol, or antacids; if you are currently taking any drugs of these types, consult your doctor about their use. If you are unsure of the type or contents of your medications, ask your doctor or pharmacist. • This drug always produces certain side effects, which may include dry mouth, blurred vision, reduced sweating, drowsiness, difficult urination, constipation, increased sensitivity to light, and palpitations. Avoid tasks that require alertness. Avoid excessive work or exercise in hot weather. To prevent oversedation, avoid taking alcohol or other drugs that have sedative properties. • Call your doctor if you notice a rash, flushing, or pain in the eye. • This drug has a slight potential for abuse, but taken as directed, there is little danger. Do not increase the dose of this drug without first consulting your doctor. • Elderly patients generally should take the smallest effective dosage of this drug.
Comments: This drug is best taken one-half to one hour before meals. • This drug does not cure ulcers, but may help them improve. • Chew gum or suck on ice chips or a piece of hard candy to reduce mouth dryness.

R_x   ## Librium sedative and hypnotic

Manufacturer: Roche Products, Inc.
Ingredient: chlordiazepoxide hydrochloride

462

Equivalent Products: A-poxide, Abbott Laboratories; Chlordiazachel, Rachelle Laboratories, Inc.; chlordiazepoxide hydrochloride, various manufacturers; Diazachel, North American Pharmacal, Inc.; Mitran, Winston Pharmaceuticals, Inc.; Murcil, Tutag Pharmaceuticals, Inc.; Reposans, Foy Laboratories, Inc.; SK-Lygen, Smith Kline & French Laboratories; Sereen, Foy Laboratories, Inc.; Tenax, Reid-Provident Laboratories, Inc.; Zetran, W. E. Hauck, Inc.

Dosage Forms: Capsule: 5 mg (green/yellow); 10 mg (green/black); 25 mg (green/white). Tablet: 5 mg; 10 mg; 25 mg (green)

Use: Relief of anxiety; nervousness; tension; muscle spasms; withdrawal symptoms of alcohol addiction

Minor Side Effects: Confusion; constipation; depression; difficult urination; dizziness; drowsiness; dry mouth; fatigue; headache; nausea; rash; slurred speech; uncoordinated movements

Major Side Effects: Blurred vision; decreased sexual drive; double vision; jaundice; low blood pressure; stimulation; tremors

Contraindications: This drug should not be used by people who are allergic to it. Consult your doctor immediately if this drug has been prescribed for you and you have such an allergy.

Warnings: This drug should be used cautiously by people who have liver or kidney disease, and by those who are pregnant. Be sure your doctor knows if you have any of these conditions. • Elderly people should use this drug cautiously, and take the smallest effective dose. • This drug has the potential for abuse and must be used with caution. Tolerance may develop quickly; do not increase the dose of this drug without first consulting your doctor. • Taken alone, this drug is safe. Do not take it with other sedative drugs, central nervous system depressants, or alcohol, however, or serious adverse reactions may develop. • This drug may cause drowsiness; avoid tasks that require alertness. • Consult your doctor if you wish to discontinue use of this drug; do not stop taking the drug suddenly. If you have been using the drug for an extended period of time, it will be necessary to reduce the dosage gradually, following medical advice.

Comments: Although this drug is effectively used to relieve nervousness, phenobarbital is often equally effective, and it may cost less. Consult your doctor. • Chew gum or suck on ice chips or a piece of hard candy to reduce mouth dryness.

℞   **Lidex steroid hormone**

Manufacturer: Syntex Laboratories, Inc.
Ingredient: fluocinonide
Dosage Forms: Cream; Ointment: 0.05%
Use: Relief of skin inflammation associated with conditions such as eczema or poison ivy

Minor Side Effects: Burning sensation; dryness; irritation of affected area; itching; rash

Major Side Effects: Secondary infection

Contraindications: This drug should not be taken by people who are allergic to it. Consult your doctor immediately if this drug has been prescribed for you and you have such an allergy. • This drug should not be used in the eyes.

Warnings: If irritation develops, consult your doctor. If extensive areas are treated or if occlusive dressings are used, there will be increased systemic absorption of this drug and suitable precautions should be taken, especially in children and infants. • This drug should be used cautiously by pregnant women.

Comments: Topsyn steroid hormone is another product manufactured by Syntex Laboratories, Inc. Topsyn contains fluocinonide, but in a gel form. For all practical purposes, Topsyn is the same as Lidex, and they are similar in

price. The gel form, however, may produce a cooling sensation on the skin. •
If the affected area is dry or scaling, the skin may be moistened before applying the product by soaking in water or by applying water with a clean cloth.
The ointment form is probably the better product for dry skin. • Do not use
these products with an occlusive wrap of transparent plastic film unless
directed to do so by your doctor.

Lidinium sedative and anticholinergic (Spencer-Mead, Inc.), see Librax sedative and anticholinergic.

OTC   Liquifilm Tears ocular lubricant

Manufacturer: Allergan Pharmaceuticals, Inc.
Ingredients: chlorobutanol; polyvinyl alcohol; sodium chloride
Dosage Form: Solution: chlorobutanol, 0.5%; polyvinyl alcohol, 1.4%;
sodium chloride
Use: Ocular lubricant for wearers of hard contact lenses
Side Effects: Allergic reactions (rash, itching, soreness); local irritation
Contraindications: Do not use with soft contact lenses.
Comments: Do not touch the dropper or bottle top to the eye or other
tissue because contamination of the solution will result. The use of more
than one eye product at a time may cause severe irritation to the eye. Consult
your pharmacist before doing so.

OTC   Liquimat acne preparation

Manufacturer: Texas Pharmacal Company
Ingredients: alcohol; sulfur; tinted bases
Dosage Form: Lotion: alcohol, 22%; sulfur, 5%; tinted bases
Use: Treatment of acne
Side Effects: Allergy; local irritation
Warnings: Do not get product in or near eyes.
Comments: If the condition worsens, stop using this product and call your
pharmacist.

OTC   Liquiprin analgesic

Manufacturer: Norcliff Thayer Inc.
Ingredient: acetaminophen
Dosage Form: Liquid (content per 2.5 ml, or one dropperful): acetamino-
phen, 120 mg
Use: Reduction of fever and relief of pain
Side Effects: When taken in overdose: blood disorders, rash
Warnings: When taken in overdose, acetaminophen is more toxic than
aspirin. The dosage instructions listed on the package should be followed
carefully; toxicity may occur in adults or children with repeated doses.

OTC   Listerine throat lozenges

Manufacturer: Warner-Lambert Company
Ingredients: hexylresorcinol; eucalyptol; menthol
Dosage Form: Lozenge: hexylresorcinol, 2.4 mg; eucalyptol; menthol
Use: Temporary relief of dryness and minor irritation of the mouth and
throat
Contraindications: Do not give this product to children under three years of
age, unless otherwise directed by your doctor.
Warnings: A sore throat in a child under age six should never be treated
without medical supervision. Consult your doctor. • If your sore throat is

severe; is accompanied by headache, high fever, nausea, or vomiting; or lasts for more than two days, consult your doctor promptly.

Comments: The antibacterial ingredients included represent an irrational use for this product if it is recommended to treat an infection-induced sore throat. Colds are caused by viruses, and the ingredients in this product are not effective against viral infections.

Lobac analgesic (The Seatrace Co.), see Parafon Forte analgesic.

Lofene anticholinergic and antispasmodic (The Lannett Company, Inc.), see Lomotil anticholinergic and antispasmodic.

Loflo anticholinergic and antispasmodic (Spencer-Mead, Inc.), see Lomotil anticholinergic and antispasmodic.

R_x   Lomotil anticholinergic and antispasmodic

Manufacturer: Searle & Co.
Ingredients: atropine sulfate; diphenoxylate hydrochloride
Equivalent Products: Colonil, Mallinckrodt, Inc.; Diphenatol, Rugby Laboratories; Enoxa, Tutag Pharmaceuticals, Inc.; Lofene, The Lannett Company, Inc.; Loflo, Spencer-Mead, Inc.; Lonox, Geneva Generics, Inc.; Lo-Trol, Vangard Laboratories; Low-Quel, Halsey Drug Co., Inc.; Nor-Mil, North American Pharmacal, Inc.; SK-Diphenoxylate, Smith Kline & French Laboratories
Dosage Forms: Liquid (content per 5 ml); Tablet (white): atropine sulfate, 0.025 mg; diphenoxylate hydrochloride, 2.5 mg
Use: Treatment of diarrhea
Minor Side Effects: Abdominal pain; blurred vision; constipation; difficult urination; dizziness; drowsiness; dry mouth; flushing; headache; insomnia; itching; loss of the sense of taste; nausea; nervousness; rash; sedation; sweating; swollen gums; vomiting
Major Side Effects: Breathing difficulties; coma; euphoria; impotence; numbness in fingers or toes; palpitations
Contraindications: This drug should not be taken by children under the age of two. This drug should not be taken by people who have jaundice or drug-induced diarrhea, or by those who are allergic to it. Consult your doctor immediately if this drug has been prescribed for you and you have any of these conditions.
Warnings: This drug should be used cautiously by children, pregnant or nursing women, and people who have liver disease or ulcerative colitis. Be sure your doctor knows if you have any of these conditions. • This drug has the potential for abuse and must be used with caution. Tolerance to this drug may develop quickly; do not increase the dose of this drug without first checking with your doctor. • This drug may add to the effect of alcohol and other drugs with sedative properties. Do not use them without first checking with your doctor. • This drug interacts with amantidine, haloperidol, antacids, phenothiazines, and monoamine oxidase inhibitors; if you are currently taking any drugs of these types, consult your doctor about their use. If you are unsure of the type or contents of your medications, ask your doctor or pharmacist. • This drug may interfere with your ability to perform hazardous tasks such as driving. • Unless your doctor prescribes otherwise, do not take this drug for more than five days. • If you take this drug with you when traveling to a foreign country, do not use it unless you absolutely have to. Make sure that the diarrhea is not just a temporary occurrence (two to three hours). • Call your doctor if you notice a rash or a pain in the eye.
Comments: While taking this drug, drink at least nine glasses of water a day.

Lonox anticholinergic and antispasmodic (Geneva Generics, Inc.), see Lomotil anticholinergic and antispasmodic.

R_x   **Lopressor beta blocker**

Manufacturer: Geigy Pharmaceuticals
Ingredient: metoprolol tartrate
Dosage Form: Tablet: 50 mg (light red); 100 mg (light blue)
Use: Management of high blood pressure
Minor Side Effects: Constipation; diarrhea; flatulence; gastric pain; headache; heartburn; insomnia; nausea; nightmares
Major Side Effects: Cold extremities; depression; dizziness; elevated blood urea levels; hallucinations; itching; low blood pressure; rash; reversible loss of hair; shortness of breath; tiredness; visual disturbance; wheezing
Contraindications: This drug should not be used by people with certain heart diseases, including sinus bradycardia, certain heart blocks , cardiogenic shock, and overt cardiac failure. Consult your doctor immediately if this drug has been prescribed for you and you have heart disease.
Warnings: This drug should be used with caution by people with heart failure, angina, impaired kidney or liver function, asthma, diabetes, or thyroid disease. Be sure your doctor knows if you have any of these conditions. • Persons about to undergo surgery should use this drug with caution. • Pregnant women should take this drug only when clearly needed. Since most drugs are excreted in human milk, nursing mothers should not take this drug. • This drug should be used with caution in children. • This drug should not be taken with reserpine. If you are currently taking this drug, consult your doctor about its use. If you are unsure about the contents of your medications, ask your doctor or pharmacist.
Comments: This drug is a potent medication and should not be stopped abruptly. Chest pain and even deaths have occurred when this drug has been stopped suddenly. • While taking this drug, do not take any nonprescription item for cough, cold, or sinus problems without first checking with your doctor. • Your doctor may want you to take your pulse every day while you are taking this drug. Check with your doctor about this possibility. • This drug may cause drowsiness; do not take part in any activity for which you need to be alert. • Be sure to take the doses of this drug at the same time each day. • The action of this drug is similar to that of Inderal beta blocker, except that Inderal is usually taken four times a day; Lopressor is usually taken twice a day.

Loqua diuretic and antihypertensive (Columbia Medical Co.), see hydrochlorothiazide diuretic and antihypertensive.

Loquapres diuretic and antihypertensive (Columbia Medical Co.), see Hydropres diuretic and antihypertensive.

R_x   **Lotrimin antifungal agent**

Manufacturer: Schering Corporation
Ingredient: clotrimazole
Equivalent Product: Mycelex antifungal agent, Dome Division
Dosage Forms: Cream (content per gram); Solution (content per 1 ml): 10 mg
Use: Treatment of fungal infections of the skin
Minor Side Effects: Redness; stinging sensation
Major Side Effects: Blistering; irritation; peeling of the skin

Contraindications: This drug should not be used by people who are allergic to it. Consult your doctor immediately if this drug has been prescribed for you and you have such an allergy.

Warnings: This drug should be used with caution by pregnant women. • Do not use this drug in or near the eyes.

Comments: This drug should be rubbed well into the affected area and the surrounding skin. • Improvement in your condition may not be seen for one week after beginning treatment with this drug. If the condition has not improved after four weeks, consult your doctor. • This drug is also available in vaginal cream and vaginal tablet forms to treat certain fungal infections of the vagina. Mycelex-G (Dome Division) and Gyne-Lotrimin (Schering Corporation) antifungal agents are trademarked products of this type. • If you have a fungal infection of the vagina, wear cotton panties rather than those made of nylon or other "nonporous" materials while the infection is being treated. Careful attention to personal hygiene may help prevent subsequent fungal infections of the vagina.

Lo-Trol anticholinergic and antispasmodic (Vangard Laboratories), see Lomotil anticholinergic and antispasmodic.

Low-Quel anticholinergic and antispasmodic (Halsey Drug Co., Inc.), see Lomotil anticholinergic and antispasmodic.

Luminal Ovoids sedative and hypnotic (Winthrop Laboratories), see phenobarbital sedative and hypnotic.

L V Penicillin antibiotic (Paul B. Elder Company), see penicillin potassium phenoxymethyl antibiotic.

OTC   Maalox antacid

Manufacturer: William H. Rorer, Inc.

Ingredients: aluminum hydroxide; magnesium hydroxide

Dosage Form: Suspension (content per teaspoon): aluminum hydroxide, 225 mg; magnesium hydroxide, 200 mg

Use: Relief from acid indigestion, heartburn, sour stomach and/or hyperacidity associated with such conditions as peptic ulcer and hiatal hernia

Side Effects: Abdominal discomfort; constipation; diarrhea; dizziness; mouth irritation; nausea; rash; vomiting

Contraindications: Persons with kidney disease should not use this product. In persons with kidney disease, repeated daily use of this product may cause nausea, vomiting, depressed reflexes and breathing difficulties.

Warnings: Long-term (several weeks) use of this product may lead to intestinal obstruction and dehydration. • Phosphate depletion may occur leading to weakness, loss of appetite, and eventually bone pain. This may be prevented by drinking at least one glass of milk a day.

Comments: Self-treatment of severe or repeated attacks of heartburn, indigestion, or upset stomach is not recommended. If you do self-treat, limit therapy to two weeks, then call your doctor if your symptoms persist. Never self-medicate with this product if your symptoms occur regularly (two to three times or more a month); if they are particularly worse than normal; if you feel a "tightness" in your chest, have chest pains, or are sweating; or if you are short of breath. Consult your doctor. • To prevent constipation, drink at least eight glasses of water a day. If constipation persists, consult your doctor or pharmacist. • This product works best when taken one hour after meals or at bedtime, unless otherwise directed by your doctor or pharmacist. • Do not take this product within two hours of a dose of a tetracycline antibiotic. Also, if you are taking iron, a vitamin-mineral product, chlorpromazine, phenytoin, digoxin, quinidine, or warfarin, remind your doctor or pharmacist that you are taking this product. If you are unsure of the type or contents of your medications, consult your doctor or pharmacist.

OTC   Maalox #1 antacid

Manufacturer: William H. Rorer, Inc.
Ingredients: aluminum hydroxide; magnesium hydroxide
Dosage Form: Tablet: aluminum hydroxide, 200 mg; magnesium hydroxide, 200 mg
Use: Relief from acid indigestion, heartburn, sour stomach and/or hyperacidity associated with such conditions as peptic ulcer and hiatal hernia
Side Effects: Abdominal discomfort; constipation; diarrhea; dizziness; mouth irritation; nausea; rash; vomiting
Contraindications: Persons with kidney disease should not use this product. In persons with kidney disease, repeated daily use of this product may cause nausea, vomiting, depressed reflexes and breathing difficulties.
Warnings: Long-term (several weeks) use of this product may lead to intestinal obstruction and dehydration. Phosphate depletion may occur leading to weakness, loss of appetite, and eventually bone pain. This may be prevented by drinking at least one glass of milk a day.
Comments: Self-treatment of severe or repeated attacks of heartburn, indigestion, or upset stomach is not recommended. If you do self-treat, limit therapy to two weeks, then call your doctor if your symptoms persist. Never self-medicate with this product if your symptoms occur regularly (two to three times or more a month); if they are particularly worse than normal; if you feel a "tightness" in your chest, have chest pains, or are sweating; or if you are short of breath. Consult your doctor. • This product works best when taken one hour after meals or at bedtime, unless otherwise directed by your doctor or pharmacist. • Do not take this product within two hours of a dose of a tetracycline antibiotic. Also, if you are taking iron, a vitamin-mineral product, chlorpromazine, phenytoin, digoxin, quinidine, or warfarin, remind your doctor or pharmacist that you are taking this product.

OTC   Maalox #2 antacid

Manufacturer: William H. Rorer, Inc.
Ingredients: aluminum hydroxide; magnesium hydroxide
Dosage Form: Tablet: aluminum hydroxide, 400 mg; magnesium hydroxide, 400 mg
Use: Relief from acid indigestion, heartburn, sour stomach and/or hyperacidity associated with such conditions as peptic ulcer and hiatal hernia
Side Effects: Abdominal discomfort; constipation; diarrhea; dizziness; mouth irritation; nausea; rash; vomiting
Contraindications: Persons with kidney disease should not use this product. In persons with kidney disease, repeated daily use of this product may cause nausea, vomiting, depressed reflexes and breathing difficulties.
Warnings: Long-term (several weeks) use of this product may lead to intestinal obstruction and dehydration. • Phosphate depletion may occur leading to weakness, loss of appetite, and eventually bone pain. This may be prevented by drinking at least one glass of milk a day.
Comments: Self-treatment of severe or repeated attacks of heartburn, indigestion, or upset stomach is not recommended. If you do self-treat, limit therapy to two weeks, then call your doctor if your symptoms persist. Never self-medicate with this product if symptoms occur regularly (two to three

times or more a month); if they are particularly worse than normal; if you feel a "tightness" in your chest, have chest pains, or are sweating; or if you are short of breath. Consult your doctor. • This product works best when taken one hour after meals or at bedtime, unless otherwise directed by your doctor or pharmacist. • Do not take this product within two hours of a dose of a tetracycline antibiotic. Also, if you are taking iron, a vitamin-mineral product, chlorpromazine, phenytoin, digoxin, quinidine, or warfarin, remind your doctor or pharmacist that you are taking this product.

℞   **Macrodantin antibacterial**

Manufacturer: Norwich-Eaton Pharmaceuticals
Ingredient: nitrofurantoin (macrocrystals)
Equivalent Products: nitrofurantoin, various manufacturers
Dosage Form: Capsule: 25 mg (white); 50 mg (yellow/white); 100 mg (yellow)
Use: Treatment of bacterial urinary tract infections such as pyelonephritis, pyelitis, or cystitis
Minor Side Effects: Abdominal cramps; change in urine color; loss of appetite; nausea; vomiting
Major Side Effects: "Black tongue"; chest pain; cough; fever; irritation of the mouth; rash; rectal and vaginal itching; superinfection
Contraindications: This drug should not be used by persons with severe kidney disease or little or no urine production. Be sure your doctor knows if you have such a condition. • This drug should not be used by pregnant women at term or in infants under one month of age. • This drug should not be used by people who are allergic to it. Consult your doctor immediately if this drug has been prescribed for you and you have such an allergy.
Warnings: This drug should be taken cautiously; it has been associated with lung problems. If such problems occur, your doctor will discontinue this drug and appropriate measures will be taken. There have been isolated reports of pulmonary reactions as a contributing cause of death. • This drug should be used with caution in blacks and in ethnic groups of Mediterranean and near-Eastern origin, since cases of hemolytic anemia have been known to be brought about in a percentage of such persons while using this drug. Any signs of such anemia warrant discontinuance of the drug. The problem usually ceases when the drug is withdrawn. • This drug should be used with caution in pregnant women, women of childbearing age, and nursing mothers. • Use of this drug may result in nerve damage, which may become severe or irreversible; fatalities have been reported. Certain predisposing conditions, including kidney disease, anemia, diabetes, vitamin-B imbalance, electrolyte imbalance, and debilitating disease may enhance nerve damage. Be sure your doctor knows if you have any of these conditions.
Comments: This drug is similar to the generic product nitrofurantoin. However, this drug is much better tolerated (causes less nausea and stomach distress) than other nitrofurantoin products. Regular nitrofurantoin preparations (e.g., Furadantin antibacterial) are not generic equivalents. • If you have a urinary tract infection, you should drink at least nine or ten glasses of water each day. • To reduce nausea and vomiting, take this drug with a meal or glass of milk. • This drug may cause false results with urine sugar tests. • This drug may color your urine and stain your undergarments. Do not be alarmed. • This drug should be taken for at least ten full days, even if symptoms have disappeared within that time.

OTC   **magnesium citrate solution laxative**

Manufacturer: various manufacturers
Ingredient: magnesium citrate in water

Dosage Form: Liquid (quantity of ingredient not specified)
Use: Relief of constipation; cathartic
Side Effects: Excess loss of fluid; griping (cramps); mucus in feces
Contraindications: Persons with high fever (100° F or more); black or tarry stools; nausea; vomiting; abdominal pain; or children under age three should not use this product unless directed by a doctor. • Do not use this product when constipation is caused by megacolon or other diseases of the intestine, or hypothyroidism.
Warnings: Excessive use (daily for a month or more) of this product may cause diarrhea, vomiting, and loss of certain blood electrolytes.
Comments: Evacuation may occur within several hours. Never self-medicate with this product if constipation lasts longer than two weeks or if the medication does not produce a laxative effect within a week. • Limit use to seven days unless otherwise directed by your doctor since this product may cause laxative-dependence (addiction) if used for a longer time. • A glass (eight ounces) of water should be taken with each dose (if possible). • Although the directions indicate that a full bottle can be taken for a cathartic (strong effect), try taking one-half bottle to see if you get sufficient activity.

Mallergan expectorant (Mallard Incorporated), see Phenergan expectorant.

Mallergan VC with Codeine expectorant (Mallard Incorporated), see Phenergan VC with Codeine expectorant.

Mallergan with Codeine expectorant (Mallard Incorporated), see Phenergan with Codeine expectorant.

℞ Marax adrenergic, sedative, and smooth muscle relaxant

Manufacturer: Roerig
Ingredients: ephedrine sulfate; hydroxyzine hydrochloride; theophylline
Equivalent Products: Asminorel Improved, Tutag Pharmaceuticals, Inc.; E.T.H. Compound, Stayner Corporation; Hydrophed, Rugby Laboratories; Theo-Drox, Columbia Medical Co.; Theophozine, Spencer-Mead, Inc.; Theozine, Henry Schein, Inc.
Dosage Forms: Syrup (content per 5 ml): ephedrine sulfate, 6.25 mg; hydroxyzine hydrochloride, 2.5 mg; theophylline, 32.5 mg. Tablet: ephedrine sulfate, 25 mg; hydroxyzine hydrochloride, 10 mg; theophylline 130 mg (dye free)
Use: Control of asthmatic bronchospasm
Minor Side Effects: Difficult urination; drowsiness; insomnia; nausea; restlessness; stimulation; stomach pain; vomiting
Major Side Effects: Chest pain; cold and clammy skin; convulsions; difficult breathing; high blood pressure; palpitations
Contraindications: This drug should not be taken by people who have severe heart disease, hyperthyroid disease, high blood pressure, an allergy to any of the components, or who are in early pregnancy. Consult your doctor immediately if this drug has been prescribed for you and you have, or may have, any of these conditions.
Warnings: This drug should be used cautiously by elderly males and by those with enlarged prostate. Be sure your doctor knows if you have an enlarged prostate. • This drug interacts with central nervous system depressants, guanethidine, lithium carbonate, monoamine oxidase inhibitors, and propranolol; if you are currently taking any drugs of these types consult your doctor about their use. If you are unsure of the type or contents of your medications, ask your doctor or pharmacist. • This drug may cause

drowsiness; avoid tasks that require alertness. To prevent oversedation, avoid the use of alcohol or other drugs that have sedative properties. • While taking this drug, do not take any nonprescription item for cough, cold, or sinus problems without first checking with your doctor. • Never take this drug more frequently than your doctor prescribes. A serious overdose may result. • Call your doctor if you develop severe stomach pain or nausea, or insomnia and restlessness. This product may aggravate an ulcer.

Comments: Take this drug with food or milk. • Drink at least eight glasses of water daily.

OTC — Marezine antinauseant

Manufacturer: Burroughs Wellcome Co.
Ingredient: cyclizine hydrochloride
Dosage Form: Tablet: cyclizine hydrochloride, 50 mg
Use: Antinauseant for prevention or treatment of motion sickness
Side Effects: Blurred vision, drowsiness, dry mouth
Warnings: Persons with glaucoma should use this product with caution. Consult your doctor or pharmacist if you have any questions concerning the use of this drug.
Comments: Vomiting is one of the body's defense mechanisms to rid itself of toxic or poisonous substances. Do not self-medicate with this product if vomiting has occurred for two or more days. Call your doctor. • Nausea and vomiting in women, especially early in the day, are early symptoms of pregnancy. Never take this product, or any other drug, until pregnancy has been ruled out. • If your vomitus has blood in it, or if you have a headache or abdominal pain, call your doctor. • This product is recommended only for nausea or vomiting caused by motion sickness. It is less effective for other disorders. • For best results, take this medication one hour before departure. • Avoid the use of alcohol, tranquilizers, or any drug that sedates the nervous system while taking this product.

Margesic Compound No. 65 analgesic (North American Pharmacal, Inc.), see Darvon Compound-65 analgesic.

Margesic Improved analgesic (North American Pharmacal, Inc.), see Darvon analgesic.

Marnal analgesic and sedative (North American Pharmacal, Inc.), see Fiorinal analgesic and sedative.

Maruate Spantab adrenergic (North American Pharmacal, Inc.), see Tenuate adrenergic.

Maytrex antibiotic (Mayrand Incorporated), see tetracycline hydrochloride antibiotic.

OTC — Measurin analgesic

Manufacturer: Breon Laboratories, Inc.
Ingredient: aspirin
Dosage Form: Time-release tablet; aspirin, 660 mg (10 grains)
Use: Temporary relief of minor pain in conditions such as rheumatoid arthritis, osteoarthritis, bursitis; or other prolonged aches and pains such as from minor injuries or menstruation; relief of pain of headache, colds, and similar conditions
Side Effects: Dizziness; mental confusion; nausea and vomiting; ringing in

the ears; slight blood loss; sweating

Contraindications: This product may cause an increased bleeding tendency and should not be taken by persons with a history of bleeding, peptic ulcer, or stomach bleeding.

Warnings: Persons with asthma, hay fever, or other allergies should be extremely careful about using this product. The product may interfere with the treatment of gout. If you have any of these conditions, consult your doctor or pharmacist before using this medication. • Do not use this product if you are currently taking alcohol, methotrexate, oral anticoagulants, oral antidiabetics, probenecid, steroids, and/or sulfinpyrazone; if you are unsure of the type or contents of your medications, ask your doctor or pharmacist. • This product has sustained action; never take it more frequently than directed. The dosage instructions listed on the package should be followed carefully; toxicity may occur in adults or children with repeated doses.

OTC   Medi-Quik burn remedy and antiseptic

Manufacturer: Lehn & Fink Products Company
Ingredients: benzalkonium chloride; ethyl alcohol; lidocaine; isopropyl alcohol
Dosage Forms: Aerosol: benzalkonium chloride, 0.1%; ethyl alcohol, 38%; lidocaine, 2.5%; isopropyl alcohol, 12%. Pump spray: benzalkonium chloride, 0.1%; ethyl alcohol, 38%; lidocaine, 2.5%; isopropyl alcohol, 79%
Use: First-aid spray for sunburn, minor cuts, scrapes, poison ivy, burns, and insect bites
Side Effects: Allergy; local irritation
Contraindications: This product should not be used on large areas of the body because a toxic amount of the medication may be absorbed. • Do not use this product on deep wounds or serious burns.

Rx   Medrol steroid hormone

Manufacturer: The Upjohn Company
Ingredient: methylprednisolone
Equivalent Product: methylprednisolone, various manufacturers
Dosage Form: Tablet: 2 mg (pink), 4 mg (white), 8 mg (peach), 16 mg (white), 24 mg (yellow), 32 mg (peach)
Use: Relief of inflammations (e.g., arthritis, dermatitis, poison ivy); endocrine and rheumatic disorders; asthma; blood diseases; certain cancers; gastrointestinal disturbances (e.g., ulcerative colitis)
Minor Side Effects: Dizziness; headache; increased sweating; menstrual irregularities
Major Side Effects: Abdominal distention; cataracts; fluid retention; glaucoma; growth impairment in children; hemorrhage; high blood pressure; impaired wound healing; peptic ulcer; potassium loss; weakness
Contraindications: This drug should not be taken by people who have systemic fungal infections. Consult your doctor immediately if this drug has been prescribed for you and you have such a condition.
Warnings: This drug should be used cautiously by people who have peptic ulcer, tuberculosis, hypothyroidism, herpes simplex, cirrhosis, colitis, kidney disease, high blood pressure, and myasthenia gravis; and by pregnant and nursing women. Be sure your doctor knows if you have any of these conditions. • People subjected to unusual stress may need larger doses of this product. • This drug interacts with antidiabetics, aspirin, barbiturates, diuretics, estrogens, indomethacin, oral anticoagulants, and phenytoin; if you are currently taking any drugs of these types, consult your doctor about

their use. If you are unsure of the type or contents of your medications, ask your doctor or pharmacist. • While taking this drug, people should not be vaccinated for smallpox. • This drug may cause bone damage and changes in the mental or emotional state. • Blood pressure, body weight, and vision should be monitored at regular intervals. • While taking this drug, stomach x-rays are desirable for persons with suspected or known peptic ulcers. • Do not stop taking this drug without your doctor's knowledge. • If you are taking this drug for a long period of time, you should carry a notice with you that you are taking a steroid. • This drug can cause potassium loss. To help avoid potassium loss, take the drug with a glass of fresh or frozen orange juice, or eat a banana everyday. The use of Co-Salt salt substitute helps prevent potassium loss.

Comments: If your doctor tells you to take the entire daily dose of the medication at one time, take it as close to 8:00 A.M. as possible to receive optimal response. • In order to determine the lowest possible effective dose, your doctor may prescribe that this drug be taken in decreasing dosages. • When this drug is used for short periods of time, as in the treatment of allergy or poison ivy, it is often taken on a decreasing dosage schedule (i.e., one tablet four times daily for several days, then one tablet three times daily, then one tablet twice daily, then one tablet daily). • When this drug is used for long periods of time, as in the treatment of arthritis, an every-other-day dosage schedule is preferred (i.e., two tablets every other day instead of one tablet per day).

Rx   **Mellaril phenothiazine**

Manufacturer: Sandoz Pharmaceuticals
Ingredient: thioridazine hydrochloride
Dosage Forms: Liquid concentrates (content per ml): thioridazine hydrochloride, 30 mg; alcohol, 3%. Thioridazine hydrochloride, 100 mg; alcohol, 4.2%. Tablet: 10 mg (pale green); 15 mg (pink); 25 mg (buff); 50 mg (white); 100 mg (green); 150 mg (yellow); 200 mg (pink)
Use: Relief of certain types of psychoses and depression; control of agitation, aggressiveness, and hyperactivity in children
Minor Side Effects: Blurred vision; change in urine color; constipation; diarrhea; dizziness; drooling; drowsiness; dry mouth; jitteriness; menstrual irregularities; nasal congestion; nausea; rash; reduced sweating; restlessness; uncoordinated movements; vomiting
Major Side Effects: Difficulty in swallowing; enlarged or painful breasts (both sexes); fluid retention; impotence; involuntary movements of the face, mouth, tongue, or jaw; jaundice; muscle stiffness; rise in blood pressure; sore throat; tremors
Contraindications: This drug should not be taken by persons with severe heart disease. Be sure your doctor knows if you have such a condition.
Warnings: This drug should be taken with extreme caution, since it may cause convulsions, drop in white blood cell count, or eye disease. This drug should be used with caution in pregnant women. • Since this drug may cause drowsiness, tasks requiring mental alertness should be avoided. • This drug is not recommended for use in children under two years of age. • This drug interacts with alcohol, antacids, anticholinergics, and central nervous system depressants. If you are currently taking any drugs of these types, consult your doctor about their use. If you are unsure of the type or contents of your medications, ask your doctor or pharmacist.
Comments: The effects of this drug may not be apparent for at least two weeks. • This drug has persistent action; never take it more frequently than your doctor prescribes. A serious overdose may result. • While taking this drug, do not take any nonprescription item for cough, cold, or sinus problems

without first checking with your doctor. • This drug interacts with alcohol and other sedative drugs; avoid using them while taking this product. • This drug may cause dryness of the mouth. To reduce this feeling, chew gum or suck on ice chips or a piece of hard candy. • This drug reduces sweating; avoid excessive work or exercise in hot weather. • To avoid dizziness or lightheadedness when you stand, contract and relax the muscles of your legs for a few moments before rising. Do this by pushing one foot against the floor while raising the other foot slightly, alternating feet so that you are "pumping" your legs in a pedaling motion. • As with any other drug that has anti-vomiting activity, symptoms of severe disease or toxicity due to overdose of other drugs may be masked by this drug. • The liquid concentrate form of this drug should be added to 60 ml (¼ cup) or more of water, milk, juice, coffee, tea, or carbonated beverages; or to pulpy foods (applesauce, etc.) just prior to administration.

Menogen estrogen hormone (General Pharmaceutical Prods., Inc.), see Premarin estrogen hormone.

Menotab estrogen hormone (Fleming & Company), see Premarin estrogen hormone.

OTC Mentholatum Deep Heating external analgesic

Manufacturer: The Mentholatum Company
Ingredients: lanolin; menthol; methyl salicylate; eucalyptus oil; turpentine oil (ingredients vary with dosage form.)
Dosage Forms: Lotion: menthol, 6%; methyl salicylate, 20%. Ointment: menthol, 6%; methyl salicylate, 12.7% (quantities of other ingredients not specified)
Use: Temporary relief of pain in muscles and other areas
Side Effects: Allergic reactions (rash, itching, soreness); local irritation
Warnings: Do not swallow this product. • Do not use on broken or irritated skin or on large areas of the body; avoid contact with eyes. • When using this product, avoid exposure to direct sunlight, heat lamp, or sunlamp. • If condition persists, call your doctor.
Comments: This product smells good and may be attractive to a child. It should be stored safely out of the reach of children. • Be sure to rub this product well into the skin.

Rx meprobamate sedative and hypnotic

Manufacturer: various manufacturers
Ingredient: meprobamate
Equivalent Products: Bamate, Century Pharmaceuticals, Inc.; Bamo, Misemer Pharmaceuticals; Coprobate, Coastal Pharmaceutical Co., Inc.; Equanil, Wyeth Laboratories; F. M. -200, F. M. -400, Amfre-Grant, Inc., Miltown, Wallace Laboratories; Neuramate, Halsey Drug Co., Inc.; Protran, Vanguard Laboratories; Sedabamate, Mallard Incorporated; SK-Bamate, Smith Kline & French Laboratories; Tranmep, Reid-Provident Laboratories, Inc.; Tranqui-Tabs, General Pharmaceutical Prods., Inc.
Dosage Forms: Capsule; Tablet: 200 mg; 400 mg; 600 mg (variety of colors)
Use: Relief of anxiety or tension; sleeping aid
Minor Side Effects: Diarrhea; dizziness; fever; headache; nausea; palpitations; rash; sedation; sore throat; vomiting
Major Side Effect: Fainting
Contraindications: This drug should not be used by people allergic to it or by those who have porphyria. Consult your doctor immediately if this drug

has been prescribed for you and you have either condition. • This drug should not be used by children under age six.

Warnings: This drug should be used cautiously by people with epilepsy, or liver and kidney diseases. Pregnant or nursing women should try to avoid using this drug. Be sure your doctor knows if you have any of these conditions. • This drug should be used cautiously by older children and the elderly. This drug adds to the effect of other sedative drugs. If you are currently taking any other sedatives, consult your doctor about their use. If you are unsure of the type or contents of your medications, ask your doctor or pharmacist. • This drug may cause drowsiness; avoid tasks that require alertness. To prevent oversedation, avoid the use of alcohol. • This drug has the potential for abuse and must be used with caution. Tolerance may develop quickly; do not increase the dose of this drug without first consulting your doctor. • Call your doctor if you get a rash, sore throat, or fever while taking this drug. • If you have been taking this drug for two to three months, do not stop taking it abruptly. Talk to your doctor about tapering off slowly.

Meprogesic analgesic (Premo Pharmaceutical Laboratories, Inc.), see Equagesic analgesic.

Mequin sedative and hypnotic (Lemmon Company), see Quaalude sedative and hypnotic.

OTC   Mercurochrome external anti-infective

Manufacturer: Consumer Products
Ingredient: merbromin
Dosage Form: Liquid: merbromin, 2%
Use: Promotes healing of cuts and abrasions, minor burns, skin irritations
Side Effects: Allergic reactions (rash, itching, soreness); local irritation
Comments: Apply this product at least three times daily to maintain effectiveness. • If the infection does not clear in two to three weeks, consult your doctor or pharmacist. • This product has a low order of effectivensss. For serious skin infections another product should be chosen. Consult your pharmacist.

OTC   merthiolate (thimerosal) tincture

Manufacturer: Eli Lilly and Company
Ingredient: thimerosal
Dosage Form: Liquid: thimerosal, 0.1% in alcohol
Use: To disinfect minor burns, cuts, and scrapes on skin
Side Effects: Burning; itching; stinging. If swallowed may cause abdominal cramping; diarrhea; nausea; vomiting.
Warnings: Do not swallow this product. • Keep this product out of the reach of children.
Comments: This product is not as effective a skin disinfectant as iodine tincture. • This product is also available in a water solution; merthiolate in water does not burn or sting as much as merthiolate in alcohol, but it is also less effective as a disinfectant.

OTC   Metamucil laxative

Manufacturer: Searle Consumer Products
Ingredients: citric acid; psyllium hydrophilic mucilloid; sodium bicarbonate; sucrose; dextrose (ingredients vary with dosage form)

Dosage Forms: Instant mix (content per packet): citric acid; psyllium hydrophilic mucilloid, 3.5 g; sodium bicarbonate equivalent to 250 mg sodium; sucrose. Regular powder: dextrose, 50%; psyllium hydrophilic mucilloid, 50%. (Also available in an "orange-flavored" product.)

Use: Relief of constipation

Contraindications: Persons with high fever (100° F or more); black or tarry stools; nausea; vomiting; abdominal pain; or children under age three should not use this product unless directed by a doctor. • Do not use this product when constipation is caused by megacolon or other diseases of the intestine, or hypothyroidism. • Persons with intestinal ulcers, intestinal obstruction, fecal impaction, or difficulty in swallowing should not use this product.

Warnings: Excessive use (daily for a month or more) of this product may cause diarrhea, vomiting, and loss of certain blood electrolytes. • Pregnant women should not use this product except on the advice of a doctor.

Comments: Evacuation may not occur for 12 to 72 hours. Never self-medicate with this product if constipation lasts longer than two weeks or if the medication does not produce a laxative effect within a week. • This product must be completely mixed in water or juice before taking; a glass (eight ounces) of water should be drunk immediately afterwards. • If you are taking other drugs do not take this product until you have checked with your doctor or pharmacist. • Limit use to seven days unless directed otherwise by your doctor; this product may cause laxative-dependence (addiction) if used for a longer period.

Metandren steroid hormone (CIBA Pharmaceutical Co., Inc.), see methyltestosterone steroid hormone.

Metho-500 muscle relaxant (Mallard Inc.), see Robaxin muscle relaxant.

℞   **methotrexate antimetabolite**

Manufacturer: Lederle Laboratories
Ingredient: methotrexate (formerly A-methopterin)
Equivalent Product: Mexate (injectable only), Bristol Laboratories
Dosage Form: Tablet: 2.5 mg (yellow)
Use: Treatment of certain types of cancer, severe psoriasis
Minor Side Effects: Abdominal distress; diarrhea; nausea; vomiting
Major Side Effects: Abnormal tissue changes; acne; back pain; bleeding; blood disorders; blurred vision; convulsions; death; depigmentation; dental problems; diabetes; drowsiness; headache; infertility; itching; kidney failure; liver damage; loss of hair; lung damage; menstrual dysfunction; mouth sores; numbness in fingers and toes; paralysis; rash; sunlight sensitivity

Contraindications: This drug should not be taken by people with severe kidney, liver, or blood disease, or by women who are pregnant. Be sure your doctor knows if you have any of these conditions.

Warnings: This drug should be used very cautiously by people who have infections, peptic ulcer, kidney disease, ulcerative colitis, or debility. Be sure your doctor knows if you have any of these conditions. • This drug should be used with caution by children and the elderly. • Since this drug is excreted principally by the kidneys, its use in the presence of impaired kidney function may result in an accumulation of toxic amounts or even additional kidney damage. Therefore, the patient's kidney status should be carefully determined prior to and during the use of this drug. • Various lab tests should be performed prior to therapy with this drug, at appropriate periods during therapy, and after stoppage of the therapy. • This drug has been reported to suppress the immune system. • This drug interacts with salicylates, sulfonamides, phenylbutazone, phenytoin, tetracycline, chloramphenicol, anticoagulants, folic acid, probenecid, and para-aminobenzoic acid (PABA). If you are currently taking any drugs of these types, consult your doctor about their use. If you are unsure of the type or contents of your medications, ask your doctor or pharmacist.

Comments: While taking this drug, do not begin taking any over-the-counter vitamin product without your doctor's knowledge. • Pharmacists are advised by the manufacturer that a maximum of seven day's therapy be dispensed at any one time. This is to help prevent severe toxicity if too many tablets are taken. • Never increase the dose of this drug without the permission of your doctor. • This drug should never be taken for psoriasis unless other treatments have been tried and have failed.

R_X   **methyltestosterone steroid hormone**

Manufacturer: various manufacturers
Ingredient: methyltestosterone
Equivalent Products: Android, Brown Pharmaceutical Co., Inc.; Metandren, CIBA Pharmaceutical Co., Inc.; Oreton Methyl, Schering Corporation
Dosage Forms: Buccal tablet: 5 mg; 10 mg. Capsule: 10 mg. Tablet: 10 mg; 25 mg. Timed-release capsule: 10 mg
Use: Treatment of various sex-hormone-related disorders and impotency in the male; certain kinds of breast cancer and postpartum breast pain and engorgement in the female
Minor Side Effects: Acne; diarrhea; excitation; habituation; increased or decreased libido; nausea; persistent erection (enlarged penis or increased frequency of erection in prepubertal males); skin flushing; sleeplessness; vomiting
Major Side Effects: Bleeding in patients taking anticoagulants; chills; edema; enlarged breasts; growth impairment in children; impotence; leukopenia; occasional liver toxicity; reproductive system dysfunctions; symptoms of peptic ulcer; hirsutism; male-pattern baldness; deepening of voice; clitoral enlargement in females
Contraindications: This drug should not be taken by males with known or suspected prostatic cancer, breast cancer, or prostatic hypertrophy or by people with heart, kidney, or liver disease. Be sure your doctor knows if you have any of these conditions. • This drug should not be taken by people with high serum calcium, by the elderly, or by young children. • Pregnant or lactating women should not take this drug. • This drug should not be taken by people who are allergic to it. Consult your doctor immediately if this drug has been prescribed for you and you have any of these conditions.
Warnings: Female patients using this drug should be watched closely for symptoms or signs of virilization, such as hoarseness, deepening of the voice, oily skin, acne, enlarged clitoris, or menstrual irregularities. Some of these signs may be irreversible even after the drug is stopped. • This drug should be used cautiously by immobilized patients and in patients with breast cancer, since hypercalcemia may result. If this occurs, the drug should be discontinued. • This drug should also be discontinued if cholestatic hepatitis with jaundice appears or if liver tests become abnormal. • This drug should be stopped if vaginal bleeding, lowered sperm count, or fluid retention occurs. • Serum cholesterol may increase or decrease when administering this drug. • This drug should be used with caution by people with known acute intermittent porphyria or thyroid disease. This drug should not be taken with anticoagulants, adrenal steroids, or ACTH. If you are taking any of these drug types, consult your doctor about their use. If you are unsure of the con-

tents of your medications, ask your doctor or pharmacist. • This drug should not be taken with glucose-tolerance tests.

Comments: Buccal tablets should not be swallowed whole or chewed. They should be placed deep in the cheek pouch (against the gum) to dissolve there, or, less preferably, under the tongue. Avoid eating, drinking, or smoking while the tablet is in place and for several minutes afterwards. Buccal tablets allow twice as much medication to get to the bloodstream as the tablets or capsules. • Call your doctor if you develop hoarseness, deep voice, abnormal hair growth, acne, swollen tissues (edema), jaundice, or menstrual irregularities. • Testosterone is also known as the "male sex hormone," and it is produced naturally in the body. • Take the oral tablets with food or milk. This drug should be taken only under close medical supervision.

Meticorten steroid hormone (Schering Corporation), see prednisone steroid hormone.

Mexate antimetabolite (Bristol Laboratories), see methotrexate antimetabolite.

OTC   **Mexsana Medicated Powder rash remedy**

Manufacturer: Plough, Inc.
Ingredients: camphor; cornstarch; eucalyptus oil; kaolin; triclosan; zinc oxide
Dosage Form: Powder (quantities of ingredients not specified)
Use: For keeping skin dry; soothing diaper rash, prickly heat, and chafing
Side Effects: Allergy; local irritation
Comments: While using this product, be careful not to inhale any of the powder.

OTC   **Microsyn acne preparation**

Manufacturer: Syntex Laboratories, Inc.
Ingredients: camphor; colloidal alumina; menthol; resorcinol; salicylic acid; sodium thiosulfate
Dosage Form: Lotion: resorcinol, 2%; salicylic acid, 2%; sodium thiosulfate, 8% (quantities of other ingredients not specified)
Use: Treatment of acne
Side Effects: Allergy; local irritation
Warnings: Do not get product in or near the eyes.
Comments: If the condition worsens, stop using this product and call your pharmacist.

Midatane DC expectorant (Vangard Laboratories), see Dimetane DC expectorant.

Midatane expectorant (Vangard Laboratories), see Dimetane expectorant.

Midatap antihistamine (Vangard Laboratories), see Dimetapp antihistamine.

Migrastat migraine remedy (Winston Pharmaceuticals, Inc.), see Cafergot migraine remedy.

OTC   **milk of magnesia**

Manufacturer: various manufacturers

Ingredient: magnesium hydroxide
Dosage Form: Liquid: magnesium hydroxide, 7% to 8.5%
Use: Symptomatic relief of constipation; acid indigestion
Side Effects: Diarrhea; nausea
Contraindications: This product should not be used if symptoms of appendicitis are present (e.g., abdominal pain, nausea, vomiting).
Warnings: This product should not be used by persons with kidney disease, except under the supervision of a doctor. • Magnesium can produce numerous side effects, including sedation, if absorbed by the body. Only a small amount of magnesium is absorbed with each dose of this product, however, and this product is safe for occasional use. • Magnesium may interfere with the absorption of tetracycline antibiotics; if you are currently taking tetracycline, check with your doctor or pharmacist before taking this product. You will probably be advised to separate the dosages of the two drugs by a few hours.
Comments: Shake the liquid well before using. • Do not store the liquid in the freezer. • If you are taking this product for its laxative effects, take each dose with at least one full glass of water. • This product is also referred to as magnesium magma and as cream of magnesium. • If you take this product regularly and are also taking other drugs, be sure to inform your doctor and pharmacist of all your medications.

Miltown sedative and hypnotic (Wallace Laboratories), see meprobamate sedative and hypnotic.

OTC   **mineral oil**

Manufacturer: various manufacturers
Ingredient: mineral oil
Dosage Form: Liquid
Use: To relieve constipation by lubricating and softening the stool
Contraindications: This product should not be used by persons with abdominal pain, nausea, or vomiting; black or tarry stools; or high fever (100° F or more). • Do not give this product to children under age three unless directed otherwise by a doctor. • This product should not be used when constipation is caused by megacolon or other diseases of the intestine, or hypothyroidism.
Warnings: Excessive use (daily for a month or more) of this product may cause diarrhea, vomiting, and loss of certain blood electrolytes. • A type of pneumonia could occur if this product is used daily for more than two months. • Mineral oil may interfere with the body's absorption of calcium, phosphate, and vitamins A and D. • Limit the use of this product to seven continuous days unless directed otherwise by your doctor. Consult your doctor if constipation lasts longer than two weeks or if the medication does not produce a laxative effect within a week. • If you are taking mineral oil, do not take any additional stool-softening products.
Comments: For best results, take mineral oil at bedtime; do not take your dose with meals. Drink a full glass (eight ounces) of water with each dose of mineral oil. • Evacuation may occur within several hours. • If mineral oil leaks through the rectum, reduce the dose until this symptom disappears. • Mineral oil is available in light or heavy form; neither form has been shown to possess significant advantages over the other.

Rx   **Minipress antihypertensive**

Manufacturer: Pfizer Laboratories Division
Ingredient: prazosin hydrochloride

Dosage Form: Capsule: 1 mg (white); 2 mg (pink/white); 5 mg (blue/white)

Use: Treatment of high blood pressure

Minor Side Effects: Abdominal pain; constipation; diarrhea; dizziness; drowsiness; dry mouth; headache; impotence; itching; nasal congestion; nausea; palpitations; rash; ringing in the ears; tingling in fingers and toes; tiredness; vomiting; weakness

Major Side Effects: Blurred vision; depression; fainting; low blood pressure; nosebleed

Warnings: This drug should be used with caution in conjunction with other antihypertensive drugs and with beta-blocker drugs such as propranolol. If you are currently taking either of these drug types, consult your doctor about their use. If you are unsure of the type or contents of your medications, ask your doctor or pharmacist. • This drug should be used very cautiously by pregnant women and children. • Persons taking this drug should try to avoid situations where injury could result should dizziness occur. • Patients should always be started on the 1 mg capsule. The 2 mg and 5 mg capsules are not indicated for initial therapy.

Comments: The effects of this drug may not be apparent for at least two weeks. • Mild side effects (e.g., nasal congestion) are most noticeable during the first two weeks of therapy and become less bothersome after this period. • Initial doses of this drug may be given under supervision in order to adjust dosages to control side effects. • Do not drive or operate machinery for four hours after taking the first dose of this drug. • Do not discontinue this medication unless your doctor directs you to do so. • While taking this drug, do not take any nonprescription item for cough, cold, or sinus problems without first checking with your doctor. • While taking this drug, you should limit your consumption of alcoholic beverages in order to prevent dizziness or light-headedness. • To avoid dizziness or light-headedness when you stand, contract and relax the muscles of your legs for a few moments before rising. Do this by pushing one foot against the floor while raising the other foot slightly, alternating feet so that you are "pumping" your legs in a pedaling motion. • If you are taking this drug and begin therapy with another antihypertensive drug, your doctor will probably reduce the dosage of Minipress to 1 or 2 mg three times a day, then recalculate your correct dose over the next couple of weeks.

℞   **Minocin antibiotic**

Manufacturer: Lederle Laboratories

Ingredient: minocycline hydrochloride

Equivalent Product: Vectrin, Parke-Davis

Dosage Forms: Capsule: 50 mg (orange), 100 mg (purple/orange); Syrup (content per 5 ml): 50 mg

Use: Treatment of a wide variety of bacterial infections

Minor Side Effects: Diarrhea; dizziness; increased sensitivity to light; loss of appetite; nausea; vomiting

Major Side Effects: Anemia; "black tongue;" irritation of the mouth; itching; rash; sore throat; superinfection; rectal and vaginal itching

Contraindications: Anyone who has demonstrated an allergy to any of the tetracyclines should not take this drug. Consult your doctor immediately if this drug has been prescribed for you and you have such a history.

Warnings: This drug should be used cautiously by people who have liver and kidney diseases, children under age nine, and women who are nursing or pregnant. Be sure your doctor knows if you fit any of these descriptions. • This drug may impair your ability to perform hazardous tasks. • This drug can cause permanent discoloration of the teeth when taken by children under eight. When taken during the last half of pregnancy, it can cause discoloration of the fetus's teeth. • Call the doctor if you develop a fever, headache, sore throat, or nausea while taking this drug. • This drug interacts with penicillin, anticoagulants, barbiturates, carbamazepine, dairy products, diuretics, and phenytoin. If you are currently taking any drugs of these types, consult your doctor about their use. If you are unsure of the type or contents of your medications, ask your doctor or pharmacist. • Do not take this drug within two hours of the time you take an antacid or an iron preparation. • This drug should be taken for at least ten days even if symptoms have disappeared. • This drug may affect tests for syphilis. Make sure your doctor knows you are taking this drug if you are scheduled for this test. • This drug is taken once or twice a day. Never increase the dosage unless your doctor tells you to do so.

Comments: Try to take this drug on an empty stomach (one hour before or two hours after a meal). If you find the drug upsets your stomach, you may try taking it with food. • While taking this drug, avoid prolonged exposure to sunlight.

Mi-Pilo ophthalmic solution (Barnes-Hines Pharmaceuticals, Inc.) see Isopto Carpine ophthalmic solution.

Mistura ophthalmic solution (Lederle Laboratories), see Isopto Carpine ophthalmic solution.

Mitran sedative and hypnotic (Winston Pharmaceuticals, Inc.), see Librium sedative and hypnotic.

Mity-Quin steroid hormone and anti-infective (Reid-Provident Laboratories, Inc.), see Vioform-Hydrocortisone steroid hormone and anti-infective.

OTC   **Modane Bulk laxative**

Manufacturer: Warren-Teed Laboratories
Ingredients: psyllium hydrophilic mucilloid; dextrose
Dosage Form: Powder: psyllium hydrophilic mucilloid, 50%; dextrose, 50%
Use: Relief of constipation
Side Effects: Abdominal cramps; occasional nausea and vomiting
Contraindications: Persons with high fever (100° F or more); black or tarry stools; nausea; vomiting; abdominal pain; or children under age three should not use this product unless directed by a doctor. • Do not use this product when constipation is caused by megacolon or other diseases of the intestine, or hypothyroidism. • Persons with intestinal ulcers, intestinal obstruction, fecal impaction, difficulty in swallowing or those on a salt-free diet should not use this product.
Warnings: This product may combine with other drugs. If you are currently taking salicylates (including aspirin) or any prescription drug, do not take this product without first checking with your doctor. Excessive use (daily for a month or more) of this product may cause diarrhea, vomiting, and loss of certain blood electrolytes. • Pregnant women should not use this product except on the advice of a doctor.
Comments: Evacuation may not occur for 12 to 72 hours. Never self-medicate with this product if constipation lasts longer than two weeks or if the medication does not produce a laxative effect within a week. • This product must be completely mixed in water or juice before taking; a glass (eight ounces) of water should be drunk immediately afterwards. • If you are taking other drugs do not take this product until you have checked with your doctor

or pharmacist. • Limit use to seven days unless directed otherwise by your doctor; this product may cause laxative-dependence (addiction) if used for a longer period.

OTC Modane laxative, Modane Mild laxative

Manufacturer: Warren-Teed Laboratories
Ingredients: danthron; alcohol
Dosage Forms: Liquid (content per 5 ml): alcohol, 5%; danthron, 37.5 mg. Tablet, Modane: danthron, 75 mg. Tablet, Modane Mild: danthron, 37.5 mg
Use: Relief of constipation
Side Effects: Excess loss of fluid; griping (cramps); mucus in feces
Contraindications: Persons with high fever (100° F or more); black or tarry stools; nausea; vomiting; abdominal pain; or children under age three should not use these products unless directed by a doctor. • Do not use this product when constipation is caused by megacolon or other diseases of the intestine, or hypothyroidism.
Warnings: Excessive use (daily for a month or more) of these products may cause diarrhea, vomiting, and loss of certain blood electrolytes. • Hypokalemia may impair the effectiveness of this product. • Pregnant women should not use these products except on the advice of a doctor.
Comments: These products may discolor the urine. • Evacuation may occur within 6 to 12 hours. Never self-medicate with these products if constipation lasts longer than two weeks or if the medication does not produce a laxative effect within a week. • Limit use to seven days unless directed otherwise by a doctor since these products may cause laxative-dependence (addiction) if used for a longer time. • Modane Bulk laxative (Warren-Teed Laboratories) contains different ingredients than these products. It is not the same.

Rx Monistat 7 antifungal agent

Manufacturer: Ortho Pharmaceutical Corporation
Ingredient: miconazole nitrate
Dosage Form: Vaginal cream: 2%
Use: Treatment of fungal infections of the vagina
Minor Side Effects: Burning; irritation; itching
Major Side Effects: Headache; hives; pelvic cramps; skin rash
Contraindications: This drug should not be taken by people who are allergic to it. Consult your doctor immediately if this drug has been prescribed for you and you have such an allergy.
Warnings: This drug should be used with caution by pregnant women in the first trimester of their pregnancy. Be sure your doctor knows if you are pregnant. • Notify your doctor immediately if sensitization, burning, itching, or irritation occurs during use of this drug.
Comments: Usually, one seven-day course of this drug is sufficient, but it may be repeated for another seven days. • This drug is effective in the treatment of fungal infections in pregnant and nonpregnant women, as well as in women taking oral contraceptives. However, because small amounts of the drug may be absorbed through the vaginal wall, this drug generally should not be used during the first three months of pregnancy. • This drug should be used until the prescribed amount is gone. • Avoid sexual intercourse, or ask your partner to use a condom, until treatment is complete to avoid reinfection. • Wear cotton panties rather than those made of silk or other "nonporous" materials while treating fungal infections.

℞   **Motrin anti-inflammatory**

Manufacturer: The Upjohn Company
Ingredient: ibuprofen
Dosage Form: Tablet: 300 mg (white); 400 mg (orange); 600 mg (peach)
Use: Reduction of pain and swelling due to arthritis; relief of menstrual pain, dental pain, postoperative pain, and musculoskeletal pain
Minor Side Effects: Bloating; cramps; diarrhea; drowsiness; flatulence; headache; heartburn; nausea; ringing in the ears; vomiting
Major Side Effects: Blood in stools; depression; fluid retention; hearing loss; jaundice; palpitations; tremors; visual disturbances
Contraindications: This drug should not be taken by people who are allergic to it or to aspirin. Consult your doctor immediately if this drug has been prescribed for you and you have such an allergy.
Warnings: This drug should be used with extreme caution in patients with a history of ulcers, or gastrointestinal disease. Peptic ulcers and gastrointestinal bleeding, sometimes severe, have been reported in persons taking this drug. Make sure your doctor knows if you have or have had either condition. • This drug should be used with caution in persons with anemia, heart disease, bleeding disease, liver disease, or kidney disease. Be sure your doctor knows if you have any of these conditions. • Should any eye problems arise while taking this drug, notify your doctor immediately. • This drug should be used with extreme caution in pregnant women, by nursing mothers, and in children. • Use of this drug has been reported to bring about fluid retention, skin rash, edema, and weight gain. Patients exhibiting any of these symptoms should immediately consult their doctor. • This drug should be used with caution when a person is also on anticoagulants, since this drug has been found to prolong bleeding time, even in normal subjects. • This drug interacts with anticoagulants, aspirin, oral antidiabetics, phenytoin, and sulfonamides. If you are currently taking any drugs of these types, consult your doctor about their use. If you are unsure of the type or contents of your medications, ask your doctor or pharmacist.
Comments: In numerous tests, this drug has been shown to be as effective as aspirin in the treatment of arthritis, but aspirin is still the drug of choice for the disease. Because of the high cost of this drug, consult your doctor about prescribing proper doses of aspirin instead. • Do not take aspirin or alcohol while taking this drug without first consulting your doctor. • You should note improvement in your condition soon after you start using this drug; however, full benefit may not be obtained for as long as a month. It is important not to stop taking this drug even though symptoms have diminished or disappeared. • This drug is not a substitute for rest, physical therapy, or other measures recommended by your doctor to treat your condition.

M-Tetra 250 antibiotic (Misemer Pharmaceuticals, Inc.), see tetracycline hydrochloride antibiotic.

OTC   **Multicebrin multivitamin**

Manufacturer: Eli Lilly and Company
Ingredients: vitamin A; vitamin D; vitamin E; ascorbic acid (vitamin C); thiamine hydrochloride (vitamin B_1); riboflavin (vitamin B_2); niacin; pyridoxine hydrochloride (vitamin B_6); cyanocobalamin (vitamin B_{12})
Dosage Form: Capsule: vitamin A, 10,000 IU; vitamin D, 400 IU; vitamin E, 6.6 IU; ascorbic acid, 75 mg; thiamine hydrochloride, 3 mg; riboflavin, 3 mg; niacin, 25 mg; pyridoxine hydrochloride, 1.2 mg; cyanocobalamin, 3 mcg

Use: Dietary supplement

Warnings: This product contains ingredients that accumulate and are stored in the body. The recommended dose should not be exceeded for long periods (several weeks to months) except by doctor's orders.

Comments: If large doses are taken, this product may interfere with the results of urine tests. Inform your doctor and pharmacist you are taking this product.

Murcil sedative and hypnotic (Tutag Pharmaceuticals, Inc.), see Librium sedative and hypnotic.

OTC   Murine eyedrops

Manufacturer: Cooper Vision Pharmaceuticals, Inc.

Ingredients: benzalkonium chloride; edetate disodium; glycerin; monobasic and dibasic sodium phosphate; methylcellulose; potassium chloride; sodium chloride

Dosage Form: Drop: benzalkonium chloride, 0.01%; edetate disodium, 0.05%; methylcellulose; monobasic and dibasic sodium phosphate; potassium chloride; sodium chloride

Use: Relief from minor eye irritation

Side Effects: Allergic reactions (rash, itching, soreness); local irritation; momentary blurred vision

Contraindications: Do not use this product if you have glaucoma.

Warnings: Do not use this product for more than two days without checking with your doctor.

Comments: Use this product only for minor eye irritations. • Do not touch the dropper or bottle top to the eye or other tissue because contamination of the solution will result. • The use of more than one eye product at a time may cause severe irritation to the eye. Consult your pharmacist before doing so.

OTC   Murine Plus decongestant eyedrops

Manufacturer: Cooper Vision Pharmaceuticals, Inc.

Ingredients: tetrahydrozoline hydrochloride; edetate disodium; benzalkonium chloride; boric acid; sodium acetate

Dosage Form: Drop: tetrahydrozoline hydrochloride, 0.05%; edetate disodium, 0.1%; benzalkonium chloride, 0.01%; boric acid; sodium acetate

Use: To soothe and remove redness in eyes

Side Effects: Allergic reactions (rash, itching, soreness); local irritation; momentary blurred vision

Contraindications: This product should not be used by persons who have glaucoma or other serious eye diseases.

Warnings: If redness or pain persists or becomes worse, discontinue use of this product and consult a doctor; this product should not be used for more than two consecutive days without checking with your doctor. • The use of more than one eye product at a time may cause severe irritation to the eye. Consult your pharmacist before using this product in conjunction with any other eye product. • Keep this product out of the reach of children; if swallowed, this drug is likely to cause overstimulation in children. Call your doctor immediately if this product is accidentally swallowed.

Comments: This product contains boric acid, a toxic substance that many medical authorities believe should not be used. Follow package directions carefully. • Do not touch the tip of the bottle to your eye or any surface; contamination of the solution may result.

Myadec multivitamin and mineral supplement

Manufacturer: Parke-Davis

Ingredients: vitamin A; vitamin D; vitamin E; vitamin C; folic acid; thiamine; riboflavin; niacin; vitamin B_6; vitamin B_{12}; pantothenic acid; iodine; iron; magnesium; copper; zinc; manganese

Dosage Form: Tablet: vitamin A, 10,000 IU; vitamin D, 400 IU; vitamin E, 30 IU; vitamin C, 250 mg; folic acid, 0.4 mg; thiamine, 10 mg; riboflavin, 10 mg; niacin (as niacinamide), 100 mg; vitamin B_6, 5 mg; vitamin B_{12}, 6 mcg; pantothenic acid, 20 mg; iodine, 150 mcg; iron, 20 mg; magnesium, 100 mg; copper, 2 mg; zinc, 20 mg; manganese, 1.25 mg

Use: Dietary supplement

Side Effects: Constipation; diarrhea; nausea; stomach pain

Contraindications: This product should not be used by persons who have active peptic ulcer or ulcerative colitis.

Warnings: The minerals in this product interact with oral tetracycline antibiotics and reduce the absorption of the antibiotics. If you are currently taking tetracycline, consult your doctor or pharmacist before taking this product. If you are unsure of the type or contents of your medications, ask your doctor or pharmacist. • Alcoholics and persons who have chronic liver or pancreatic disease should use this product with special caution; such persons may have enhanced iron absorption and are therefore more likely than others to experience iron toxicity. • Accidental iron poisoning is common in children; be sure to keep this product safely out of their reach. • This product contains vitamin B_6 in an amount great enough that it may interact with levodopa (L-dopa). If you are currently taking L-dopa, check with your doctor before taking this product. • This product contains ingredients that accumulate and are stored in the body. The recommended dose should not be exceeded for long periods (several weeks to months) except by a doctor's orders.

Comments: Most people do not require the high dosages of the ingredients contained in this product. • Because of its iron content, this product may cause constipation, diarrhea, nausea, or stomach pain. These symptoms usually disappear or become less severe after two to three days. Taking your dose with food or milk may help minimize these side effects. If they persist, ask your pharmacist to recommend another product. • Black, tarry stools are a normal consequence of iron therapy. If your stools are not black and tarry, this product may not be working for you. Ask your pharmacist to recommend another product. • If two or more tablets are taken daily, this product may interfere with the results of urine tests. Inform your doctor and pharmacist you are taking this product.

Mycelex antifungal agent (Dome Division), see Lotrimin antifungal agent.

Mycelex-G antifungal agent (Dome Division), see Lotrimin antifungal agent.

OTC   **Mycitracin external anti-infective**

Manufacturer: The Upjohn Company

Ingredients: bacitracin; neomycin sulfate; polymyxin B sulfate

Dosage Form: Ointment (content per gram): bacitracin, 500 units; neomycin sulfate, 5 mg; polymyxin B sulfate, 5,000 units

Use: Prevents infection from cuts and abrasions; treats impetigo

Side Effects: Allergic reactions (rash, itching, soreness); local irritation

Comments: Apply this product at least three times daily to maintain effectiveness. • If the infection does not clear in two to three days, consult your doctor or pharmacist.

R̽ Mycolog steroid hormone and anti-infective

Manufacturer: E. R. Squibb & Sons, Inc.
Ingredients: gramicidin; neomycin sulfate; nystatin; triamcinolone acetonide
Dosage Forms: Cream; Ointment (content per gram): gramicidin, 0.25 mg; neomycin sulfate, equivalent to 2.5 mg neomycin base; nystatin, 100,000 units; triamcinolone acetonide, 1 mg
Use: Relief of skin inflammations associated with conditions such as dermatitis, eczema, or poison ivy
Minor Side Effects: Burning sensation; dryness; irritation; itching; rash
Contraindications: This drug should not be used for viral diseases of the skin, for most fungal lesions of the skin, or in circumstances when circulation is markedly impaired. • This drug should not be used in the eyes or in the external ear canals of patients with perforated eardrums. Be sure your doctor knows if you have any of these conditions. • This drug should not be used by people who are allergic to any of its ingredients. Consult your doctor immediately if this drug has been prescribed for you and you have such an allergy.
Warnings: Prolonged use of large amounts of this drug should be avoided in the treatment of skin infections following extensive burns and other conditions where absorption of neomycin is possible. Prolonged use of this drug may result in secondary infection. • If extensive areas are treated or if an occlusive bandage is used, the possibility exists of increased absorption of this drug into the bloodstream. • If irritation develops, discontinue use of this drug and notify your doctor immediately. • This drug should not be used extensively on pregnant women, in large amounts, or for prolonged periods.
Comments: If the affected area is extremely dry or is scaling, the skin may be moistened before applying the medication by soaking in water or by applying water with a clean cloth and then drying thoroughly. The ointment form is probably better for dry skin. • Do not use this product with an occlusive wrap of transparent plastic film unless instructed to do so by your doctor.

R̽ Mycostatin antifungal agent

Manufacturer: E. R. Squibb & Sons, Inc.
Ingredient: nystatin
Equivalent Products: Candex, Dome Division; Korostatin, Holland-Rantos Company, Inc.; Nilstat, Lederle Laboratories
Dosage Forms: Cream; Ointment; Powder (per gram): 100,000 units. Oral suspension (per 1 ml): 100,000 units. Oral tablet: 500,000 units. Vaginal tablet: 100,000 units
Use: Treatment of fungal infections
Minor Side Effects: Diarrhea; itching; nausea; rash (topical and vaginal forms); vomiting (oral forms)
Contraindications: This drug should not be used by people who are allergic to it. Contact your doctor immediately if this drug has been prescribed for you, and you have such an allergy.
Warnings: If you suffer allergic reactions (e.g., rash) from taking this drug, consult your doctor; use of the drug will probably be discontinued.
Comments: If you are using the powder form of this drug to treat a foot infection, sprinkle the powder liberally into your shoes and socks. • Moist lesions or sores are best treated with the powder form of this drug. • If you are using the oral suspension form of this drug to treat an infection in the mouth,

rinse the drug around in your mouth as long as possible before swallowing. • If you are using this drug to treat a vaginal infection, avoid sexual intercourse or ask your partner to wear a condom until treatment is completed; these measures will help prevent reinfection. • The vaginal tablets are supplied with an applicator that should be used to insert the tablets high into the vagina. • Unless instructed otherwise by your doctor, do not douche two to three weeks before or after you use vaginal tablets, or during the treatment period. • Use the vaginal tablets continuously, including during a menstrual period, until your doctor tells you to stop. • Wear cotton panties rather than those made of nylon or other nonporous materials while fungal infections of the vagina are being treated. • You may wish to wear a sanitary napkin while using the vaginal tablets to prevent soiling of your underwear.

OTC Mylanta antacid and antiflatulent

Manufacturer: Stuart Pharmaceuticals
Ingredients: aluminum hydroxide, magnesium hydroxide; simethicone
Dosage Forms: Suspension (content per teaspoon); Tablet: aluminum hydroxide, 200 mg; magnesium hydroxide, 200 mg; simethicone, 20 mg
Use: Relief of acid indigestion, heartburn, sour stomach, and accompanying painful gas symptoms
Side Effects: Abdominal discomfort; constipation; diarrhea; dizziness; mouth irritation; nausea; rash; vomiting
Contraindications: Persons with kidney disease should not use this product. In persons with kidney disease, repeated daily use of this product may cause nausea, vomiting, depressed reflexes and breathing difficulties.
Warnings: Long-term (several weeks) use of this product may lead to intestinal obstruction and dehydration. • Phosphate depletion may occur leading to weakness, loss of appetite, and eventually bone pain. This may be prevented by drinking at least one glass of milk a day.
Comments: Self-treatment of severe or repeated attacks of heartburn, indigestion, or upset stomach is not recommended. If you do self-treat, limit therapy to two weeks, then call your doctor if your symptoms persist. Never self-medicate with this product if symptoms occur regularly (two to three times or more a month); if they are particularly worse than normal; if you feel a "tightness" in your chest, have chest pains, or are sweating; or if you are short of breath. Consult your doctor. • This product works best when taken one hour after meals or at bedtime, unless otherwise directed by your doctor or pharmacist. • To prevent constipation, drink at least eight glasses of water a day. If constipation persists, consult your doctor or pharmacist. • The suspension form of this product is superior to the tablet form and should be used unless you have been specifically directed to use the tablet. Do not take this product within two hours of a dose of a tetracycline antibiotic. Also, if you are taking iron, a vitamin-mineral product, chlorpromazine, phenytoin, digoxin, quinidine, or warfarin, remind your doctor or pharmacist that you are taking this product. • Simethicone is included to relieve bloating and gas formation by enhancing belching or flatus formation. If you do not suffer from these symptoms, use a product without simethicone to save money.

OTC Mylanta-II antacid and antiflatulent

Manufacturer: Stuart Pharmaceuticals
Ingredients: aluminum hydroxide; magnesium hydroxide; simethicone
Dosage Forms: Suspension (content per teaspoon); Tablet: aluminum hydroxide, 400 mg; magnesium hydroxide, 400 mg; simethicone, 30 mg
Use: For relief of acid indigestion, heartburn, sour stomach, and accompanying painful gas symptoms

Side Effects: Abdominal discomfort; constipation; diarrhea; dizziness; mouth irritation; nausea; rash; vomiting

Contraindications: Persons with kidney disease should not use this product. In persons with kidney disease, repeated daily use of this product may cause nausea, vomiting, depressed reflexes and breathing difficulties.

Warnings: Long-term (several weeks) use of this product may lead to intestinal obstruction and dehydration. • Phosphate depletion may occur leading to weakness, loss of appetite, and eventually bone pain. This may be prevented by drinking at least one glass of milk a day.

Comments: Self-treatment of severe or repeated attacks of heartburn, indigestion, or upset stomach is not recommended. If you do self-treat, limit therapy to two weeks, then call your doctor if your symptoms persist. Never self-medicate with this product if symptoms occur regularly (two to three times or more a month); if they are particularly worse than normal; if you feel a "tightness" in your chest, have chest pains, or are sweating; or if you are short of breath. Consult your doctor. • This product works best when taken one hour after meals or at bedtime, unless otherwise directed by your doctor or pharmacist. • To prevent constipation, drink at least eight glasses of water a day. If constipation persists, consult your doctor or pharmacist. • The suspension form of this product is superior to the tablet form and should be used unless you have been specifically directed to use the tablet. • Do not take this product within two hours of a dose of a tetracycline antibiotic. Also, if you are taking iron, a vitamin-mineral product, chlorpromazine, phenytoin, digoxin, quinidine, or warfarin, remind your doctor or pharmacist that you are taking this product. • Simethicone is included to relieve bloating and gas formation by enhancing belching or flatus formation. If you do not suffer from these symptoms, use a product without simethicone to save money.

OTC   Mylicon; Mylicon-80 antiflatulents

Manufacturer: Stuart Pharmaceuticals
Ingredient: simethicone
Dosage Forms: Chewable tablet: simethicone, 40 mg; 80 mg. Drop (content per 0.6 ml): simethicone, 40 mg
Use: Symptomatic relief of flatulence and excessive, pain-causing gas in the digestive tract
Side Effects: Minor nausea and vomiting (rare)
Warnings: Self-treatment of severe or repeated attacks of gas is not recommended. If you do self-treat, limit therapy to two weeks, and call your doctor if symptoms persist.

Comments: This product works by helping gas bubbles in the stomach and intestines to burst; thus the gas is freed and is eliminated more easily by belching or passing flatus. • The tablets should be chewed thoroughly before being swallowed. • Simethicone is available in tablet form as Silain antiflatulent (A. H. Robins Company). Silain contains 50 mg simethicone per tablet.

Myobid smooth muscle relaxant (Laser, Inc.), see Pavabid Plateau Caps smooth muscle relaxant.

℞   Naldecon adrenergic and antihistamine

Manufacturer: Bristol Laboratories
Ingredients: chlorpheniramine maleate; phenylephrine hydrochloride; phenylpropanolamine hydrochloride; phenyltoloxamine citrate
Equivalent Products: Col-Decon, Columbia Medical Co.; Quadra-Hist, Henry Schein, Inc.; Tri-Phen-Chlor, Rugby Laboratories; Triphenyl Plus,

Spencer-Mead, Inc.; Tudecon T.D., Tutag Pharmaceuticals, Inc.

Dosage Forms: Pediatric drops (content per 1 ml); syrup (content per 5 ml): chlorpheniramine maleate, 0.5 mg; phenylephrine hydrochloride, 1.25 mg; phenylpropanolamine hydrochloride, 5.0 mg; phenyltoloxamine citrate, 2.0 mg. Sustained-action tablet (white with red specks); Syrup (content per 5 ml): chlorpheniramine maleate, 2.5 mg; phenylephrine hydrochloride, 5.0 mg; phenylpropanolamine hydrochloride, 20 mg; phenyltoloxamine citrate, 7.5 mg

Use: Relief of symptoms of hay fever and other allergies; sinusitis; upper respiratory tract infections

Minor Side Effects: Blurred vision; confusion; constipation; diarrhea; difficult urination; dizziness; drowsiness; dry mouth; headache; heartburn; insomnia; loss of appetite; nasal congestion; nausea; palpitations; rash; reduced sweating; restlessness; vomiting; weakness

Major Side Effects: Chest pain; high blood pressure; low blood pressure; severe abdominal pain; sore throat

Contraindications: This drug should not be taken by people who are allergic to any of its components. Consult your doctor immediately if this drug has been prescribed for you and you have such an allergy.

Warnings: This drug should be used cautiously by people who have high blood pressure, heart disease, diabetes, thyroid disease, glaucoma, vessel disease, or enlarged prostate. Be sure your doctor knows if you have any of these conditions. • This drug should not be used in conjunction with guanethidine or monoamine oxidase inhibitors; if you are currently taking any drugs of these types, consult your doctor about their use. If you are unsure of the type or contents of your medications, ask your doctor or pharmacist. • While taking this drug, do not take any nonprescription item for cough, cold, or sinus problems without first checking with your doctor. • This drug may cause drowsiness; avoid tasks that require alertness. To prevent oversedation, avoid the use of alcohol or other drugs that have sedative properties. • Because this drug reduces sweating, avoid excessive work or exercise in hot weather. • The tablet form of this drug has sustained action; never increase your dose or take it more frequently than your doctor prescribes. A serious overdose could result.

Comments: The tablet form of this drug must be swallowed whole. • Chew gum or suck on ice chips or a piece of hard candy to reduce mouth dryness.

R_X   **Nalfon anti-inflammatory**

Manufacturer: Dista Products Company
Ingredient: fenoprofen calcium
Dosage Forms: Capsule: 300 mg (yellow/ocher). Tablet: 600 mg (yellow)
Use: Relief of pain and swelling due to arthritis

Minor Side Effects: Bloating; cramps; diarrhea; drowsiness; flatulence; headache; heartburn; nausea; ringing in the ears; vomiting

Major Side Effects: Blood in stools; depression; fluid retention; hearing loss; jaundice; palpitations; tremors; visual disturbances

Contraindications: This drug should not be given to persons who are allergic to this drug or to aspirin. Consult your doctor immediately if this drug has been prescribed for you and you have such an allergy.

Warnings: This drug should be given with caution to patients with a history of upper gastrointestinal tract disease. Gastrointestinal bleeding, sometimes severe, has been reported in persons receiving this drug. Be sure your doctor knows if you have had such a problem. • This drug should be used cautiously in persons with peptic ulcer, anemia, heart disease, bleeding diseases, liver disease, or kidney disease. Be sure your doctor knows if you have any of these conditions. • This drug should be used with caution in pregnant women, nursing mothers, and children. • Dosage adjustment of this drug may have to be made if the patient also is taking phenobarbital. • Since this drug may cause drowsiness, tasks requiring alertness should be avoided while taking this drug. • Patients with impaired hearing who take this drug for a long time should have periodic hearing tests of auditory function. • Use of this drug may prolong bleeding times, so persons taking anticoagulants in addition to this drug should use this drug with extreme caution. It is desirable to have periodic kidney, liver, and eye tests while receiving this drug. This drug interacts with aspirin, anticoagulants, oral antidiabetics, phenytoin, and sulfonamides. If you are currently taking any drugs of these types, consult your doctor about their use. If you are unsure of the type or contents of your medications, ask your doctor or pharmacist.

Comments: In numerous tests, this drug has been shown to be as effective as aspirin in the treatment of arthritis, but aspirin is still the drug of choice for the disease. Because of the high cost of this drug, consult your doctor about prescribing proper doses of aspirin instead. • Do not take aspirin or alcohol while taking this drug without first consulting your doctor. • You should note improvement in your condition soon after you start using this drug; however, full benefit may not be obtained for as long as a month. It is important not to stop taking this drug even though symptoms have diminished or disappeared. • This drug is not a substitute for rest, physical therapy, or other measures recommended by your doctor to treat your condition. • This drug should be taken 30 minutes before or two hours after meals during the daytime.

℞   **Naprosyn anti-inflammatory**

Manufacturer: Syntex Puerto Rico, Inc.
Ingredient: naproxen
Dosage Form: Tablet: 250 mg (yellow)
Use: Relief of pain and swelling due to rheumatoid arthritis
Minor Side Effects: Bloating; cramps; diarrhea; drowsiness; flatulence; headache; heartburn; nausea; ringing in the ears; vomiting
Major Side Effects: Blood in stools; depression; fluid retention; hearing loss; jaundice; palpitations; tremors; visual disturbances
Contraindications: This drug should not be taken by people who are allergic to it or to aspirin. Consult your doctor immediately if this drug has been prescribed for you and you have such an allergy.
Warnings: This drug should be used with caution in pregnant women, nursing mothers, and children. This drug should be used with caution in persons with anemia, ulcers, heart disease, or kidney disease. Be sure your doctor knows if you have any of these conditions. • This drug should be given under close supervision to patients prone to upper gastrointestinal tract disease. Gastrointestinal bleeding, sometimes severe, and occasionally fatal, has been reported in patients receiving this drug. • It is recommended that persons taking this drug for a long time have eye tests performed periodically. • This drug may cause drowsiness, dizziness, or depression; avoid activities that require alertness. • This drug may prolong bleeding times, so persons also taking anticoagulants should use this drug with extreme caution. • Periodic blood tests and urine tests are recommended for persons taking this drug. • This drug interacts with anticoagulants, aspirin, oral antidiabetics, phenytoin, and sulfonamides. If you are currently taking any drugs of these types, consult your doctor about their use. If you are unsure about the type or contents of your medications, ask your doctor or pharmacist.
Comments: In numerous tests, this drug has been shown to be as effective as aspirin in the treatment of arthritis, but aspirin is still the drug of choice for the disease. Because of the high cost of this drug, consult your doctor

about prescribing proper doses of aspirin instead. • You should note improvement in your condition soon after you start using this drug; however, full benefit may not be obtained for as long as a month. It is important not to stop taking this drug even though symptoms have diminished or disappeared. • This drug is not a substitute for rest, physical therapy, or other measures recommended by your doctor to treat your condition. • Do not take aspirin or alcohol while taking this drug without first consulting your doctor.

OTC   Nature's Remedy laxative

Manufacturer: Norcliff Thayer, Inc.
Ingredients: aloe; cascara sagrada
Dosage Form: Tablet (regular and candy-coated): aloe, 143 mg; cascara sagrada, 127 mg
Use: Relief of constipation
Side Effects: Excess loss of fluid; griping (cramps); mucus in feces
Contraindications: Persons with high fever (100° F or more); black or tarry stools; nausea; vomiting; abdominal pain; or children under age three should not use this product unless directed by a doctor. • Do not use this product if constipation is caused by megacolon or other diseases of the intestine, or hypothyroidism.
Warnings: Excessive use (daily for a month or more) of this product may cause diarrhea, vomiting, and loss of certain blood electrolytes. • Pregnant women should not use this product except on the advice of a doctor.
Comments: This product may discolor the urine. • Evacuation may occur within 6 to 12 hours. Never self-medicate with this product if constipation lasts longer than two weeks or if the medication does not produce a laxative effect within a week. • Limit use to seven days unless directed otherwise by a doctor since this product may cause laxative-dependence (addiction) if used for a longer time.

Rx   Nembutal Sodium hypnotic

Manufacturer: Abbott Laboratories
Ingredient: pentobarbital
Equivalent Product: pentobarbital, various manufacturers (see "Comments")
Dosage Forms: Capsule: 30 mg (yellow); 50 mg (white/orange); 100 mg (yellow). Elixir (content per 5 ml): 18.2 mg with alcohol, 18%
Use: Relief of anxiety, tension; sleeping aid
Minor Side Effects: Drowsiness; nausea; vomiting
Major Side Effects: Cold and clammy skin; difficult breathing; rash or other allergic reaction
Contraindications: This drug should not be used by people who have porphyria or an allergy to it. Consult your doctor if this drug has been prescribed for you and you have either condition.
Warnings: This drug should be used cautiously by people who have liver, kidney, or lung diseases; those in a state of shock; and by pregnant women. Be sure your doctor knows if you have any of these conditions. • This drug has the potential for abuse and must be used with caution. Tolerance may develop quickly; do not increase the dose of this drug without first consulting your doctor. • This drug interacts with alcohol, central nervous system depressants, griseofulvin, oral anticoagulants, phenytoin, steroids, sulfonamides, tetracyclines, and tricyclic antidepressants; if you are currently taking any drugs of these types, consult your doctor about their use. If you are unsure of the type or contents of your medications, ask your doctor or pharmacist. • This drug may cause drowsiness and affect your ability to perform

hazardous tasks; avoid tasks that require alertness.

Comments: Drugs used for sleep should be taken one-half to one hour before bedtime. • Butisol Sodium hypnotic (sodium butabarbital), manufactured by McNeil Laboratories, and Seconal Sodium hypnotic, manufactured by Eli Lilly and Company, have uses, side effects, warnings, and comments generally identical to those of this drug.

Neocurtasal salt substitute (Winthrop Laboratories), see Co-Salt salt substitute.

OTC   Neoloid laxative

Manufacturer: Lederle Laboratories
Ingredient: castor oil
Dosage Form: Emulsion: castor oil, 36.4%
Use: Relief of isolated bouts of constipation
Side Effects: Excess loss of fluid; griping (cramps); mucus in feces
Contraindications: Persons with high fever (100° F or more); black or tarry stools; nausea; vomiting; abdominal pain; or children under age three should not use this product unless directed by a doctor. • Do not use this product when constipation is caused by megacolon or other diseases of the intestine, or hypothyroidism.
Warnings: Excessive use (daily for a month or more) of this product may cause diarrhea, vomiting, and loss of certain blood electrolytes. • Pregnant women should not use this product except on the advice of their doctor.
Comments: Generally, castor oil is not recommended for treatment of constipation. • Evacuation may occur within 6 to 12 hours. Never self-medicate with this product if constipation lasts longer than two weeks or if the medication does not produce a laxative effect within a week. • Limit use to seven days unless directed otherwise by a doctor since this product may cause laxative-dependence (addiction) if used for a longer time. • Limit use to one dose per each infrequent bout of constipation.

OTC   Neo-Polycin Ointment external anti-infective

Manufacturer: Dow Pharmaceuticals
Ingredients: bacitracin zinc; fuzene base; light liquid petrolatum; neomycin sulfate; polyethylene glycol distearate; polymyxin B sulfate; synthetic glyceride wax; white petrolatum
Dosage Form: Ointment (content per gram): bacitracin zinc, 400 units; neomycin sulfate, 3 mg; polymyxin B sulfate, 5000 units (quantities of other ingredients not specified)
Use: Prevention of infection from cuts and abrasions; treatment of impetigo
Side Effects: Allergic reactions (rash, itching, soreness); local irritation
Comments: Apply this product at least three times daily to maintain effectiveness. • If the infection does not clear in two to three weeks, consult your doctor or pharmacist.

℞   Neosporin antibiotic ophthalmic solution

Manufacturer: Burroughs Wellcome Co.
Ingredients: gramicidin; neomycin sulfate; polymyxin B sulfate; alcohol; thimerosal
Dosage Form: Drop (content per cc): gramicidin, 0.025 mg; neomycin sulfate, 2.5 mg (equivalent to 1.75 mg neomycin base); polymyxin B sulfate, 5,000 units; alcohol, 0.5%; thimerosal, 0.001%

Use: Short-term treatment of superficial bacterial infections of the eye
Minor Side Effects: Blurred vision; burning; stinging
Major Side Effects: Worsening of the condition
Contraindications: This drug should not be taken by people with known sensitivity to any of its ingredients. Make sure your doctor knows if you have such sensitivity if this drug is prescribed for you.
Warnings: Prolonged use of this drug may result in secondary infection. Culture and susceptibility testing should be performed during treatment.
Comments: Minor side effects will go away quickly. Be careful about the contamination of solutions used for the eyes. Wash your hands before administering eyedrops. Do not touch the dropper to your eye. Do not wash or wipe the dropper before replacing it in the bottle. Close the bottle tightly to keep out moisture.

OTC   Neosporin Ointment external anti-infective

Manufacturer: Burroughs Wellcome Co.
Ingredients: bacitracin zinc; neomycin sulfate; polymyxin B sulfate; white petrolatum
Dosage Form: Ointment (content per gram): bacitracin zinc, 400 units; neomycin sulfate, 5 mg; polymyxin B sulfate, 5,000 units; white petrolatum
Use: Prevention of infection from cuts and abrasions; treatment of impetigo
Side Effects: Allergic reactions (rash, itching, soreness); local irritation
Comments: Apply this product at least three times daily to maintain effectiveness. • If the infection does not clear in two to three weeks, consult your doctor or pharmacist.

OTC   Neo-Synephrine Compound decongestant cold remedy

Manufacturer: Winthrop Laboratories
Ingredients: phenylephrine hydrochloride; thenyldiamine hydrochloride; acetaminophen; caffeine
Dosage Form: Tablet: phenylephrine hydrochloride, 5 mg; thenyldiamine hydrochloride, 7.5 mg; acetaminophen, 150 mg; caffeine, 15 mg
Use: Temporary relief of nasal congestion, fever, aches, pains, and general discomfort of colds
Side Effects: Anxiety; blurred vision; chest pain; confusion; constipation; difficult and painful urination; dizziness; drowsiness; headache; increased blood pressure; insomnia; loss of appetite; nausea; nervousness; palpitations; rash; sweating; tension; tremor; vomiting
Contraindications: This product should not be used by persons who have severe heart disease or severe high blood pressure. This product should not be given to newborn or premature infants.
Warnings: This product should be used with special caution by the elderly or debilitated, and by persons who have asthma, diabetes, enlarged prostate, glaucoma (certain types), heart disease, high blood pressure, kidney disease, obstructed bladder, obstructed intestine, peptic ulcer, or thyroid disease. If you have any of these conditions, consult your doctor before taking this product. • This product may cause drowsiness. Do not take it if you must drive, operate heavy machinery, or perform other tasks requiring mental alertness. To prevent oversedation, avoid the use of alcohol or other drugs that have sedative properties. • This product interacts with alcohol, guanethidine, monoamine oxidase inhibitors, sedative drugs, and tricyclic antidepressants. If you are currently taking any drugs of these types, check with your doctor before taking this product. If you are unsure of the type or contents of your medications, ask your doctor or pharmacist. • Because this product reduces sweating, avoid excessive work or exercise in hot weather. • When taken in

overdose, acetaminophen is more toxic than aspirin. Follow dosage instructions carefully.

Comments: Many other conditions (some serious) mimic the common cold. If symptoms persist beyond one week or if they occur regularly without regard to season, consult your doctor. • The effectiveness of this product may diminish after being taken regularly for seven to 10 days; consult your pharmacist about substituting another product containing a different antihistamine if this product begins to lose its effectiveness for you. • Chew gum or suck on ice chips or a piece of hard candy to reduce mouth dryness.

OTC   Neo-Synephrine Intranasal nasal decongestant

Manufacturer: Winthrop Laboratories

Ingredients: phenylephrine hydrochloride; benzalkonium chloride; phenylmercuric acetate; thimerosal; methylparaben; propylparaben; sodium bisulfite

Dosage Forms: Drop: phenylephrine hydrochloride, 0.125%; 0.25%; 0.5%; 1%; benzalkonium chloride, 0.125%; methylparaben; propylparaben; sodium bisulfite. Jelly: phenylephrine hydrochloride, 0.5%; phenylmercuric acetate. Nasal spray: phenylephrine hydrochloride, 0.25%; 0.5%; benzalkonium chloride, 0.02%; thimerosal, 0.001%

Use: Temporary relief of nasal congestion due to colds, sinusitis, hay fever, or other upper respiratory allergies

Side Effects: Blurred vision; burning, dryness of nasal mucosa; increased nasal congestion or discharge; sneezing, and/or stinging; dizziness; drowsiness; headache; insomnia; nervousness; palpitations; slight increase in blood pressure; stimulation

Contraindications: This product should not be used by persons who have glaucoma (certain types).

Warnings: This product should be used with special caution by persons who have diabetes, advanced hardening of the arteries, heart disease, high blood pressure, or thyroid disease. If you have any of these conditions, consult your doctor before taking this product. • This product interacts with guanethidine, monoamine oxidase inhibitors, and thyroid preparations. If you are currently taking any drugs of these types, check with your doctor before taking this product. If you are unsure of the type or contents of your medications, ask your doctor or pharmacist. • To avoid side effects such as burning, sneezing, or stinging, and a "rebound" increase in nasal congestion and discharge, do not exceed the recommended dosage and do not use this product for more than three or four continuous days. • This product should not be used by more than one person; sharing the dispenser may spread infection.

Comments: The spray form of this product, although slightly more expensive than the drops and jelly, is preferred for adult use. The spray penetrates far back into the nose, covering the nasal area more completely, and is more convenient to use. The drops are preferable for administration to children. Winthrop Laboratories also produces Neo-Synephrine II nasal decongestant (nasal spray and drops). This product contains xylometazoline hydrochloride and has a duration of action of approximately 12 hours. Because of this product's dosing schedule, it is less likely to cause "rebound" congestion during use than nasal decongestants that do not contain this ingredient.

Neo-Synephrine II nasal decongestant (Winthrop Laboratories), see Neo-Synephrine Intranasal nasal decongestant.

OTC   Neoxyn poison ivy remedy

Manufacturer: William H. Rorer, Inc.

Ingredients: acetanilid; acetic acid; benzethonium chloride; hydrogen peroxide; propylparaben

Dosage Form: Liquid: acetanilid, 0.0169%; acetic acid, 1.15%; benzethonium chloride, 0.26%; hydrogen peroxide, 2.85%; propylparaben, 0.02%
Use: Relief of itching due to poison ivy and poison oak
Side Effects: Local irritation
Comments: This product requires that the skin first be scraped with a stick that is provided. When used correctly, this remedy is effective.

OTC   **Nervine Nightime Sleep-Aid**

Manufacturer: Miles Laboratories, Inc.
Ingredient: pyrilamine maleate
Dosage Form: Capsule-shaped tablet: pyrilamine maleate, 25 mg
Use: To induce drowsiness and assist in falling asleep
Side Effects: Blurred vision; confusion; constipation; difficult urination; dizziness; drowsiness; dry mouth and respiratory passages; headache; insomnia; low blood pressure; nausea; nervousness; palpitations; rash; restlessness; vomiting. Children may react with primary symptoms of excitement (convulsions; flushed skin; nervousness; tremors; twitching of muscles; uncoordinated movements).
Contraindications: This product should not be given to children under 12 years of age. • Do not take this product if you are pregnant or nursing.
Warnings: This product must be used with extreme caution by persons who have asthma, glaucoma, or enlarged prostate. If you have any of these conditions, do not take this product without first consulting your doctor. • This product may interact with other drugs; if you are currently taking any other prescription or over-the-counter medication, do not take this product without first consulting your doctor or pharmacist. • Tolerance to this drug may develop; do not increase the recommended dosage of this drug unless your doctor directs you to do so. • This drug may cause drowsiness; avoid driving, operating heavy machinery, or performing other tasks requiring mental alertness. To prevent oversedation, avoid the use of alcohol and other sedative drugs.
Comments: Insomnia may be a symptom of a serious illness; consult a doctor if sleeplessness lasts for more than two weeks.

Neuramate sedative and hypnotic (Halsey Drug Co., Inc.), see meprobamate sedative and hypnotic.

Niac vitamin supplement (O'Neal, Jones & Feldman Pharmaceuticals), see nicotinic acid vitamin supplement.

Nicalex vitamin supplement (Merrell-National Laboratories), see nicotinic acid vitamin supplement.

NICL vitamin supplement (Saran Pharmacal Corp.), see nicotinic acid vitamin supplement.

Nicobid vitamin supplement (Armour Pharmaceutical Corp.), see nicotinic acid vitamin supplement.

Nicocap vitamin supplement (ICN Pharmaceuticals, Inc.), see nicotinic acid vitamin supplement.

Nico-400 Plateau Caps vitamin supplement (Marion Laboratories, Inc.), see nicotinic acid vitamin supplement.

Niconyl antitubercular (Parke-Davis), see isoniazid antitubercular.

nico-Span vitamin supplement (Key Pharmaceuticals, Inc.), see nicotinic acid vitamin supplement.

Rₓ   nicotinic acid vitamin supplement

Manufacturer: various manufacturers
Ingredient: nicotinic acid
Equivalent Products: Diacin, Lemmon Company; Niac, O'Neal, Jones & Feldman Pharmaceuticals; Nicalex, Merrell-National Laboratories; NICL, Saran Pharmacal Corp.; Nicobid, Armour Pharmaceutical Corp.; Nicocap, ICN Pharmaceuticals, Inc.; Nico-400 Plateau Caps, Marion Laboratories, Inc.; nico-Span, Key Pharmaceuticals Inc.; SK-Niacin, Smith Kline & French Laboratories; Tega-Span, Ortega Pharmaceutical Co., Wampocap, Wallace Laboratories
Dosage Forms: Capsule; Liquid; Tablet; Time-release capsule (various dosages and colors)
Use: To correct niacin deficiency; lower blood cholesterol levels
Minor Side Effects: Dizziness; dryness of skin; flushing and warmth; headache; itching; nausea; palpitations; tingling in fingers and toes; vomiting
Major Side Effects: Activation of peptic ulcers
Contraindications: This drug should not be used by people who are hemorrhaging or by people who are allergic to niacin (nicotinic acid). Consult your doctor immediately if this drug has been prescribed for you and you have either condition.
Warnings: This drug should be used cautiously by people who have diabetes, glaucoma, liver disease, or peptic ulcer, and by those who are pregnant. Be sure your doctor knows if you have any of these conditions. • If you are taking this drug as a nutritional supplement rather than as a vasodilator, consult your doctor about taking niacinamide instead. Niacinamide does not cause flushing and other cardiovascular effects, but it may not lower blood cholesterol. • Toniacol vasodilator (Roche Products, Inc.) contains nicotinyl alcohol and has been classified as "possibly effective" in conditions associated with deficient blood flow.
Comments: Nicotinic acid is also known as vitamin B_3 or niacin. • Flushing, warmth, and dizziness produced by this drug usually go away after several days of continuous therapy. To avoid dizziness or light-headedness when you stand, contract and relax the muscles of your legs for a few moments before rising. Do this by pushing one foot against the floor while raising the other foot slightly, alternating feet so that you are "pumping" your legs in a pedaling motion.

Nilstat antifungal agent (Lederle Laboratories), see Mycostatin antifungal agent.

Nitrine-TDC antianginal (Paddock Laboratories), see Nitro-Bid Plateau Caps antianginal.

Nitro antianginal (Spencer-Mead, Inc.), see Nitro-Bid Plateau Caps antianginal.

Rₓ   Nitro-Bid Plateau Caps antianginal

Manufacturer: Marion Laboratories, Inc.
Ingredient: nitroglycerin
Equivalent Products: Ang-O-Span, Scrip-Physician Supply Co.; Dialex, Trimen Laboratories, Inc.; Gly-Trate Meta-Kaps, Sutliff & Case Co., Inc.;

496

Nitrine-TDC, Paddock Laboratories; Nitro, Spencer-Mead, Inc.; Nitrobon-TR, Forest Laboratories, Inc.; Nitrocap T.D., North American Pharmacal, Inc.; Nitrocels Diacels, Winston Pharmaceuticals, Inc.; Nitrocot, Truxton, Inc., Co.; nitroglycerin, various manufacturers; Nitrospan, USV (P.R.) Development Corp.; Nitrosule Pellsules, Misemer Pharmaceuticals, Inc.; Nitro T.D., Fleming & Co.; Nitrotym, Everett; Trates Granucaps, Tutag Pharmaceuticals, Inc.; Vasoglyn Unicelles, Reid-Provident Laboratories, Inc.

Dosage Form: Time-release capsule: 2.5 mg (purple/white with white beads); 6.5 mg (blue/yellow with white beads); 9 mg (yellow/green with white beads)

Use: Prevention of chest pain (angina) due to heart disease; possibly effective for management of attacks of angina

Minor Side Effects: Dizziness; flushing of face; headache

Major Side Effects: Palpitations

Contraindications: This drug should not be taken by people who have low blood pressure, severe anemia, glaucoma; or by those who have recently suffered a heart attack and those who are allergic to this drug. Consult your doctor immediately if this drug has been prescribed for you and you have any of these conditions.

Warnings: If you develop blurred vision or dry mouth, contact your doctor. • Do not drink alcohol unless your doctor has told you you may. • This drug may not continue to relieve chest pain after one to three months because tolerance to nitroglycerin develops quickly. Discuss the merits of this drug with your doctor before accepting a prescription.

Comments: This drug must be swallowed; do not crush or break the capsules. • Side effects generally disappear after two to three weeks of continued therapy. • To avoid dizziness or light-headedness when you stand, contract and relax the muscles of your legs for a few moments before rising. Do this by pushing one foot against the floor while raising the other foot slightly, alternating feet so that you are "pumping" your legs in a pedaling motion.

Nitrobon-TR antianginal (Forest Laboratories, Inc.), see Nitro-Bid Plateau Caps antianginal.

Nitrocap T.D. antianginal (North American Pharmacal, Inc.), see Nitro-Bid Plateau Caps antianginal.

Nitrocels Diacels antianginal (Winston Pharmaceuticals, Inc.), see Nitro-Bid Plateau Caps antianginal.

Nitrocot antianginal (Truxton, Inc. Co.), see Nitro-Bid Plateau Caps antianginal.

Nitrospan antianginal (USV [P.R.] Development Corp.), see Nitro-Bid Plateau Caps antianginal.

℞   Nitrostat antianginal

Manufacturer: Parke-Davis

Ingredient: nitroglycerin

Dosage Form: Sublingual tablet: 0.15 mg; 0.3 mg; 0.4 mg; 0.6 mg (all are white)

Use: Relief of chest pain (angina) due to heart disease

Minor Side Effects: Dizziness; flushing of face; headache

Major Side Effects: Fainting; palpitations

Contraindications: This drug should not be used by people who have severe anemia or by those who have suffered a head injury or recent heart attack. Consult your doctor immediately if this drug has been prescribed for you and you have any of these conditions.

Warnings: This drug should be used cautiously by people who have liver or kidney disease and by pregnant women. Be sure your doctor knows if you have any of these conditions. • If you develop blurred vision or dry mouth, contact your doctor. • This drug interacts with alcohol and other vasodilators. Consult your doctor about their use. If you are unsure of the type or contents of your medications, ask your doctor or pharmacist. • If you require more tablets than usual to relieve chest pain, contact your doctor. You may have developed a tolerance to the drug, or the drug may not be working effectively because of interference with other medication. • If this drug does not relieve pain, or if pain arises from a different location or differs in severity, call your doctor immediately. • Before using this drug to relieve pain, be certain the pain arises from the heart and is not due to a muscle spasm or indigestion.

Comments: Frequently chest pain will be relieved in two to five minutes simply by sitting down. • When you take this drug, sit down, lower your head, and breathe deeply. • Do not swallow this drug. The tablets must be placed under the tongue. Do not drink water or swallow for five minutes after taking this drug. • Side effects caused by this drug are most bothersome the first two weeks after starting therapy. • This drug must be stored in a tightly capped glass container. Never store the tablets in a metal box, plastic vial, or in the refrigerator.

Nitrosule Pellsules antianginal (Misemer Pharmaceuticals, Inc.), see Nitro-Bid Plateau Caps antianginal.

Nitro T.D. antianginal (Fleming & Co.), see Nitro-Bid Plateau Caps antianginal.

Nitrotym antianginal (Everett), see Nitro-Bid Plateau Caps antianginal.

Norafed adrenergic and antihistamine (North American Pharmacal, Inc.), see Actifed adrenergic and antihistamine.

Nordryl antihistamine (North American Pharmacal, Inc.), see Benadryl antihistamine.

Norfranil antidepressant (North American Pharmacal, Inc.), see Tofranil antidepressant.

R_x   **Norgesic analgesic**

Manufacturer: Riker Laboratories, Inc.

Ingredients: aspirin, caffeine, orphenadrine citrate, phenacetin

Dosage Form: Tablet: aspirin, 225 mg or 450 mg; caffeine, 30 mg or 60 mg; orphenadrine citrate, 25 mg or 50 mg; phenacetin, 160 mg or 320 mg (both tri-layered green/white/yellow)

Use: Relief of mild to moderate pain in muscles or joints

Minor Side Effects: Blurred vision; confusion; constipation; diarrhea; dilation of pupils; dizziness; drowsiness; dry mouth; headache; nausea; rash; ringing in the ears; slight blood loss; sweating; vomiting; weakness

Major Side Effects: Palpitations; rapid heartbeat; urinary hesitancy or retention

Contraindications: This drug should not be used in patients with glaucoma, intestinal obstruction, difficult swallowing, enlarged prostate, obstructions of the bladder, or myasthenia gravis. Be sure your doctor knows if you have any of these conditions. • This drug should not be taken by persons allergic to any of its ingredients. Contact your doctor immediately if this drug has been prescribed for you and you have such an allergy.

Warnings: This drug may cause drowsiness; avoid engaging in potentially hazardous activities, such as operating machinery or driving a motor vehicle. • This drug should be used cautiously by pregnant women, nursing mothers, and in women of childbearing age. • This drug is not recommended for use in children under 12 years of age. • This drug should be used with caution in persons with kidney problems, irregular heartbeat, peptic ulcers, or coagulation problems. Be sure your doctor knows if you have any of these conditions. • If this drug is prescribed for a long period, periodic monitoring of blood, urine, and liver function is recommended.

Comments: This drug is not a substitute for rest, physical therapy, or other measures recommended by your doctor to treat your condition. • This drug should be taken with food or milk. • If you hear buzzing or ringing, if your ears feel strange, or if your stomach hurts, your dosage may need adjustment. Call your doctor. • Chew gum or suck on ice chips or a piece of hard candy to reduce mouth dryness.

Normatane antihistamine (North American Pharmacal, Inc.), see Dimetapp antihistamine.

Normatane DC expectorant (North American Pharmacal, Inc.), see Dimetane DC expectorant.

Normatane expectorant (North American Pharmacal, Inc.), see Dimetane expectorant.

Nor-Mil anticholinergic and antispasmodic (North American Pharmacal, Inc.), see Lomotil anticholinergic and antispasmodic.

Noroxine thyroid hormone (North American Pharmacal, Inc.), see Synthroid thyroid hormone.

℞   **Norpace antiarrhythmic**

Manufacturer: Searle Laboratories
Ingredient: disopyramide phosphate
Dosage Form: Capsule: 100 mg (white/orange); 150 mg (brown/orange)
Use: Treatment of some heart arrhythmias
Minor Side Effects: Bleeding; blurred vision; diarrhea; difficult urination; dizziness; dry mouth; dry nose, eyes, throat; gas; headache; loss of appetite; muscle weakness; nausea; nervousness; pain; rash; vomiting
Major Side Effects: Chest pain; edema and weight gain; fainting; low blood pressure; low blood sugar; psychosis; shortness of breath
Contraindications: This drug should not be taken by persons who have certain types of heart disease. This drug should not be taken by people who are allergic to it. Consult your doctor immediately if this drug has been prescribed for you and you have such an allergy or condition.
Warnings: This drug should be used with caution, since its use may cause low blood pressure and heart failure. • This drug should be used cautiously in conjunction with certain other antiarrhythmic agents, such as quinidine or procainamide, and/or propranolol. If you are currently taking any drugs of these types, consult your doctor about their use. If you are unsure of the type or contents of your medications, ask your doctor or pharmacist. • Patients receiving more than one antiarrhythmic drug must be carefully monitored. • This drug should be used with caution in persons with glaucoma, urinary re-

tention, low blood potassium (hypokalemia), liver and kidney disease, pregnancy; and by nursing mothers. Be sure your doctor knows if any of these conditions relate to you. • This drug should be used with caution in children.

Comments: This drug is similar in action to procainamide and to quinidine sulfate. • While taking this drug, do not take any nonprescription item for cough, cold, or sinus problems without first checking with your doctor.

Norpanth anticholinergic (North American Pharmacal, Inc.), see ProBanthine anticholinergic.

Nor-Pres antihypertensive (North American Pharmacal, Inc.), see Apresoline antihypertensive.

Nor-Tet antibiotic (North American Pharmacal, Inc.), see tetracycline hydrochloride antibiotic.

OTC   Novahistine cold and allergy remedy

Manufacturer: Dow Pharmaceuticals

Ingredients: phenylpropanolamine hydrochloride; chlorpheniramine maleate; alcohol (liquid form only)

Dosage Forms: Liquid (content per 5 ml, or one teaspoon): phenylpropanolamine hydrochloride, 18.75 mg; chlorpheniramine maleate, 2 mg; alcohol, 5%. Tablet: phenylpropanolamine hydrochloride, 18.75 mg; chlorpheniramine maleate, 2 mg

Use: Temporary relief of nasal congestion and other symptoms of colds, "flu," and upper respiratory allergies

Side Effects: Anxiety; blurred vision; chest pain; confusion; constipation; difficult and painful urination; dizziness; drowsiness; headache; increased blood pressure; insomnia; loss of appetite; nausea; nervousness; palpitations; rash; reduced sweating; tension; tremor; vomiting

Contraindications: This product should not be used by persons who have severe heart disease or severe high blood pressure. • This product should not be given to newborn or premature infants.

Warnings: This product should be used with special caution by the elderly or debilitated, and by persons who have asthma, diabetes, enlarged prostate, glaucoma (certain types), heart disease, high blood pressure, kidney disease, obstructed bladder, obstructed intestine, peptic ulcer, or thyroid disease. If you have any of these conditions, consult your doctor before taking this product. • This product may cause drowsiness. Do not take it if you must drive, operate heavy machinery, or perform other tasks requiring mental alertness. To prevent oversedation, avoid the use of alcohol or other drugs that have sedative properties. • This product interacts with alcohol, guanethidine, monoamine oxidase inhibitors, sedative drugs, and tricyclic antidepressants. If you are currently taking any drugs of these types, check with your doctor before taking this product. If you are unsure of the type or contents of your medications, ask your doctor or pharmacist. • Because this product reduces sweating, avoid excessive work or exercise in hot weather.

Comments: Many other conditions (some serious) mimic the common cold. If symptoms persist beyond one week or if they occur regularly without regard to season, consult your doctor. • The effectiveness of this product may diminish after being taken regularly for seven to ten days; consult your pharmacist about substituting another product containing a different antihistamine if this product begins to lose its effectiveness for you. • Chew gum or suck on ice chips or a piece of hard candy to reduce mouth dryness.

OTC   Novahistine DH expectorant cough remedy

Manufacturer: Dow Pharmaceuticals

Ingredients: codeine phosphate; phenylpropanolamine hydrochloride; chlorpheniramine maleate; alcohol

Dosage Form: Liquid (content per 5 ml, or one teaspoon): codeine phosphate, 10 mg; phenylpropanolamine hydrochloride, 18.75 mg; chlorpheniramine maleate, 2 mg; alcohol, 5%

Use: Temporary relief of cough, nasal congestion, and other symptoms of colds or "flu"; also to convert a dry, nonproductive cough to a productive phlegm-producing cough

Side Effects: Anxiety; blurred vision; chest pain; confusion; constipation; diarrhea; difficult and painful urination; dizziness; drowsiness; dry mouth; headache; heartburn; increased blood pressure; insomnia; loss of appetite; low blood pressure; nasal congestion; nausea; nervousness; palpitations; rash; reduced sweating; severe abdominal pain; sore throat; tension; tremor; vomiting

Contraindications: This product should not be used by persons who have severe heart disease or severe high blood pressure. • This product should not be given to newborn or premature infants.

Warnings: This product should be used with special caution by the elderly or debilitated, and by persons who have asthma or respiratory disease, diabetes, enlarged prostate, glaucoma (certain types), heart disease, high blood pressure, kidney disease, obstructed bladder, obstructed intestine, peptic ulcer, or thyroid disease. If you have any of these conditions, consult your doctor before taking this product. • This product may cause drowsiness. Do not take it if you must drive, operate heavy machinery, or perform other tasks requiring mental alertness. To prevent oversedation, avoid the use of alcohol or other drugs that have sedative properties. • This product interacts with alcohol, guanethidine, monoamine oxidase inhibitors, sedative drugs, and tricyclic antidepressants. If you are currently taking any drugs of these types, check with your doctor before taking this product. If you are unsure of the type or contents of your medications, ask your doctor or pharmacist. • Because this product reduces sweating, avoid excessive work or exercise in hot weather. • Because this product contains codeine, it has the potential for abuse and must be used with caution. It usually should not be taken for more than seven to ten days. Tolerance may develop quickly, but do not increase the dose without consulting your doctor.

Comments: Many other conditions (some serious) mimic the common cold. If symptoms persist beyond one week or if they occur regularly without regard to season, consult your doctor. • Do not use this product to treat chronic coughs, such as those from smoking or asthma. • Do not use this product to treat productive (hacking) coughs that produce phlegm. • If you require an expectorant, you need more moisture in your environment. Drink eight to ten glasses of water daily. The use of a vaporizer or humidifier may also be beneficial. Consult your doctor. • Chew gum or suck on ice chips or a piece of hard candy to reduce mouth dryness. • Over-the-counter sale of this product may not be permitted in some states.

OTC   Novahistine DMX cough remedy

Manufacturer: Dow Pharmaceuticals

Ingredients: dextromethorphan hydrobromide; pseudoephedrine hydrochloride; guaifenesin; alcohol

Dosage Form: Liquid (content per 5 ml, or one teaspoon): dextromethorphan hydrobromide, 10 mg; pseudoephedrine hydrochloride, 30 mg; guaifenesin, 100 mg; alcohol, 10%

Use: Temporary relief of cough and nasal congestion due to colds or "flu"; also to convert a dry, nonproductive cough to a productive, phlegm-producing cough

Side Effects: Drowsiness; mild stimulation; nausea; vomiting

Warnings: This product should be used with special caution by children under two years of age, and by persons who have diabetes, heart disease, high blood pressure, or thyroid disease. If you have any of these conditions, consult your doctor before taking this product. • This product interacts with guanethidine and monoamine oxidase inhibitors; if you are currently taking any drugs of these types, check with your doctor before taking this product. If you are unsure of the type or contents of your medications, ask your doctor or pharmacist.

Comments: Do not use this product to treat chronic coughs, such as those from smoking or asthma. • Do not use this product to treat productive (hacking) coughs that produce phlegm. • If you require an expectorant, you need more moisture in your environment. Drink eight to ten glasses of water daily. The use of a vaporizer or humidifier may also be beneficial. Consult your doctor.

OTC   Novahistine Expectorant cough remedy

Manufacturer: Dow Pharmaceuticals

Ingredients: alcohol; codeine phosphate; guaifenesin; phenylpropanolamine hydrochloride

Dosage Form: Liquid (content per 5 ml, or one teaspoon): alcohol, 7.5%; codeine phosphate, 10 mg; guaifenesin, 100 mg; phenylpropanolamine hydrochloride, 18.75 mg

Use: Temporary relief of cough, nasal congestion, and other symptoms of colds or "flu"; also to convert a dry, nonproductive cough to a productive, phlegm-producing cough

Side Effects: Anxiety; chest pain; confusion; constipation; diarrhea; dizziness; drowsiness; headache; heartburn; increased blood pressure; insomnia, loss of appetite; nausea; nervousness; palpitations; rash; severe abdominal pain; sweating; tension; tremor; vomiting

Contraindications: This product should not be used by persons who have severe heart disease or severe high blood pressure. • This product should not be given to newborn or premature infants.

Warnings: This product should be used with special caution by the elderly or debilitated, and by persons who have asthma or respiratory disease, diabetes, enlarged prostate, glaucoma (certain types), heart disease, high blood pressure, kidney disease, obstructed bladder, obstructed intestine, peptic ulcer, or thyroid disease. If you have any of these conditions, consult your doctor before taking this product. • This product may cause drowsiness. Do not take it if you must drive, operate heavy machinery, or perform other tasks requiring mental alertness. To prevent oversedation, avoid the use of alcohol or other drugs that have sedative properties. • This product interacts with alcohol, guanethidine, monoamine oxidase inhibitors, and sedative drugs. If you are currently taking any drugs of these types, check with your doctor before taking this product. If you are unsure of the type or contents of your medications, ask your doctor or pharmacist. • Because this product contains codeine, it has the potential for abuse and must be used with caution. It usually should not be taken for more than seven to ten days. Tolerance may develop quickly, but do not increase the dose without consulting your doctor.

Comments: Many other conditions (some serious) mimic the common cold. If symptoms persist beyond one week or if they occur regularly without regard to season, consult your doctor. • Do not use this product to treat chronic coughs, such as those from smoking or asthma. • Do not use this product to treat productive (hacking) coughs that produce phlegm. • If you require an expectorant, you need more moisture in your environment. Drink eight to ten glasses of water daily. The use of a vaporizer or humidifier may also be beneficial. Consult your doctor. • Over-the-counter sale of this product may not be permitted in some states.

OTC Noxzema Medicated burn remedy and antiseptic

Manufacturer: Noxell Corporation
Ingredients: camphor; clove oil; eucalyptus oil; lime water; menthol; phenol; water-dispersible base
Dosage Forms: Cream; Lotion: phenol, less than 0.5% (quantities of other ingredients not specified)
Use: Treatment of sunburn; minor cuts; scrapes; poison ivy; burns; and insect bites
Side Effects: Allergy; local irritation
Warnings: Do not use this product on broken skin. • This product should not be used on large areas of the body because a toxic amount of the medication can be absorbed.
Comments: Remember that ointments that are put on serious (second- or third-degree) burns will have to be taken off before definitive treatment can be given. Consult your doctor or pharmacist if you have any questions concerning the use of this product.

OTC NP-27 athlete's foot remedy

Manufacturer: Norwich-Eaton Pharmaceuticals
Ingredients: 8-hydroxyquinoline benzoate; undecylenic acid; salicylic acid; zinc undecylenate (Ingredients vary with dosage form; see below.)
Dosage Forms: Cream: 8-hydroxyquinoline benzoate; benzoic acid; salicylic acid. Liquid: orthochloromercuriphenol, 0.02%; benzoic acid; salicylic acid; propyl alcohol; isopropyl alcohol, 30%. Powder: salicylic acid; boric acid; propylparaben; benzoic acid. Spray powder: zinc undecylenate; alcohol, 20.5%.
Use: Treatment of athlete's foot (all dosage forms); treatment of ringworm of the body exclusive of the nails and scalp (cream and liquid only)
Side Effects: Allergy; local irritation
Warnings: Diabetics should not use this product without first consulting a physician; persons with impaired circulation should not use the liquid form without first consulting a physician. • Do not apply this product to mucous membranes, scraped skin, or to large areas of skin. • If your condition worsens, or if irritation occurs, stop using this product and consult your pharmacist. • When using the aerosol form of this product, be careful not to inhale any of the powder.
Comments: Some lesions take months to heal, so it is important not to stop treatment too soon. • If foot lesions are consistently a problem, check the fit of your shoes. • Wash your hands thoroughly after applying this product. • The cream and liquid forms of this product are preferable to the powders for effectiveness; the best action of the powders may be in drying the infected area. • When using the liquid form of this product, avoid contaminating the contents of the bottle by pouring some of the liquid into a separate container for each use. • The liquid form may sting temporarily after application. • The aerosol powder may be more expensive than the other forms of this product; check prices before paying for convenience you do not need.

NTZ nasal decongestant

Manufacturer: Winthrop Laboratories
Ingredients: phenylephrine hydrochloride; thenyldiamine hydrochloride; benzalkonium chloride
Dosage Form: Drop: phenylephrine hydrochloride, 0.5%; thenyldiamine hydrochloride, 0.1%; benzalkonium chloride, 1:5000
Use: Temporary relief of nasal congestion due to colds, sinusitis, and hay fever or other upper respiratory allergies
Side Effects: Burning, dryness of nasal mucosa; increased nasal congestion or discharge; sneezing, and/or stinging; blurred vision; dizziness; drowsiness; headache; insomnia; nervousness; palpitations; slight increase in blood pressure; stimulation
Contraindications: This product should not be used by persons who have glaucoma (certain types).
Warnings: This product should be used with special caution by persons who have diabetes, advanced hardening of the arteries, heart disease, high blood pressure, or thyroid disease. If you have any of these conditions, consult your doctor before taking this product. • This product interacts with guanethidine, monoamine oxidase inhibitors, and thyroid preparations. If you are currently taking any drugs of these types, check with your doctor before taking this product. If you are unsure of the type or contents of your medications, ask your doctor or pharmacist. • To avoid side effects such as burning, sneezing, or stinging, and a "rebound" increase in nasal congestion and discharge, do not exceed the recommended dosage and do not use this product for more than three or four continuous days. • This product should not be used by more than one person; sharing the dispenser may spread infection.
Comments: Although slightly more expensive, nasal decongestants in spray form are preferred to this product for adult use. Nasal sprays penetrate far back into the nose, covering the nasal area more completely, and are more convenient to use. Many other brands of nasal decongestants that contain the same or similar ingredients to this product are available in spray form. For administration to children, however, drops are preferable.

OTC **Nujol laxative**

Manufacturer: Plough, Inc.
Ingredient: mineral oil
Dosage Form: Liquid (quantity of ingredient not specified)
Use: Stool softener
Contraindications: Persons with high fever (100° F or more); black or tarry stools; nausea; vomiting; abdominal pain; or children under age six should not use this product unless directed by a doctor. • Do not use this product when constipation is caused by megacolon or other diseases of the intestine, or hypothyroidism.
Warnings: Excessive use (daily for a month or more) of this product may cause diarrhea, vomiting, and loss of certain blood electrolytes. • A type of pneumonia may occur after prolonged (more than two months) and repeated (daily) use. • Pregnant women should not use this product except on the advice of a doctor.
Comments: Evacuation may occur within six to eight hours. Never self-medicate with this product if constipation lasts longer than two weeks or if the medication does not produce a laxative effect within a week. • Mineral oil may interfere with the absorption of vitamins A and D, calcium, and phosphate. If you take mineral oil longer than seven days, consult your doctor. • This laxative is best taken at bedtime; it should not be taken at mealtime. • If this product leaks through the rectum, the dose should be reduced until this

symptom disappears. • Do not take a stool softener product at the same time as you are taking this product. • Limit use to seven days; this product may cause laxative-dependence (addiction) if used for a longer period.

OTC　　　Nupercainal hemorrhoidal preparation

Manufacturer: CIBA Pharmaceutical Company
Ingredients: acetone sodium bisulfite; dibucaine NF
Dosage Form: Ointment: acetone sodium bisulfite, 0.5%; dibucaine NF, 1%
Use: Relief of pain and itching of hemorrhoids and other irritated skin conditions
Warnings: Sensitization (continued itching and redness) may occur with long-term and repeated use.
Comments: Hemorrhoidal (pile) preparations relieve itching, reduce pain and inflammation, and check bleeding, but do not heal, dry up, or give lasting relief from hemorrhoids. • Certain ingredients in this product may cause an allergic reaction; do not use for longer than seven days at a time unless your doctor has advised you otherwise. • Never self-medicate for hemorrhoids if pain is continuous or throbbing, if bleeding or itching is excessive, or if you feel a large pressure within the rectum.

OTC　　　Nupercainal hemorrhoidal preparation

Manufacturer: CIBA Pharmaceutical Company
Ingredients: cocoa butter; acetone sodium bisulfite; bismuth subgallate; dibucaine; zinc oxide
Dosage Form: Suppository: acetone sodium bisulfite, 0.05%; bismuth subgallate; cocoa butter; dibucaine, 2.5 mg; zinc oxide
Use: Relief of pain and itching of hemorrhoids
Warnings: Sensitization (continued itching and redness) may occur with long-term use.
Comments: Hemorrhoidal (pile) preparations relieve itching, reduce pain and inflammation, and check bleeding, but do not heal, dry up, or give lasting relief from the hemorrhoids. • Certain ingredients in this product may cause an allergic reaction; do not use for longer than seven days at a time unless your doctor has advised you otherwise. • The suppository is not recommended for external hemorrhoids or bleeding internal hemorrhoids. Use the ointment form. Use caution when inserting applicator. • Never self-medicate for hemorrhoids if pain is continuous or throbbing, if bleeding or itching is excessive, or if you feel a large pressure within the rectum.

OTC　　　Nupercainal local anesthetic

Manufacturer: CIBA Pharmaceutical Company
Ingredients: acetone sodium bisulfite; dibucaine
Dosage Forms: Cream: acetone sodium bisulfite, 0.37%; dibucaine, 0.5%. Ointment: acetone sodium bisulfite, 0.5%; dibucaine, 1%
Use: Relief of pain and itching from sunburn, nonpoisonous insect bites, minor burns, cuts, and scratches
Side Effects: Allergy; local irritation
Contraindications: Do not use this product on broken skin. • This product should not be used on large areas of the body because a toxic amount of the medication may be absorbed.
Warnings: Do not put this product in or near the eyes.
Comments: Remember that ointments that are put on serious (second- or third-degree) burns will have to be taken off before definitive treatment can be

given. Consult your doctor or pharmacist if you have any questions concerning the use of this product.

Nydrazid antitubercular (E. R. Squibb & Sons), see isoniazid antitubercular.

OTC   **Nyquil cough remedy**

Manufacturer: Vicks Health Care Division
Ingredients: dextromethorphan hydrobromide; ephedrine sulfate; doxylamine succinate; acetaminophen; alcohol
Dosage Form: Liquid (content per 30 ml, or two tablespoons): dextromethorphan hydrobromide, 15 mg; ephedrine sulfate, 8 mg; doxylamine succinate, 7.5 mg; acetaminophen, 600 mg; alcohol, 25%
Use: Temporary relief of cough, nasal congestion, fever, aches, and pains due to colds or "flu"
Side Effects: Anxiety; blurred vision; chest pain; confusion; constipation; difficult and painful urination; dizziness; drowsiness; headache; increased blood pressure; insomnia; loss of appetite; nausea; nervousness; palpitations; rash; reduced sweating; tension; tremor; vomiting
Contraindications: Do not give this product to children under ten years of age except with your doctor's approval.
Warnings: This product should be used with special caution by persons who have diabetes, heart disease, high blood pressure, or thyroid disease. If you have any of these conditions, consult your doctor before taking this product. • This product may cause drowsiness. Do not take it if you must drive, operate heavy machinery, or perform other tasks requiring mental alertness. To prevent oversedation, avoid the use of alcohol or other drugs that have sedative properties. • This product interacts with alcohol, guanethidine, monoamine oxidase inhibitors, sedative drugs, and tricyclic antidepressants. If you are currently taking any drugs of these types, check with your doctor before taking this product. If you are unsure of the type or contents of your medications, ask your doctor or pharmacist. • When taken in overdose, acetaminophen is more toxic than aspirin. Follow dosage instructions carefully. • Because this product reduces sweating, avoid excessive work or exercise in hot weather.
Comments: Do not use this product to treat chronic coughs, such as those from smoking or asthma. • Do not use this product to treat productive (hacking) coughs that produce phlegm.

OTC   **Nytol Tablets sleeping aid**

Manufacturer: Block Drug Company, Inc.
Ingredient: pyrilamine maleate
Dosage Form: Tablet: 25 mg; capsule: 50 mg
Use: To induce drowsiness and assist in falling asleep
Side Effects: Blurred vision; confusion; constipation; difficult urination; dizziness; drowsiness; dry mouth and respiratory passages; headache; insomnia; low blood pressure; nausea; nervousness; palpitations; rash; restlessness; vomiting. Children may react with primary symptoms of excitement (convulsions; flushed skin; nervousness; tremors; twitching of muscles; uncoordinated movements).
Contraindications: This product must be used with extreme caution by persons who have asthma, glaucoma, or enlarged prostate. If you have any of these conditions, do not take this product without first consulting your doctor. • This product may interact with other drugs; if you are currently taking any other prescription or over-the-counter medication, do not take this prod-

uct without first consulting your doctor or pharmacist. • Tolerance to this drug may develop; do not increase the recommended dosage of this drug unless your doctor directs you to do so. • This drug may cause drowsiness; avoid driving, operating heavy machinery, or performing other tasks requiring mental alertness. To prevent oversedation, avoid the use of alcohol and other sedative drugs.

Comments: Insomnia may be a symptom of a serious illness; consult a doctor if sleeplessness lasts for more than two weeks.

o.b.c.t. adrenergic (Pharmics, Inc.), see Tenuate adrenergic.

OTC   Ocusol Drops eye decongestant

Manufacturer: Norwich-Eaton Pharmaceuticals
Ingredients: benzalkonium chloride; boric acid; methylcellulose; phenylephrine hydrochloride; tetrahydrozoline; sodium borate; sodium chloride
Dosage Form: Drops: phenylephrine hydrochloride, 0.02%
Use: Relief of minor eye irritation
Side Effects: Allergic reactions (rash, itching, soreness); local irritation; momentary blurred vision
Contraindications: Do not use this product if you have glaucoma.
Warnings: Do not use this product for more than two consecutive days without checking with your doctor.
Comments: Do not touch the dropper or bottle top to the eye or other tissue because contamination of the solution will result. • This product contains boric acid which many medical authorities believe should not be used because it is toxic. Follow the directions on package. • The use of more than one eye product at a time may cause severe irritation to the eye. Consult your pharmacist before doing so.

Omnipen antibiotic (Wyeth Laboratories), see ampicillin antibiotic.

OTC   One-A-Day multivitamin

Manufacturer: Miles Laboratories, Inc.
Ingredients: vitamin A; vitamin E; vitamin C; folic acid; thiamine; riboflavin; niacin; vitamin B6; vitamin B12; vitamin D
Dosage Form: Tablet: vitamin A, 5000 IU; vitamin E, 15 IU; vitamin C, 60 mg; folic acid, 0.4 mg; thiamine, 1.5 mg; riboflavin, 1.7 mg; niacin, 20 mg; vitamin B6, 2 mg; vitamin B12, 6 mcg; vitamin D, 400 IU
Use: Dietary supplement
Warnings: This product contains ingredients that accumulate and are stored in the body. The recommended dose should not be exceeded for long periods (several weeks to months) except by doctor's orders.
Comments: If large doses are taken, this product may interfere with the results of urine tests. Inform your doctor and pharmacist you are taking this product.

OTC   One-A-Day Plus Iron multivitamin and iron supplement

Manufacturer: Miles Laboratories, Inc.
Ingredients: vitamin A; vitamin E; vitamin C; folic acid; thiamine; riboflavin; niacin; vitamin B6; vitamin B12; vitamin D; iron
Dosage Form: Tablet: vitamin A, 5000 IU; vitamin E, 15 IU; vitamin C, 60 mg; folic acid, 0.4 mg; thiamine, 1.5 mg; riboflavin, 1.7 mg; niacin, 20 mg; vitamin B6, 2 mg; vitamin B12, 6 mcg; vitamin D, 400 IU; iron, 18 mg
Use: Dietary supplement
Side Effects: Constipation; diarrhea; nausea; stomach pain

Contraindications: This product should not be used by persons who have active peptic ulcer or ulcerative colitis.

Warnings: The iron in this product interacts with oral tetracycline antibiotics and reduces the absorption of the antibiotics. If you are currently taking tetracycline, consult your doctor or pharmacist before taking this product. If you are unsure of the type or contents of your medications, ask your doctor or pharmacist. • Alcoholics and persons who have chronic liver or pancreatic disease should use this product with special caution; such persons may have enhanced iron absorption and are therefore more likely than others to experience iron toxicity. • Accidental iron poisoning is common in children; be sure to keep this product safely out of their reach. • This product contains ingredients that accumulate and are stored in the body. The recommended dose should not be exceeded for long periods (several weeks to months) except by doctor's orders.

Comments: Because of its iron content, this product may cause constipation, diarrhea, nausea, or stomach pain. These symptoms usually disappear or become less severe after two to three days. Taking your dose with food or milk may help minimize these side effects. If they persist, ask your pharmacist to recommend another product. • Black, tarry stools are a normal consequence of iron therapy. If your stools are not black and tarry, this product may not be working for you. Ask your pharmacist to recommend another product. • If large doses are taken, this product may interfere with the results of urine tests. Inform your doctor and pharmacist you are taking this product.

OTC **One-A-Day Plus Minerals multivitamin and mineral supplement**

Manufacturer: Miles Laboratories, Inc.

Ingredients: vitamin A; vitamin E; vitamin C; folic acid; thiamine; riboflavin; niacin; vitamin B_6; vitamin B_{12}; vitamin D; pantothenic acid; iron; calcium; phosphorus; iodine; magnesium; copper; zinc

Dosage Form: Tablet: vitamin A, 5000 IU; vitamin E, 15 IU; vitamin C, 60 mg; folic acid, 0.4 mg; thiamine, 1.5 mg; riboflavin, 1.7 mg; niacin, 20 mg; vitamin B_6, 2 mg; vitamin B_{12}, 6 mcg; vitamin D, 400 IU; pantothenic acid, 10 mg; iron, 18 mg; calcium, 100 mg; phosphorus, 100 mg; iodine, 150 mcg; magnesium, 100 mg; copper, 2 mg; zinc, 15 mg

Use: Dietary supplement

Side Effects: Constipation; diarrhea; nausea; stomach pain

Contraindications: This product should not be used by persons who have active peptic ulcer or ulcerative colitis.

Warnings: The minerals in this product interact with oral tetracycline antibiotics and reduce the absorption of the antibiotics. If you are currently taking tetracycline, consult your doctor or pharmacist before taking this product. If you are unsure of the type or contents of your medications, ask your doctor or pharmacist. • Alcoholics and persons who have chronic liver or pancreatic disease should use this product with special caution; such persons may have enhanced iron absorption and are therefore more likely than others to experience iron toxicity. • Accidental iron poisoning is common in children; be sure to keep this product safely out of their reach. • This product contains ingredients that accumulate and are stored in the body. The recommended dose should not be exceeded for long periods (several weeks to months) except by doctor's orders.

Comments: Because of its iron content, this product may cause constipation, diarrhea, nausea, or stomach pain. These symptoms usually disappear or become less severe after two to three days. Taking your dose with food or milk may help minimize these side effects. If they persist, ask your pharmacist to recommend another product. • Black, tarry stools are a normal consequence of iron therapy. If your stools are not black and tarry, this product may not be working for you. Ask your pharmacist to recommend another product. • If large doses are taken, this product may interfere with the results of urine tests. Inform your doctor and pharmacist you are taking this product.

OTC — Orajel toothache and sore gums remedy

Manufacturer: Commerce Drug Co.
Ingredients: benzocaine; polyethylene glycol-like base
Dosage Form: Cream (quantities of ingredients not specified)
Use: Relief of pain of toothache and sore gums
Warnings: If you have an oral ulcer which does not heal within three weeks, see your dentist.
Comments: This product is useful for toothache only when the nerve is exposed. • Teething lotions and toothache preparations are the same.

Rx — oral contraceptives

Oral contraceptives is a descriptive term.
Examples: Brevicon oral contraceptive, Norinyl oral contraceptive (Syntex [F.P.] Inc.); Demulen oral contraceptive, Enovid oral contraceptive, Ovulen oral contraceptive (Searle & Co.); Loestrin oral contraceptive, Norlestrin oral contraceptive (Parke-Davis); Lo/Ovral oral contraceptive, Micronor oral contraceptive , Ovral oral contraceptive , Ovrette oral contraceptive (Wyeth Laboratories); Modicon oral contraceptive, Ortho-Novum oral contraceptive (Ortho Pharmaceutical Corporation); Ovcon oral contraceptive (Mead Johnson Pharmaceutical Division); Zorane oral contraceptive (Lederle Laboratories)
Dosage Form: Tablets in packages. Some contain 20 or 21 tablets; others 28. When 28 are present, 7 are blank or contain iron (see Comments).
Use: Birth control
Minor Side Effects: Abdominal cramps; diarrhea; dizziness; nausea; nervousness; vomiting
Major Side Effects: Blood clots; breakthrough bleeding (spotting); cancer; changes in menstrual flow; depression; elevated blood sugar; enlarged or tender breasts; eye damage; fluid retention; gallbladder disease; high blood pressure; increase or decrease in hair growth; jaundice; migraine; reduced ability to conceive after drug is stopped; painful menstruation; rash; skin color changes; stroke; weight changes
Contraindications: This type of drug should not be used by people with certain types of heart disease, liver disease, blood disease, vaginal bleeding, clots, or history of blood disease, clots, or stroke. Be sure your doctor knows if you have or have had any of these conditions. • This type of drug should not be taken by people who smoke cigarettes.
Warnings: This type of drug has been known or suspected to cause cancer. If you have a family history of cancer, you should inform your doctor of it before taking oral contraceptives. • This type of drug should be used cautiously by women over age 30. • Oral contraceptives are known to cause an increased risk of clotting disorders, blood diseases, eye disease, cancer, birth defects, diabetes, high blood pressure, headache, bleeding disorders, and poor production of breast milk. • Caution should be observed while taking oral contraceptives if you have uterine tumors, mental depression, epilepsy, migraine, asthma, heart or kidney disease, jaundice, or vitamin deficiency. Be sure your doctor knows if you have any of these conditions. Oral contraceptives interact with oral anticoagulants, rifampin, and steroids. Contact your doctor immediately if you are currently taking any drugs of these types. If you are unsure of the type or contents of your medications, ask your doctor or pharmacist.

Comments: Oral contraceptives currently are considered the most effective available method of birth control. The table below shows various methods of birth control and their effectiveness.

Birth Control Method	Effectiveness*
Oral contraceptive	less than 1
Intrauterine device (IUD)	up to 6
Diaphragm	up to 20
Aerosol foam	up to 29
Condom	up to 36
Gel or cream	up to 36
Rhythm	up to 47

*Pregnancies per 100 women years.

Take an oral contraceptive at the same time every day to get into the habit of taking the pills. If you skip one day, take a tablet for the day you missed as soon as you think of it and another tablet at the regular time. • Missing a day increases your chances of pregnancy; use other methods of contraception for the rest of the cycle and continue taking the tablets. • If you do not start to menstruate on schedule at the end of the pill cycle, begin the next cycle of pills at the prescribed time, anyway. Many women taking oral contraceptives have irregular menstruation. Do not be alarmed, but consult your doctor. • Stop taking oral contraceptive tablets at least three months before you wish to become pregnant. Use another type of contraceptive during this three-month period. • Some oral contraceptive packets contain 28 tablets rather than the usual 20 or 21 tablets. The 28-tablet packets contain seven placebos (sugar pills) or iron tablets. The placebos help you remember to take a tablet each day even while you are menstruating, and the iron tablets help replace the iron that is lost in menstruation. • Nausea is common, especially during the first two or three months, but may be prevented by taking the tablets at bedtime. If nausea persists for more than three months, consult your doctor. • Although many brands of oral contraceptives are available, most differ in only minor ways, and you may have to try several brands before you find the product that is ideal for you. • Your pharmacist will give you a booklet explaining birth control pills with every prescription. Read this booklet carefully. It contains exact directions on how to use the medication correctly. • If you use oral contraceptives, you should not smoke cigarettes; taking oral contraceptives and smoking may cause heart disease. • You should visit your doctor for a checkup at least twice a year while you are taking oral contraceptives.

Orapav Timecelles smooth muscle relaxant (W. E. Hauck, Inc.), see Pavabid Plateau Caps smooth muscle relaxant.

Orasone steroid hormone (Rowell Laboratories, Inc.), see prednisone steroid hormone.

Oretic diuretic and antihypertensive (Abbott Laboratories), see hydrochlorothiazide diuretic and antihypertensive.

Oreton Methyl steroid hormone (Schering Corporation), see methyltestosterone steroid hormone.

℞ **Orinase oral antidiabetic**

Manufacturer: The Upjohn Company
Ingredient: tolbutamide
Equivalent Product: tolbutamide, various manufacturers
Dosage Form: Tablet: 250 mg; 500 mg (both white)

Use: Treatment of diabetes mellitus

Minor Side Effects: Diarrhea; dizziness; fatigue; headache; loss of appetite; nausea; rash; vomiting; weakness

Major Side Effects: Low blood pressure; jaundice; sore throat

Contraindications: This drug should not be used to treat diabetes complicated by acidosis, ketosis, or coma; it should not be used by people who have severe kidney diseases. Consult your doctor immediately if this drug has been prescribed for you and you have any of these conditions.

Warnings: This drug should not be used to treat juvenile-onset diabetes unless insulin is also administered. • This drug should be used cautiously by people who have severe infections, those who have suffered severe trauma or are about to undergo surgery, or by those who are pregnant or malnourished. Be sure your doctor knows if you have any of these conditions. • This drug is not an oral form of insulin. • Studies have shown that a good diet and exercise program may be just as effective as oral antidiabetic drugs. However, these drugs allow diabetics more leeway in their lifestyles. Persons taking this drug should carefully watch their diet and exercise program. • Persons taking this drug should visit the doctor at least once a week for the first six weeks of therapy. They should check their urine for sugar and ketones at least three times a day, and they should know how to recognize the first signs of low blood sugar. • People taking this drug will have to switch to insulin therapy if complications develop (e.g., ketoacidosis, severe trauma, severe infection, diarrhea, nausea or vomiting, or the need for major surgery). • Do not drink alcohol and do not take any other drugs unless directed to do so by your doctor while you are taking this drug. Be especially careful with nonprescription cold remedies. • This drug interacts with anabolic steroids, anticoagulants, aspirin, chloramphenicol, guanethidine, propranolol, monoamine oxidase inhibitors, phenylbutazone, steroids, tetracycline, thiazide diuretics, and thyroid hormones; if you are currently taking any drugs of these types, consult your doctor about their use. If you are unsure of the type or contents of your medications, ask your doctor or pharmacist. • Avoid long exposure to sunlight while taking this drug.

Comments: Take this drug at the same time everyday. • Recent evidence indicates that not all generic forms of tolbutamide are equivalent. Ask your pharmacist for a product that is bioequivalent.

OTC   Ornacol Capsules, Ornacol Liquid cough remedies

Manufacturer: Menley & James Laboratories

Ingredients: dextromethorphan hydrobromide (capsule form only); phenylpropanolamine hydrochloride; alcohol (liquid form only)

Dosage Forms: Capsule: dextromethorphan hydrobromide, 30 mg; phenylpropanolamine hydrochloride, 25 mg. Liquid (content per 5 ml, or one teaspoon) dextromethorphan hydrobromide, 15 mg; phenylpropanolamine hydrochloride, 12.5 mg; alcohol, 8%

Use: Temporary relief of cough and nasal congestion due to colds or "flu"

Side Effects: Drowsiness; mild stimulation; nausea; vomiting

Warnings: This product should be used with special caution by children under two years of age, and by persons who have diabetes, heart disease, high blood pressure, or thyroid disease. If you have any of these conditions, consult your doctor before taking this product. • This product interacts with guanethidine and monoamine oxidase inhibitors. If you are currently taking any drugs of these types, check with your doctor before taking this product. If you are unsure of the type or contents of your medications, ask your doctor.

Comments: Do not use this product to treat chronic coughs, such as from smoking or asthma. • Do not use this product to treat productive (hacking) coughs that produce phlegm.

℞ **Ornade Spansule antihistamine, anticholinergic, and adrenergic**

Manufacturer: Smith Kline & French Laboratories
Ingredients: chlorpheniramine maleate; isopropamide iodide; phenylpropanolamine hydrochloride
Equivalent Products: Allernade, Rugby Laboratories; Capade, Spencer-Mead, Inc.
Dosage Form: Capsule: chlorpheniramine maleate, 8 mg; isopropamide iodide, 2.5 mg; phenylpropanolamine hydrochloride, 50 mg (blue/clear with red and white beads)
Use: Symptomatic relief of upper respiratory tract congestion
Minor Side Effects: Blurred vision; confusion; constipation; diarrhea; difficult urination; dizziness; drowsiness; dry mouth; headache; heartburn; insomnia; loss of appetite; nasal congestion; nausea; palpitations; rash; reduced sweating; restlessness; vomiting; weakness
Major Side Effects: Chest pain; high blood pressure; low blood pressure; severe abdominal pain; sore throat
Contraindications: This drug should not be taken by people who are allergic to any of its components. The drug should not be taken by people who are using monoamine oxidase inhibitors (ask your pharmacist if you are unsure), or by those who have asthma, heart disease, severe high blood pressure, obstructed bladder, obstructed intestine, or ulcer (certain types). Consult your doctor immediately if this drug has been prescribed for you and you have any of these conditions. • This drug should not be given to children under six years of age.
Warnings: This drug should be used cautiously by people who have glaucoma, heart disease, thyroid disease, or enlarged prostate; and by women who are pregnant or nursing. Be sure your doctor knows if you have any of these conditions. • This drug should not be taken in conjunction with guanethidine or monoamine oxidase inhibitors; if you are currently taking any drugs of these types, consult your doctor about their use. If you are unsure of the type or contents of your medications, ask your doctor or pharmacist. • While taking this drug, do not take any nonprescription item for cough, cold, or sinus problems without first checking with your doctor. • This drug may cause drowsiness; avoid tasks that require alertness. To prevent oversedation, avoid the use of alcohol or other drugs that have sedative properties. • Because this drug reduces sweating, avoid excessive work or exercise in hot weather. • This drug has sustained action; never increase your dose or take it more frequently than your doctor prescribes. A serious overdose could result. • This drug may alter the results of thyroid function tests; remind your doctor that you are taking the drug if you are scheduled for a thyroid test.
Comments: Chew gum or suck on ice chips or a piece of hard candy to reduce mouth dryness.

OTC **Ornade 2 for Children cold and allergy remedy**

Manufacturer: Smith Kline & French Laboratories
Ingredients: phenylpropanolamine hydrochloride; chlorpheniramine maleate; alcohol
Dosage Form: Liquid (content per 5 ml, or one teaspoon): phenylpropanolamine hydrochloride, 12.5 mg; chlorpheniramine maleate, 2 mg; alcohol, 5%
Use: Temporary relief of symptoms of colds and upper respiratory allergies
Side Effects: Anxiety; blurred vision; chest pain; confusion; constipation; difficult and painful urination; dizziness; drowsiness; headache; increased blood pressure; insomnia; loss of appetite; nausea; nervousness; palpitations; rash; sweating; tension; tremor; vomiting

Contraindications: This product should not be used by persons who have severe heart disease or severe high blood pressure. • This product should not be given to newborn or premature infants.

Warnings: This product should be used with special caution by persons who have asthma, diabetes, enlarged prostate, glaucoma (certain types), heart disease, high blood pressure, kidney disease, obstructed bladder, obstructed intestine, peptic ulcer, or thyroid disease. If your child has any of these conditions, consult your doctor before administering this product. • This product interacts with alcohol, guanethidine, monoamine oxidase inhibitors, sedative drugs, and tricyclic antidepressants. If your child is currently taking any drugs of these types, check with your doctor before administering this product. If you are unsure of the type or contents of your child's medications, ask your doctor or pharmacist.

Comments: Many other conditions (some serious) mimic the common cold. If symptoms persist beyond one week or if they occur regularly without regard to season, consult your doctor. • The effectiveness of this product may diminish after being taken regularly for seven to ten days; consult your pharmacist about substituting another product containing a different antihistamine if this product begins to lose its effectiveness for your child. • Have your child chew gum or suck on ice chips or a piece of hard candy to reduce mouth dryness.

OTC   Ornex cold remedy

Manufacturer: Menley & James Laboratories
Ingredients: phenylpropanolamine hydrochloride; acetaminophen
Dosage Form: Capsule: phenylpropanolamine hydrochloride, 18 mg; acetaminophen, 325 mg
Use: Temporary relief of nasal congestion, fever, aches, pains, and general discomfort due to colds or "flu"
Side Effects: Mild to moderate stimulation; nausea; vomiting
Warnings: This product should be used with special caution by persons who have diabetes, heart disease, high blood pressure, or thyroid disease. If you have any of these conditions, consult your doctor before taking this product. • This product interacts with alcohol, guanethidine, monoamine oxidase inhibitors, sedative drugs, and tricyclic antidepressants. If you are currently taking any drugs of these types, check with your doctor before taking this product. If you are unsure of the type or contents of your medications, ask your doctor or pharmacist. • When taken in overdose, acetaminophen is more toxic than aspirin. Follow dosage instructions carefully.
Comments: Many other conditions (some serious) mimic the common cold. If symptoms persist beyond one week or if they occur regularly without regard to season, consult your doctor. • The effectiveness of this product may diminish after being taken regularly for seven to ten days; consult your pharmacist about substituting another medication if this product begins to lose its effectiveness for you.

OTC   Ortho-Creme contraceptive

Manufacturer: Ortho Pharmaceutical Corporation
Ingredient: nonoxynol-9
Dosage Form: Vaginal cream: nonoxynol-9, 2%
Use: Used with diaphragm for prevention of pregnancy
Side Effects: Allergy of user or partner; local irritation to user or partner
Comments: Be sure to insert a new dose of this product for each intercourse. • Do not douche for at least six hours after intercourse. • This product should be used with a diaphragm; used alone, it is not as effective as when it is combined with a diaphragm.

Ortho-Gynol contraceptive jelly

Manufacturer: Ortho Pharmaceutical Corporation
Ingredient: p-diisobutylphenoxypolyethoxyethanol
Dosage Form: Vaginal jelly: p-diisobutylphenoxypolyethoxyethanol, 1%
Use: Used with diaphragm for prevention of pregnancy
Side Effects: Allergy of user or partner; local irritation to user or partner
Comments: Be sure to insert a new dose of this product for each intercourse. • Do not douche for at least six hours after intercourse. • This product should be used with a diaphragm; used alone, it is not as effective as when it is combined with a diaphragm.

Otobione otic suspension (Schering Corporation), see Cortisporin otic solution/suspension.

Oto otic solution (North American Pharmacal, Inc.), see Auralgan otic solution.

OTC   Outgro ingrown toenail remedy

Manufacturer: Whitehall Laboratories
Ingredients: chlorobutanol; tannic acid; isopropyl alcohol
Dosage Form: Liquid: chlorobutanol, 5%; tannic acid, 25%; isopropyl alcohol, 83%
Use: Temporary relief of pain, swelling, and inflammation from ingrown toenails
Side Effects: Burning; minor rash; stinging. (If swallowed, may cause abdominal cramping; diarrhea; nausea; vomiting.)
Contraindications: This product should not be used by persons who have diabetes or impaired circulation. Do not apply this product to an infected toe.
Warnings: Do not apply this product to any area other than immediately around the ingrown nail.
Comments: This product does not affect the growth, shape, or position of the ingrown nail, but it toughens the surrounding skin, allowing the nail to be cut.

Ovest estrogen hormone (Trimen Laboratories, Inc.), see Premarin estrogen hormone.

Oxalid anti-inflammatory (USV [P.R.] Development Corp.), see Butazolidin anti-inflammatory.

Oxlopar antibiotic (Parke-Davis), see Terramycin antibiotic.

Oxybiotic antibiotic (Star Pharmaceuticals, Inc.), see Terramycin antibiotic.

OTC   Oxy-5 and Oxy-10 acne preparations

Manufacturer: Norcliff Thayer Inc.
Ingredient: benzoyl peroxide
Dosage Form: Lotion, Oxy-5: benzoyl peroxide, 5%; Oxy-10: benzoyl peroxide, 10%
Use: Treatment of acne
Side Effects: Allergy; local irritation
Warnings: This product should not be used by patients with known sensitivity to benzoyl peroxide.
Comments: If the condition worsens, stop using this product and call your

pharmacist. • These acne preparations may be especially active on fair-skinned people. • Wash area gently with warm water and pat dry before apply-ing this product. • Avoid exposure to heat lamps, sunlamps, or direct sunlight when using these acne preparations. • This product may damage certain fabrics including rayon.

Oxy-Tetrachel antibiotic (Rachelle Laboratories, Inc.), see Ter-ramycin antibiotic.

OTC   PAC analgesic

Manufacturer: The Upjohn Company
Ingredients: aspirin; phenacetin; caffeine
Dosage Form: Tablet: aspirin, 228 mg (3½ grains); phenacetin, 163 mg; caf-feine, 32 mg
Use: Relief of pain of headache, toothache, sprains, muscular aches, nerve inflammation, menstruation; relief of discomforts and fever of colds; tem-porary relief of minor aches and pains of arthritis and rheumatism
Side Effects: Dizziness; hemolytic anemias; jaundice; kidney damage; men-tal confusion; nausea and vomiting; ringing in the ears; slight blood loss; sweating
Contraindications: This product may cause an increased bleeding ten-dency and should not be taken by persons with a history of bleeding, peptic ulcer, or stomach bleeding.
Warnings: Persons with kidney disease, asthma, hay fever, or other allergies should be extremely careful about using this product. The product may interfere with the treatment of gout. If you have any of these conditions, consult your doctor or pharmacist before using this medication. • Do not use this product if you are currently taking alcohol, methotrexate, oral anti-coagulants, oral antidiabetics, probenecid, steroids, and/or sulfinpyrazone; if you are unsure of the type or contents of your medications, ask your doctor or pharmacist. • The dosage instructions listed on the package should be followed carefully; toxicity may occur in adults or children with repeated doses.
Comments: You can save money by taking plain aspirin instead of this product; there is no evidence that combinations of ingredients are more ef-fective than similar doses of a single-ingredient product. The caffeine in this product may have a slight stimulant effect but has no pain-relieving value.

OTC   Pain-A-Lay toothache,
sore throat, and sore gums remedy

Manufacturer: Roberts Proprietaries, Inc.
Ingredients: boric acid; cresol
Dosage Form: Liquid (quantities of ingredients not specified)
Use: Relieves pain of toothache, sore throat, and sore gums
Warnings: If you have an oral ulcer which does not heal within three weeks, see your dentist.
Comments: This product is useful for toothache only when the nerve is ex-posed. • Teething lotions and toothache preparations are the same.

Paltet antibiotic (Palmedico, Inc.), see tetracycline hydrochloride antibiotic.

Panasol steroid hormone (The Seatrace Co.), see prednisone steroid hormone.

Panazid antitubercular (Panray Division), see isoniazid antitubercular.

Pan-Kloride potassium chloride replacement (Panray Co., Inc.), see potassium chloride replacement.

Panmycin antibiotic (The Upjohn Company), see tetracycline hydrochloride antibiotic.

Panwarfin anticoagulant (Abbott Laboratories), see Coumadin anticoagulant.

Pap-Kaps-150 Meta-Kaps smooth muscle relaxant (Sutliff & Case Co., Inc.), see Pavabid Plateau Caps smooth muscle relaxant.

Parachlor analgesic (Stayner Corporation), see Parafon Forte analgesic.

Paracort steroid hormone (Parke-Davis), see prednisone steroid hormone.

℞   Parafon Forte analgesic

Manufacturer: McNeil Laboratories
Ingredients: acetaminophen; chlorzoxazone
Equivalent Products: Chlorofon-F, Rugby Laboratories; Chlorzone Forte, Henry Schein, Inc.; chlorzoxazone w/APAP, various manufacturers; Lobac, The Seatrace Co.; Parachlor, Stayner Corporation; Tuzon, Tutag Pharmaceuticals, Inc.
Dosage Form: Tablet: acetaminophen, 300 mg; chlorzoxazone, 250 mg (green)
Use: Relief of pain from strained muscles
Minor Side Effects: Change in urine color; diarrhea; dizziness; drowsiness; fatigue; light-headedness; nausea; overstimulation; rash
Major Side Effects: Jaundice
Contraindications: This drug should not be taken by people allergic to either of its components. Consult your doctor immediately if this drug has been prescribed for you and you have such an allergy.
Warnings: This drug should be used cautiously by people who have liver disease and by those who are pregnant. Be sure your doctor knows if you have either condition. • This drug may cause allergic reactions. Contact your doctor if you develop a rash. • This drug may color the urine orange or reddish purple. This side effect is usually not serious and persists only as long as the drug is taken. • This drug is not a substitute for rest, physical therapy, or other measures recommended by your doctor. • This drug may cause drowsiness; avoid tasks that require alertness. To prevent oversedation, avoid the use of alcohol or other drugs that have sedative properties.

Paragesic-65 analgesic (Parmed Pharmaceuticals, Inc.), see Darvon analgesic.

℞   paregoric antidiarrheal

Manufacturer: various manufacturers
Ingredient: paregoric (camphorated tincture of opium)
Dosage Form: Liquid (content per 5 ml, or one teaspoon): the equivalent of 2 mg morphine
Use: Symptomatic relief of diarrhea; occasionally used for its sedative-hypnotic or its analgesic narcotic effects

Minor Side Effects: Constipation; drowsiness; dry mouth; euphoria; flushing; light-headedness; nausea; palpitations; rash; sweating; uncoordinated movements; urine retention; vomiting

Major Side Effects: Breathing difficulty; faintness; rapid heartbeat; tremors

Contraindications: This drug should not be taken by persons who are allergic to opium derivatives. Consult your doctor immediately if this drug has been prescribed for you and you have such an allergy.

Warnings: This drug should be used with extreme caution by the elderly, and by pregnant or nursing women. This drug should be used cautiously by people who have asthma and other respiratory problems; epilepsy; head injuries; diseases of the liver, kidney, prostate, or thyroid; or an acute abdominal condition. Be sure your doctor knows if you have any of these conditions. • This drug should be used with caution by people who are taking central nervous system depressants. Be sure your doctor is aware of every medication you use. • This drug has the potential for abuse and must be used with caution. Tolerance may develop quickly; do not increase the dose of the drug without first consulting your doctor. • This drug may cause drowsiness; avoid tasks that require alertness. To prevent oversedation, avoid the use of alcohol or other drugs that have sedative properties. • This drug may cause a drop in blood pressure and should be used cautiously by people with heart disease. • This drug should not be used in conjunction with alcohol, monoamine oxidase inhibitors, phenothiazines, and antidepressants; if you are currently taking any drugs of these types, consult your doctor about their use. If you are unsure of the type or contents of your medications, ask your doctor or pharmacist. • Because it contains a narcotic, this drug should not be used for more than seven to ten days.

Comments: To avoid dizziness or light-headedness when you stand, contract and relax the muscles of your legs for a few moments before rising. Do this by pushing one foot against the floor while raising the other foot slightly, alternating feet so that you are "pumping" your legs in a pedaling motion. • This drug may be mixed in water to help improve the taste.

OTC   Parepectolin diarrhea remedy

Manufacturer: William H. Rorer, Inc.

Ingredients: alcohol; kaolin; paregoric; pectin

Dosage Form: Liquid (content per ounce): alcohol, 0.69%; kaolin, 5.4 g; paregoric, 3.6 mg; pectin, 162 mg

Use: For treatment of common diarrhea

Side Effects: Blurred vision; constipation after long-term use (seven days to two months); coughing and sore throat; difficult urination; dizziness; drowsiness; dry mouth; faintness; fever; flushing of face; headaches; loss of appetite; mental confusion; nervousness; palpitations; sedation; skin rash; warm skin; weakness

Contraindications: Persons with glaucoma, myasthenia gravis, certain types of heart, liver, or kidney disease should not use this product. • This product or any other product should not be used to self-medicate without first consulting a doctor if the person is under age three or over age 60, has a history of asthma, heart disease, peptic ulcer, or is pregnant.

Warnings: Persons with heart, liver, lung, or thyroid disease should use with caution. Consult your doctor or pharmacist if you have any questions concerning the use of this product.

Comments: Over-the-counter sale of this product may not be permitted in some states. • Diarrhea should stop in two to three days. If it persists longer, recurs frequently or in presence of high fever, call your doctor and be sure to tell him of any drugs you are taking. Be sure to drink at least eight glasses of water each day. • This product contains a narcotic but when used as directed, you need not worry about addiction to it. • If you are taking other drugs, do not take this product until you have first checked with your doctor or pharmacist. Avoid excessive use of alcohol, tranquilizers, or any drug that sedates the nervous system if you are taking large and repeated doses of this product.

Parest sedative and hypnotic (Parke-Davis), see Quaalude sedative and hypnotic.

Pargesic Compound 65 analgesic (Parmed Pharmaceuticals, Inc.), see Darvon Compound-65 analgesic.

Partrex antibiotic (Parmed Pharmaceuticals. Inc.), see tetracycline hydrochloride antibiotic.

℞ **Pavabid Plateau Caps smooth muscle relaxant**

Manufacturer: Marion Laboratories, Inc.
Ingredient: papaverine hydrochloride
Equivalent Products: Blupav, Bluco Incorporated; Cerespan, USV (P.R.) Development Corp.; Delapav, Dunhall Pharmaceuticals, Inc.; Dilart, Trimen Laboratories, Inc.; Dipav, Lemmon Company; Kavrin, Hyrex Pharmaceuticals; K-Pava, Kay Pharmacal Company, Inc.; Lapav Graduals, Amfre-Grant, Inc.; Myobid, Laser, Inc.; Orapav Timecelles, W. E. Hauck, Inc.; papaverine hydrochloride, various manufacturers; Pap-Kaps-150 Meta-Kaps, Sutliff & Case Co., Inc.; Pava-2, General Pharmaceutical Prods., Inc.; Pavacap Unicelles, Reid-Provident Laboratories, Inc.; Pavacels, Winston Pharmaceuticals, Inc.; Pavacen Cenules, The Central Pharmacal Co.; Pavacot T. D., C. O. Truxton, Inc.; Pavacron, H. R. Cenci Laboratories, Inc.; Pavadur, Century Pharmaceuticals, Inc.; Pavadyl, Bock Drug Co., Inc.; Pavakey, Key Pharmaceuticals, Inc.; Pava-Mead, Spencer-Mead, Inc.; Pava-Par, Parmed Pharmaceuticals Inc.; Pava-RX, Blaine Co., Inc.; Pavased, Mallard Incorporated; Pavasule, Misemer Pharmaceuticals, Inc.; Pavatran, Mayrand Incorporated; Pavatym, Everett Laboratories, Inc.; Paverine Spancaps, North American Pharmacal, Inc.; Pava-Wol, Wolins Pharmacal Corp., Paverolan, The Lannett Company, Inc.; Sustaverine, ICN Pharmaceuticals, Inc.; Tri-Pavasule, Tri-State Pharmaceutical Co., Inc.; Vasal Granucaps, Tutag Pharmaceuticals, Inc.; Vasocap-150, Keene Pharmaceuticals, Inc.; Vasospan, Ulmer Pharmacal Co.
Dosage Form: Time-release capsule: 150 mg (black/clear)
Use: To promote blood flow to the heart muscle and brain
Minor Side Effects: Abdominal distress; constipation; diarrhea; dizziness; drowsiness; fatigue; headache; loss of appetite; nausea; rash; sweating
Warnings: This drug should be used cautiously by people who have glaucoma or liver disease. Be sure your doctor knows if you have either condition. • This drug may cause drowsiness; avoid tasks that require alertness. To prevent oversedation, avoid the use of alcohol or other drugs that have sedative properties. • While taking this drug, do not take any nonprescription item for cough, cold, or sinus problems without first checking with your doctor.
Comments: This drug and many of its equivalents are also available as capsules which do not provide sustained action. • This drug increases the flow of blood to the brain and heart muscle, but this activity has not been shown to alleviate chest pain or the aftereffects of a stroke. In addition, the AMA Drug Evaluations (1980) states that no objective study has proven this drug effective in peripheral blood vessel disease. • Discuss the merits of this drug with your doctor before starting therapy.

Pavacap Unicelles smooth muscle relaxant (Reid-Provident Laboratories, Inc.), see Pavabid Plateau Caps smooth muscle relaxant.

Pavacels smooth muscle relaxant (Winston-Pharmaceuticals, Inc.), see Pavabid Plateau Caps smooth muscle relaxant.

Pavacen Cenules smooth muscle relaxant (The Central Pharmacal Co.), see Pavabid Plateau Caps smooth muscle relaxant.

Pavacot T.D. smooth muscle relaxant (C. O. Truxton, Inc.), see Pavabid Plateau Caps smooth muscle relaxant.

Pavacron smooth muscle relaxant (H. R. Cenci Laboratories, Inc.), see Pavabid Plateau Caps smooth muscle relaxant.

Pavadon analgesic (Coastal Pharmaceutical Co., Inc.), see Tylenol with Codeine analgesic.

Pavadur smooth muscle relaxant (Century Pharmaceuticals, Inc.), see Pavabid Plateau Caps smooth muscle relaxant.

Pavadyl smooth muscle relaxant (Bock Drug Co., Inc.), see Pavabid Plateau Caps smooth muscle relaxant.

Pavakey smooth muscle relaxant (Key Pharmaceuticals, Inc.), see Pavabid Plateau Caps smooth muscle relaxant.

Pava-Mead smooth muscle relaxant (Spencer-Mead, Inc.), see Pavabid Plateau Caps smooth muscle relaxant.

Pava-Par smooth muscle relaxant (Parmed Pharmaceuticals Inc.), see Pavabid Plateau Caps smooth muscle relaxant.

Pava-RX smooth muscle relaxant (Blaine Co., Inc.), see Pavabid Plateau Caps smooth muscle relaxant.

Pavased smooth muscle relaxant (Mallard Incorporated), see Pavabid Plateau Caps smooth muscle relaxant.

Pavasule smooth muscle relaxant (Misemer Pharmaceuticals, Inc.), see Pavabid Plateau Caps smooth muscle relaxant.

Pavatran smooth muscle relaxant (Mayrand Incorporated), see Pavabid Plateau Caps smooth muscle relaxant.

Pava-2 smooth muscle relaxant (General Pharmaceutical Prods., Inc.), see Pavabid Plateau Caps smooth muscle relaxant.

Pavatym smooth muscle relaxant (Everett Laboratories, Inc.), see Pavabid Plateau Caps smooth muscle relaxant.

Pava-Wol smooth muscle relaxant (Wolins Pharmacal Corp.), see Pavabid Plateau Caps smooth muscle relaxant.

Paverine Spancaps smooth muscle relaxant (North American Pharmacal, Inc.), see Pavabid Plateau Caps smooth muscle relaxant.

Paverolan smooth muscle relaxant (The Lannett Company, Inc.), see Pavabid Plateau Caps smooth muscle relaxant.

PBR/12 sedative and hypnotic (Scott-Alison Pharmaceuticals, Inc.), see phenobarbital sedative and hypnotic.

Pediamycin antibiotic (Ross Laboratories), see erythromycin antibiotic.

OTC　　　　Pediaquil cough remedy for children

Manufacturer: Philips Roxane Laboratories, Inc.
Ingredients: phenylephrine hydrochloride; guaifenesin; alcohol; squill; sorbitol; corn syrup; currant and caramel flavors
Dosage Form: Liquid (contents per 30 ml, or two tablespoons): phenylephrine hydrochloride, 15 mg; guaifenesin, 300 mg; alcohol, 5%; squill, 105 mg; sorbitol; corn syrup; currant and caramel flavors
Use: Temporary relief of cough and nasal congestion due to colds or "flu"
Side Effects: Mild stimulation; occasional nausea, vomiting
Warnings: This product should be used with special caution by children under two years of age, and by persons who have diabetes, heart disease, high blood pressure, or thyroid disease. If you have any of these conditions, consult your doctor before taking this product. • This product interacts with guanethidine and monoamine oxidase inhibitors. If you are currently taking any drugs of these types, check with your doctor before taking this product. If you are unsure of the type or contents of your medications, ask your doctor or pharmacist.
Comments: Do not use this product to treat chronic coughs, such as those from smoking or asthma. • Do not use this product to treat productive (hacking) coughs that produce phlegm. • If your child requires an expectorant, he needs more moisture in his environment. Have your child drink eight to ten glasses of water daily. The use of a vaporizer or humidifier may also be beneficial. Consult your doctor.

Pen A antibiotic (Pfipharmecs Division), see ampicillin antibiotic.

Penapar VK antibiotic (Parke-Davis), see penicillin potassium phenoxymethyl antibiotic.

Penbritin antibiotic (Ayerst Laboratories), see ampicillin antibiotic.

R︎x　　　　　　　penicillin G antibiotic

Manufacturer: various manufacturers
Ingredient: penicillin G
Equivalent Products: Pentids, E. R. Squibb & Sons, Inc.; Pfizerpen G, Pfipharmecs Division; G-Recillin, Reid-Provident Laboratories, Inc.; K-Pen, Kay Pharmacal Company, Inc.; SK-Penicillin G, Smith Kline & French Laboratories
Dosage Forms: Liquid; Tablet (various dosages and various colors)
Use: Treatment of a wide variety of bacterial infections
Minor Side Effects: Diarrhea; nausea; vomiting
Major Side Effects: "Black tongue;" cough; irritation of the mouth; rash; rectal and vaginal itching; severe diarrhea; superinfection
Contraindications: This drug should not be taken by people who are allergic to any penicillin drug. Consult your doctor immediately if this drug has been prescribed for you and you have such an allergy.
Warnings: This drug should be used cautiously by people who have asthma or other significant allergies. Be sure your doctor knows if you have any type of allergy. • This drug interacts with chloramphenicol, erythromycin, and tetracycline; if you are currently taking any drugs of these types, consult your

doctor about their use. If you are unsure of the type or contents of your medications, ask your doctor or pharmacist. • This drug is readily destroyed by acids in the stomach; do not drink orange juice or other beverages with high acidic content when you take this medication.

Comments: This drug is almost identical in nature and action to amoxicillin and ampicillin. • Severe allergic reactions to this drug (indicated by breathing difficulties or a drop in blood pressure) have been reported, but are rare when the drug is taken orally. • This drug should be taken for at least ten full days, even if symptoms disappear within that time. • The liquid form of this drug should be stored in the refrigerator. • Take this drug on an empty stomach (one hour before or two hours after a meal). • Diabetics using Clinitest urine test may get a false high sugar reading while taking this drug. Change to Clinistix or Tes-Tape urine test to avoid this problem.

℞　　　penicillin potassium phenoxymethyl antibiotic

Manufacturer: various manufacturers
Ingredients: penicillin potassium phenoxymethyl
Equivalent Products: Betapen-VK, Bristol Laboratories; Cocillin V-K, Coastal Pharmaceutical Co., Inc.; Deltapen-VK, Trimen Laboratories, Inc.; Genecillin-VK-400, General Pharmaceutical Prods., Inc.; Ledercillin VK, Lederle Laboratories; L V Penicillin, Paul B. Elder Company; Penapar VK, Parke-Davis; Pen-Vee K, Wyeth Laboratories; Pfizerpen VK, Pfipharmecs Division; Repen-VK, Reid-Provident Laboratories, Inc.; Robicillin VK, A. H. Robins Company; SK-Penicillin VK, Smith Kline & French Laboratories; Uticillin VK, The Upjohn Company; V-Cillin K, Eli Lilly and Company; Veetids '250', E. R. Squibb & Sons, Inc.
Dosage Forms: Liquid; Tablet (various dosages and various colors)
Use: Treatment of a wide variety of bacterial infections
Minor Side Effects: Diarrhea; nausea; vomiting
Major Side Effects: "Black tongue;" cough; irritation of the mouth; rash; rectal and vaginal itching; severe diarrhea; superinfection
Contraindications: This drug should not be used by people allergic to any penicillin drug. Consult your doctor immediately if this drug has been prescribed for you and you have such an allergy.
Warnings: This drug should be used cautiously by people who have asthma or other significant allergies. Be sure your doctor knows if you have any type of allergy. • Contact your doctor if you develop a fever, rash, or sore throat. • This drug interacts with chloramphenicol, erythromycin, and tetracycline; if you are currently taking any drugs of these types, consult your doctor about their use. If you are unsure of the type or contents of your medications, ask your doctor or pharmacist.
Comments: "Penicillin V" is another name for this drug. • This drug has approximately the same antibacterial activity as the less expensive product penicillin G. However, this drug is more stable in the stomach and is worth the extra cost. • This drug is almost identical in nature and action to amoxicillin and ampicillin. • Severe allergic reactions to this drug (indicated by breathing difficulties or a drop in blood pressure) have been reported, but are rare when the drug is taken orally. • This drug should be taken for at least ten full days, even if symptoms disappear within that time. • The liquid form of this drug should be stored in the refrigerator. • Take this drug on an empty stomach (one hour before or two hours after a meal). • Diabetics using Clinitest urine test may get a false high sugar reading while taking this drug. Change to Clinistix or Tes-Tape urine test to avoid this problem.

Pensyn antibiotic (The Upjohn Company), see ampicillin antibiotic.

Pentazine expectorant (Century Pharmaceuticals, Inc.), see Phenergan expectorant.

Pentazine with Codeine expectorant (Century Pharmaceuticals, Inc.), see Phenergan with Codeine expectorant.

Pentids antibiotic (E. R. Squibb & Sons, Inc.), see penicillin G antibiotic.

Pen-Vee K antibiotic (Wyeth Laboratories), see penicillin potassium phenoxymethyl antibiotic.

OTC   Pepto-Bismol diarrhea remedy

Manufacturer: Norwich-Eaton Pharmaceuticals
Ingredients: bismuth subsalicylate
Dosage Form: Liquid: bismuth subsalicylate
Use: For treatment of common diarrhea
Side Effects: Constipation after long-term use (seven days to two months)
Contraindications: This product or any other product for diarrhea should not be used to self-medicate without first consulting a doctor if the person is under age three or over age 60, has a history of asthma, heart disease, peptic ulcer, or is pregnant.
Comments: Diarrhea should stop in two to three days. If it persists longer, recurs frequently or in presence of high fever, call your doctor and be sure to tell him of any drugs you are taking. • Be sure to drink at least eight glasses of water each day. • If you are taking other drugs, do not take this product until you have first checked with your doctor or pharmacist. • This product is believed by some to relieve nausea and vomiting. However, its value for the relief of these symptoms has never been shown. • This product may discolor the feces and tongue.

R̽   Percodan analgesic

Manufacturer: Endo Laboratories, Inc
Ingredients: aspirin; caffeine; oxycodone hydrochloride; oxycodone terephthalate; phenacetin
Dosage Form: Tablet: aspirin, 224 mg; caffeine, 32 mg; oxycodone hydrochloride, 4.50 mg; oxycodone terephthalate, 0.38 mg; phenacetin, 160 mg (yellow)
Use: Relief of moderate to moderately severe pain
Minor Side Effects: Constipation; dizziness; dry mouth; flushing; itching; light-headedness; nausea; odd movements; palpitations; rash; ringing in the ears; sedation; sweating; vomiting
Major Side Effects: Jaundice; kidney disease; low blood sugar; rapid heartbeat; tremors
Contraindications: This drug should not be taken by people who are allergic to any of its components. Consult your doctor immediately if this drug has been prescribed for you and you have such an allergy.
Warnings: This drug can produce drug dependence of the morphine type and, therefore, has the potential for abuse. Psychological dependence, physical dependence, and tolerance may develop upon repeated administration of this drug. • This drug may cause drowsiness; avoid tasks requiring alertness, such as driving a car or operating machinery. • This drug should be used cautiously in persons with peptic ulcer, abdominal disease, head injury, liver disease, kidney disease, thyroid disease, or prostate disease. Be sure your doctor knows if you have any of these conditions. • Use of this drug may

cause blood coagulation problems and potentiation with other depressant drugs. • This drug should be used cautiously in pregnant women, the elderly, children, and debilitated persons. • This drug should not be taken with alcohol, ammonium chloride, methotrexate, oral anticoagulants, oral antidiabetics, probenecid, steroids, aspirin, or sulfinpyrazone. If you are currently taking any drugs of these types, consult your doctor about their use. If you are unsure of the type or contents of your medications, ask your doctor or pharmacist. • This drug has the potential for abuse and must be used with caution. Tolerance may develop quickly; do not increase the dose of this drug without first consulting your doctor.

Comments: Products containing narcotics (e.g., oxycodone) are usually not used for more than seven to ten days. • This drug interacts with alcohol; avoid alcohol while taking this product. • If you are also taking an anticoagulant ("blood thinner"), remind your doctor. • Take this drug with food or milk. • If your ears feel strange, if you hear buzzing or ringing, or if your stomach hurts, your dosage may need adjustment. Call your doctor. • There is a half-strength form of this drug available. It is called Percodan-Demi, and is also made by Endo Laboratories, Inc. (Only the oxycodone components are half strength.)

Percodan-Demi analgesic (Endo Laboratories, Inc.), see Percodan analgesic.

OTC   Percogesic analgesic

Manufacturer: Endo Laboratories, Inc.
Ingredients: acetaminophen; phenyltoloxamine citrate
Dosage Form: Tablet: acetaminophen, 325 mg; phenyltoloxamine citrate, 30 mg
Use: Relief of pain of headache, toothache, sprains, muscular aches, nerve inflammation, menstruation; relief of discomforts and fever of colds; temporary relief of minor aches and pains of arthritis and rheumatism
Side Effects: Blurred vision; confusion; constipation; difficult urination; dizziness; drowsiness; dry mouth and respiratory passages; headache; insomnia; low blood pressure; nausea; nervousness; palpitations; rash; restlessness; vomiting. Children may react with convulsions; flushed skin; nervousness; tremor; twitching of muscles; and/or uncoordinated movements.
Warnings: When taken in overdose, this product is more toxic than aspirin. The dosage instructions listed on the package should be followed carefully; toxicity may occur in adults or children with repeated doses. • This product may cause drowsiness. Do not take it if you must drive, operate heavy machinery, or perform other tasks requiring mental alertness. To prevent oversedation, avoid the use of alcohol or other drugs that have sedative properties.
Comments: This product may not work as well after seven to ten days as it did when you began taking it. Consult your pharmacist about using another product if the effectiveness of this medication diminishes. • Chew gum or suck on ice chips or a piece of hard candy to reduce mouth dryness.

Rx   Periactin antihistamine

Manufacturer: Merck Sharp & Dohme
Ingredient: cyproheptadine hydrochloride
Equivalent Products: Cyprodine, Spencer-Mead, Inc.; cyproheptadine hydrochloride, various manufacturers
Dosage Forms: Syrup (content per 5 ml): 2 mg. Tablet: 4 mg (white)
Use: Relief of hay fever symptoms; itching; rash

Minor Side Effects: Blurred vision; confusion; diarrhea; difficult urination; dizziness; drowsiness; dry mouth; headache; heartburn; insomnia; loss of appetite; nasal congestion; nausea; nervousness; palpitations; rash; reduced sweating; restlessness; vomiting; weakness

Major Side Effects: Low blood pressure; rash from exposure to sunlight; severe abdominal pain; sore throat

Contraindications: This drug should not be taken by people who have asthma, glaucoma (certain types), ulcer (certain types), enlarged prostate, obstructed bladder, or obstructed intestine. It should not be taken by infants, nursing mothers, those who are allergic to it, or those who are taking monoamine oxidase inhibitors. Consult your doctor immediately if this drug has been prescribed for you and you have any of these conditions or fit into any of these categories.

Warnings: This drug should be used cautiously by pregnant women and the elderly. The elderly are more likely to suffer side effects, especially sedation, from this drug than are other people. • Children under 12 who take this drug may become excited or restless. • This drug may add to the effects of alcohol, other sedatives, and central nervous system depressants. Avoid using drugs of these types while taking this product. If you are unsure of the type of your medications, ask your doctor or pharmacist. • This drug may cause drowsiness; avoid tasks that require alertness. • This drug may cause the following conditions to worsen; asthma, glaucoma, thyroid disease, heart disease, high blood pressure. Consult your doctor if you have any of these conditions and this drug has been prescribed for you. • While taking this drug, do not take any nonprescription item for cough, cold, or sinus problems without first checking with your doctor.

Comments: Chew gum or suck on ice chips or a piece of hard candy to reduce mouth dryness. • Because this drug reduces sweating, avoid excessive work or exercise in hot weather.

OTC   Peri-Colace laxative

Manufacturer: Mead Johnson Nutritional Division

Ingredients: casanthranol; docusate sodium (dioctyl sodium sulfosuccinate)

Dosage Forms: Capsule: casanthranol, 30 mg; docusate sodium, 100 mg. Syrup (content per teaspoon): casanthranol, 10 mg; docusate sodium, 20 mg

Use: Relief of constipation and stool softener

Side Effects: Excess loss of fluid; griping (cramps); mucus in feces

Contraindications: Persons with high fever (100° F or more); black or tarry stools; nausea; vomiting; abdominal pain; or children under age three should not use this product unless directed by a doctor. • Do not use this product when constipation is caused by megacolon or other diseases of the intestine, or hypothyroidism.

Warnings: Excessive use (daily for a month or more) of this product may cause diarrhea, vomiting, and loss of certain blood electrolytes. • Pregnant women should not use this product except on the advice of a doctor.

Comments: This product may discolor the urine. • Evacuation may occur within 6 to 12 hours. Never self-medicate with this product if constipation lasts longer than two weeks or if the medication does not produce a laxative effect within a week. • Limit use to seven days unless directed otherwise by a doctor since this product may cause laxative-dependence (addiction) if used for a longer time. • An ingredient in this product is referred to as a stool softener. This product is recommended for prevention of constipation when the stool is hard and dry. Do not take another product containing mineral oil at the same time as you are taking this product. • Take the syrup form of this product in one-half glass of milk or fruit juice to help mask the taste.

Perphenyline phenothiazine and antidepressant (Henry Schein, Inc.), see Triavil phenothiazine and antidepressant.

℞ Persantine antianginal

Manufacturer: Boehringer Ingelheim Ltd.
Ingredient: dipyridamole
Dosage Form: Tablet: 25 mg; 50 mg; 75 mg (all orange)
Use: Prevention of chronic chest pain (angina) due to heart disease
Minor Side Effects: Dizziness; fainting; flushing; headache; nausea; rash; weakness
Major Side Effects: Worsening of chest pain (mainly at start of therapy)
Warnings: This drug should be used cautiously in patients with low blood pressure. This drug may cause allergic-type reactions, particularly in persons with aspirin hypersensitivity. Be sure your doctor knows if you have low blood pressure or such sensitivity.
Comments: The effectiveness of this drug for prevention of chronic angina is controversial. This drug is more frequently prescribed to prevent blood clot formation, although use of the drug for this purpose is not approved by the FDA. • This drug should be taken on an empty stomach (one hour before or two hours after a meal) and taken only in the prescribed amount. • The effects of this drug may not be apparent for at least two months. • This drug will not stop chest pain from angina that has already begun. It is used only to prevent such pain from occurring. • To avoid dizziness or light-headedness when you stand, contract and relax the muscles of your legs for a few moments before rising. Do this by pushing one foot against the floor while raising the other foot slightly, alternating feet so that you are "pumping" your legs in a pedaling motion.

OTC Pertussin 8-Hour Cough Formula

Manufacturer: Chesebrough-Pond's Inc.
Ingredients: dextromethorphan hydrobromide; alcohol
Dosage Form: Liquid (content per 20 ml, or 4 teaspoons): dextromethorphan hydrobromide, 30 mg; alcohol, 9.5%
Use: Temporary suppression of coughs
Side Effects: Drowsiness; nausea; vomiting
Warnings: This product interacts with monoamine oxidase inhibitors; if you are currently taking any drugs of this type, check with your doctor before taking this product. If you are unsure of the type or contents of your medications, ask your doctor or pharmacist.
Comments: Do not use this product to treat chronic coughs, such as from smoking or asthma. • Do not use this product to treat productive (hacking) coughs that produce phlegm.

Pethadol analgesic (Halsey Drug Co., Inc.), see Demerol analgesic.

Pfiklor potassium chloride replacement (Pfizer Laboratories, Inc.), see potassium chloride replacement.

Pfizer-E antibiotic (Pfipharmecs Division), see erythromycin antibiotic.

Pfizerpen G antibiotic (Pfipharmecs Division), see penicillin G antibiotic.

Pfizerpen VK antibiotic (Pfipharmecs Division), see penicillin potassium phenoxymethyl antibiotic.

Phedral antiasthmatic (North American Pharmacal, Inc.), see Tedral antiasthmatic.

Phen-Amin antihistamine (Scrip-Physician Supply Co.), see Benadryl antihistamine.

Phenaphen with Codeine analgesic (A. H. Robins Company), see Tylenol with Codeine analgesic.

Phenazodine analgesic (The Lannett Company, Inc.), see Pyridium analgesic.

Rx   **Phenergan expectorant**

Manufacturer: Wyeth Laboratories
Ingredients: citric acid; potassium guaiacolsulfonate; promethazine hydrochloride; sodium citrate
Equivalent Products: Mallergan, Mallard Incorporated; Pentazine, Century Pharmaceuticals, Inc.; Proclan, H.R. Cenci Laboratories, Inc.; Promethazine Hydrochloride, Lederle Laboratories; Promex, Lemmon Company; Prothazine, North American Pharmacal, Inc.
Dosage Form: Liquid (content per 5 ml): citric acid, 60 mg; potassium guaiacolsulfonate, 44 mg; promethazine hydrochloride, 5 mg; sodium citrate, 197 mg; alcohol, 7%
Use: Symptomatic relief of coughing
Minor Side Effects: Blurred vision; change in urine color; confusion; constipation; diarrhea; difficult urination; dizziness; drowsiness; dry mouth; headache; insomnia; loss of appetite; nasal congestion; nausea; nervousness; palpitations; rash; reduced sweating; restlessness; trembling; vomiting; weakness
Major Side Effects: Jaundice; low blood pressure; rash from exposure to sunlight; severe abdominal pain; sore throat
Contraindications: This drug should not be taken by people who are allergic to any of its components. Consult your doctor immediately if this drug has been prescribed for you and you have such an allergy.
Warnings: This drug interacts with amphetamine, anticholinergics, levodopa, antacids, and trihexyphenidyl; if you are currently taking any drugs of these types, consult your doctor about their use. If you are unsure of the type or contents of your medications, ask your doctor or pharmacist. • While taking this drug, do not take any nonprescription item for cough, cold, or sinus problems without first checking with your doctor. • This drug may cause drowsiness; avoid tasks that require alertness. To prevent oversedation, avoid the use of alcohol or other drugs that have sedative properties. • Because this drug reduces sweating, avoid excessive work or exercise in hot weather.
Comments: If you need an expectorant, you need more moisture in your environment. Drink nine to ten glasses of water daily. The use of a humidifier or vaporizer may also be beneficial. • Consult your doctor. Chew gum or suck on ice chips or a piece of hard candy to reduce mouth dryness.

Rx   **Phenergan VC expectorant**

Manufacturer: Wyeth Laboratories
Ingredients: citric acid; phenylephrine hydrochloride; potassium guaiacolsulfonate; promethazine hydrochloride; sodium citrate
Equivalent Products: J-Gan-VC, J. Pharmacal Co.; Proclan VC, H. R. Cenci Laboratories, Inc.
Dosage Form: Liquid (content per 5 ml): citric acid, 60 mg; phenylephrine

hydrochloride, 5 mg; potassium guaiacolsulfonate, 44 mg; promethazine hydrochloride, 5 mg; sodium citrate, 197 mg; alcohol, 7%

Use: Symptomatic relief of coughing and congestion

Minor Side Effects: Blurred vision; change in urine color; confusion; constipation; diarrhea; difficult urination; dizziness; drowsiness; dry mouth; headache; heartburn; insomnia; loss of appetite; nasal congestion; nausea; palpitations; rash; reduced sweating; restlessness; trembling; vomiting; weakness

Major Side Effects: Chest pain; high blood pressure; jaundice; low blood pressure; severe abdominal pain; sore throat

Contraindications: This drug should not be taken by people who are allergic to any of its components.

Warnings: This drug should be used cautiously by people who have high blood pressure, blood vessel or heart disease, thyroid disease, or diabetes. Be sure your doctor knows if you have any of these conditions. • This drug interacts with amphetamine, anticholinergics, trihexyphenidyl, guanethidine, levodopa, monoamine oxidase inhibitors, antacids, and antidepressants; if you are currently taking any drugs of these types, consult your doctor about their use. If you are unsure of the type or contents of your medications, ask your doctor or pharmacist. • While taking this drug, do not take any nonprescription item for cough, cold, or sinus problems without first checking with your doctor. • This drug may cause drowsiness; avoid tasks that require alertness. To prevent oversedation, avoid the use of alcohol or other drugs that have sedative properties. • Because this drug reduces sweating, avoid excessive work or exercise in hot weather.

Comments: If you need an expectorant, you need more moisture in your environment. Drink nine to ten glasses of water daily. The use of a humidifier or vaporizer may also be beneficial. Consult your doctor. • Chew gum or suck on ice chips or a piece of hard candy to reduce mouth dryness.

Rx   **Phenergan VC with Codeine expectorant**

Manufacturer: Wyeth Laboratories

Ingredients: citric acid; codeine phosphate; phenylephrine hydrochloride; potassium guaiacolsulfonate; promethazine hydrochloride; sodium citrate

Equivalent Products: HRC-Proclan VC with Codeine, H.R. Cenci Laboratories, Inc.; Mallergan VC with Codeine, Mallard Incorporated; Promethazine Hydrochloride VC with Codeine, Lederle Laboratories

Dosage Form: Liquid (content per 5 ml): citric acid, 60 mg; codeine phosphate, 10 mg; phenylephrine hydrochloride, 5 mg; potassium guaiacolsulfate, 44 mg; promethazine hydrochloride, 5 mg; sodium citrate, 197 mg; alcohol, 7%

Use: Relief of symptoms of the common cold

Minor Side Effects: Blurred vision; change in urine color; confusion; constipation; diarrhea; difficult urination; dizziness; drowsiness; dry mouth; headache; heartburn; insomnia; loss of appetite; nasal congestion; nausea; palpitations; rash; reduced sweating; restlessness; trembling; vomiting; weakness

Major Side Effects: Chest pain; high blood pressure; jaundice; low blood pressure; severe abdominal pain; sore throat

Contraindications: This drug should not be taken by people who are allergic to any of its components.

Warnings: This drug should be used cautiously by people who have high blood pressure, blood vessel or heart disease, thyroid disease, or diabetes. Be sure your doctor knows if you have any of these conditions. This drug interacts with amphetamine, anticholinergics, trihexyphenidyl, guanethidine, levodopa, monoamine oxidase inhibitors, and antacids; if you are currently taking any drugs of these types, consult your doctor about their use. If you are unsure of the type or contents of your medications, ask your doctor or pharmacist. • While taking this drug, do not take any nonprescription item for cough, cold, or sinus problems without first checking with your doctor. • This drug may cause drowsiness; avoid tasks that require alertness. To prevent oversedation, avoid the use of alcohol or other drugs that have sedative properties. • Because this product contains codeine, it has the potential for abuse and must be used with caution. It usually should not be taken for more than ten days. Tolerance may develop quickly, but do not increase the dose without consulting your doctor. • Because this drug reduces sweating, avoid excessive work or exercise in hot weather.

Comments: If you need an expectorant, you need more moisture in your environment. Drink nine to ten glasses of water daily. The use of a humidifier or vaporizer may also be beneficial. Consult your doctor. • Chew gum or suck on ice chips or a piece of hard candy to reduce mouth dryness.

℞   **Phenergan with Codeine expectorant**

Manufacturer: Wyeth Laboratories

Ingredients: citric acid; codeine phosphate; potassium guaiacolsulfonate; promethazine hydrochloride; sodium citrate

Equivalent Products: HRC-Proclan with Codeine, H.R. Cenci Laboratories, Inc.; K-Phen with Codeine, Kay Pharmacal Company, Inc.; Mallergan with Codeine, Mallard Incorporated; Pentazine with Codeine, Century Pharmaceuticals, Inc.; Promethazine Hydrochloride with Codeine, Lederle Laboratories; Promex with Codeine, Lemmon Company; Prothazine with Codeine, North American Pharmacal, Inc.

Dosage Form: Liquid (content per 5 ml): citric acid, 60 mg; codeine phosphate, 10 mg; potassium guaiacolsulfonate, 44 mg; promethazine hydrochloride, 5 mg; sodium citrate, 197 mg; alcohol, 7%

Use: Cough suppressant

Minor Side Effects: Blurred vision; change in urine color; confusion; constipation; diarrhea; difficult urination; dizziness; drowsiness; dry mouth; headache; insomnia; loss of appetite; nasal congestion; nausea; nervousness; palpitations; rash; reduced sweating; restlessness; trembling; vomiting; weakness

Major Side Effects: Jaundice; low blood pressure; rash from exposure to sunlight; severe abdominal pain; sore throat

Contraindications: This drug should not be taken by people who are allergic to any of its components. Consult your doctor immediately if this drug has been prescribed for you and you have such an allergy.

Warnings: This drug interacts with amphetamine, anticholinergics, levodopa, antacids, and trihexyphenidyl; if you are currently taking any drugs of these types, consult your doctor about their use. If you are unsure of the type or contents of your medications, ask your doctor or pharmacist. • While taking this drug, do not take any nonprescription item for cough, cold, or sinus problems without first checking with your doctor. • This drug may cause drowsiness; avoid tasks that require alertness. To prevent oversedation, avoid the use of alcohol or other drugs that have sedative properties. • Because this product contains codeine, it has the potential for abuse and must be used with caution. It usually should not be taken for more than ten days. Tolerance may develop quickly, but do not increase the dosage without consulting your doctor. • Because this drug reduces sweating, avoid excessive work or exercise in hot weather.

Comments: If you need an expectorant, you need more moisture in your environment. Drink nine to ten glasses of water daily. The use of a vaporizer or humidifier may also be beneficial. Consult your doctor. • Chew gum or suck on ice chips or a piece of hard candy to reduce mouth dryness.

℞   **phenobarbital sedative and hypnotic**

Manufacturer: various manufacturers
Ingredient: phenobarbital
Equivalent Products: Barbita, North American Pharmacal, Inc.; Eskabarb, Smith Kline & French Laboratories; Henotal, Bowman Pharmaceuticals; Luminal Ovoids, Winthrop Laboratories; PBR/12, Scott-Alison Pharmaceuticals, Inc.; Pheno-Squar, Mallard Incorporated; SK-Phenobarbital, Smith Kline & French Laboratories; Solfoton, Wm. P. Poythress & Co. Inc.
Dosage Forms: Capsule; Drops; Liquid; Tablet; Time-release capsules (various dosages and various colors)
Use: Control of convulsions; relief of anxiety or tension; sleeping aid
Minor Side Effects: Drowsiness; nausea; vomiting
Major Side Effects: Breathing difficulty; cold and clammy skin; other allergic reactions
Contraindications: This drug should not be used by people who are allergic to it, or who have porphyria or a history of drug abuse. Consult your doctor immediately if this drug has been prescribed for you and you fit any of these categories.
Warnings: This drug should be used cautiously by people who have liver or kidney disease, certain lung diseases, and by women who are pregnant or nursing. Be sure your doctor knows if you have any of these conditions. • This drug interacts with alcohol, central nervous system depressants, griseofulvin, oral anticoagulants, phenytoin, steroids, sulfonamides, tetracycline, and antidepressants; if you are currently taking any drugs of these types, consult your doctor about their use. If you are unsure of the type or contents of your medications, ask your doctor or pharmacist. • This drug may cause drowsiness; avoid tasks that require alertness. To prevent oversedation, avoid the use of alcohol or other drugs that have sedative properties. • This drug has the potential for abuse and must be used with caution. Tolerance may develop quickly; do not increase the dose of this drug without first consulting your doctor. If you are taking an anticoagulant ("blood thinner") in addition to this drug, remind your doctor.

Pheno-Squar sedative and hypnotic (Mallard Incorporated), see phenobarbital sedative and hypnotic.

OTC   **Phillips' Milk of Magnesia laxative and antacid**

Manufacturer: Glenbrook Laboratories
Ingredients: magnesium hydroxide, peppermint oil
Dosage Forms: Liquid (content per 30 ml, or two tablespoons): magnesium hydroxide, 2.28 to 2.61 g; peppermint oil, 1.14 mg. Tablet: magnesium hydroxide, 311 mg; peppermint oil, 1.166 mg
Use: Relief of constipation and symptoms associated with gastric hyperacidity
Side Effects: Diarrhea
Contraindications: Persons with kidney disease should not use this product. In persons with kidney disease, repeated (daily) use of this product may cause nausea, vomiting, depressed reflexes, and breathing difficulties. • Persons with high fever (100° F or more); black or tarry stools; nausea; vomiting; abdominal pain; or children under age three should not use this product unless directed to do so by a doctor. • Do not use this product when constipation is caused by megacolon or other diseases of the intestine, or hypothyroidism. • Pregnant women should use this product only on the advice of a doctor.
Warnings: Excessive use (daily for a month or more) of this product may

cause diarrhea, vomiting, and loss of certain blood electrolytes.

Comments: Evacuation may occur within several hours after using this product. • A glass (eight ounces) of water should be taken with each dose. • Never self-medicate with this product for constipation if the condition lasts longer than two weeks or if the medication does not produce a laxative effect within a week. • Self-treatment of severe or repeated attacks of heartburn, indigestion, or upset stomach is not recommended. If you do self-treat, limit therapy to two weeks, then call your doctor if symptoms persist. Never self-medicate with this product if your symptoms occur regularly (two to three times or more a month); if they are particularly worse than normal; if you feel a "tightness" in your chest, have chest pains, are sweating, or are short of breath. Consult your doctor. • As an antacid, this product works best when taken one hour after meals or at bedtime, unless otherwise directed by your doctor or pharmacist. • The liquid form of this product is superior to the tablet form and should be used unless you have been specifically directed to use the tablet. • If you are currently taking a tetracycline antibiotic, do not take this product within two hours of a dose of the tetracycline. The magnesium in this product interacts with tetracycline and interferes with the body's absorption of the drug. Consult your doctor or pharmacist if you have questions about separating your dosages, or if you are unsure of the type or contents of your other medications. This product also interacts with iron, some vitamin-mineral products, chlorpromazine, phenytoin, digoxin, quinidine, and warfarin. If you are currently taking any drugs of these types, do not take this product without first consulting your doctor or pharmacist. • Limit use to seven consecutive days; this product may cause laxative-dependence (addiction) if used for a longer period.

OTC   pHisoDan dandruff remedy

Manufacturer: Winthrop Laboratories
Ingredients: cholesterols; entsufon sodium; lanolin; petrolatum; precipitated sulfur; salicylic acid
Dosage Form: Shampoo: precipitated sulfur, 5%; salicylic acid, 0.5% (quantities of other ingredients not specified)
Use: Control of dandruff
Side Effects: Burning of the skin; discoloration of hair; dryness or oiliness of hair or scalp; eye irritation
Warnings: Do not use this product if the skin is broken.
Comments: Although this shampoo has not been reported to cause serious toxicity, if you swallow any, call your doctor or pharmacist immediately. • Leave the shampoo on the scalp for a few minutes before rinsing.

Rx   pHisoHex detergent cleanser

Manufacturer: Winthrop Laboratories
Ingredient: hexachlorophene
Equivalent Products: Soy-Dome Cleanser, Dome Laboratories; WescoHEX, West Chemical Products, Inc.
Dosage Form: Liquid: 3%
Use: Antibacterial skin cleanser
Minor Side Effects: Rare, but redness and/or mild scaling or dryness of the skin
Major Side Effects: Allergic reactions; brain damage; convulsions; dermatitis; irritability; sensitivity to sunlight. Swallowing this drug may cause abdominal cramps, dehydration, diarrhea, hypotension, loss of appetite, shock, and—in some instances—death.
Contraindications: This drug should not be used on burned or denuded

530

skin. • This drug should not be used with an occlusive dressing or on a wet pack. Nor should it be used routinely for total body bathing. • This drug should not be used as a vaginal pack or tampon, or on any mucous membrane. • Persons who are allergic to its components should not use this drug. Consult your doctor immediately if this drug has been prescribed for you and you have such an allergy.

Warnings: After using this drug, rinse it off thoroughly with water, especially from sensitive areas such as the scrotum. • This drug is for external use only. If swallowed, this drug is harmful, especially to infants and children. Rapid absorption of this drug may occur, especially in infants, when it is applied to certain skin lesions, resulting in toxic blood levels. • This drug should be discontinued promptly if signs of cerebral irritability occur. • This drug should not be used routinely for bathing infants and should not be used in conjunction with baby-skin products containing alcohol. • This drug should be washed out promptly and thoroughly if it accidently comes in contact with the eyes. • This drug should be used with caution by pregnant women.

Comments: This drug was formerly available OTC. It was switched to a prescription drug because of the possibility of blood toxicity reported after absorption. However, when this drug is used as directed, it is safe to use. • This drug should not be poured into measuring cups, medicine bottles, or similar containers, since it may be mistaken for baby formula or other medications. • Prolonged direct exposure of this drug to strong light may cause brownish surface discoloration, but such discoloration does not affect its antibacterial or detergent properties.

Pilocar ophthalmic solution (Smith, Miller & Patch), see Isopto Carpine ophthalmic solution.

Pilomiotin ophthalmic solution (Smith, Miller & Patch), see Isopto Carpine ophthalmic solution.

Piracaps antibiotic (Tutag Pharmaceuticals, Inc.), see tetracycline hydrochloride antibiotic.

℞   Polaramine antihistamine

Manufacturer: Schering Corporation
Ingredient: dexchlorpheniramine maleate
Dosage Forms: Liquid (content per 5 ml, or one teaspoon): dexchlorpheniramine maleate, 2 mg; alcohol, 6%. Repeat-action tablet: 4 mg (light red); 6 mg (bright red). Tablet: 2 mg (red)
Use: Prevention and relief of allergic symptoms
Minor Side Effects: Blurred vision; confusion; diarrhea; difficult urination; dizziness; drowsiness; dry mouth; headache; heartburn; insomnia; loss of appetite; nasal congestion; nausea; nervousness; palpitations; rash; restlessness; vomiting; weakness
Major Side Effects: Low blood pressure; rash from exposure to sunlight; severe abdominal pain; sore throat
Warnings: Drowsiness may occur from use of this drug; patients should avoid tasks requiring alertness, such as driving a motor vehicle. • This drug in liquid form should be used cautiously in persons with high blood pressure. Be sure your doctor knows if you have this condition. • This drug should not be taken with alcohol or other central nervous system depressants. If you are presently taking any drugs of these types, consult your doctor about their use. If you are unsure of the type or contents of your medication, ask your doctor or pharmacist.

Comments: The 4-mg and 6-mg repeat-action tablets must be swallowed whole. • Never take the repeat-action-tablet form more frequently than your doctor prescribes. A serious overdose may result. Whereas sedation is the usual response to overdosage in adults, children may experience symptoms of excitation leading to convulsions or death. • This drug may cause dryness of the mouth. To reduce this feeling, chew gum or suck on ice chips or a piece of hard candy. • While taking this drug, do not take any nonprescription item for cough, cold, or sinus problems without first checking with your doctor. • This drug reduces sweating; avoid excessive work or exercise in hot weather.

Polycillin antibiotic (Bristol Laboratories), see ampicillin antibiotic.

Polymox antibiotic (Bristol Laboratories), see amoxicillin antibiotic.

OTC Polysporin Ointment external anti-infective

Manufacturer: Burroughs Wellcome Co.
Ingredients: bacitracin zinc; polymyxin B sulfate; white petrolatum
Dosage Form: Ointment (content per gram): bacitracin zinc, 500 units; polymyxin B sulfate, 10,000 units; white petrolatum
Use: Prevention of infection from cuts and abrasions; treatment of impetigo
Side Effects: Allergic reactions (rash, itching, soreness); local irritation
Comments: Apply this product at least three times daily to maintain effectiveness. If the infection does not clear in two to three weeks, consult your doctor or pharmacist.

Rx Poly-Vi-Flor vitamin and fluoride supplement

Manufacturer: Mead Johnson Nutritional Division
Ingredients: vitamins A, D, E, C; folic acid; thiamine; riboflavin; niacin; vitamins B_6, B_{12}; fluoride
Dosage Forms: Chewable tablet: vitamin A, 2500 I.U.; vitamin D, 400 I.U.; vitamin E, 15 I.U.; vitamin C, 60 mg; folic acid, 0.3 mg; thiamine, 1.05 mg; riboflavin, 1.2 mg; niacin, 13.5 mg; vitamin B_6, 1.05 mg; vitamin B_{12}, 4.5 mcg; fluoride, 1.0 mg. Drops (content per ml): vitamin A, 1500 I.U.; vitamin D, 400 I.U.; vitamin E, 5 I.U.; vitamin C, 35 mg; thiamine, 0.5 mg; riboflavin, 0.6 mg; niacin, 8 mg; vitamin B_6, 0.4 mg; vitamin B_{12}, 2 mcg; fluoride, 0.5 mg
Use: Protection against tooth decay and vitamin deficiencies in children
Minor Side Effects: Rash (rare)
Contraindications: This product should not be used when fluoride content of drinking water is 0.7 parts per million or more. The drops form should not be used by infants from birth to two years of age in areas where the drinking water contains 0.3 parts per million or more of fluoride. • This product should not be used in the presence of frank dental fluorosis.
Warnings: The recommended dose should not be exceeded or other fluoride-containing drugs given concurrently, since prolonged excessive fluoride intake may cause dental fluorosis in children.
Comments: This product should never be referred to as candy or "candy-flavored vitamins." Your child may take you literally and swallow too many. • If you are unsure of the fluoride content of your drinking water, ask your doctor, or call your County Health Department. • Mead Johnson Nutritional Division also manufacturers a similar product, Tri-Vi-Flor vitamin and fluoride supplement, which contains only vitamins A, C, and D, and sodium fluoride. • The chewable tablets and drops discussed here are very similar to each other, but they do not contain exactly the same kind and amounts of vitamins. There are no products that are identical to this product. However, other products are similar and they may be cheaper. Talk to your doctor.

OTC   **Poly-Vi-Sol multivitamin**

Manufacturer: Mead Johnson Nutritional Division
Ingredients: vitamin A; vitamin D; vitamin E; vitamin C; folic acid (tablet form only); thiamine; riboflavin; niacin; vitamin B_6; vitamin B_{12}
Dosage Forms: Chewable tablet: vitamin A, 2500 IU; vitamin D, 400 IU; vitamin E, 15 IU; vitamin C, 60 mg; folic acid, 0.3 mg; thiamine, 1.05 mg; riboflavin, 1.2 mg; niacin, 13.5 mg; vitamin B_6, 1.05 mg; vitamin B_{12}, 4.5 mcg. Drop (content per 1.0-ml dropper): vitamin A, 1500 IU; vitamin D, 400 IU; vitamin E, 5 IU; vitamin C, 35 mg; thiamine, 0.5 mg; riboflavin, 0.6 mg; niacin, 8 mg; vitamin B_6, 0.4 mg; vitamin B_{12}, 2 mcg
Use: Dietary supplement
Warnings: This product contains ingredients that accumulate and are stored in the body. The recommended dose should not be exceeded for long periods (several weeks to months) except by doctor's orders.
Comments: If large doses are taken, this product may interfere with the results of urine tests. Inform your doctor and pharmacist you are taking this product. • Chewable tablets should never be referred to as "candy" or as "candy-flavored" vitamins. Your child may take you literally and swallow toxic amounts.

OTC   **Porox7 acne preparation**

Manufacturer: Commerce Drug Co., Inc.
Ingredient: benzoyl peroxide
Dosage Form: Cream: benzoyl peroxide, 7%
Use: Treatment of acne
Side Effects: Allergy, local irritation
Contraindications: Persons having known hypersensitity to benzoyl peroxide should not use this product.
Warnings: Do not get this product in or near the eyes.
Comments: If the condition worsens, stop using this product and call your pharmacist. • Wash the area gently with warm water and pat dry before applying this acne preparation. • Avoid exposure to heat lamps, sunlamps, or direct sunlight when using this product. This preparation may be especially active on fair-skinned people. • This product may damage certain fabrics including rayon.

Potasalan potassium chloride replacement (The Lannett Company, Inc.), see potassium chloride replacement.

℞   **potassium chloride replacement**

Manufacturer: various manufacturers
Ingredient: potassium chloride
Equivalent Products: Kaochlor, Warren-Teed Laboratories; Kaochlor-Eff, Warren-Teed Laboratories; Kaon-Cl, Warren-Teed Laboratories; Kay Ciel, Berlex Laboratories Inc.; KEFF, Lemmon Company; K-Lor, Abbott Laboratories; KLOR, Upsher-Smith Laboratories, Inc.; KLOR-CON, Upsher-Smith Laboratories, Inc.; Kloride, Amfre-Grant, Inc.; Klorvess, Dorsey Laboratories; K-Lyte/Cl, Mead Johnson Pharmaceutical Division; K-10, H.R. Cenci Laboratories, Inc.; Pan-Kloride, Panray Co., Inc.; Pfiklor, Pfizer Laboratories Division; Potasalan, The Lannett Company, Inc.; Rum-K, Fleming & Co.; Slow-K, CIBA Pharmaceutical Company
Dosage Forms: Effervescent tablet; Liquid; Powder; Slow-release tablet (various dosages and various colors)
Use: Prevention or treatment of potassium deficiency, especially that caused by diuretics

Minor Side Effects: Diarrhea; nausea; vomiting

Major Side Effects: Confusion; numbness or tingling in arms or legs

Contraindications: This drug should not be used by people who have severe kidney disease, high blood levels of potassium, or by those suffering acute dehydration or heat cramps. Consult your doctor immediately if this drug has been prescribed for you and you have any of these conditions.

Warnings: This drug should be used cautiously by people who have heart disease (certain types). Be sure your doctor knows if you have such a condition. This drug interacts with spironolactone and triamterene; if you are currently taking any drugs of these types, consult your doctor about their use. If you are unsure of the type or contents of your medications, ask your doctor or pharmacist. • Follow your doctor's dosage instructions exactly and do not stop taking this medication without first consulting your doctor.

Comments: This drug should be taken with food. • The liquid and powder forms of this drug may be added to one-half or one full glass of cold water, then swallowed. The effervescent tablet form of this drug must be completely dissolved in a full glass of water before being swallowed. Do not crush or chew the slow-release tablets; this form of the drug must be swallowed whole. • Ask your doctor about using a salt substitute instead of potassium chloride; salt substitutes are similar, less expensive, and more convenient.

℞   **Povan anthelmintic**

Manufacturer: Parke-Davis

Ingredient: pyrvinium pamoate

Dosage Forms: Liquid (content per 5 ml): 50 mg. Tablet: 50 mg (red)

Use: Treatment of pinworm infection (enterobiasis)

Minor Side Effects: Cramping; diarrhea; nausea; vomiting

Major Side Effects: Allergic reactions, including itching, photosensitivity, rash

Warnings: This drug should be used with caution by pregnant women. Be sure your doctor knows if you are pregnant.

Comments: Vomiting and the other gastrointestinal reactions are more frequently seen in older children and adults who have received large doses of this drug. These reactions are more common with the liquid form of this drug than with the tablet form. • Care should be given not to spill the liquid form of this drug because it will stain most materials, including the skin and clothing. • This drug will color the stool dark red. This reaction is not harmful, so do not discontinue the use of this drug should this effect occur. • This drug is given as a single dose. If necessary, the dose may be repeated once, in two to three weeks. • Pinworms are easily transmitted to other persons. Observe strict sanitary procedures. If pinworm infection is detected in one member of the household, every family member should receive a treatment. • The drug pyrantel pamoate (Antiminth, Roerig Pharmaceuticals) is another drug used to treat pinworms. It is also effective against roundworms, and is given as a single dose. • Antepar (piperazine, Burroughs Wellcome) is an older drug used to treat pinworms. It must be taken as several doses each day and it causes more side effects than Povan. Ask your doctor if you can take Povan.

Poxy Compound-65 analgesic (Sutliff & Case Co., Inc.), see Darvon Compound-65 analgesic.

Prednicen-M steroid hormone (The Central Pharmacal Co.), see prednisone steroid hormone.

℞   **prednisone steroid hormone**

Manufacturer: various manufacturers

Ingredient: prednisone
Equivalent Products: Cortan, Halsey Drug Co., Inc.; Deltasone, The Upjohn Company; Fernisone, Ferndale Laboratories, Inc.; Meticorten, Schering Corporation; Orasone, Rowell Laboratories, Inc.; Panasol, The Seatrace Co.; Paracort, Parke-Davis; Prednicen-M, The Central Pharmacal Co.; Ropred, Robinson Laboratory, Inc.; Sterapred, Mayrand Incorporated
Dosage Form: Tablet: 1 mg; 2.5 mg; 5 mg; 10 mg; 20 mg; 50 mg (various colors)
Use: Treatment of endocrine or rheumatic disorders; asthma; blood diseases; certain cancers; gastrointestinal disturbances such as ulcerative colitis; inflammations such as arthritis, dermatitis, or poison ivy
Minor Side Effects: Dizziness; headache; increased sweating; increased susceptibility to infection; menstrual irregularities
Major Side Effects: Abdominal enlargement; cataracts; fluid retention; glaucoma; growth impairment in children; hemorrhage; high blood pressure; impaired healing of wounds; peptic ulcer; potassium loss; weakness
Contraindications: This drug should not be taken by people who are allergic to it, or who have systemic fungal infections. Consult your doctor if this drug has been prescribed for you and you have either of these conditions.
Warnings: This drug should be used cautiously by people who have thyroid disease, cirrhosis, ulcerative colitis, kidney disease, high blood pressure, osteoporosis, myasthenia gravis, eye damage or disease, peptic ulcer, or tuberculosis; and by pregnant or nursing women. Be sure your doctor knows if you have any of these conditions. • This drug should be used cautiously in children and infants; their growth must be carefully observed if they receive prolonged treatment with the drug. • People using this drug should not be vaccinated against smallpox, and should not receive any other immunizations. • This drug may cause sudden fluctuations in mood, personality changes, and can intensify psychotic tendencies and/or emotional instability. • This drug interacts with antidiabetics, aspirin, barbiturates, diuretics, estrogens, indomethacin, oral anticoagulants, and phenytoin; if you are currently taking any drugs of these types, consult your doctor about their use. If you are unsure of the type or contents of your medications, ask your doctor or pharmacist. • Blood pressure, body weight, and vision should be checked at regular intervals. Stomach x-rays are advised for persons with suspected or known peptic ulcers. • Do not stop taking this drug without your doctor's knowledge. • To help avoid potassium loss while using this drug, take your dose with a glass of fresh or frozen orange juice, and eat a banana each day. The use of Co-Salt salt substitute also helps prevent potassium loss.
Comments: This drug is often taken on a decreasing-dosage schedule (four times a day for several days, then three times a day, etc.). For long-term treatment, taking the drug every other day (e.g., 10 mg every other day rather than 5 mg daily) is preferred. Generally, taking the entire dose at one time (about 8:00 A.M.) gives the best results. Ask your doctor about alternate-day dosing and the best hour of the day to take this drug. • If you are using this drug chronically, you should wear or carry a notice that you are taking a steroid.

R̥   **Preludin anorectic**

Manufacturer: Boehringer Ingelheim Ltd.
Ingredient: phenmetrazine hydrochloride
Dosage Forms: Sustained-release tablet: 50 mg (white); 75 mg (pink). Tablet: 25 mg (white)
Use: Short-term treatment of obesity
Minor Side Effects: Constipation; diarrhea; dizziness; dry mouth; euphoria;

headache; insomnia; nausea; palpitations; rash; restlessness; tremor; unpleasant taste in mouth; vomiting

Major Side Effects: Changes in libido; chest pain; high blood pressure; impotence; overstimulation of nerves

Contraindications: This drug should not be used by people with heart disease, high blood pressure, glaucoma, history of drug abuse, hypothyroidism, hypersensitivity to sympathomimetic amines; or those in agitated states. Be sure your doctor knows if you have any of these conditions.

Warnings: This drug should be used with caution by pregnant women, nursing mothers, and children under 12 years of age. This drug should not be taken by women who may become pregnant. Be sure your doctor knows if you fit into any of these categories. • This drug has the potential for abuse and must be used with caution. Tolerance may develop within a few weeks. Do not increase the dose of this drug without first consulting your doctor. If tolerance should occur, notify your doctor, because the drug should be discontinued. • Abrupt cessation following prolonged high dosage administration of this drug results in extreme fatigue and mental depression. Chronic intoxication with this drug can result in psychosis. Acute overdosage of this drug can result in psychological disturbances, circulatory collapse, or even death. • This drug interacts with central nervous system depressants, antidiabetic drugs, monoamine oxidase inhibitors, guanethidine, and other adrenergics. Consult your doctor immediately about their use if you are taking any of these drugs. If you are unsure about the type or contents of your medications, ask your doctor or pharmacist. • This drug may mask symptoms of extreme fatigue and decrease your ability to perform potentially dangerous or hazardous tasks, such as driving or operating machinery. Use appropriate caution.

Comments: The sustained-release tablet form of this drug, called Endurets, must not be chewed or crushed, but swallowed whole. • Weight loss is greatest during the first three weeks of taking this drug. • To be effective, therapy with this drug must be accompanied by a low-calorie diet. • The effects of this drug on appetite control wear off; do not take this drug for more than three weeks at a time. One way to get full benefit from this drug is to take it for three weeks, stop for three weeks, then resume taking the drug again. Consult your doctor about this regimen. • While taking this drug, do not take any nonprescription item for cough, cold, or sinus problems without first checking with your doctor. Do not take an Enduret (sustained-release tablet) later than 3:00 P.M. to avoid sleeplessness. • Never take the sustained-release tablet form of this drug more frequently than your doctor prescribes. A serious overdose may result.

℞   **Premarin estrogen hormone**

Manufacturer: Ayerst Laboratories

Ingredient: conjugated estrogens

Equivalent Products: Congens No. 1, Blaine Co., Inc.; conjugated estrogens, various manufacturers; Estroate, Kay Pharmacal Company, Inc.; Estrocon, Mallard Incorporated; Kestrin, Hyrex Pharmaceuticals; Menogen, General Pharmaceutical Prods., Inc.; Menotab, Fleming & Company; Ovest, Trimen Laboratories, Inc.; Sodestrin, Tutag Pharmaceuticals, Inc.

Dosage Form: Tablet: 0.3 mg (green); 0.625 mg (maroon); 1.25 mg (yellow); 2.5 mg (purple)

Use: Estrogen replacement therapy; treatment of enlarged breasts after childbirth; symptoms due to menopause; prostatic cancer in men; uterine bleeding; and some cases of breast cancer

Minor Side Effects: Bleeding; bloating; cramps; loss of appetite; nausea; tender breasts; vomiting

Major Side Effects: Allergic rash; gallbladder disease; high blood pressure; skin color changes; severe headache; vision changes; weight gain (more than two pounds per week)

Contraindications: This drug should not be used by pregnant women, or by people who have blood clotting disorders, endometrial cancer, or vaginal bleeding. In most cases this drug should not be used by people who have breast cancer. Consult your doctor immediately if this drug has been prescribed for you and you have any of these conditions.

Warnings: Studies have shown that estrogens increase the risk of cancer. In three independent studies, the rate of endometrial cancer development was 4.5 to 13.9 times greater in estrogen users than in nonusers. Your pharmacist has a brochure that describes the benefits and risks involved with estrogen therapy. He is required by law to give you a copy each time he fills a prescription for this drug. Read this material carefully. • This drug should be used cautiously by people who have asthma, diabetes, epilepsy, gallbladder disease, heart disease, high blood levels of calcium, high blood pressure, kidney disease, liver disease, migraine, uterine fibroid tumors, a history of depression, and by nursing women. Be sure your doctor knows if you have any of these conditions. • This drug may retard bone growth, and therefore should be used cautiously in young patients who have not yet completed puberty. • This drug interacts with oral anticoagulants and steroids; if you are currently taking any drugs of these types, consult your doctor about their use. If you are unsure of the type of your medications, ask your doctor or pharmacist. • Notify your doctor immediately if you experience any of the following symptoms: abnormal vaginal bleeding, breast lumps, pains in the calves or chest, sudden shortness of breath, coughing of blood, severe headache, dizziness, faintness, changes in vision or skin color. • This drug may affect a number of laboratory tests; remind your doctor that you are taking it if you are scheduled for any tests. • You should have a complete physical examination at least once a year while you are on this medication.

Comments: This drug is usually taken for 21 days followed by a 7-day rest.

OTC   Preparation H hemorrhoidal preparation

Manufacturer: Whitehall Laboratories

Ingredients: live yeast cell derivative; phenylmercuric nitrate; shark liver oil

Dosage Forms: Ointment; Suppository: live yeast cell derivative supplying 2,000 units of skin respiratory factor; phenylmercuric nitrate, 0.01%; shark liver oil, 3%

Use: Relief of pain, burning, and itching of hemorrhoids

Warnings: Sensitization (continued itching and redness) may occur with long-term and repeated use.

Comments: Hemorrhoidal (pile) preparations relieve itching, reduce pain and inflammation, and check bleeding, but do not heal, dry up, or give lasting relief from the hemorrhoids. • Certain ingredients in this product may cause an allergic reaction; do not use for longer than seven days at a time unless your doctor has advised you otherwise. • The suppository is not recommended for external hemorrhoids or bleeding internal hemorrhoids. Use the ointment form. Use caution when inserting the applicator. • Never self-medicate for hemorrhoids if pain is continuous or throbbing, if bleeding or itching is excessive, or if you feel a large pressure within the rectum.

Presamine antidepressant (USV [P.R.] Development Corp.), see Tofranil antidepressant.

OTC   Primatene M asthma remedy

Manufacturer: Whitehall Laboratories

Ingredients: ephedrine hydrochloride; pyrilamine maleate; theophylline
Dosage Form: Tablet: ephedrine hydrochloride, 24 mg; pyrilamine maleate, 16 mg; theophylline, 130 mg
Use: For relief and control of attacks of bronchial asthma and associated hay fever
Side Effects: Anxiety; blurred vision; chest pain; confusion; constipation; dizziness; drowsiness; dry mouth and respiratory passages; increased blood pressure; increased frequency of urination; insomnia; loss of appetite; nausea; nervousness; palpitations; rash; restlessness; sweating; tension; tremor; vomiting. Children may react with primary symptoms of excitement (convulsions, flushed skin, nervousness, tremor, twitching of muscles, and uncoordinated movements).
Warnings: Persons with glaucoma should use this product with caution. Consult your doctor or pharmacist if you have any questions concerning the use of this product. • Persons with high blood pressure, diabetes, thyroid, or heart disease should use this product only on the advice of their doctor. • Overdose may result in convulsions, coma, and cardiovascular collapse.
Comments: While taking this product, avoid the use of sedative drugs or alcohol, guanethidine, monoamine oxidase inhibitors, or tricyclic antidepressants. If you are taking any medication of these types, or if you are unsure of the type of medication you are taking, consult your doctor.

OTC   **Primatene P asthma remedy**

Manufacturer: Whitehall Laboratories
Ingredients: ephedrine hydrochloride; phenobarbital; theophylline
Dosage Form: Tablet: ephedrine hydrochloride, 24 mg; phenobarbital, 8 mg; theophylline, 130 mg
Use: For relief and control of attacks of bronchial asthma and associated hay fever
Side Effects: Anxiety; chest pain; dizziness; headache; increased blood pressure; increased frequency of urination; insomnia; loss of appetite; nausea; nervousness; palpitations; sweating; tension; tremor; vomiting.
Warnings: Persons with high blood pressure, diabetes, thyroid, or heart disease should use this product only on the advice of a doctor. • Overdose may result in convulsions, coma, and cardiovascular collapse.
Comments: Over-the-counter sale of this product may not be permitted in some states. • While taking this product, avoid the use of guanethidine, monoamine oxidase inhibitors, or tricyclic antidepressants. If you are taking medication of this type, or if you are unsure of the type of medication you are taking, consult your doctor. • Do not worry about addiction to this product if you follow directions for use.

Principen antibiotic (E. R. Squibb & Sons), see ampicillin antibiotic.

OTC   **Privine nasal decongestant**

Manufacturer: CIBA Pharmaceutical Company
Ingredients: naphazoline hydrochloride; benzalkonium chloride
Dosage Forms: Drop; Nasal spray: naphazoline hydrochloride, 0.05%; benzalkonium chloride, 1:5000
Use: Temporary relief of nasal congestion due to colds, sinusitis, hay fever, or other upper respiratory allergies
Side Effects: Blurred vision; burning, dryness of nasal mucosa; increased nasal congestion or discharge; sneezing, and/or stinging; dizziness; drowsiness; headache; insomnia; nervousness; palpitations; slight increase in blood pressure; stimulation

Contraindications: This product should not be used by persons who have glaucoma (certain types).

Warnings: This product should be used with special caution by children under 12 years of age and by persons who have diabetes, advanced hardening of the arteries, heart disease, high blood pressure, or thyroid disease. If you have any of these conditions, consult your doctor before taking this product. • This product interacts with monoamine oxidase inhibitors, thyroid preparations, and tricyclic antidepressants. If you are currently taking any drugs of these types, check with your doctor before taking this product. If you are unsure of the type or contents of your medications, ask your doctor or pharmacist. • To avoid side effects such as burning, sneezing, or stinging, and a "rebound" increase in nasal congestion and discharge, do not exceed the recommended dosage and do not use this product for more than three or four continuous days. • This product should not be used by more than one person; sharing the dispenser may spread infection.

Comments: The spray form of this product, although slightly more expensive than the drops, is preferred. The spray penetrates far back into the nose, covering the nasal area more completely, and is more convenient to use. • Do not transfer the contents of this product into an atomizer that has aluminum parts because the drug may decompose and lose its effectiveness. • If the solution becomes discolored, it should be discarded.

Probalan uricosuric (The Lannett Company, Inc.), see Benemid uricosuric.

℞   **Pro-Banthine anticholinergic**

Manufacturer: Searle Pharmaceuticals Inc.

Ingredient: propantheline bromide

Equivalent Products: Norpanth, North American Pharmacal, Inc.; propantheline bromide, various manufacturers; Ropanth, Tutag Pharmaceuticals, Inc.

Dosage Form: Tablet: 7.5 mg (white); 15 mg (peach)

Use: Treatment of peptic ulcer; irritable bowel syndrome

Minor Side Effects: Blurred vision; constipation; difficult urination; dizziness; drowsiness; dry mouth; headache; increased sensitivity to light; insomnia; loss of the sense of taste; nausea; nervousness; palpitations; reduced sweating; vomiting

Major Side Effects: Impotence; rash

Contraindications: This drug should not be taken by people who have glaucoma, enlarged prostate, severe ulcerative colitis, severe hemorrhage, obstructed bladder, obstructed intestine, myasthenia gravis, or hiatal hernia. Consult your doctor immediately if this drug has been prescribed for you and you have any of these conditions.

Warnings: This drug should be used cautiously by the elderly, and by people who have high blood pressure, thyroid disease, liver or kidney disease, or heart disease; and by those who are pregnant. Be sure your doctor knows if you have any of these conditions. • People who have ulcerative colitis should be especially careful about taking this drug, and should never increase the dosage unless told to do so by their doctor. • This drug interacts with amantadine, antacids, haloperidol, and phenothiazines; if you are currently taking any drugs of these types, consult your doctor about their use. If you are unsure of the type or contents of your medications, ask your doctor or pharmacist. • This drug always produces certain side effects, which may include dry mouth, blurred vision, drowsiness, reduced sweating, difficult urination, constipation, increased sensitivity to light, and palpitations. Avoid tasks that require alertness. Avoid excessive work or exercise in hot weather. To prevent oversedation, avoid taking alcohol or other drugs that have sedative properties. • Call your doctor if you have diarrhea, or develop pain in the eye, or a rash. • Never take this drug more frequently than prescribed; a serious overdose could result, especially if you use the sustained-action form.

Comments: This drug is best taken one-half to one hour before meals. • This drug does not cure ulcers, but may help them improve. • Chew gum or suck on ice chips or a piece of hard candy to reduce mouth dryness. • A product combining Pro-Banthine anticholinergic with phenobarbital is available for persons who are especially nervous or anxious. Despite the phenobarbital content, this formulation has not been shown to have high potential for abuse.

Probenimead uricosuric (Spencer-Mead, Inc.), see Benemid uricosuric.

Procamide antiarrhythmic (Amfre-Grant, Inc.), see Pronestyl antiarrhythmic.

Prochlor-Iso anticholinergic and phenothiazine (Henry Schein, Inc.), see Combid Spansule anticholinergic and phenothiazine.

Proclan expectorant (H. R. Cenci Laboratories, Inc.), see Phenergan expectorant.

Proclan VC expectorant (H. R. Cenci Laboratories, Inc.), see Phenergan VC expectorant.

Progesic Compound-65 analgesic (Ulmer Pharmacal Company), see Darvon Compound-65 analgesic.

Progesic-65 analgesic (Ulmer Pharmacal Company), see Darvon analgesic.

OTC   Prolamine appetite suppressant

Manufacturer: Thompson Medical Company, Inc.
Ingredients: caffeine; phenylpropanolamine hydrochloride
Dosage Form: Capsule: caffeine, 140 mg; phenylpropanolamine hydrochloride, 50 mg
Use: Aid in diet control
Side Effects: Diarrhea; dizziness; headache; insomnia; nervousness; palpitations; increase in blood pressure, blood sugar, heart rate, and thyroid activity; in larger than the recommended dose: irregular heartbeat, nasal dryness, upset stomach
Contraindications: Persons with heart disease, high blood pressure, diabetes, kidney or thyroid disease, and/or pregnant or nursing women should not use this product. Consult your doctor.
Warnings: Avoid use of this drug if taking prescription antihypertension and antidepressive drugs containing monoamine oxidase inhibitors or other medication containing sympathomimetic amines. • Avoid continuous use for longer than three months. • Discontinue use of this product if rapid pulse, dizziness or palpitations occur.
Comments: During the first week of taking this product, expect increased frequency of urination. • Many medical authorities believe that the ingredient phenylpropanolamine does not help in weight loss programs. The FDA Review Panel has reported that it is effective. If you want to use this product, remember that you become tolerant to any beneficial effects after a couple of weeks. After each two weeks of use, stop for one week, then resume. • The primary value in products of this nature is in following the caloric reduction plan that goes with it.

R_x   **Proloid thyroid hormone**

Manufacturer: Parke-Davis
Ingredient: thyroglobulin
Equivalent Products: thyroglobulin, various manufacturers
Dosage Form: Tablet: 32 mg; 65 mg; 100 mg; 130 mg; 200 mg (all grey)
Use: Thyroid replacement therapy
Minor Side Effects: None when drug is used as directed
Major Side Effects: Chest pain; diarrhea; headache; heat intolerance; insomnia; palpitations; sweating; weight loss
Contraindications: This drug should not be used by people whose adrenal glands are not functioning. Consult your doctor immediately if this drug has been prescribed for you and you have such a condition.
Warnings: This drug should be used cautiously by people who have heart disease. Be sure your doctor knows if you have such a condition. • This drug interacts with cholestyramine, digitalis, oral anticoagulants, oral antidiabetics, and phenytoin; if you are currently taking any drugs of these types, consult your doctor about their use. If you are unsure of the type or contents of your medications, ask your doctor or pharmacist. • This drug alters the results of thyroid function tests; remind your doctor that you are taking it if you are scheduled to have such a test. • If you are undergoing thyroid replacement therapy, do not take any nonprescription item for cough, cold, or sinus problems without first checking with your doctor. • If you are taking digitalis in addition to this drug, watch carefully for symptoms of increased toxicity (e.g., nausea, blurred vision, palpitations) and notify your doctor immediately if they occur. • Be sure to follow your doctor's dosage instructions exactly. Most side effects from this drug can be controlled by dosage adjustment; consult your doctor if you experience side effects.
Comments: Generic thyroid hormone tablets (see the profile on thyroid hormone) may work as well as this drug and are often less expensive. Check with your doctor.

Promapar phenothiazine (Parke-Davis), see Thorazine phenothiazine.

Promethazine Hydrochloride expectorant (Lederle Laboratories), see Phenergan expectorant.

Promethazine Hydrochloride VC with Codeine expectorant (Lederle Laboratories), see Phenergan VC with Codeine expectorant.

Promethazine Hydrochloride with Codeine expectorant (Lederle Laboratories), see Phenergan with Codeine expectorant.

Promex expectorant (Lemmon Company), see Phenergan expectorant.

Promex with Codeine expectorant (Lemmon Company), see Phenergan with Codeine expectorant.

R_x   **Pronestyl antiarrhythmic**

Manufacturer: E. R. Squibb & Sons, Inc.
Ingredient: procainamide hydrochloride
Equivalent Products: Procamide, Amfre-Grant, Inc.; procainamide hydrochloride, various manufacturers; Sub-Quin, Scrip-Physician Supply Co.
Dosage Forms: Capsule: 250 mg (yellow); 375 mg (orange/white); 500 mg (yellow/orange). Tablet: 250 mg (yellow); 375 mg (deep orange); 500 mg (red)
Use: Treatment of some heart arrhythmias

Minor Side Effects: Bitter taste in the mouth; diarrhea; itching; loss of appetite; nausea; rash; vomiting

Major Side Effects: Chills; depression; fever; giddiness; pain in the joints; weakness

Contraindications: This drug should not be taken by people who are allergic to it or to procaine and related drugs. • The drug should not be taken by people who have myasthenia gravis, or certain types of heart disease. Consult your doctor immediately if this drug has been prescribed for you and you fit into any of these categories.

Warnings: People who have liver or kidney disease, or certain types of heart disease should use this drug with caution. Be sure your doctor knows if you have any of these conditions. • While taking this drug, do not take any non-prescription item for cough, cold, or sinus problems without first checking with your doctor. • This drug may cause symptoms of lupus (e.g., arthritis or breathing pains); notify your doctor if you experience such symptoms. • Follow your doctor's dosage instructions carefully; it is especially important that this drug be taken on time. • Do not break or crush the capsules or tablets; they must be swallowed whole.

Prothazine expectorant (North American Pharmacal, Inc.), see Phenergan expectorant.

Prothazine with Codeine expectorant (North American Pharmacal, Inc.), see Phenergan with Codeine expectorant.

Protran sedative and hypnotic (Vanguard Laboratories), see meprobamate sedative and hypnotic.

R_x   **Provera progesterone hormone**

Manufacturer: The Upjohn Company
Ingredient: medroxyprogesterone acetate
Equivalent Product: Amen, Carnrick Laboratories
Dosage Form: Tablet: 2.5 mg (peach); 10 mg (white)
Use: Treatment of abnormal menstrual bleeding, difficult menstruation, or lack of menstruation

Minor Side Effects: Acne

Major Side Effects: Cessation of menstrual flow; itching; migraine; rash; spotting or breakthrough or unusual vaginal bleeding; tender breasts; visual disturbances; weight gain or loss

Contraindications: This drug should not be taken by people who have cancer of the breast or genitals, clotting disorders or a history of clotting disorders, vaginal bleeding of unknown cause, liver disease; or by those who are pregnant. The drug should not be used by anyone with a history of missed abortion (retention of a dead fetus in the uterus for a number of weeks). Consult your doctor immediately if this drug has been prescribed for you and you have any of these conditions. • This drug should not be used as a test to determine pregnancy.

Warnings: This drug should be used cautiously by people who have epilepsy, migraines, asthma, heart or kidney disease, depression, or diabetes. Be sure your doctor knows if you have any of these conditions. • Watch for early signs of clotting disorders, cancer, loss of vision, or headache and report any such signs to your doctor immediately. Notify your doctor if any unusual vaginal bleeding occurs. • If you took this drug and later discovered that you were pregnant while using the medication, consult your doctor immediately. • This drug should not be used in conjunction with oral anticoagulants or steroids; if you are currently taking any drugs of these types, consult your doctor about their use. If you are unsure about the type or contents of your medications, ask your doctor or pharmacist.

Proxagesic analgesic (Tutag Pharmaceuticals, Inc.), see Darvon analgesic.

Proxagesic Compound-65 analgesic (Tutag Pharmaceuticals, Inc.), see Darvon Compound-65 analgesic.

Proxene analgesic (Bowman Pharmaceuticals), see Darvon analgesic.

Puretane DC expectorant (Purepac Pharmaceutical Co.), see Dimetane DC expectorant.

Puretane expectorant (Purepac Pharmaceutical Co.), see Dimetane expectorant.

P.V. Carpine Liquifilm ophthalmic solution (Allergan Pharmaceuticals), see Isopto Carpine ophthalmic solution.

Pyridiate analgesic (Rugby Laboratories), see Pyridium analgesic.

℞ **Pyridium analgesic**

Manufacturer: Parke-Davis
Ingredient: phenazopyridine hydrochloride
Equivalent Products: Azodine, North American Pharmacal; Azo-100, Scruggs Pharmacal Company, Inc.; Azo-Standard, Webcon Pharmaceuticals; Azo-Stat, O'Neal, Jones & Feldman; Di-Azo, Kay Pharmacal Company, Inc.; Phenazodine, The Lannett Company, Inc.; phenazopyridine hydrochloride, various manufacturers; Pyridiate, Rugby Laboratories; Urodine, Robinson Laboratory, Inc.
Dosage Form: Tablet: 100 mg; 200 mg (both dark maroon)
Use: Symptomatic relief of the burning and pain of urinary tract disorders
Minor Side Effects: Change in urine color; nausea; vomiting
Major Side Effects: Anemia; jaundice
Contraindications: This drug should not be taken by people who have severe kidney disease. Consult your doctor immediately if this drug has been prescribed for you and you have this condition.
Comments: Take this drug with at least a full glass of water. Drink at least nine glasses of water daily. • This drug will cause your urine to become orange-red in color. Do not be alarmed by this side effect. The urine will return to its normal color soon after the drug has been discontinued. • This drug should not be used for pain other than that associated with the urinary tract. • Diabetics may get a false reading for sugar or ketones while using this drug.

℞ **Quaalude sedative and hypnotic**

Manufacturer: Lemmon Company
Ingredient: methaqualone
Equivalent Products: Mequin, Lemmon Company; Parest, Parke-Davis; Sopor, Arnar-Stone Laboratories, Inc.
Dosage Form: Tablet: 150 mg; 300 mg (both white)
Use: Sleeping aid
Minor Side Effects: Anxiety; diarrhea; dizziness; dry mouth; fatigue; hangover; headache; loss of appetite; nausea; numbness of the fingers or toes; rash; reduced sweating; vomiting
Major Side Effects: Sore throat

Contraindications: This drug should not be used by people who are allergic to it or by pregnant women. Consult your doctor immediately if this drug has been prescribed for you and you have such an allergy or are pregnant.

Warnings: This drug should be used cautiously by people who have liver disease. Be sure your doctor knows if you have any of these conditions. • This drug should not be used by children. • This drug interacts with central nervous system depressants; to prevent oversedation, avoid the use of alcohol or other drugs that have sedative properties. If you are currently taking any depressant or sedative drugs, consult your doctor about their use. If you are unsure of the type or contents of your medications, ask your doctor or pharmacist. • Because this drug may produce drowsiness within 10 to 20 minutes, it should be taken only at bedtime. Do not attempt to drive, operate heavy machinery, or perform other tasks that require alertness directly after taking this drug. • This drug has the potential for abuse and must be used with caution; it may cause dependence, and therefore is intended for short-term use only. Tolerance may develop quickly; do not increase the dose of this drug without first consulting your doctor.

Quadra-Hist adrenergic and antihistamine (Henry Schein, Inc.), see Naldecon adrenergic and antihistamine.

℞ Quibron expectorant and smooth muscle relaxant

Manufacturer: Mead Johnson Pharmaceutical Division
Ingredients: guaifenesin; theophylline
Equivalent Products: Cerylin, Spencer-Mead, Inc.; Glyceryl-T, Rugby Laboratories; Lanophyllin-GG, The Lannett Company, Inc.; Slo-Phyllin, Dooner Laboratories, Inc.; Theo-Col, Columbia Medical Co.
Dosage Forms: Capsule: guaifenesin, 180 mg; theophylline, 300 mg (yellow). Liquid (content per 15 ml): guaifenesin, 90 mg; theophylline, 150 mg
Use: Prevention and treatment of asthmatic attacks or related conditions
Minor Side Effects: Mild stimulation; nausea; vomiting
Major Side Effects: Convulsions; difficult breathing; palpitations
Contraindications: This drug should not be taken by people who are allergic to either of its components or to any xanthine derivative. Consult your doctor immediately if this drug has been prescribed for you and you have such an allergy.
Warnings: Excessive doses of this drug are toxic, so follow your doctor's dosage instructions exactly. This drug should not be taken more frequently than once every six hours or within 12 hours of any similar product given rectally. Be sure to take your dose at exactly the right time. • This drug should be used cautiously by people over age 55, and by people who have heart disease, thyroid disease, high blood pressure, liver or kidney disease, alcoholism, or a history of peptic ulcer; and by those who are pregnant or nursing. Be sure your doctor knows if you have any of these conditions. • This drug interacts with lithium carbonate, propranolol, furosemide, reserpine, chlordiazepoxide, some antibiotics, and other xanthines; if you are currently taking any drugs of these types, consult your doctor about their use. If you are unsure of the type or contents of your medications, ask your doctor or pharmacist. • While taking this drug, do not use any nonprescription item for asthma without first checking with your doctor. • Avoid drinking coffee, tea, cola drinks, cocoa, or other beverages that contain caffeine. • Call your doctor if you have severe stomach pain, vomiting, or restlessness, because this drug may aggravate an ulcer. • This drug may affect the results of urine tests; remind your doctor that you are taking it if you are scheduled for any such tests.
Comments: While taking this drug, drink at least eight glasses of water daily. Take your dose with food or milk.

Quinidex Extentabs antiarrhythmic (A. H. Robins Company), see quinidine sulfate antiarrhythmic.

Rx **quinidine sulfate antiarrhythmic**

Manufacturer: various manufacturers
Ingredient: quinidine sulfate
Equivalent Products: Cin-Quin, Rowell Laboratories, Inc.; Quinidex Extentabs, A. H. Robins Company; Quinora, Key Pharmaceuticals, Inc. (also see Warnings)
Dosage Forms: Capsule; Sustained-release tablet; Tablet: 100 mg, 200 mg, 300 mg (various colors)
Use: Treatment of certain types of heart arrhythmias
Minor Side Effects: Abdominal pain; diarrhea; headache; nausea; vomiting
Major Side Effects: Anemia; blurred vision; dizziness; lightheadedness; ringing in the ears
Contraindications: This drug should not be used by people who are allergic to it, or by those who have a blood disease or digitalis poisoning. Consult your doctor immediately if this drug has been prescribed for you and you fit into any of these categories.
Warnings: This drug should be used cautiously by people who are also taking digitalis, and by those who have liver or kidney disease, low blood levels of potassium, certain types of heart disease, and by pregnant women. Be sure your doctor knows if you have any of these conditions. • This drug interacts with acetazolamide, anticholinergics, antacids, oral anticoagulants, sodium bicarbonate, and potassium. If you are currently taking any drugs of these types, consult your doctor about their use. If you are unsure of the type or contents of your medications, ask your doctor or pharmacist. • If you are being treated for a heart arrhythmia, do not take any nonprescription item for cough, cold, or sinus problems without first checking with your doctor. • If you develop ringing or thumping in your ears, light-headedness, or blurred vision, contact your doctor immediately; these may be symptoms of toxicity of this drug. • Although many quinidine sulfate products are on the market, they are not all bioequivalent; that is, they may not all be absorbed into the bloodstream at the same rate or have the same overall pharmacologic activity. Don't change brands of this drug without consulting your doctor or pharmacist to make sure you are receiving an identically functioning product.

Quinora antiarrhythmic (Key Pharmaceuticals, Inc.), see quinidine sulfate antiarrhythmic.

Racet steroid hormone and anti-infective (Lemmon Company), see Vioform-Hydrocortisone steroid hormone and anti-infective.

Raurine antihypertensive (O'Neal, Jones & Feldman Pharmaceuticals), see reserpine antihypertensive.

Rau-Sed antihypertensive (E. R. Squibb & Sons, Inc.), see reserpine antihypertensive.

Rx **Rauzide diuretic and antihypertensive**

Manufacturer: E. R. Squibb & Sons, Inc.
Ingredients: bendroflumethiazide; powdered rauwolfia serpentina
Dosage Form: Tablet: bendroflumethiazide, 4 mg; powdered rauwolfia serpentina, 50 mg (green)
Use: Treatment of high blood pressure

Minor Side Effects: Cramps; diarrhea; dizziness; headache; itching; loss of appetite; nasal congestion; nausea; palpitations; rash; restlessness; tingling in fingers and toes; vomiting

Major Side Effects: Chest pain; depression; drowsiness; elevated blood sugar; elevated uric acid; glaucoma; muscle spasms; nightmares; sore throat

Contraindications: This drug should not be used in patients who are allergic to either of its ingredients or to sulfa drugs. Consult your doctor immediately if this drug has been prescribed for you and you have such an allergy. • This drug should not be taken by persons suffering from anuria (no urine), mental depression (especially suicidal tendencies), active peptic ulcer, or ulcerative colitis; and persons undergoing electroshock therapy. This drug should not be used routinely in otherwise healthy pregnant women. Consult your doctor immediately if this drug has been prescribed for you and you have any of these conditions.

Warnings: This drug should be used with caution in patients with severe kidney disease, bronchial asthma, allergies, diabetes, gallstones, or liver disease. Be sure your doctor knows if you have any of these conditions. • Use of this drug may cause lupus erythematosus, depression, suicide attempts, low blood potassium level, low sodium level, gout, or ulcerative colitis. Persons taking this drug should have periodic blood and urine tests. • This drug may affect the results of thyroid tests. • This drug interacts with curare, digitalis, quinidine, amphetamine, antidiabetics, colestipol hydrochloride, decongestants, levodopa, lithium carbonate, monoamine oxidase inhibitors, and steroids. If you are currently taking any drugs of these types, consult your doctor about their use. If you are unsure of the type or contents of your medication, ask your doctor or pharmacist. • This drug should be used with caution in pregnant women and nursing mothers.

Comments: A doctor should probably not prescribe this drug or other "fixed dose" combination products as the first choice in the treatment of high blood pressure. The patient should receive each of the individual ingredients singly, and if response is adequate to the fixed doses contained in this product, it can then be substituted. The advantage of a combination product such as this drug is based on increased convenience to the patient. • Take this drug with food or milk. • This drug causes frequent urination. Expect this effect; it should not alarm you. • The effects of therapy with this drug may not be apparent for at least two weeks. • Mild side effects (e.g., nasal congestion) are most noticeable during the first two weeks of therapy and become less bothersome after this period. • This drug can cause potassium loss. To help avoid potassium loss, take this drug with a glass of fresh or frozen orange juice. You may also eat a banana each day. The use of Co-Salt salt substitute helps prevent potassium loss. • This drug may cause drowsiness or depression; to prevent oversedation, avoid the use of alcohol or other sedative drugs. If you feel continually tired or depressed, consult your doctor. • While taking this product (as with many drugs that lower blood pressure), you should limit your consumption of alcoholic beverages in order to prevent dizziness or light-headedness. • To avoid dizziness or light-headedness when you stand, contract and relax the muscles of your legs for a few moments before rising. Do this by pushing one foot against the floor while raising the other foot slightly, alternating feet so that you are "pumping" your legs in a pedaling motion. • Persons taking digitalis in addition to this product should watch carefully for symptoms of increased toxicity (e.g., nausea, blurred vision, palpitations), and notify their doctor immediately if symptoms occur. While taking this drug, do not take any nonprescription item for cough, cold, or sinus problems without first checking with your doctor. • If you are allergic to a sulfa drug, you may likewise be allergic to this drug. • This drug can affect your ability to drive or operate machinery.

Rx Regroton diuretic and antihypertensive

Manufacturer: USV (P.R.) Development Corp.
Ingredients: chlorthalidone; reserpine
Dosage Form: Tablet: chlorthalidone, 50 mg; reserpine, 0.25 mg (pink)
Use: Treatment of high blood pressure
Minor Side Effects: Constipation; cramps; diarrhea; headache; itching; loss of appetite; nasal congestion; nausea; numbing or tingling of fingers or toes; palpitations; vomiting
Major Side Effects: Chest pain; depression; dizziness; drowsiness; elevated blood sugar; glaucoma; impotence; muscle spasms; nightmares; restlessness; sore throat
Contraindications: This drug should not be used by persons with mental depression and most kinds of severe kidney or liver disease. • This drug should not be used by people who are allergic to either of its ingredients. Consult your doctor immediately if this drug has been prescribed for you and you have any of these conditions or such an allergy.
Warnings: This drug should be used with caution in persons with severe kidney disease, liver disease, asthma, allergies, or ulcer. Be sure your doctor knows if you have any of these conditions. • This drug should be used cautiously, since it may cause suicide attempts, low potassium level, low sodium level, diabetes, gout, colitis, gallstones, asthma, or ulcer. • Persons using this drug should have periodic urine and blood tests. • The use of this drug can affect thyroid tests and anesthetics. • The use of this drug should be discontinued in patients developing mental depression. In patients who have had depression, the drug should not be started. • Patients undergoing electroshock therapy should not take this drug, since severe and even fatal reactions have occurred. This drug should be stopped at least seven days before giving electroshock therapy. • This drug should be used with caution in pregnant women and nursing mothers. • This drug should be used with caution in persons undergoing emergency surgery. • This drug should not be taken with other blood pressure drugs, amphetamine, colestipol hydrochloride, decongestants, digitalis, levodopa, lithium carbonate, monoamine oxidase inhibitors, oral antidiabetics, or steroids. If you are currently taking any drugs of these types, consult your doctor about their use. If you are unsure of the type or contents of your medications, ask your doctor or pharmacist.
Comments: A doctor probably should not prescribe this drug or other "fixed dose" products as the first choice in the treatment of high blood pressure. The patient should receive each of the ingredients individually, and if response is adequate to the fixed doses contained in this drug, this product can then be substituted. The advantage of a combination product such as this drug is based on increased convenience to the patient. • Take this drug with food or milk. • This drug causes frequent urination. Expect this effect; it should not alarm you. • The effects of therapy with this drug may not be apparent for at least two weeks. • Mild side effects (e.g., nasal congestion) are most noticeable during the first two weeks of therapy and become less bothersome after this period. • This drug can cause potassium loss. To help avoid potassium loss, take this drug with a glass of fresh or frozen orange juice. You may also eat a banana each day. The use of a salt substitute helps prevent potassium loss. • This drug may cause drowsiness; to prevent oversedation, avoid the use of other sedative drugs. • If you feel continually tired or depressed, consult your doctor. While taking this product (as with many drugs that lower blood pressure), you should limit your consumption of alcoholic beverages in order to prevent dizziness or light-headedness. • To avoid dizziness or light-headedness when you stand, contract and relax the muscles of your legs for a few moments before rising. Do this by pushing one foot against the floor while raising the other foot slightly, alternating feet so

that you are "pumping" your legs in a pedaling motion. • Persons taking this product and digitalis should watch carefully for symptoms of increased toxicity (e.g., nausea, blurred vision, palpitation). • While taking this drug, do not take any nonprescription item for cough, cold, or sinus problems without first checking with your doctor. • If you are allergic to sulfa drugs, you may likewise be allergic to this drug. • This drug causes cancer in rats. It has not been shown to cause cancer in people. • This drug affects driving. • A product called Demi-Regroton diuretic and antihypertensive is identical, except it is half the strength.

OTC   Regutol laxative

Manufacturer: Plough, Inc.
Ingredient: docusate sodium (dioctyl sodium sulfosuccinate)
Dosage Form: Tablet: docusate sodium, 100 mg
Use: Relief of constipation and stool softener
Contraindications: Persons with high fever (100° F or more); black or tarry stools; nausea; vomiting; abdominal pain; or children under age three should not use this product unless directed by a doctor. • Do not use this product when constipation is caused by megacolon or other diseases of the intestine, or hypothyroidism.
Warnings: Excessive use (daily for a month or more) of this product may cause diarrhea, vomiting, and loss of certain blood electrolytes. • Pregnant women should not use this product except on the advice of a doctor.
Comments: Evacuation may occur within 72 hours. • Never self-medicate with this product if constipation lasts longer than two weeks or if the medication does not produce a laxative effect within a week. • This product is referred to as a stool softener and is recommended for prevention of constipation when the stool is hard and dry. Do not take another product containing mineral oil at the same time as you are taking this product. • Limit use to seven days unless directed otherwise by a doctor.

Repen-VK antibiotic (Reid-Provident Laboratories, Inc.), see penicillin potassium phenoxymethyl antibiotic.

Reposans sedative and hypnotic (Foy Laboratories, Inc.), see Librium sedative and hypnotic.

Repro Compound 65 analgesic (Reid-Provident Laboratories, Inc.), see Darvon Compound-65 analgesic.

Rx   reserpine antihypertensive

Manufacturer: various manufacturers
Ingredient: reserpine
Equivalent Products: Hiserpia, Bowman Pharmaceuticals; Raurine, O'Neal, Jones & Feldman Pharmaceuticals; Rau-Sed, E. R. Squibb & Sons, Inc.; Reserpoid, The Upjohn Company; Rolserp, Robinson Laboratory, Inc.; Sandril, Eli Lilly and Company; Serpalan, The Lannett Company, Inc.; Serpasil, CIBA Pharmaceutical Company; Serpate, The Vale Chemical Co., Inc; Vio-Serpine, Rowell Laboratories, Inc.
Dosage Forms: Liquid; Tablet (various dosages and colors)
Use: Treatment of high blood pressure
Minor Side Effects: Diarrhea; itching; loss of appetite; nasal congestion; nausea; palpitations; rash; vomiting
Major Side Effects: Chest pain; depression; drowsiness; glaucoma; nightmares

548

Contraindications: This drug should not be taken by people who are allergic to it, or by those who have active peptic ulcer, ulcerative colitis, mental depression, or who are receiving electroshock therapy. Consult your doctor immediately if this drug has been prescribed for you and you have any of these conditions.

Warnings: This is a powerful drug that may persist in the body for several months after the medication is discontinued, and patients must be watched for signs of drug-induced depression which might lead to suicide. If you feel continually tired or depressed, consult your doctor. • This drug should be used cautiously by pregnant women and by people who are taking monoamine oxidase inhibitors (ask your pharmacist if you are unsure), or who have kidney disease, or a history of ulcer, gallstones, or colitis. Be sure your doctor knows if you have any of these conditions. • Nursing women who must take this drug should stop nursing. • This drug interacts with amphetamine, decongestants, levodopa, and monoamine oxidase inhibitors; if you are currently taking any drugs of these types, consult your doctor about their use. If you are unsure of the type or contents of your medications, ask your doctor or pharmacist. • This drug must be used cautiously with digitalis and quinidine; be sure your doctor knows if you are taking either of these drugs. Watch for symptoms of increased toxicity (e.g., nausea, blurred vision, palpitations) and notify your doctor if they occur. • While taking this drug, do not take any nonprescription item for cough, cold, or sinus problems without first checking with your doctor. • This drug may cause drowsiness; avoid tasks that require alertness. To prevent oversedation, avoid the use of alcohol or other drugs that have sedative properties. • Reserpine causes cancer in rats. It has not been shown to cause cancer in people.

Comments: The effects of therapy with this drug may not be apparent for at least two weeks. • Take your dose with food or milk. • Mild side effects (e.g., nasal congestion) are most noticeable during the first two weeks of drug therapy and become less bothersome after this period. • To avoid dizziness or light-headedness when you stand, contract and relax the muscles of your legs for a few moments before rising. Do this by pushing one foot against the floor while raising the other foot slightly, alternating feet so that you are "pumping" your legs in a pedaling motion.

Reserpoid antihypertensive (The Upjohn Company), see reserpine antihypertensive.

Retet antibiotic (Reid-Provident Laboratories, Inc.), see tetracycline hydrochloride antibiotic.

℞   **Retin-A acne preparation**

Manufacturer: Ortho Pharmaceutical Corporation
Ingredient: tretinoin (retinoic acid; vitamin A acid)
Dosage Forms: Cream: 0.1%; 0.05%. Gel: 0.025%; 0.01%. Liquid: 0.05%. Swab: 0.05%
Use: Topical application in treatment of acne vulgaris
Minor Side Effect: Localized rash
Major Side Effects: Blistering or crusting of the skin; heightened susceptibility to sunlight; peeling; temporary hyperpigmentation or hypopigmentation of the skin
Contraindications: This drug should not be used by people who are allergic to it. Consult your doctor immediately if this drug has been prescribed for you and you have such an allergy.
Warnings: This drug should not be used in conjunction with other ointments (peeling agents), particularly those containing sulfur, resorcinol, ben-

zoyl peroxide, or salicylic acid. • While using this drug, exposure to sunlight (or sunlamps), wind, and/or cold should be minimized or totally avoided to prevent skin irritation. • This drug should be used with extreme caution in persons suffering from eczema. • Medicated or abrasive soaps and cosmetics that have a strong drying effect, along with locally applied products containing high amounts of alcohol, spices, or lime, should be used with caution because of a possible negative interaction with the drug.

Comments: This drug should be kept away from the eyes, the mouth, the angles of the nose, and the mucous membranes. • A temporary feeling of warmth or a slight stinging may be noted following application of this drug. This effect is normal and not dangerous. • The liquid form of this drug may be applied with a fingertip, gauze pad, or cotton swab. If gauze or cotton is used, do not oversaturate so that the liquid runs onto areas that are not intended for treatment. • During the early weeks of using this drug, there may be an apparent increase in skin lesions. This is usually not a reason to discontinue its use. However, your doctor may wish to modify the concentration of the drug. Therapeutic effects may be noted within two to three weeks, although more than six weeks may be required before definite benefits are seen.

OTC   Rezamid acne preparation

Manufacturer: Dermik Laboratories, Inc.
Ingredients: alcohol; chloroxylenol; microsize sulfur; resorcinol
Dosage Form: Lotion: alcohol, 28.5%; chloroxylenol, 0.5%; microsize sulfur, 5%; resorcinol, 2%
Use: Treatment of acne
Side Effects: Allergy; local irritation
Warnings: Do not get product in or near the eyes.
Comments: This preparation may stain the skin. • If the condition worsens, stop using this product and call your pharmacist.

OTC   Rhulicream poison ivy remedy

Manufacturer: Lederle Laboratories
Ingredients: benzocaine; camphor; isopropyl alcohol; menthol; methylparaben; propylparaben; zirconium oxide
Dosage Form: Ointment: benzocaine, 1%; camphor, 0.3%; isopropyl alcohol, 8.8%; menthol, 0.7%; methylparaben, 0.08%; propylparaben, 0.02%; zirconium oxide, 1%
Use: For temporary relief of itching, pain, and discomfort of poison ivy and poison oak; insect bites; mild sunburn; minor skin irritations
Side Effects: Allergic reactions (rash, itching, soreness); local irritation
Warnings: Avoid application of this product around the eyes and genitalia or on infected wounds.
Comments: To prevent irritation and secondary infection, avoid scratching. • Before applying medication, soak the area in warm water or apply towels soaked in water for five to ten minutes. Dry the area gently by patting with a soft towel, then apply medication.

OTC   Rhulihist poison ivy remedy

Manufacturer: Lederle Laboratories
Ingredients: alcohol; benzocaine; benzyl alcohol; calamine USP; camphor USP; menthol; methylparaben; propylparaben; tripelennamine HCl USP; zirconium oxide
Dosage Form: Lotion: alcohol, 28.76%; benzocaine, 1%; benzyl alcohol, 0.674%; calamine USP, 1%; camphor USP, 0.1%; menthol, 0.1%; methylpara-

ben, 0.08%; propylparaben, 0.02%; tripelennamine HCl USP, 1%; zirconium oxide, 1%

Use: Temporary relief of itching, pain and discomfort of poison ivy and oak; insect bites; mild sunburn; minor skin irritations

Side Effects: Allergic reactions (rash, itching, soreness); local irritation

Warnings: Avoid application of this product around the eyes and genitalia or on infected wounds.

Comments: To prevent irritation and secondary infection, avoid scratching. • Before applying medication, soak the area in warm water or apply towels soaked in water for five to ten minutes. Dry the area gently by patting with a soft towel, then apply medication.

OTC   Rid antilouse preparation

Manufacturer: Pfipharmecs Division

Ingredients: benzyl alcohol; petroleum distillate; piperonyl butoxide; pyrethrins

Dosage Form: Liquid: benzyl alcohol, 2.4%; petroleum distillate, 1.2%; piperonyl butoxide, 3%; pyrethrins, 0.3%

Use: Kills body lice; head lice; pubic lice; and their eggs

Side Effects: If swallowed: coma; convulsions; nausea; restlessness; vomiting

Contraindications: Persons with asthma or those sensitive to ragweed should not use this product.

Warnings: Avoid contact with mucous membranes. • Do not get this product into eyes. Flush eyes with copious amounts of water if eyes are accidentally contaminated and call your doctor. • If skin irritation or signs of infection are present, call your doctor. • Consult your doctor if infestation of eyebrows or eyelashes occurs. • This product is harmful if swallowed. Do not inhale.

Comments: Follow directions. Do not exceed recommended dosage. • In order to prevent reinfestation with lice, all clothing and bedding must be sterilized or treated at the same time as using this product.

OTC   Riopan antacid

Manufacturer: Ayerst Laboratories

Ingredient: magaldrate

Dosage Forms: Chewable tablet; Suspension (content per teaspoon); Tablet: magaldrate, 400 mg

Use: For relief from acid indigestion, heartburn, and/or sour stomach

Side Effects: Constipation; diarrhea

Contraindications: Persons with kidney disease should not use this product. In persons with kidney disease, repeated (daily) use of this product may cause nausea, vomiting, depressed reflexes, and breathing difficulties.

Warnings: Long-term (several weeks) use of this product may lead to intestinal obstruction and dehydration. • Phosphate depletion may occur leading to weakness, loss of appetite, and eventually bone pain. This may be prevented by drinking at least one glass of milk a day.

Comments: Self-treatment of severe or repeated attacks of heartburn, indigestion, or upset stomach is not recommended. If you do self-treat, limit therapy to two weeks, then call your doctor if symptoms persist. • Never self-medicate if your symptoms occur regularly (two to three times or more a month); if they are particularly worse than normal; if you feel a "tightness" in your chest, have chest pains, or are sweating; of if you are short of breath. Consult your doctor. • This product works best when taken one hour after meals or at bedtime, unless otherwise directed by your doctor or pharmacist. • The suspension form of this product is superior to the tablet form and should be used unless you have been specifically directed to use the tablet. • Do not take this product within two hours of a dose of a tetracycline antibiotic. Also, if you are taking iron, a vitamin-mineral product, chlorpromazine, phenytoin, digoxin, quinidine, or warfarin, remind your doctor or pharmacist that you are taking this product.

℞ Ritalin adrenergic

Manufacturer: CIBA Pharmaceutical Company
Ingredient: methylphenidate hydrochloride
Equivalent Products: methylphenidate hydrochloride, various manufacturers
Dosage Form: Tablet: 5 mg (yellow); 10 mg (green); 20 mg (peach)
Use: Treatment of hyperactivity in children; treatment of narcolepsy; relief of mild depression
Minor Side Effects: Headache; insomnia; nausea; nervousness; palpitations; rash; vomiting
Major Side Effects: Chest pain; high blood pressure. In children: abdominal pain; impairment of growth; weight loss
Contraindications: This drug should not be taken by persons with marked anxiety, tension, or agitation, since it may aggravate these symptoms. This drug should not be taken by people who are allergic to it. Consult your doctor immediately if this drug has been prescribed for you and you have any of these conditions or such an allergy. • This drug should not be taken by people with glaucoma. Be sure your doctor knows if you have this condition.
Warnings: This drug is not recommended for use in children under six years of age, since suppression of growth has been reported with long-term use. The long-term effects of this drug in children have not been well established. • This drug should be used cautiously in persons with severe depression, epilepsy, high blood pressure, or eye disease. Be sure your doctor knows if you have any of these conditions. • This drug should not be used for the prevention or treatment of normal fatigue. • This drug should be used with caution in pregnant women. • This drug should be given cautiously to emotionally unstable patients, such as those with a history of drug dependence or alcoholism, because such patients may increase dosage on their own accord. Chronic abuse of this drug can lead to tolerance and psychological dependence, with varying degrees of abnormal behavior. • Periodic blood tests are recommended for patients on long-term therapy with this drug. • This drug interacts with acetazolamide, guanethidine, monoamine oxidase inhibitors, phenothiazines, sodium bicarbonate, antidepressants, anticoagulants, anticonvulsants, and phenylbutazone. If you are currently taking any drugs of these types, consult your doctor about their use. If you are unsure of the type or contents of your medications, ask your doctor or pharmacist.
Comments: This drug should not be taken later than 3:00 P.M. to avoid sleeplessness. • While taking this drug, do not take any nonprescription item for cough, cold, or sinus problems without first checking with your doctor. • This drug may mask symptoms of fatigue and pose serious danger; never take this drug as a stimulant to keep awake. • This drug has the potential for abuse and must be used with caution. Tolerance may develop quickly; do not increase the dose of this drug without first consulting your doctor. • If your child's teacher tells you your child is hyperkinetic (hyperactive), take the child to a physician for a thorough diagnosis. If the hyperkinetic child needs to take a dose of this drug at noontime, make arrangements with the school nurse.

Robamox antibiotic (A. H. Robins Company), see amoxicillin antibiotic.

℞   **Robaxin muscle relaxant**

Manufacturer: A. H. Robins Company
Ingredient: methocarbamol
Equivalent Products: Delaxin, Ferndale Laboratories, Inc.; Forbaxin, Forest Laboratories, Inc.; methocarbamol, various manufacturers; Metho-500, Mallard Incorporated; Spenaxin, Spencer-Mead, Inc.; Tumol-750, Tutag Pharmaceuticals, Inc.
Dosage Form: Tablet: 500 mg; 750 mg (white)
Use: Relief of pain in muscles or joints
Minor Side Effects: Blurred vision; dizziness; drowsiness; headache; lightheadedness; nasal congestion; nausea; rash
Major Side Effect: Fever
Contraindications: This drug should not be used by people who are allergic to it. Consult your doctor immediately if this drug has been prescribed for you and you have such an allergy.
Warnings: This drug should be used cautiously by women who are pregnant or nursing. Be sure your doctor knows if you are pregnant or nursing. • This drug should be used cautiously by children under 12 years of age; the drug's safety for children has not been established. • This drug may alter the results of some lab tests; if you are scheduled for any tests, remind your doctor that you are taking this drug. • This drug interacts with central nervous system depressants; if you are currently taking any drugs of this type, consult your doctor about their use. If you are unsure of the type of your medications, ask your doctor or pharmacist. • This drug may cause drowsiness; avoid tasks that require alertness. To prevent oversedation, avoid the use of alcohol or other drugs that have sedative properties. • This drug is not a substitute for rest, physical therapy, or other measures recommended by your doctor to treat your condition.
Comments: This drug is available combined with aspirin for additional analgesic effect; the combination product is marketed generically as methocarbamol with aspirin, or is available in trademarked form as Robaxisal muscle relaxant and analgesic (A. H. Robins Company).

Robaxisal muscle relaxant and analgesic (A. H. Robins Company), see Robaxin muscle relaxant.

Robenecid uricosuric (Robinson Laboratory, Inc.), see Benemid uricosuric.

Robicillin VK antibiotic (A. H. Robins Company), see penicillin potassium phenoxymethyl antibiotic.

Robimycin antibiotic (A. H. Robins Co.), see erythromycin antibiotic.

Robitet '250' antibiotic (A. H. Robins Company), see tetracycline hydrochloride antibiotic.

OTC   **Robitussin A-C cough remedy**

Manufacturer: A. H. Robins Company
Ingredients: codeine phosphate; guaifenesin; alcohol
Dosage Form: Liquid (content per 5 ml, or one teaspoon): codeine phosphate, 10 mg; guaifenesin, 100 mg; alcohol, 3.5%
Use: Temporary relief of cough due to colds or "flu"; also to convert a dry, nonproductive cough to a productive, phlegm-producing cough

Side Effects: Blurred vision; confusion; constipation; difficult or painful urination; dizziness; drowsiness; dry mouth and respiratory passages; headache; insomnia; low blood pressure; nausea; nervousness; palpitations; rash; restlessness; vomiting. Children may react with primary symptoms of excitement (convulsions; flushed skin; nervousness; tremors; twitching of muscles; uncoordinated movements).

Warnings: This product should be used with caution by persons who have asthma or other respiratory diseases. If you have such a condition, consult your doctor before taking this product. • Because this product contains codeine, it has the potential for abuse and must be used with caution. It usually should not be taken for more than seven to ten days. Tolerance may develop quickly, but do not increase the dose without consulting your doctor. • This product interacts with alcohol, guanethidine, monoamine oxidase inhibitors, sedative drugs, and tricyclic antidepressants. If you are currently taking any drugs of these types, check with your doctor before taking this product. If you are unsure of the type or contents of your medications, ask your doctor or pharmacist.

Comments: Do not use this product to treat chronic coughs, such as from smoking or asthma. Do not use this product to treat productive (hacking) coughs that produce phlegm. • If you require an expectorant, you need more moisture in your environment. Drink eight to ten glasses of water daily. The use of a vaporizer or humidifier may also be beneficial. Consult your doctor. • Over-the-counter sale of this product may not be permitted in some states.

OTC Robitussin-CF cough remedy

Manufacturer: A. H. Robins Company
Ingredients: dextromethorphan hydrobromide; guaifenesin; phenylpropanolamine hydrochloride; alcohol
Dosage Form: Liquid (content per 5 ml, or one teaspoon): dextromethorphan hydrobromide, 10 mg; guaifenesin, 100 mg; phenylpropanolamine hydrochloride, 12.5 mg; alcohol, 1.4%
Use: Temporary relief of cough and nasal congestion due to colds or "flu"; also to convert a dry, nonproductive cough to a productive, phlegm-producing cough
Side Effects: Drowsiness; mild stimulation; nausea; vomiting
Warnings: This product should be used with special caution by children under two years of age, and by persons who have diabetes, heart disease, high blood pressure, or thyroid disease. If you have any of these conditions, consult your doctor before taking this product. • This product interacts with guanethidine and monoamine oxidase inhibitors. If you are currently taking any drugs of these types, check with your doctor before taking this product. If you are unsure of the type or contents of your medications, ask your doctor or pharmacist.

Comments: Do not use this product to treat chronic coughs, such as from smoking or asthma. • Do not use this product to treat productive (hacking) coughs that produce phlegm. • If you require an expectorant, you need more moisture in your environment. Drink eight to ten glasses of water daily. The use of a vaporizer or humidifier may also be beneficial. Consult your doctor.

OTC Robitussin cough remedy

Manufacturer: A. H. Robins Company
Ingredients: guaifenesin; alcohol
Dosage Form: Liquid (content per 5 ml, or one teaspoon): guaifenesin, 100 mg; alcohol, 3.5%
Use: Temporary relief of cough due to colds or "flu"; also to convert a dry,

nonproductive cough to a productive, phlegm-producing cough

Side Effects: Occasional nausea, vomiting

Contraindications: Do not give this product to children under two years of age unless directed otherwise by your doctor.

Comments: Do not use this product to treat chronic coughs, such as from smoking or asthma. • Do not use this product to treat productive (hacking) coughs that produce phlegm. • If you require an expectorant, you need more moisture in your environment. Drink eight to ten glasses of water daily. The use of a vaporizer or humidifier may also be beneficial. Consult your doctor.

OTC   Robitussin-DM Cough Calmers cough remedy

Manufacturer: A. H. Robins Company

Ingredients: dextromethorphan hydrobromide; guaifenesin

Dosage Form: Lozenge: dextromethorphan hydrobromide, 7.5 mg; guaifenesin, 50 mg

Use: Temporary suppression or relief of cough by converting a dry, nonproductive cough to a productive, phlegm-producing cough

Side Effects: Drowsiness; nausea; vomiting

Contraindications: Do not give this product to children under six years of age unless directed otherwise by your doctor.

Warnings: This product interacts with monoamine oxidase inhibitors; if you are currently taking any drugs of this type, check with your doctor before taking this product. If you are unsure of the type or contents of your medications, ask your doctor or pharmacist.

Comments: Do not use this product to treat chronic coughs, such as from smoking or asthma. • Do not use this product to treat productive (hacking) coughs that produce phlegm. • If you require an expectorant, you need more moisture in your environment. Drink eight to ten glasses of water daily. The use of a vaporizer or humidifier may also be beneficial. Consult your doctor.

OTC   Robitussin-DM cough remedy

Manufacturer: A. H. Robins Company

Ingredients: dextromethorphan hydrobromide; guaifenesin; phenylpropanolamine hydrochloride; alcohol

Dosage Form: Liquid (content per 5 ml, or one teaspoon): dextromethorphan hydrobromide, 15 mg; guaifenesin, 100 mg; alcohol, 1.4%

Use: Temporary relief of cough and nasal congestion due to colds or "flu"; also to convert a dry, nonproductive cough to a productive, phlegm-producing cough

Side Effects: Drowsiness; mild stimulation; nausea; vomiting

Warnings: This product should be used with special caution by children under two years of age, and by persons who have diabetes, heart disease, high blood pressure, or thyroid disease. If you have any of these conditions, consult your doctor before taking this product. • This product interacts with guanethidine and monoamine oxidase inhibitors. If you are currently taking any drugs of these types, check with your doctor before taking this product. If you are unsure of the type or contents of your medications, ask your doctor or pharmacist.

Comments: Do not use this product to treat chronic coughs, such as from smoking or asthma. • Do not use this product to treat productive (hacking) coughs that produce phlegm. • If you require an expectorant, you need more moisture in your environment. Drink eight to ten glasses of water daily. The use of a vaporizer or humidifier may also be beneficial. Consult your doctor.

Robitussin-PE cough remedy

Manufacturer: A. H. Robins Company
Ingredients: guaifenesin; pseudoephedrine hydrochloride; alcohol; sucrose
Dosage Form: Liquid (content per 5 ml, or one teaspoon): guaifenesin, 100 mg; pseudoephedrine hydrochloride, 30 mg; alcohol, 1.4%; sucrose, 3.57 g
Use: Temporary relief of cough and nasal congestion due to colds or "flu"; also to convert a dry, nonproductive cough to a productive, phlegm-producing cough
Side Effects: Mild stimulation; occasional nausea, vomiting
Warnings: This product should be used with special caution by children under two years of age, and by persons who have diabetes, heart disease, high blood pressure, or thyroid disease. If you have any of these conditions, consult your doctor before taking this product. • This product interacts with guanethidine and monoamine oxidase inhibitors. If you are currently taking any drugs of these types, check with your doctor before taking this product. If you are unsure of the type or contents of your medications, ask your doctor or pharmacist.
Comments: Do not use this product to treat chronic coughs, such as from smoking or asthma. • Do not use this product to treat productive (hacking) coughs that produce phlegm. • If you require an expectorant, you need more moisture in your environment. Drink eight to ten glasses of water daily. The use of a vaporizer or humidifier may also be beneficial. Consult your doctor.

Ro-Chlorozide diuretic and antihypertensive (Robinson Laboratory, Inc.), see Diuril diuretic and antihypertensive.

Rocinolone steroid hormone (Robinson Laboratory, Inc.), see Aristocort steroid hormone.

Ro-Cloro-Serp-500 diuretic and antihypertensive (Robinson Laboratory, Inc.), see Diupres diuretic and antihypertensive.

Ro-Diet adrenergic (Robinson Laboratory, Inc.), see Tenuate adrenergic.

OTC   **Rolaids antacid**

Manufacturer: Warner-Lambert Company
Ingredient: dihydroxyaluminum sodium carbonate
Dosage Form: Tablet: dihydroxyaluminum sodium carbonate, 334 mg
Use: For relief from acid indigestion, heartburn, and/or sour stomach
Side Effects: Constipation
Contraindications: Persons with kidney disease or those on a salt-free diet should not use this product. In persons with kidney disease, repeated (daily) use of this product may cause nausea, vomiting, depressed reflexes, and breathing difficulties.
Warnings: Long-term (several weeks) use of this product may lead to intestinal obstruction and dehydration. • Phosphate depletion may occur leading to weakness, loss of appetite, and eventually bone pain. These side effects can be prevented by drinking at least one glass of milk a day.
Comments: Self-treatment of severe or repeated attacks of heartburn, indigestion, or upset stomach is not recommended. If you do self-treat, limit therapy to two weeks, then call your doctor if symptoms persist. Never self-medicate with this product if your symptoms occur regularly (two to three times or more a month); if they are particularly worse than normal; if you feel

"tightness" in your chest, have chest pains, or are sweating; or if you are short of breath. Consult your doctor. • To prevent constipation, drink at least eight glasses of water a day. If constipation persists, consult your doctor or pharmacist. • Do not take this product within two hours of a dose of a tetracycline antibiotic. Also, if you are taking iron, a vitamin-mineral product, chlorpromazine, phenytoin, digoxin, quinidine, or warfarin, remind your doctor or pharmacist that you are taking this product.

Rolazine antihypertensive (Robinson Laboratory, Inc.), see Apresoline antihypertensive.

Rolserp antihypertensive (Robinson Laboratory, Inc.), see reserpine antihypertensive.

OTC   Romilar CF cough remedy
   Manufacturer: Block Drug Company, Inc.
   Ingredients: dextromethorphan hydrobromide; ammonium chloride; alcohol
   Dosage Form: Liquid (content per 5 ml, or one teaspoon): dextromethorphan hydrobromide, 15 mg; ammonium chloride, 1%; alcohol, 20%
   Use: Temporary relief of coughs due to colds or minor throat and bronchial irritations
   Side Effects: Drowsiness; nausea; vomiting
   Warnings: This product interacts with monoamine oxidase inhibitors. If you are currently taking any drugs of this type, check with your doctor before taking this product. If you are unsure of the type or contents of your medications, ask your doctor or pharmacist.
   Comments: Do not use this product to treat chronic coughs, such as from smoking or asthma. • Do not use this product to treat productive (hacking) coughs that produce phlegm.

Romycin antibiotic (W. E. Hauck, Inc.), see erythromycin antibiotic.

Roniacol vasodilator (Roche Products, Inc.), see nicotinic acid vitamin supplement.

Ropanth anticholinergic (Tutag Pharmaceuticals, Inc.), see Pro-Banthine anticholinergic.

Ropred steroid hormone (Robinson Laboratory, Inc.), see prednisone steroid hormone.

Rosoxol antibacterial (Robinson Laboratory, Inc.), see Gantrisin antibacterial.

Ro-Thyroxine thyroid hormone (Robinson Laboratory, Inc.), see Synthroid thyroid hormone.

Rozolamide diuretic (Robinson Laboratory, Inc.), see Diamox diuretic.

RP-Mycin antibiotic (Reid-Provident Laboratories, Inc.), see erythromycin antibiotic.

Rum-K potassium chloride replacement (Fleming & Co.), see potassium chloride replacement.

**Salutensin-Demi diuretic and antihypertensive (Bristol Laboratories),
see Salutensin diuretic and antihypertensive.**

℞   **Salutensin diuretic and antihypertensive**

Manufacturer: Bristol Laboratories
Ingredients: hydroflumethiazide, reserpine
Dosage Form: Tablet: hydroflumethiazide, 50 mg; reserpine, 0.125 mg
(green)
Use: Treatment of high blood pressure
Minor Side Effects: Abdominal pain; constipation; diarrhea; dizziness;
headache; itching; loss of appetite; nasal congestion; nausea; palpitations;
rash; tingling in fingers and toes
Major Side Effects: Blurred vision; depression; drowsiness; glaucoma;
muscle spasms; nightmares; sedation; weakness
Contraindications: This drug should not be taken by persons allergic to
either of its components or to sulfa drugs. Consult your doctor immediately if
this drug has been prescribed for you and you have such an allergy. • This
drug should not be taken by persons suffering from anuria (no urine), peptic
ulcer, ulcerative colitis, or severe depression. This drug should not be given
to patients undergoing electroshock therapy. Consult your doctor immediately if this drug has been prescribed for you and you have any of these
conditions.
Warnings: This drug should be used with caution in persons with kidney
disease, liver disease, allergies, or asthma. Be sure your doctor knows if you
have any of these conditions. • Use of this drug could cause low potassium
and sodium levels, gout, diabetes, high calcium levels, ulcers, colitis, gallstones, asthma, or suicide attempts. • Persons taking this drug should have
periodic blood and urine tests. • This drug could affect thyroid tests and
anesthetics. • This drug should not be taken with amphetamine, other blood
pressure drugs, colestipol hydrochloride, decongestants, digitalis, curare,
levodopa, lithium carbonate, quinidine, monoamine oxidase inhibitors, oral
antidiabetics, or steroids. If you are currently taking any drugs of these types,
consult your doctor about their use. If you are unsure of the type or contents
of your medications, ask your doctor or pharmacist. • This drug should be
used with caution in pregnant women and nursing mothers.
Comments: A doctor probably should not prescribe this drug or other
"fixed dose" products as the first choice in the treatment of high blood pressure. The patient should receive each of the ingredients individually, and if
response is adequate to the fixed doses contained in this drug, this product
can then be substituted. The advantage of a combination product such as
this drug is based on increased convenience to the patient. • Take this drug
with food or milk. • This drug causes frequent urination. Expect this effect; it
should not alarm you. • The effects of therapy with this drug may not be apparent for at least two weeks. • Mild side effects (e.g., nasal congestion) are
most noticeable during the first two weeks of therapy and become less
bothersome after this period. • This drug can cause potassium loss. To help
avoid potassium loss, take this drug with a glass of fresh or frozen orange
juice. You may also eat a banana each day. The use of a salt substitute helps
prevent potassium loss. • This drug may cause drowsiness or depression; to
prevent oversedation, avoid the use of other sedative drugs. If you feel continually tired or depressed, consult your doctor. • While taking this product (as
with many drugs that lower blood pressure), you should limit your consumption of alcoholic beverages in order to prevent dizziness or light-headedness.
To avoid dizziness or light-headedness when you stand, contract and relax
the muscles of your legs for a few moments before rising. Do this by pushing
one foot against the floor while raising the other foot slightly, alternating feet

so that you are "pumping" your legs in a pedaling motion. • Persons taking this product and digitalis should watch carefully for symptoms of increased toxicity (e.g., nausea, blurred vision, palpitations). • While taking this drug, do not take any nonprescription item for cough, cold, or sinus problems without first checking with your doctor. • Products equivalent to this drug are available and vary widely in cost. Ask your doctor to prescribe a generic preparation; then ask your pharmacist to fill it with the least expensive brand. • Reserpine causes cancer in rats. It has not been shown to cause cancer in people.• This drug affects driving or operating machinery.• Salutensin-Demi diuretic and antihypertensive is identical to this product, except that it has 25 mg hydroflumethiazide instead of 50 mg. The reserpine content is the same. • If you are allergic to a sulfa drug, you may likewise be allergic to this drug.

Sandril antihypertensive (Eli Lilly and Company), see reserpine antihypertensive.

Scrip-Dyne Compound analgesic (Scrip-Physician Supply Co.), see Darvon Compound-65 analgesic.

Seconal Sodium hypnotic (Eli Lilly and Company), see Nembutal Sodium hypnotic.

Sedabamate sedative and hypnotic (Mallard Incorporated), see meprobamate sedative and hypnotic.

Sedralex sedative and anticholinergic (Kay Pharmacal Co., Inc.), see Donnatal sedative and anticholinergic.

OTC Selsun Blue dandruff remedy

Manufacturer: Abbott Laboratories
Ingredients: selenium sulfide; surfactants
Dosage Form: Shampoo or lotion: selenium sulfide, 1%; surfactants
Use: Control of dandruff
Side Effects: Burning of the skin; discoloration of hair; dryness or oiliness of hair or scalp; eye irritation
Warnings: Do not use this product if the skin is broken.
Comments: Although this shampoo has not been reported to cause serious toxicity, if you swallow any, call your doctor or pharmacist immediately. • Selsun dandruff remedy (Abbott Laboratories) is a stronger product available on prescription only. • Leave the shampoo on the scalp for a few minutes before rinsing.

Rx Selsun seborrheic shampoo

Manufacturer: Abbott Laboratories
Ingredient: selenium sulfide
Equivalent Products: Exsel, Herbert Laboratories; Iosel 250, Owen Drug Company
Dosage Form: Shampoo: selenium sulfide, 2.5%
Use: Treatment of dandruff or dermatitis of the scalp
Minor Side Effects: Discoloration or increased loss of hair (rare), dryness or oiliness of hair and scalp
Contraindications: This product should not be used by people who are allergic to it. • This product should not be used for infants. • This product should not be used by people who have a scalp inflammation. Consult your doctor immediately if this drug has been prescribed for you and you fit into any of these categories.

Warnings: Be careful to keep the shampoo out of your eyes to avoid eye irritation. • Discontinue use of this product if it causes your scalp or surrounding skin to become irritated. • To avoid or minimize hair discoloration or loss, be sure to rinse the shampoo out thoroughly after use; this is especially important if your hair is bleached, colored, or has a permanent wave. • Although there have been no reports of serious toxicity if this drug is swallowed, call your doctor or pharmacist immediately if this occurs.

Comments: After shampooing with this product, wash your hair and scalp again, using a regular shampoo. Otherwise, a disagreeable odor may persist on the scalp. • Selsun Blue (Abbott Laboratories) and Sul-Blue (Columbia Medical Co.) seborrheic shampoos are weaker formulations of this drug; they can be purchased without a prescription.

OTC   Semicid contraceptive

Manufacturer: Whitehall Laboratories
Ingredient: nonoxynol-9
Dosage Form: Vaginal suppository: nonoxynol-9, 100 mg
Use: Prevention of pregnancy
Side Effects: Local irritation to user or partner
Contraindications: This product should not be used if either partner has an allergy to nonoxynol.

Warnings: If you or your partner experiences irritation from using this product, discontinue its use and switch to another brand or method of contraception.

Comments: Be sure to insert a new dose of contraceptive each time intercourse is repeated. • Do not douche for six to eight hours after intercourse. • Used alone, this product is not as effective as when it is combined with a diaphragm.

OTC   Senokot laxative

Manufacturer: The Purdue Frederick Company
Ingredients: senna concentrate; senna concentrate extract
Dosage Forms: Granules (content per teaspoon): senna concentrate, 326 mg. Liquid (content per 5 ml, or one teaspoon): senna concentrate extract, 218 mg. Suppository: senna concentrate, 652 mg. Tablet: senna concentrate, 187 mg
Use: Relief of chronic or occasional constipation
Side Effects: Excess loss of fluid; griping (cramps); mucus in feces
Contraindications: Persons with high fever (100° F or more); black or tarry stools; nausea; vomiting; abdominal pain; or children under age three should not use this product unless directed to do so by a doctor. • Do not use this product when constipation is caused by megacolon or other diseases of the intestine, or hypothyroidism.

Warnings: Excessive use (daily for a month or more) of this product may cause diarrhea, vomiting, and loss of certain blood electrolytes.

Comments: This product may discolor the urine. • Evacuation may occur within six to twelve hours. Never self-medicate with this product if constipation lasts longer than two weeks or if the medication does not produce a laxative effect within a week. • Limit use to seven consecutive days unless directed otherwise by a doctor; this product may cause laxative-dependence (addiction) if used for a longer time.

Septra antibacterial (Burroughs Wellcome Co.), see Bactrim antibacterial.

560

Ser-Ap-Es diuretic and antihypertensive

Rx

Manufacturer: CIBA Pharmaceutical Company
Ingredients: hydralazine hydrochloride; hydrochlorothiazide; reserpine
Equivalent Products: Thia-Serpa-Line, Robinson Laboratory, Inc.; Tri-Hydroserpine, Rugby Laboratories; Unipres, Reid-Provident Laboratories, Inc.
Dosage Form: Tablet: hydralazine hydrochloride, 25 mg; hydrochlorothiazide, 15 mg; reserpine, 0.1 mg (salmon pink)
Use: Treatment of high blood pressure
Minor Side Effects: Abdominal pains; constipation; diarrhea; dizziness; headache; loss of appetite; nasal congestion; nausea; palpitations; tingling in fingers or toes; vomiting
Major Side Effects: Blurred vision; depression; drowsiness; joint tenderness; muscle spasms; rash; sedation; weakness
Contraindications: This drug should not be taken by people who are allergic to any of its components or to sulfa drugs. • The drug should not be taken by those who have active peptic ulcer, ulcerative colitis, heart disease, anuria (inability to urinate), mental depression or suicidal tendencies; and by people receiving electroshock therapy. Consult your doctor immediately if this drug has been prescribed for you and you have any of these conditions.
Warnings: This drug should be used cautiously by pregnant women and by people who are taking monoamine oxidase inhibitors (ask your pharmacist if you are unsure), or who have asthma or allergies, kidney or liver disease, diabetes, blood disease, or a history of ulcers, gallstones, colitis, or heart disease. Be sure your doctor knows if you have any of these conditions. • Nursing women who must take this drug should stop nursing. • This drug interacts with amphetamine, colestipol hydrochloride, decongestants, digitalis, levodopa, lithium carbonate, monoamine oxidase inhibitors, oral antidiabetics, and steroids; if you are currently taking any drugs of these types, consult your doctor about their use. If you are unsure of the type or contents of your medications, ask your doctor or pharmacist. • This drug may affect the potency of, or the patient's need for, other blood pressure drugs and antidiabetics; dosage adjustment may be necessary. • This drug must be used cautiously with digitalis and quinidine; be sure your doctor knows if you are taking either of these drugs. Watch for symptoms of increased toxicity (e.g., nausea, blurred vision, palpitations) and notify your doctor immediately if they occur. • Notify your doctor if this drug makes you feel unusually depressed. • While taking this drug, do not take any nonprescription item for cough, cold, or sinus problems without first checking with your doctor. • This drug may cause drowsiness, dizziness, or light-headedness; avoid tasks that require alertness. To prevent oversedation, avoid the use of alcohol or other drugs that have sedative properties. • To help avoid potassium loss while using this product, take your dose with a glass of fresh or frozen orange juice and eat a banana each day. The use of a salt substitute also helps prevent potassium loss. • This drug may influence the results of thyroid function tests; if you are scheduled to have such a test, remind your doctor that you are taking this drug. • This drug may cause gout, high blood levels of calcium, lupus, nerve damage, blood diseases, or the onset of diabetes that has been latent. Contact your doctor if any unexplained symptoms of generalized tiredness, weakness, fever, aching joints, or chest pain (angina) occur. Periodic blood tests are advisable while you are on this drug. • One of the components of this product, reserpine, causes cancer in rats. It has not been shown to cause cancer in people.
Comments: This product combines three antihypertensive ingredients in a single tablet. A doctor probably should not prescribe this or other "fixed dose" combination products as the first choice in the treatment of high blood pressure. The patient should receive each of the ingredients individually. If

response is adequate to the fixed doses contained in this product, it may then be substituted. The advantage of a combination product such as this one is based on increased convenience to the patient. • Take your dose with food or milk. • The effects of therapy with this drug may not be apparent for at least two weeks. • Mild side effects (e.g., nasal congestion or headache) are most noticeable during the first two weeks of drug therapy and become less bothersome after this period. • This drug causes frequent urination. Expect this effect; it should not alarm you. • If you experience numbness or tingling in your fingers or toes while using this drug, your doctor may recommend that you take vitamin B6 (pyridoxine) to relieve the symptoms. To avoid dizziness or light-headedness when you stand, contract and relax the muscles of your legs for a few moments before rising. Do this by pushing one foot against the floor while raising the other foot slightly, alternating feet so that you are "pumping" your legs in a pedaling motion.

R_X   **Serax sedative and hypnotic**

Manufacturer: Wyeth Laboratories
Ingredient: oxazepam
Dosage Forms: Capsule: 10 mg (pink/white); 15 mg (red/white); 30 mg (maroon/white). Tablet: 15 mg (yellow)
Use: Relief of anxiety, nervousness, tension; relief of muscle spasms; withdrawal from alcohol addiction
Minor Side Effects: Confusion; constipation; depression; difficult urination; dizziness; drowsiness; dry mouth; fatigue; headache; nausea; rash; slurred speech; uncoordinated movements
Major Side Effects: Blurred vision; decreased sexual drive; double vision; jaundice; low blood pressure; stimulation; tremors
Contraindications: This drug should not be used by persons allergic to it. Consult your doctor immediately if this drug has been prescribed for you and you have such an allergy. • This drug should not be used to treat persons with psychoses.
Warnings: This drug should be used with caution in pregnancy during the first trimester, since there may be an increased risk of congenital malformations associated with its use. Patients who become pregnant during drug therapy or intend to become pregnant should consult with their doctor about the desirability of discontinuing this drug. • This drug should be used with caution in patients in whom a drop in blood pressure might lead to heart problems; particularly so in the elderly patient. • Withdrawal symptoms have been noted on discontinuance of drug administration in some patients exhibiting drug dependency through chronic overdose with this drug. Dosage of this drug should be reduced gradually rather than abruptly stopped. Withdrawal symptoms following abrupt stoppage are similar to those seen with barbiturates. • Excessive and prolonged use in susceptible persons, for example, alcoholics, former drug addicts, and others, may result in dependence or habituation to this drug. • Persons taking this drug should not drive a motor vehicle or operate dangerous machinery. • Persons taking this drug should avoid taking alcoholic beverages, since their tolerance to alcohol may be lowered. • This drug is not recommended for children under six years of age and should be used with caution in children between six and twelve years of age. • Persons taking this drug should have periodic liver function and blood count tests. • This drug should not be taken with other sedatives, alcohol, or central nervous system depressants. If you are currently taking any drugs of these types, consult your doctor about their use. If you are unsure of the type or contents of your medications, ask your doctor or pharmacist. • This drug taken alone is a safe drug; when it is combined with other sedative drugs or alcohol, serious adverse reactions may develop. • This drug has the potential

for abuse and must be used with caution. Tolerance may develop quickly; do not increase the dose of this drug without first consulting your doctor.

Comments: This drug currently is used by many people to relieve nervousness. It is effective for this purpose, but it is important to try to remove the cause of the anxiety as well. Phenobarbital is also effective for this purpose, and it is less expensive. Consult your doctor. • This drug may cause dryness of the mouth. To reduce this feeling, chew gum or suck on ice chips or a piece of hard candy.

Sereen sedative and hypnotic (Foy Laboratories, Inc.), see **Librium** sedative and hypnotic.

Serpalan antihypertensive (The Lannett Company, Inc.), see **reserpine** antihypertensive.

Serpasil antihypertensive (CIBA Pharmaceutical Company), see **reserpine** antihypertensive.

Serpate antihypertensive (The Vale Chemical Co., Inc.), see **reserpine** antihypertensive.

OTC   Serutan laxative

Manufacturer: The J. B. Williams Company, Inc.

Ingredient: vegetable hemicellulose derived from Plantago Ovata

Dosage Forms: Granules: vegetable hemicellulose derived from Plantago Ovata, 45%. Powder: vegetable hemicellulose derived from Plantago Ovata, 39%

Use: Relief of constipation

Contraindications: Persons with high fever (100° F or more); black or tarry stools; nausea; vomiting; abdominal pain; intestinal ulcers; difficulty in swallowing; or children under age three should not use this product unless directed by a doctor. • Do not use this product when constipation is caused by megacolon or other diseases of the intestine, or hypothyroidism.

Warnings: Excessive use (daily for a month or more) of this product may cause diarrhea, vomiting, and loss of certain blood electrolytes. • Pregnant women should not use this product except on the advice of their doctor.

Comments: Evacuation may not occur for 12 to 72 hours. Never self-medicate with this product if constipation lasts longer than two weeks or if the medication does not produce a laxative effect within a week. • This product must be mixed in water or juice before taking; a glass (eight ounces) of water should be drunk immediately afterwards. • If you are taking other drugs do not take this product until you have checked with your doctor or pharmacist. • Limit use to seven days unless directed otherwise by your doctor; this product may cause laxative-dependence (addiction) if used for a longer time.

Setamine sedative and anticholinergic (Tutag Pharmaceuticals, Inc.), see **Donnatal** sedative and anticholinergic.

Sherafed adrenergic and antihistamine (Sheraton Laboratories, Inc.), see **Actifed** adrenergic and antihistamine.

Sherafed-C expectorant (Sheraton Laboratories, Inc.), see **Actifed-C** expectorant.

Silain antiflatulent (A. H. Robins Company), see **Mylicon** antiflatulent.

OTC   Silence is Golden cough remedy

Manufacturer: Bristol-Myers Products

Ingredients: dextromethorphan hydrobromide; honey flavor

Dosage Form: Liquid (content per 5 ml, or one teaspoon): dextromethorphan hydrobromide, 10 mg; honey flavor

Use: Temporary relief of coughs due to colds or minor throat and bronchial irritations

Side Effects: Drowsiness; nausea; vomiting

Warnings: This product interacts with monoamine oxidase inhibitors. If you are currently taking any drugs of this type, check with your doctor before taking this product. If you are unsure of the type or contents of your medications, ask your doctor or pharmacist.

Comments: Do not use this product to treat chronic coughs, such as from smoking or asthma. • Do not use this product to treat productive (hacking) coughs that produce phlegm.

OTC   Sinarest cold and allergy remedy

Manufacturer: Pharmacraft Division

Ingredients: acetaminophen; chlorpheniramine maleate; phenylpropanolamine hydrochloride

Dosage Forms: Tablet: acetaminophen, 325 mg; chlorpheniramine maleate, 2 mg; phenylpropanolamine hydrochloride, 18.7 mg. Extra-strength tablet: acetaminophen, 500 mg; chlorpheniramine maleate, 2 mg; phenylpropanolamine hydrochloride, 18.7 mg

Use: Temporary relief of nasal congestion, fever, aches, pains, and general discomfort due to colds and upper respiratory allergies

Side Effects: Anxiety; blurred vision; chest pain; confusion; constipation; difficult and painful urination; dizziness; drowsiness; headache; increased blood pressure; insomnia; loss of appetite; nausea; nervousness; palpitations; rash; reduced sweating; tension; tremor; vomiting

Contraindications: This product should not be used by persons who have severe heart disease or severe high blood pressure. • This product should not be given to newborn or premature infants.

Warnings: This product should be used with special caution by the elderly or debilitated, and by persons who have asthma, diabetes, enlarged prostate, glaucoma (certain types), heart disease, high blood pressure, kidney disease, obstructed bladder, obstructed intestine, peptic ulcer, or thyroid disease. If you have any of these conditions, consult your doctor before taking this product. • This product may cause drowsiness. Do not take it if you must drive, operate heavy machinery, or perform other tasks requiring mental alertness. To prevent oversedation, avoid the use of alcohol or other drugs that have sedative properties. • This product interacts with alcohol, guanethidine, monoamine oxidase inhibitors, sedative drugs, and tricyclic antidepressants. If you are currently taking any drugs of these types, check with your doctor before taking this product. If you are unsure of the type or contents of your medications, ask your doctor or pharmacist. • Because this product reduces sweating, avoid excessive work or exercise in hot weather. • When taken in overdose, acetaminophen is more toxic than aspirin. Follow dosage instructions carefully.

Comments: Many other conditions (some serious) mimic the common cold. If symptoms persist beyond one week or if they occur regularly without regard to season, consult your doctor. • The effectiveness of this product may diminish after being taken regularly for seven to ten days; consult your pharmacist about substituting another product containing a different antihistamine if this product begins to lose its effectiveness for you. • Chew gum

564

or suck on ice chips or a piece of hard candy to reduce mouth dryness.

OTC   Sine-Aid analgesic

Manufacturer: McNeil Consumer Products Company
Ingredients: acetaminophen; phenylpropanolamine hydrochloride
Dosage Form: Tablet: acetaminophen, 325 mg; phenylpropanolamine hydrochloride, 25 mg
Use: Relief of sinus headache pain and pressure caused by sinusitis
Side Effects: Mild to moderate stimulation; nausea; vomiting
Warnings: Persons with high blood pressure, heart disease, diabetes, or thyroid disease should be extremely careful about using this product. If you have any of these conditions, consult your doctor or pharmacist before using this medication. • Do not use this product if you are currently taking antihypertensives and/or monoamine oxidase inhibitors; if you are unsure of the type or contents of your medications, ask your doctor or pharmacist. • When taken in overdose, this product is more toxic than aspirin. The dosage instructions listed on the package should be followed carefully; toxicity may occur in adults or children with repeated doses.

Rx   Sinemet antiparkinson drug

Manufacturer: Merck Sharp & Dohme
Ingredients: carbidopa; levodopa
Dosage Form: Tablet: carbidopa, 10 mg; levodopa, 100 mg (dark, dapple-blue); carbidopa, 25 mg; levodopa, 100 mg (yellow); carbidopa, 25 mg; levodopa, 250 mg (aqua)
Use: Treatment of symptoms of Parkinson's disease
Minor Side Effects: Abdominal pain; agitation; bitter taste in the mouth; confusion; constipation; diarrhea; difficult urination; dizziness; dry mouth; excessive salivation; faintness; headache; hiccups; insomnia; loss of appetite; nausea; numbness; vomiting; weakness
Major Side Effects: Blood clots; blood disorders; convulsions; double vision; euphoria; gastrointestinal bleeding; grinding of teeth; high blood pressure; involuntary movements; irregular heartbeats; loss of hair; mental changes; nightmares; palpitations; persistent erection; skin rash; suicidal tendencies; weight gain or loss
Contraindications: Monoamine oxidase inhibitors and this drug should not be taken together. These inhibitors must be discontinued at least two weeks prior to starting therapy with this drug. Be sure your doctor knows about all the medications you take. • This drug should not be taken by people with narrow-angle glaucoma or hypersensitivity to either of the drug's ingredients. This drug should not be taken by people with certain cancers or skin diseases. Consult your doctor immediately if this drug has been prescribed for you and you fit into any of these categories.
Warnings: This drug should be used with caution by people with heart, lung, kidney, liver, or glandular diseases or ulcers. Be sure your doctor knows if you have any of these conditions. • Pregnant women, nursing mothers, and children should use this drug with caution. • People taking this drug should be observed for signs of depression or suicidal tendencies or abnormal movements. People with past or current psychoses should use this drug cautiously. • Periodic evaluations of the hepatic, hematopoietic, cardiovascular, and renal functions are recommended during extended therapy with this drug. • This drug should be taken with caution in people on antihypertensive drugs. When this drug is started, dosage adjustment of the antihypertensive drug may be required. • This drug interacts with hypoglycemics, monoamine oxidase inhibitors, antipsychotics, phenytoin, papaverine, adrenergics, and

antidepressants. If you are currently taking any drugs of these types, consult your doctor about their use. If you are unsure about the type or contents of your medications, ask your doctor or pharmacist.

Comments: When administered to patients currently taking levodopa (L-dopa), the levodopa must be discontinued at least eight hours before therapy with Sinemet is begun. Persons taking levodopa products are told to avoid taking vitamin B6 (pyridoxine) products, and to avoid eating foods rich in this vitamin. This precaution is not necessary with Sinemet antiparkinson drug. This drug causes beneficial effects in Parkinson's disease similar to levodopa. Because of its ingredient, carbidopa, lower doses of levodopa contained in the tablet give better results than if the levodopa were taken alone. • If dizziness or light-headedness occurs when you stand up, contract and relax the muscles of your legs for a few moments before rising. Do this by pushing one foot against the floor while raising the other foot slightly, alternating feet so that you are "pumping" your legs in a pedaling motion.

OTC   Sine-Off cold and allergy remedy

Manufacturer: Menley & James Laboratories

Ingredients: chlorpheniramine maleate; phenylpropanolamine hydrochloride; aspirin

Dosage Form: Tablet: chlorpheniramine maleate, 2 mg; phenylpropanolamine hydrochloride, 18.75 mg; aspirin, 325 mg (5 grains)

Use: Temporary relief of nasal congestion, fever, aches, pains, and general discomfort due to colds or upper respiratory allergies

Side Effects: Anxiety; blurred vision; chest pain; confusion; constipation; difficult and painful urination; dizziness; drowsiness; headache; increased blood pressure; insomnia; loss of appetite; nausea; nervousness; palpitations; rash; reduced sweating; ringing in the ears; slight blood loss; tension; tremor; vomiting

Contraindications: This product should not be used by persons who have aspirin sensitivity, asthma, blood-clotting disease, gout, severe heart disease, severe high blood pressure, significant drug or food allergies, or vitamin-K deficiency. This product should not be given to newborn or premature infants.

Warnings: This product should be used with special caution by the elderly or debilitated, and by persons who have diabetes, enlarged prostate, glaucoma (certain types), heart disease, high blood pressure, kidney disease, obstructed bladder, obstructed intestine, peptic ulcer, or thyroid disease. If you have any of these conditions, consult your doctor before taking this product. • This product may cause drowsiness. Do not take it if you must drive, operate heavy machinery, or perform other tasks requiring mental alertness. To prevent oversedation, avoid the use of alcohol or other drugs that have sedative properties. • This product interacts with alcohol, ammonium chloride, guanethidine, methotrexate, monoamine oxidase inhibitors, oral anticoagulants, oral antidiabetics, probenecid, sedative drugs, steroids, sulfinpyrazone, tricyclic antidepressants, and vitamin C. If you are currently taking any drugs of these types, check with your doctor before taking this product. If you are unsure of the type or contents of your medications, ask your doctor or pharmacist. • Because this product reduces sweating, avoid excessive work or exercise in hot weather.

Comments: Many other conditions (some serious) mimic the common cold. If symptoms persist beyond one week or if they occur regularly without regard to season, consult your doctor. • The effectiveness of this product may diminish after being taken regularly for seven to ten days; consult your pharmacist about substituting another product containing a different antihistamine if this product begins to lose its effectiveness for you. • Chew gum or suck on ice chips or a piece of hard candy to reduce mouth dryness.

OTC   Sine-Off Once-A-Day nasal decongestant

Manufacturer: Menley & James Laboratories
Ingredients: xylometazoline hydrochloride; thimerosal; menthol; eucalyptol; camphor; methyl salicylate
Dosage Form: Nasal spray: xylometazoline hydrochloride, 0.1%; thimerosal, 0.001%; menthol; eucalyptol; camphor; methyl salicylate
Use: Temporary relief of nasal congestion due to colds, sinusitis, hay fever, or other upper respiratory allergies
Side Effects: Blurred vision; burning, dryness of nasal mucosa; increased nasal congestion or discharge; sneezing, and/or stinging; dizziness; drowsiness; headache; insomnia; nervousness; palpitations; slight increase in blood pressure; stimulation
Contraindications: This product should not be used by persons who have glaucoma (certain types).
Warnings: This product should be used with special caution by persons who have diabetes, advanced hardening of the arteries, heart disease, high blood pressure, or thyroid disease. If you have any of these conditions, consult your doctor before taking this product. • This product interacts with monoamine oxidase inhibitors, thyroid preparations, and tricyclic antidepressants. If you are currently taking any drugs of these types, check with your doctor before taking this product. If you are unsure of the type or contents of your medications, ask your doctor or pharmacist. • To avoid side effects such as burning, sneezing, or stinging, and a "rebound" increase in nasal congestion and discharge, do not exceed the recommended dosage and do not use this product for more than three or four continuous days. • This product should not be used by more than one person; sharing the dispenser may spread infection.
Comments: This product has a duration of action of approximately 12 hours. Because it needs to be administered only twice per day (morning and at bedtime), this product is less likely to cause "rebound" congestion than nasal products containing different ingredients.

Rx   Sinequan antidepressant

Manufacturer: Pfizer Laboratories Division
Ingredient: doxepin hydrochloride
Equivalent Product: Adapin, Pennwalt Prescription Products
Dosage Forms: Capsule: 10 mg (red/pink); 25 mg (blue/pink); 50 mg (light pink/pink); 75 mg (light brown); 100 mg (blue/light pink); 150 mg (blue). Oral concentrate liquid (content per 1 ml): 10 mg
Use: Relief of depression and anxiety
Minor Side Effects: Diarrhea; difficult urination; dizziness; drowsiness; fatigue; hair loss; headache; loss of appetite; nausea; numbness in fingers or toes; palpitations; photosensitivity; rash; uncoordinated movements; vomiting; weakness
Major Side Effects: Enlarged or painful breasts (in both sexes); fatigue; imbalance; heart attack; high or low blood pressure; impotence; jaundice; mild stomach upset; mouth sores; nervousness; ringing in the ears; sleep disorders; sore throat; stroke; tremors; weight gain
Contraindications: This drug should not be used by people who are allergic to it. Consult your doctor immediately if this drug has been prescribed for you and you have such an allergy. • This drug should not be used in persons with glaucoma or with a tendency to urinary retention, particularly in older patients. Be sure your doctor knows if you have such conditions.
Warnings: The dosage of this drug should be carefully adjusted in patients

with intercurrent illness or patients taking other medications. • The dosage of this drug for elderly patients should be carefully adjusted based on the patient's condition. • This drug should be used cautiously in pregnant women, nursing mothers, and children under 12. • Serious side effects have been reported when this drug has been used in conjunction with monoamine oxidase inhibitors or alcohol, as well as with amphetamine, barbiturates, epinephrine, guanethidine, oral anticoagulants, phenylephrine, clonidine, or central nervous system depressants. If you are currently taking any drugs of these types, consult your doctor about their use. If you are unsure of the type or contents of your medications, ask your doctor or pharmacist. • This drug may cause drowsiness; avoid tasks requiring alertness. • During the early course of therapy, patients should be carefully observed for any suicidal tendencies; prescriptions should be written for the smallest feasible amounts. Should increased symptoms of psychosis or shift to manic symptoms occur while taking this drug, it may be necessary to reduce the dosage or add a major tranquilizer to the dosage regime.

Comments: The effects of this drug may not be apparent for at least two weeks. • While taking this drug, do not take any nonprescription item for cough, cold, or sinus problems without first checking with your doctor. • Do not stop or start any other drug. • This drug interacts with sedative drugs or alcohol. Avoid using them while taking Sinequan antidepressant. • This drug may cause dryness of the mouth. To reduce this feeling, chew gum or suck on ice chips or a piece of hard candy. • This drug reduces sweating; avoid excessive work or exercise in hot weather. • Products equivalent to this drug are available and vary widely in cost. Ask your doctor to prescribe a generic preparation; then ask your pharmacist to fill it with the least expensive brand. • Avoid long sun exposure while taking this drug. Immediately before taking the oral concentrate liquid, it should be diluted in about a half-glassful of water, juice or milk. Do not mix your dosage until just before you take it. • Call your doctor if eye pain, sore throat, fever, or unusual bruising or bleeding occur.

OTC   **Sinex Long-Acting nasal decongestant**

Manufacturer: Vicks Health Care Division
Ingredients: xylometazoline hydrochloride; thimerosal
Dosage Form: Nasal spray: xylometazoline hydrochloride, 0.1%; thimerosal, 0.001%
Use: Temporary relief of nasal congestion due to colds, sinusitis, hay fever, or other upper respiratory allergies
Side Effects: Blurred vision; burning, dryness of nasal mucosa, increased nasal congestion or discharge, sneezing, and/or stinging; dizziness; drowsiness; headache; insomnia; nervousness; palpitations; slight increase in blood pressure; stimulation
Contraindications: This product should not be used by persons who have glaucoma (certain types).
Warnings: This product should be used with special caution by persons who have diabetes, advanced hardening of the arteries, heart disease, high blood pressure, or thyroid disease. If you have any of these conditions, consult your doctor before taking this product. • This product interacts with monoamine oxidase inhibitors, thyroid preparations, and tricyclic antidepressants. If you are currently taking any drugs of these types, check with your doctor before taking this product. If you are unsure of the type or contents of your medications, ask your doctor or pharmacist. • To avoid side effects such as burning, sneezing, or stinging, and a "rebound" increase in nasal congestion and discharge, do not exceed the recommended dosage and do not use this product for more than three or four continuous days. •

This product should not be used by more than one person; sharing the dispenser may spread infection.

Comments: This product has a duration of action of approximately 12 hours. Because it needs to be administered only twice per day, this product is less likely to cause "rebound" congestion than nasal products containing different ingredients.

OTC   **Sinex nasal decongestant**

Manufacturer: Vicks Health Care Division
Ingredients: phenylephrine hydrochloride; cetylpyridinium chloride; thimerosal; menthol; eucalyptol; camphor; methyl salicylate
Dosage Form: Nasal spray: phenylephrine hydrochloride, 0.5%; cetylpyridinium chloride, 0.04%; thimerosal, 0.001%; menthol; eucalyptol; camphor; methyl salicylate
Use: Temporary relief of nasal congestion due to colds, sinusitis, hay fever, or other upper respiratory allergies
Side Effects: Blurred vision; burning, dryness of nasal mucosa; increased nasal congestion or discharge; sneezing, and/or stinging; dizziness; drowsiness; headache; insomnia; nervousness; palpitations; slight increase in blood pressure; stimulation
Contraindications: This product should not be used by persons who have glaucoma (certain types).
Warnings: This product should be used with special caution by persons who have diabetes, advanced hardening of the arteries, heart disease, high blood pressure, or thyroid disease. If you have any of these conditions, consult your doctor before taking this product. • This product interacts with guanethidine, monoamine oxidase inhibitors, and thyroid preparations. If you are currently taking any drugs of these types, check with your doctor before taking this product. If you are unsure of the type or contents of your medications, ask your doctor or pharmacist. • To avoid side effects such as burning, sneezing, or stinging, and a "rebound" increase in nasal congestion and discharge, do not exceed the recommended dosage and do not use this product for more than three or four continuous days. • This product should not be used by more than one person; sharing the dispenser may spread infection.

OTC   **Sinutab cold and allergy remedy**

Manufacturer: Warner-Lambert Company
Ingredients: acetaminophen; phenylpropanolamine hydrochloride; phenyltoloxamine citrate
Dosage Form: Tablet: acetaminophen, 325 mg; phenylpropanolamine hydrochloride, 25 mg; phenyltoloxamine citrate, 22 mg
Use: Temporary relief of nasal congestion, fever, aches, pains, and general discomfort due to colds or upper respiratory allergies
Side Effects: Anxiety; blurred vision; chest pain; confusion; constipation; difficult and painful urination; dizziness; drowsiness; headache; increased blood pressure; insomnia; loss of appetite; nausea; nervousness; palpitations; rash; reduced sweating; tension; tremor; vomiting
Contraindications: This product should not be used by persons who have severe heart disease or severe high blood pressure. • This product should not be given to newborn or premature infants.
Warnings: This product should be used with special caution by the elderly or debilitated, and by persons who have asthma, diabetes, enlarged prostate, glaucoma (certain types), heart disease, high blood pressure, kidney disease, obstructed bladder, obstructed intestine, peptic ulcer, or thyroid disease. If you have any of these conditions, consult your doctor before taking this prod-

569

uct. • This product may cause drowsiness. Do not take it if you must drive, operate heavy machinery, or perform other tasks requiring mental alertness. To prevent oversedation, avoid the use of alcohol or other drugs that have sedative properties. • This product interacts with alcohol, guanethidine, monoamine oxidase inhibitors, sedative drugs, and tricyclic antidepressants. If you are currently taking any drugs of these types, check with your doctor before taking this product. If you are unsure of the type or contents of your medications, ask your doctor or pharmacist. • Because this product reduces sweating, avoid excessive work or exercise in hot weather. • When taken in overdose, acetaminophen is more toxic than aspirin. Follow dosage instructions carefully.

Comments: Many other conditions (some serious) mimic the common cold. If symptoms persist beyond one week or if they occur regularly without regard to season, consult your doctor. • The effectiveness of this product may diminish after being taken regularly for seven to ten days; consult your pharmacist about substituting another product containing a different antihistamine if this product begins to lose its effectiveness for you. • Chew gum or suck on ice chips or a piece of hard candy to reduce mouth dryness.

OTC   Sinutab Long-Lasting nasal decongestant

Manufacturer: Warner-Lambert Company
Ingredients: xylometazoline hydrochloride; benzalkonium chloride
Dosage Form: Nasal spray: xylometazoline hydrochloride, 0.1%; benzalkonium chloride
Use: Temporary relief of nasal congestion due to colds, sinusitis, hay fever, or other upper respiratory allergies
Side Effects: Blurred vision; burning, dryness of nasal mucosa; increased nasal congestion or discharge; sneezing, and/or stinging; dizziness; drowsiness; headache; insomnia; nervousness; palpitations; slight increase in blood pressure; stimulation
Contraindications: This product should not be used by persons who have glaucoma (certain types).   ·
Warnings: This product should be used with special caution by persons who have diabetes, advanced hardening of the arteries, heart disease, high blood pressure, or thyroid disease. If you have any of these conditions, consult your doctor before taking this product. • This product interacts with monoamine oxidase inhibitors, thyroid preparations, and tricyclic antidepressants. If you are currently taking any drugs of these types, check with your doctor before taking this product. If you are unsure of the type or contents of your medications, ask your doctor or pharmacist. • To avoid side effects such as burning, sneezing, or stinging, and a "rebound" increase in nasal congestion and discharge, do not exceed the recommended dosage and do not use this product for more than three or four continuous days. • This product should not be used by more than one person; sharing the dispenser may spread infection.
Comments: This product has a duration of action of approximately ten hours. Because it needs to be administered only twice per day, this product is less likely to cause "rebound" congestion than nasal products containing different ingredients.

OTC   Sinutab-II cold and allergy remedy

Manufacturer: Warner-Lambert Company
Ingredients: acetaminophen; phenylpropanolamine hydrochloride
Dosage Form: Tablet: acetaminophen, 325 mg; phenylpropanolamine hydrochloride, 25 mg

Use: Temporary relief of nasal congestion, fever, aches, pains, and general discomfort due to colds or upper respiratory allergies

Side Effects: Mild to moderate stimulation; nausea; vomiting

Warnings: This product should be used with special caution by persons who have diabetes, heart disease, high blood pressure, or thyroid disease. If you have any of these conditions, consult your doctor before taking this product. • This product interacts with alcohol, guanethidine, monoamine oxidase inhibitors, sedative drugs, and tricyclic antidepressants. If you are currently taking any drugs of these types, check with your doctor before taking this product. If you are unsure of the type or contents of your medications, ask your doctor or pharmacist. • When taken in overdose, acetaminophen is more toxic than aspirin. Follow dosage instructions carefully.

Comments: Many other conditions (some serious) mimic the common cold. If symptoms persist beyond one week or if they occur regularly without regard to season, consult your doctor. •

SK-Ampicillin antibiotic (Smith Kline & French Laboratories), see ampicillin antibiotic.

SK-APAP with Codeine analgesic (Smith Kline & French Laboratories), see Tylenol with Codeine analgesic.

SK-Bamate sedative and hypnotic (Smith Kline & French Laboratories), see meprobamate sedative and hypnotic.

SK-Diphenhydramine antihistamine (Smith Kline & French Laboratories), see Benadryl antihistamine.

SK-Diphenoxylate anticholinergic and antispasmodic (Smith Kline & French Laboratories), see Lomotil anticholinergic and antispasmodic.

SK-Erythromycin, antibiotic (Smith Kline & French Laboratories), see erythromycin antibiotic.

SK-Lygen sedative and hypnotic (Smith, Kline & French Laboratories), see Librium sedative and hypnotic.

SK-Niacin vitamin supplement (Smith Kline & French Laboratories), see nicotinic acid vitamin supplement.

SK-Penicillin G antibiotic (Smith Kline & French Laboratories), see penicillin G antibiotic.

SK-Penicillin VK antibiotic (Smith Kline & French Laboratories), see penicillin potassium phenoxymethyl antibiotic.

SK-Phenobarbital sedative and hypnotic (Smith Kline & French Laboratories), see phenobarbital sedative and hypnotic.

SK-Pramine antidepressant (Smith Kline & French Laboratories), see Tofranil antidepressant.

SK-65 analgesic (Smith Kline & French Laboratories), see Darvon analgesic.

SK-65 Compound analgesic (Smith Kline & French Laboratories), see Darvon Compound-65 analgesic.

SK-Soxazole antibacterial (Smith Kline & French Laboratories), see Gantrisin antibacterial.

SK-Tetracycline antibiotic (Smith Kline & French Laboratories), see tetracycline hydrochloride antibiotic.

SK-Triamcinolone steroid hormone (Smith Kline & French Laboratories), see Aristocort steroid hormone.

OTC **Sleep-Eze sleeping aid**

Manufacturer: Whitehall Laboratories
Ingredient: pyrilamine maleate
Dosage Form: Tablet: pyrilamine maleate, 25 mg
Use: To induce drowsiness and assist in falling asleep
Side Effects: Blurred vision; confusion; constipation; difficult urination; dizziness; drowsiness; dry mouth and respiratory passages; headache; insomnia; low blood pressure; nausea; nervousness; palpitations; rash; restlessness; vomiting. Children may react with primary symptoms of excitement (convulsions; flushed skin; nervousness; tremors; twitching of muscles; uncoordinated movements).
Contraindications: This product should not be given to children under 12 years of age. • Do not take this product if you are pregnant or nursing.
Warnings: This product must be used with extreme caution by persons who have asthma, glaucoma, or enlarged prostate. If you have any of these conditions, do not take this product without first consulting your doctor. • This product may interact with other drugs; if you are currently taking any other prescription or over-the-counter medication, do not take this product without first consulting your doctor or pharmacist. • Tolerance to this drug may develop; do not increase the recommended dosage of this drug unless your doctor directs you to do so. • This drug may cause drowsiness; avoid driving, operating heavy machinery, or performing other tasks requiring mental alertness. To prevent oversedation, avoid the use of alcohol and other sedative drugs.
Comments: Insomnia may be a symptom of a serious illness; consult a doctor if sleeplessness lasts for more than two weeks.

OTC **Slim-Line Candy appetite suppressant**

Manufacturer: Thompson Medical Company, Inc.
Ingredients: benzocaine; citric acid; corn glucose syrup; methylcellulose; natural and artificial flavoring; sugar
Dosage Form: Hard candy: benzocaine, 5 mg; citric acid; corn glucose syrup; methylcellulose, 45 mg; natural and artificial flavoring; sugar
Use: Aid in diet control
Side Effects: Allergic reactions (rash, itching, soreness); diarrhea
Comments: The primary value in products of this nature is in following the caloric reduction plan that goes with it.

Slo-Phyllin expectorant and smooth muscle relaxant (Dooner Laboratories, Inc.), see Quibron expectorant and smooth muscle relaxant.

Slow-K potassium chloride replacement (CIBA Pharmaceutical Company), see potassium chloride replacement.

Sodestrin estrogen hormone (Tutag Pharmaceuticals, Inc.), see Premarin estrogen hormone.

℞   Sodium Sulamyd ophthalmic solution and ointment

Manufacturer: Schering Corporation
Ingredient: sulfacetamide sodium
Dosage Forms: Drop: 10%; 30%. Ointment: 10%
Use: Treatment of conjunctivitis, corneal ulcers, and certain other eye infections caused by microorganisms
Minor Side Effects: Local irritation; transient stinging or burning (usually associated only with 30% drops)
Contraindications: This drug should not be used by people who are allergic to it. Consult your doctor immediately if this drug has been prescribed for you and you have such an allergy.
Warnings: This drug should not be used in conjunction with products containing silver. • The use of the ointment form of this product may retard the healing of the cornea of the eye. • Certain organisms that are not susceptible to this drug, such as fungi, may proliferate during its use. • If any pus is produced during the use of this product, the pus may inactivate the effectiveness of the drug.
Comments: Be careful about the contamination of eyedrops. Wash your hands before administering eyedrops. Do not touch the dropper to the eye. Do not wash or wipe the dropper before replacing it in the bottle. Close the bottle tightly to keep out moisture. • Like other eye products, this drug may cause some clouding or blurring of vision. This symptom will go away quickly.

OTC   Solarcaine burn remedy and antiseptic

Manufacturer: Plough, Inc.
Ingredients: benzocaine; camphor; menthol; triclosan; isopropyl alcohol (spray forms); phenol (pump spray)
Dosage Forms: Cream; Lotion (quantities of ingredients not specified). Spray, aerosol: benzocaine, 9.4%; camphor; isopropyl alcohol, 24%; menthol; triclosan, 0.18%. Spray, pump: benzocaine, 2%; camphor; isopropyl alcohol, 31%; menthol; phenol, 0.3%; triclosan, 0.1%
Use: Temporary relief of sunburn pain; minor burns; cuts; scrapes; poison ivy; nonpoisonous insect bites; detergent hands; chapping
Side Effects: Allergy; local irritation
Warnings: Do not use this product on broken skin. • This product should not be used on large areas of the body because a toxic amount of the medication can be absorbed. • The aerosol spray is flammable; do not spray while smoking or near fire. Avoid inhalation. Keep away from eyes.
Comments: Remember that ointments that are put on serious (second- or third-degree) burns will have to be taken off before definitive treatment can be given. Consult your doctor or pharmacist if you have any questions.

Solfoton sedative and hypnotic (Wm. P. Poythress & Co., Inc.), see phenobarbital sedative and hypnotic.

℞   Soma Compound muscle relaxant and analgesic

Manufacturer: Wallace Laboratories
Ingredients: caffeine, carisoprodol, phenacetin
Equivalent Product: Soprodol Compound, Henry Schein, Inc.
Dosage Form: Tablet: caffeine, 32 mg; carisoprodol, 200 mg; phenacetin, 160 mg (orange)

Use: Relief of pain in muscles and joints

Minor Side Effects: Diarrhea; dizziness; drowsiness; fatigue; light-headedness; nausea; rash; ringing in the ears; vomiting

Major Side Effects: Fainting; flushing; kidney disease; palpitations; rapid heartbeat

Contraindications: This drug should not be taken by people with acute intermittent porphyria or allergy to any of its components. Consult your doctor immediately if this drug has been prescribed for you and you have such a condition or such an allergy.

Warnings: This product, if taken in large doses for long periods in combination with other analgesics, is associated with severe kidney disease. On rare occasions, the first dose of this drug has been followed by idiosyncratic symptoms appearing within minutes or hours. Symptoms usually subside over the next several hours, though hospitalization may be necessary. • This drug should be used with caution in pregnant women, nursing mothers, and children. • This drug is not recommended for use in children under age five. • This drug may cause drowsiness; avoid tasks requiring alertness, such as driving a motor vehicle or operating machinery. • Extreme caution should be exercised when taking this drug along with other central nervous system depressants, including alcohol. If you are currently taking any drugs of these types, consult your doctor about their use. If you are unsure of the type or contents of your medications, ask your doctor or pharmacist. • Restlessness and excitement may occur when this drug is abruptly withdrawn. • Psychological dependence to the caffeine in this drug has been reported. • This drug should be used with caution in addiction-prone persons and in persons with anemia, heart disease, lung disease, liver disease, or kidney disease. Be sure your doctor knows if you have any of these conditions.

Comments: This drug may cause drowsiness; to prevent oversedation, avoid the use of other sedative drugs or alcohol. • This drug is not a substitute for rest, physical therapy, or other measures recommended by your doctor to treat your condition. • This drug has the potential for abuse and must be used with caution. Tolerance may develop quickly; do not increase the dose of the drug without first consulting your doctor. • Products equivalent to this drug are available and vary widely in cost. Ask your doctor to prescribe a generic preparation; then ask your pharmacist to fill it with the least expensive brand.

OTC   Sominex sleeping aid

Manufacturer: The J. B. Williams Company, Inc.

Ingredient: pyrilamine maleate

Dosage Form: Tablet: pyrilamine maleate, 25 mg

Use: To induce drowsiness and assist in falling asleep

Side Effects: Blurred vision; confusion; constipation; difficult urination; dizziness; drowsiness; dry mouth and respiratory passages; headache; insomnia; low blood pressure; nausea; nervousness; palpitations; rash; restlessness; vomiting. Children may react with primary symptoms of excitement (convulsions; flushed skin; nervousness; tremors; twitching of muscles; uncoordinated movements).

Contraindications: This product should not be given to children under 12 years of age. • Do not take this product if you are pregnant or nursing.

Warnings: This product must be used with extreme caution by persons who have asthma, glaucoma, or enlarged prostate. If you have any of these conditions, do not take this product without first consulting your doctor. • This product may interact with other drugs; if you are currently taking any other prescription or over-the-counter medications, do not take this product without first consulting your doctor or pharmacist. • Tolerance to this drug may develop; do not increase the recommended dosage of this drug unless your doctor directs you to do so. • This drug may cause drowsiness; avoid driving, operating heavy machinery, or performing other tasks requiring mental alertness. To prevent oversedation, avoid the use of alcohol and other sedative drugs.

Comments: Insomnia may be a symptom of a serious illness; consult a doctor if sleeplessness lasts for more than two weeks.

Somophyllin bronchodilator (Fisons Corporation), see aminophylline bronchodilator.

Somophyllin-T bronchodilator (Fisons Corporation), see Elixophyllin bronchodilator.

Sopor sedative and hypnotic (Arnar-Stone Laboratores, Inc.), see Quaalude sedative and hypnotic.

Soprodol Compound muscle relaxant and analgesic (Henry Schein, Inc.), see Soma Compound muscle relaxant and analgesic.

OTC   **Sopronol athlete's foot remedy**

Manufacturer: Wyeth Laboratories
Ingredients: sodium propionate; sodium caprylate; zinc caprylate; zinc propionate
Dosage Forms: Liquid: sodium propionate, 12.3%; sodium caprylate, 10%. Ointment: sodium propionate, 12.3%; sodium caprylate, 10%; zinc caprylate, 5%. Powder: sodium propionate, 5%; sodium caprylate, 10%; zinc propionate, 5%
Use: Treatment of athlete's foot
Side Effects: Allergy; local irritation
Warnings: Do not apply this product to mucous membranes, scraped skin, or to large areas of skin. • If your condition worsens, or if irritation occurs, stop using this product and consult your pharmacist.
Comments: Some lesions take months to heal, so it is important not to stop treatment too soon. • If foot lesions are consistently a problem, check the fit of your shoes. • Wash your hands thoroughly after applying this product. • The liquid and ointment forms of this product are preferable to the powder for effectiveness; the best action of the powder may be in drying the infected area. • When using the liquid form of this product, avoid contaminating the contents of the bottle by pouring some of the liquid into a separate container for each use.

Sorate antianginal (Trimen Laboratories), see Isordil antianginal.

Sorbide antianginal (Mayrand, Inc.), see Isordil antianginal.

Sorbitrate antianginal (Stuart Pharmaceuticals), see Isordil antianginal.

Soy-Dome Cleanser detergent cleanser (Dome Laboratories), see pHisoHex detergent cleanser.

Spalix sedative and anticholinergic (Reid-Provident Laboratories, Inc.), see Donnatal sedative and anticholinergic.

Spasmolin sedative and anticholinergic (Spencer-Mead, Inc.), see Donnatal sedative and anticholinergic.

Spastyl antispasmodic (Vangard Laboratories), see Bentyl antispasmodic.

Spenaxin muscle relaxant (Spencer-Mead, Inc.), see Robaxin muscle relaxant.

Spengine vasodilator (Spencer-Mead, Inc.), see Hydergine vasodilator.

Spentane DC expectorant (Spencer-Mead, Inc.), see Dimetane DC expectorant.

Spentane expectorant (Spencer-Mead, Inc.), see Dimetane expectorant.

℞   Stelazine phenothiazine

Manufacturer: Smith Kline & French Laboratories
Ingredient: trifluoperazine hydrochloride
Dosage Forms: Liquid concentrate (content per ml): trifluoperazine hydrochloride, 10 mg; sodium tartrate, 4.75 mg; sodium biphosphate, 11.6 mg; sodium saccharin, 0.3 mg; benzyl alcohol, 0.75%. Tablet: 1 mg; 2 mg; 5 mg; 10 mg (all blue)
Use: Management of certain psychotic disorders; relief of excessive anxiety or tension
Minor Side Effects: Blurred vision; change in urine color; constipation; diarrhea; drooling; drowsiness; dry mouth; jitteriness; menstrual irregularities; nasal congestion; nausea; rash; restlessness; uncoordinated movements; vomiting
Major Side Effects: Difficulty in swallowing; enlarged or painful breasts (in both sexes); fluid retention; impotence; involuntary movements of the face, mouth, tongue, or jaw; jaundice; muscle stiffness; rise in blood pressure; sore throat; tremors
Contraindications: This drug should not be taken by persons who have drug-induced depression, or have cases of existing blood disease, bone-marrow depression, or liver damage. Consult your doctor immediately if this drug has been prescribed for you and you fit into any of these categories.
Warnings: This drug should be used with caution in patients who have exhibited hypersensitivity to a phenothiazine. Consult your doctor immediately if this drug has been prescribed for you and you have exhibited such hypersensitivity. • This drug may impair mental and/or physical abilities; avoid tasks that require alertness, especially during the first few days of therapy with this drug. • This drug should be used cautiously in pregnant women. • Use of this drug may cause blood disease, jaundice, liver damage, or motor restlessness. • This drug should be used with extreme caution in persons with heart disease. Large doses of this drug should be avoided in patients with impaired cardiovascular systems. • Problems with the retina of the eye could result from using this drug; notify your doctor immediately if you experience visual disturbances. The drug should be discontinued if eye examination indicates such problems. • The antivomiting effects of this drug may mask signs of overdose of toxic drugs or obscure the diagnosis of conditions such as intestinal obstruction and brain tumor. • This drug interacts with other depressant drugs, antacids, alcohol, or anticholinergics. If you are currently taking any drugs of these types, consult your doctor about their use. If you are unsure of the type or contents of your medications, ask your doctor or pharmacist. • There is a possibility of cumulative effects when this drug is taken for extended periods.
Comments: The effects of therapy with this drug may not be apparent for at

least two weeks. • This drug has sustained action; never take it more frequently than your doctor prescribes. A serious overdose may result. • While taking this drug, do not take any nonprescription item for cough, cold, or sinus problems without first checking with your doctor. • This drug may cause dryness of mouth. To reduce this feeling, chew gum or suck on ice chips or a piece of hard candy. • This drug reduces sweating; avoid excessive work or exercise in hot weather. • The liquid concentrate form of this drug should be added to 60 ml (¼ cup) or more of water, milk, juice, coffee, tea, or carbonated beverages; or to pulpy foods (applesauce, etc.) just prior to administration. • To avoid dizziness or light-headedness when you stand, contract and relax the muscles of your legs for a few moments before rising. Do this by pushing one foot against the floor while raising the other foot slighty, alternating feet so that you are "pumping" your legs in a pedaling motion.

Sterapred steroid hormone (Mayrand Incorporated), see prednisone steroid hormone.

OTC   Stresscaps multivitamin

Manufacturer: Lederle Laboratories
Ingredients: thiamine mononitrate (vitamin B₁); riboflavin (vitamin B₂); pyridoxine hydrochloride (vitamin B₆); cyanocobalamin (vitamin B₁₂); ascorbic acid (vitamin C); niacinamide; calcium pantothenate (pantothenic acid)
Dosage Form: Capsule: thiamine mononitrate, 10 mg; riboflavin, 10 mg; pyridoxine hydrochloride, 2 mg; cyanocobalamin, 6 mcg; ascorbic acid, 300 mg; niacinamide, 100 mg; calcium pantothenate, 20 mg
Use: Dietary supplement
Comments: Do not be misled by the name of this product; there is no proof that high doses of B and C vitamins will prevent or relieve stress. • If two or more capsules are taken daily, this product may interfere with the results of urine tests. Inform your doctor and pharmacist you are taking this product.

OTC   Stresstabs 600 multivitamin

Manufacturer: Lederle Laboratories
Ingredients: alpha tocopheryl acetate (vitamin E); ascorbic acid (vitamin C); thiamine mononitrate (vitamin B₁); riboflavin (vitamin B₂); niacinamide; pyridoxine hydrochloride (vitamin B₆); cyanocobalamin (vitamin B₁₂); calcium pantothenate (pantothenic acid)
Dosage Form: Tablet: alpha tocopheryl acetate, 30 IU; ascorbic acid, 600 mg; thiamine mononitrate, 15 mg; riboflavin, 15 mg; niacinamide, 100 mg; pyridoxine hydrochloride, 5 mg; cyanocobalamin, 12 mcg; calcium pantothenate, 20 mg
Use: Dietary supplement
Warnings: This product contains vitamin B₆ in an amount great enough that it may interact with levodopa (L-dopa). If you are currently taking L-dopa, check with your doctor before taking this product.
Comments: Do not be misled by the name of this product; there is no proof that high doses of B and C vitamins will prevent or relieve stress. • This product may interfere with the results of urine tests. Inform your doctor and pharmacist you are taking this product.

OTC   Stri-Dex acne preparation

Manufacturer: Lehn and Fink Products Co.
Ingredients: alcohol; salicylic acid; citric acid, fragrance, simethicone, sodium carbonate and sulfonated alkyl benzenes as vehicle for alcohol
Dosage Form: Medicated pad: alcohol, 28%; salicylic acid, 0.5%; citric

acid, fragrance, simethicone, sodium carbonate and sulfonated alkyl benzenes as vehicle for alcohol
Use: Treatment of acne
Side Effects: Allergy; local irritation
Warnings: Do not get product in or near the eyes.
Comments: If the condition worsens, stop using this product and call your pharmacist.

Sub-Quin antiarrhythmic (Scrip-Physician Supply Co.), see Pronestyl antiarrhythmic.

OTC   Sucrets throat lozenges

Manufacturer: Calgon Consumer Products Company, Inc.
Ingredients: hexylresorcinol
Dosage Form: Lozenge: hexylresorcinol, 2.4 mg
Use: Temporary relief of minor throat irritations
Contraindications: Unless directed otherwise by your doctor, do not give this product to children under three years of age.
Warnings: A sore throat in a child under age six should never be treated without medical supervision. Consult your doctor. • If your sore throat is severe; is accompanied by headache, high fever, nausea, or vomiting; or lasts for more than two days, consult your doctor promptly.
Comments: The antibacterial ingredient included represents an irrational use for this product if it is recommended to treat an infection-induced sore throat. Colds are caused by viruses, and the ingredients in this product are not effective against viral infections. The value of this product lies in its throat-soothing quality.

OTC   Sudafed cold remedy

Manufacturer: Burroughs Wellcome Co.
Ingredients: pseudoephedrine hydrochloride
Dosage Forms: Liquid (content per 5 ml, or one teaspoon); Tablet: 30 mg
Use: Temporary relief of symptoms of colds
Side Effects: Mild to moderate stimulation; nausea; vomiting
Warnings: This product should be used with special caution by persons who have diabetes, heart disease, high blood pressure, or thyroid disease. If you have any of these conditions, consult your doctor before taking this product. • This product interacts with alcohol, guanethidine, monoamine oxidase inhibitors, sedative drugs, and tricyclic antidepressants. If you are currently taking any drugs of these types, check with your doctor before taking this product. If you are unsure of the type or contents of your medications, ask your doctor or pharmacist.
Comments: Many other conditions (some serious) mimic the common cold. If symptoms persist beyond one week or if they occur regularly without regard to season, consult your doctor. • The effectiveness of this product may diminish after being taken regularly for seven to 10 days; consult your pharmacist about substituting another medication if this product begins to lose its effectiveness for you.

OTC   Sudafed Plus cold remedy

Manufacturer: Burroughs Wellcome Co.
Ingredients: pseudoephedrine hydrochloride; chlorpheniramine maleate
Dosage Forms: Liquid (content per 5 ml, or one teaspoon): pseudoephedrine hydrochloride, 30 mg; chlorpheniramine maleate, 2 mg. Tablet: pseudoephedrine hydrochloride, 60 mg; chlorpheniramine maleate, 4 mg

Use: Temporary relief of nasal congestion and other symptoms of colds

Side Effects: Anxiety; blurred vision; chest pain; confusion; constipation; difficult and painful urination; dizziness; drowsiness; headache; increased blood pressure; insomnia; loss of appetite; mild to moderate stimulation; nausea; nervousness; palpitations; rash; sweating; tension; tremor; vomiting

Contraindications: This product should not be used by persons who have severe heart disease or severe high blood pressure. • This product should not be given to newborn or premature infants.

Warnings: This product should be used with special caution by the elderly or debilitated, and by persons who have asthma, diabetes, enlarged prostate, glaucoma (certain types), heart disease, high blood pressure, kidney disease, obstructed bladder, obstructed intestine, peptic ulcer, or thyroid disease. If you have any of these conditions, consult your doctor before taking this product. • This product may cause drowsiness. Do not take it if you must drive, operate heavy machinery, or perform other tasks requiring mental alertness. To prevent oversedation, avoid the use of alcohol or other drugs that have sedative properties. • This product interacts with alcohol, guanethidine, monoamine oxidase inhibitors, sedative drugs, and tricyclic antidepressants. If you are currently taking any drugs of these types, check with your doctor before taking this product. If you are unsure of the type or contents of your medications, ask your doctor or pharmacist. • Because this product reduces sweating, avoid excessive work or exercise in hot weather.

Comments: Many other conditions (some serious) mimic the common cold. If symptoms persist beyond one week or if they occur regularly without regard to season, consult your doctor. • Chew gum or suck on ice chips or a piece of hard candy to reduce mouth dryness.

Sudahist adrenergic and antihistamine (Upsher-Smith Laboratories, Inc.), see Actifed adrenergic and antihistamine.

Suda-Prol adrenergic and antihistamine (Columbia Medical Co.), see Actifed adrenergic and antihistamine.

Sul-Blue seborrheic shampoo (Columbia Medical Co.), see Selsun seborrheic shampoo.

Suldiazo antibacterial and analgesic (Kay Pharmacal Company, Inc.), see Azo Gantrisin antibacterial and analgesic.

Sulfalar antibacterial (Parke-Davis), see Gantrisin antibacterial.

OTC   **Sulforcin acne preparation**

Manufacturer: Texas Pharmacal Company
Ingredients: alcohol; resorcinol; sulfur
Dosage Form: Lotion: alcohol, 11.65%; resorcinol, 2%; sulfur, 5%
Use: Treatment of acne
Side Effects: Allergy; local irritation
Warnings: Do not get product in or near the eyes.
Comments: This preparation may stain the skin. • If the condition worsens, stop using this product and call your pharmacist.

R×   **Sultrin vaginal anti-infective**

Manufacturer: Ortho Pharmaceutical Corporation
Ingredients: sulfabenzamide; sulfacetamide; sulfathiazole; urea
Dosage Forms: Vaginal cream: sulfabenzamide, 3.7%; sulfacetamide, 2.86%; sulfathiazole, 3.42%; urea, 0.64%. Vaginal tablet: sulfabenzamide, 184.0 mg; sulfacetamide, 143.75 mg; sulfathiazole, 172.5 mg; compounded

with urea, lactose, guar gum, starch, and magnesium stearate
Use: Treatment of vaginal infections
Minor Side Effects: Mild vaginal itching and irritation
Contraindications: This drug should not be used by people allergic to sulfa drugs. Consult your doctor immediately if this drug has been prescribed for you and you have such an allergy. • This drug should not be used by people with kidney disease. Be sure your doctor knows if you have such a condition.
Comments: Triple Sulfa vaginal cream (E. Fougera and Co.) contains the same ingredients as this drug, but at different strengths. • This drug should be used until the prescribed amount of medication is gone. • Call your doctor if you develop burning or itching. Refrain from sexual intercourse, or ask your partner to use a condom until treatment is finished, to avoid reinfection.

Sumox antibiotic (Reid-Provident Laboratories, Inc.), see amoxicillin antibiotic.

Sumycin antibiotic (E. R. Squibb & Sons, Inc.), see tetracycline hydrochloride antibiotic.

Supen antibiotic (Reid-Provident Laboratories, Inc.), see ampicillin antibiotic.

OTC　　　　**Super Odrinex appetite suppressant**

Manufacturer: Fox Pharmacal, Inc.
Ingredients: caffeine; phenylpropanolamine hydrochloride
Dosage Form: Tablet: caffeine, 100 mg; phenylpropanolamine hydrochloride, 25 mg
Use: Aid in dietary control
Side Effects: Diarrhea; drowsiness; headache; insomnia; nervousness; increase in blood pressure, blood sugar, heart rate, and thyroid activity; in larger than the recommended dose: irregular heartbeat, upset stomach
Contraindications: Persons with heart disease, high blood pressure, diabetes, or thyroid disease; children under 16 years of age; and pregnant women should not use this product. Consult your doctor.
Warnings: Do not take this product concurrently with cough, cold or allergy medications that contain a decongestant.
Comments: During the first week of taking this product, expect increased frequency of urination. • Many medical authorities believe that the ingredient phenylpropanolamine does not help in weight loss programs. The FDA Review Panel has reported that it is effective. If you want to use this product, remember that you become tolerant to any beneficial effects after a couple of weeks. After each two weeks of use, stop for one week, then resume. • The primary value in products of this nature is in following the caloric reduction plan that goes with it.

OTC　　　　**Surfak laxative**

Manufacturer: Hoechst-Roussel Pharmaceuticals Inc.
Ingredients: docusate calcium (dioctyl calcium sulfosuccinate)
Dosage Form: Capsule: docusate calcium, 50 mg; 240 mg
Use: Relief of constipation and stool softener
Side Effects: Mild, transitory cramping pains; nausea; rash
Contraindications: Persons with high fever (100° F or more); black or tarry stools; nausea; vomiting; abdominal pain; or children under age three should not use this product unless directed by a doctor. • Do not use this product when constipation is caused by megacolon or other diseases of the intestine, or hypothyroidism.

Warnings: Excessive use (daily for a month or more) of this product may cause diarrhea, vomiting, and loss of certain blood electrolytes. • Pregnant women should not use this product except on the advice of a doctor.

Comments: Evacuation may occur within 72 hours. Never self-medicate with this product if constipation lasts longer than two weeks or if the medication does not produce a laxative effect within a week. • This product is referred to as a stool softener. It is recommended for prevention of constipation when the stool is hard and dry. Do not take another product containing mineral oil at the same time as you are taking this product. • Limit use to seven days unless directed otherwise by your doctor; this product may cause laxative-dependence (addiction) if used for a longer period.

Sustaverine smooth muscle relaxant (ICN Pharmaceuticals, Inc.), see Pavabid Plateau Caps smooth muscle relaxant.

Rx   **Synalar steroid hormone**

Manufacturer: Syntex Laboratories, Inc.
Ingredient: fluocinolone acetonide
Equivalent Products: Fluonid, Herbert Laboratories; Synemol, Syntex Laboratories, Inc.
Dosage Forms: Cream: 0.025%, 0.01%. Ointment: 0.025%. Topical solution: 0.01%
Use: Relief of skin inflammation associated with such conditions as dermatitis, eczema, or poison ivy
Minor Side Effects: Burning sensation; dryness; irritation; itching; rash
Major Side Effects: Secondary infection
Contraindications: This drug should not be used by people who are allergic to it. Consult your doctor immediately if this drug has been prescribed for you and you have such an allergy. • This drug should not be used in infants under two years old.
Warnings: If irritation develops when using this drug, immediately discontinue its use and notify your doctor. • If extensive areas are treated or if an occlusive bandage is used, there will be increased systemic absorption of this drug and suitable precautions should be taken, particularly in children and infants. • This drug should be used with caution in pregnant women. • This drug is not meant for use in the eyes.
Comments: If the affected area is extremely dry or scaling, the skin may be moistened before applying the medication by soaking in water or by applying water with a clean cloth. The ointment form is probably better for dry skin. The solution form is best for hairy areas. • Do not use this drug with an occlusive wrap unless directed to do so by your doctor. If it is necessary for you to use this drug under a wrap, follow your doctor's instructions exactly; do not leave the wrap in place longer than specified.

Synalgos analgesic (Ives Laboratories, Inc.), see Synalgos·DC analgesic.

Rx   **Synalgos·DC analgesic**

Manufacturer: Ives Laboratories, Inc.
Ingredients: aspirin; caffeine; dihydrocodeine bitartrate; phenacetin; promethazine hydrochloride
Dosage Form: Capsule: aspirin, 194.4 mg; caffeine, 30 mg; dihydrocodeine bitartrate, 16 mg; phenacetin, 162 mg; promethazine hydrochloride, 6.25 mg (blue/gray)
Use: Relief of moderate to severe pain
Minor Side Effects: Blurred vision; constipation; dizziness; drowsiness; dry

mouth; flushing; itching; jitteriness; light-headedness; menstrual irregularities; nausea; nasal congestion; odd movements; palpitations; rash; ringing in the ears; sedation; sweating; vomiting

Major Side Effects: Breathing difficulties; death; fluid retention; jaundice; kidney disease; low blood sugar; muscle stiffness; rapid heartbeat; rise in blood pressure; sore throat; tremors

Contraindications: This drug should not be used by people who are allergic to any of its components. Consult your doctor immediately if this drug has been prescribed for you and you have such an allergy.

Warnings: This drug should be used with extreme caution in the presence of peptic ulcer, blood coagulation problems, certain types of heart disease, kidney disease, liver disease, prostate disease, or thyroid disease. Be sure your doctor knows if you have any of these problems. • The drug should be used with caution in pregnant women, the elderly, and children. • This drug may cause drowsiness; avoid tasks requiring alertness, such as driving a motor vehicle or operating machinery. • This drug can produce drug dependence of the codeine type and, therefore, has the potential for abuse. • Concurrent use of this drug with other depressants can have adverse effects. • This drug should not be taken with alcohol, ammonium chloride, amphetamine, methotrexate, antacids, oral anticoagulants, oral antidiabetics, probenecid, steroids, sulfinpyrazone, anticholinergics, or central nervous system depressants. If you are currently taking any drugs of these types, consult your doctor about their use. If you are unsure of the type or contents of your medications, ask your doctor or pharmacist.

Comments: Products containing narcotics (e.g., dihydrocodeine bitartrate) are usually not taken for more than seven to ten days. • While taking this drug, do not take any nonprescription item for cough, cold, or sinus problems without first checking with your doctor. • If you are also taking an anticoagulant ("blood thinner"), remind your doctor. • This drug interacts with alcohol and other sedatives; avoid using them while taking this drug. • This drug has the potential for abuse and must be used with caution. Tolerance may develop quickly; do not increase the dose of the drug without first consulting your doctor. • Although no product exactly equivalent to this drug is available, similar products are, and buying them may save you money. Consult your doctor. • Take this product with food or milk. • If your ears feel strange, if you hear buzzing or ringing, or if your stomach hurts, your dosage may need adjustment. Consult your doctor. • A product, Synalgos analgesic, is identical to Synalgos-DC analgesic except that it does not contain dihydrocodeine bitartrate.

Synemol steroid hormone (Syntex Laboratories, Inc.), see Synalar steroid hormone.

OTC   **Synthaloids throat lozenges**

Manufacturer: Buffington, Div. Otis Clapp & Son
Ingredients: benzocaine; calcium-iodine complex
Dosage Form: Lozenge (quantities of ingredients not specified)
Use: Temporary relief of minor throat irritations
Side Effects: Itching
Contraindications: Unless directed otherwise by your doctor, do not give this product to children under three years of age.
Warnings: A sore throat in a child under age six should never be treated without medical supervision. Consult your doctor. • If your sore throat is severe; is accompanied by headache, high fever, nausea, or vomiting; or lasts for more than two days, consult your doctor promptly.
Comments: The antibacterial ingredients included represent an irrational

use for this product if it is recommended to treat an infection-induced sore throat. Colds are caused by viruses, and the ingredients in this product are not effective against viral infections. The value of this product lies in its throat-soothing quality.

℞ **Synthroid thyroid hormone**

Manufacturer: Flint Laboratories
Ingredient: levothyroxine sodium.
Equivalent Products: Levoid, Nutrition Control Products; Levothroid, Armour Pharmaceutical Company; levothyroxine sodium, various manufacturers; Noroxine, North American Pharmacal, Inc.; Ro-Thyroxine, Robinson Laboratory, Inc.
Dosage Form: Tablet: 0.025 mg (orange); 0.05 mg (white); 0.1 mg (yellow); 0.15 mg (blue); 0.2 mg (pink); 0.3 mg (green)
Use: Thyroid replacement therapy
Major Side Effects: Chest pain; diarrhea; headache; heat intolerance; insomnia; nervousness; palpitations; sweating; weight loss
Contraindications: This drug should not be used to treat obesity.
Warnings: This drug should be used cautiously by people who have heart disease, high blood pressure, or diabetes. Be sure your doctor knows if you have any of these conditions. • This drug interacts with cholestyramine, digitalis, oral anticoagulants, oral antidiabetics, and phenytoin; if you are currently taking any drugs of these types, consult your doctor about their use. If you are unsure of the type or contents of your medications, ask your doctor or pharmacist. • While taking this drug, do not take any nonprescription item for cough, cold, or sinus problems without first checking with your doctor. • If you are taking digitalis in addition to this drug, watch carefully for symptoms of increased toxicity (e.g., nausea, blurred vision, palpitations) and notify your doctor immediately if they occur. • Be sure to follow your doctor's dosage instructions exactly. Most side effects from this drug can be controlled by dosage adjustment; consult your doctor if you experience side effects.
Comments: For most patients, generic thyroid hormone tablets (see the profile on thyroid hormone) will work as well as this drug and are less expensive. Check with your doctor.

Tagafed adrenergic and antihistamine (Tutag Pharmaceuticals, Inc.), see Actifed adrenergic and antihistamine.

℞ **Tagamet antisecretory**

Manufacturer: Smith Kline & French Laboratories
Ingredient: cimetidine
Dosage Form: Tablet: 300 mg (pale green)
Use: Treatment of duodenal ulcer; long-term treatment of excessive gastric acid secretion; prevention of recurrent ulcers
Minor Side Effects: Confusion; diarrhea; dizziness; muscle pain; rash
Major Side Effects: Blood damage; increased breast size (both sexes)
Warnings: This drug should be used with caution, since it may cause gastric cancer. • This drug should be used with caution in women of childbearing age, in pregnant women, and in nursing mothers. This drug is not recommended for use in children under 16 years of age. • This drug should be used with caution in patients with severe kidney problems. Be sure your doctor knows if you have such a condition. • This drug may affect the functioning of anticoagulants. If you are currently taking any drugs of this type, consult your doctor about their use. If you are unsure about the type or contents of your medications, ask your doctor or pharmacist.
Comments: Although this drug is classed as an histamine blocker, its only

action on histamine in the body is in the stomach and intestine. • This drug should not be crushed or chewed because cimetidine has a bitter taste and an unpleasant odor. • Antacid therapy may be continued while taking this drug. Talk to your doctor about this. • This drug is usually taken throughout the day. Some people get as much benefit from taking only one or two doses each day. Consult with your doctor. • When used as a preventive, the medication may be taken as a single dose at bedtime.

Rx   **Talwin analgesic**

Manufacturer: Winthrop Laboratories
Ingredient: pentazocine hydrochloride
Dosage Form: Tablet: 50 mg (peach)
Use: Relief of moderate to severe pain
Minor Side Effects: Constipation; diarrhea; dizziness; headache; insomnia; light-headedness; loss of appetite; nausea; vomiting
Major Side Effects: Blurred vision; euphoria; nightmares
Contraindications: This drug should not be used by people who are allergic to it. Consult your doctor immediately if this drug has been prescribed for you and you have such an allergy.
Warnings: This drug should be used with caution in persons with a history of drug abuse; there have been instances of physical and psychological dependence on it. Abrupt discontinuance following the extended use of this drug has resulted in withdrawal symptoms. Patients with a history of drug dependence should use this drug only under close supervision. • This drug should be used with extreme caution in patients with head injury or increased intracranial pressure. • This drug should be used with caution in pregnant women. • This drug is not recommended for use in children under twelve years of age. • This drug, on rare occasions, has produced hallucinations (usually visual), disorientation, and confusion in some patients, but these side effects have cleared spontaneously in a few hours. • This drug should be used with caution in persons with severe respiratory depression from any cause, severe bronchial asthma and other obstructive respiratory conditions, cyanosis, liver diseases, kidney diseases, epilepsy, or myocardial infarction (heart attack). Be sure your doctor knows if you have any of these conditions. • This drug should be used cautiously in patients about to undergo gallbladder surgery. • This drug is a mild narcotic antagonist; some patients previously given narcotics, including methadone for the daily treatment of narcotic dependence, have experienced withdrawal symptoms after receiving this drug. • Use of this drug may cause drowsiness; avoid tasks that require alertness. • This drug interacts with alcohol, narcotics, phenothiazines, and antidepressants. If you are currently taking any drugs of these types, consult your doctor about their use. If you are unsure of the type or contents of your medications, ask your doctor or pharmacist.
Comments: Tolerance to this drug may develop quickly; do not increase the dose of this drug without first consulting your doctor.

Tandearil anti-inflammatory (Geigy Pharmaceuticals), see Butazolidin anti-inflammatory.

Rx   **Tedral antiasthmatic**

Manufacturer: Parke-Davis
Ingredients: ephedrine hydrochloride; phenobarbital; theophylline
Equivalent Products: Asa-lief, Columbia Medical Co.; Phedral, North American Pharmacal, Inc.; Theodrine, Rugby Laboratories; Theofensae, Spencer-Mead, Inc.; Theophed, Bowman Pharmaceuticals; Theoral, Vangard Laboratories

Dosage Forms: Elixir (content per 5 ml): ephedrine hydrochloride, 6 mg; phenobarbital, 2 mg; theophylline, 32.5 mg. Sustained-action tablet: ephedrine hydrochloride, 48 mg; phenobarbital, 25 mg; theophylline, 180 mg (coral/mottled white). Tablet: ephedrine hydrochloride, 24 mg; phenobarbital, 8 mg; theophylline, 130 mg (white)

Use: Prevention and relief of symptoms of bronchial asthma

Minor Side Effects: Difficult urination; drowsiness; insomnia; nausea; stimulation; vomiting

Major Side Effects: Chest pain; cold and clammy skin; convulsions; difficult breathing; high blood pressure; palpitations

Contraindications: This drug should not be taken by people who are allergic to any of its components, or by those who have porphyria. Consult your doctor immediately if this drug has been prescribed for you and you have either condition.

Warnings: This drug should be used cautiously by people who have glaucoma (certain types), heart disease (certain types), enlarged prostate, thyroid disease, or high blood pressure. Be sure your doctor knows if you have any of these conditions. • This drug interacts with central nervous system depressants, griseofulvin, guanethidine, propranolol, lithium carbonate, monoamine oxidase inhibitors, oral anticoagulants, steroids, sulfonamides, tetracycline, and antidepressants; if you are currently taking any drugs of these types, consult your doctor about their use. If you are unsure of the type or contents of your medications, ask your doctor or pharmacist. • Never take this product more frequently than your doctor prescribes; a serious overdose could result. • This drug may cause drowsiness; avoid tasks that require alertness. To prevent oversedation, avoid the use of alcohol or other drugs that have sedative properties. • If you are taking an anticoagulant ("blood thinner") in addition to this drug, remind your doctor. • Call your doctor if you develop stomach pain or vomiting, because this product may aggravate ulcers. • While taking this drug, do not use any other product for asthma, cough, cold, or sinus problems without first checking with your doctor. • Because this product contains phenobarbital, it has the potential for abuse and must be used with caution. Do not take this drug more frequently than prescribed or increase the dose without consulting your doctor.

Comments: While taking this drug, drink at least eight glasses of water daily. • Take your dose with food or milk. • In many states, this product may be purchased without a prescription.

OTC   Tedral asthma remedy

Manufacturer: Warner-Lambert Company

Ingredients: ephedrine hydrochloride; phenobarbital; theophylline anhydrous

Dosage Forms: Elixir (content per 5 ml, or one teaspoon): ephedrine hydrochloride, 6 mg; phenobarbital, 2 mg; theophylline anhydrous, 32.5 mg. Suspension (content per 5 ml, or one teaspoon): ephedrine hydrochloride, 12 mg; phenobarbital, 4 mg; theophylline anhydrous, 65 mg. Tablet: ephedrine hydrochloride, 24 mg; phenobarbital, 8 mg; theophylline anhydrous, 130 mg

Use: Control of symptoms of bronchial asthma

Side Effects: Anxiety; chest pain; dizziness; headache; increased blood pressure; increased frequency of urination; insomnia; loss of appetite; nausea; nervousness; palpitations; sweating; tension; tremor; vomiting. (Overdose may result in convulsions, coma, and cardiovascular collapse.)

Comments: Over-the-counter sale of this product may not be permitted in some states • This product interacts with guanethidine, monoamine oxidase inhibitors, and tricyclic antidepressants. If you are currently taking any drugs of these types, check with your doctor before taking this product. If you are unsure of the type or contents of your medications, ask your doctor or pharmacist. • Do not worry about addiction to this product if you follow directions for use.

Tega-Span vitamin supplement (Ortega Pharmaceutical Co.), see nicotinic acid vitamin supplement.

OTC Tegrin antipsoriasis remedy

Manufacturer: Block Drug Company, Inc.
Ingredients: allantoin; coal tar extract
Dosage Forms: Shampoo; cream; lotion: allantoin, 1.7%; coal tar extract, 5%
Use: Controls flaking, itching, and scaling associated with psoriasis
Side Effects: Allergic reactions; burning of the skin; discoloration of hair; dryness or oiliness of hair or scalp; eye irritation
Warnings: Do not use this product if the skin is broken.
Comments: Although this shampoo has not been reported to cause serious toxicity, if you swallow any, call your doctor or pharmacist right away. • Leave the shampoo on the scalp for a few minutes before rinsing. • This product is often used for the treatment of psoriasis without medical supervision. However, psoriasis is a serious disease and you should consult your doctor before any treatment is tried. • Discontinue use if allergic reactions or irritation occur.

OTC Teldrin allergy remedy

Manufacturer: Menley & James Laboratories
Ingredients: chlorpheniramine maleate
Dosage Form: Timed-release capsule: chlorpheniramine maleate, 8 or 12 mg
Use: Prolonged relief of symptoms of hay fever and other upper respiratory allergies
Side Effects: Anxiety; blurred vision; chest pain; confusion; constipation; difficult and painful urination; dizziness; drowsiness; headache; increased blood pressure; insomnia; loss of appetite; mild stimulation; nausea; nervousness; palpitations; rash; reduced sweating; tension; tremor; vomiting
Contraindications: This product should not be used by pregnant women. • This product should not be given to newborn or premature infants.
Warnings: This product should be used with special caution by the elderly or debilitated, and by persons who have asthma, diabetes, enlarged prostate, glaucoma (certain types), heart disease, high blood pressure, kidney disease, liver disease, obstructed bladder, obstructed intestine, peptic ulcer, or thyroid disease. If you have any of these conditions, consult your doctor before taking this product. • This product may cause drowsiness. Do not take it if you must drive, operate heavy machinery, or perform other tasks requiring mental alertness. To prevent oversedation, avoid the use of alcohol or other drugs that have sedative properties. • This product interacts with alcohol, guanethidine, monoamine oxidase inhibitors, sedative drugs, and tricyclic antidepressants. If you are currently taking any drugs of these types, check with your doctor before taking this product. If you are unsure of the type or contents of your medications, ask your doctor or pharmacist. • Because this product reduces sweating, avoid excessive work or exercise in hot weather. • This product has sustained action; never increase the recommended dose or take it more frequently than directed. A serious overdose could result.
Comments: Many other conditions (some serious) mimic the common cold. If symptoms persist beyond one week or if they occur regularly without regard to season, consult your doctor. • The effectiveness of this product

may diminish after being taken regularly for seven to ten days; consult your pharmacist about substituting another product containing a different antihistamine if this product begins to lose its effectiveness for you. • Chew gum or suck on ice chips or a piece of hard candy to reduce mouth dryness. • Products equivalent to this one are available and vary widely in cost. Check prices; you may save money by comparison shopping.

Teline antibiotic (Winston Pharmaceuticals, Inc.), see tetracycline hydrochloride antibiotic.

OTC   **Tempra analgesic**

Manufacturer: Mead Johnson Nutritional Division
Ingredient: acetaminophen
Dosage Forms: Drop (content per 0.6 ml drop): acetaminophen, 60 mg (1 grain); alcohol, 10%. Syrup (content per 5 ml teaspoon): acetaminophen, 120 mg (2 grains); alcohol, 10%
Use: Relief of discomforts and fever following immunizations, or of colds or "flu"
Side Effects: When taken in overdose: blood disorders, rash
Warnings: When taken in overdose, this product is more toxic than aspirin. The dosage instructions listed on the package should be followed carefully; toxicity may occur with repeated doses.
Comments: This product is intended for children.

Tenax sedative and hypnotic (Reid-Provident Laboratories, Inc.), see Librium sedative and hypnotic.

Ten-Shun analgesic and sedative (Bowman Pharmaceuticals, Inc.), see Fiorinal analgesic and sedative.

Rx   **Tenuate adrenergic**

Manufacturer: Merrell-National Laboratories
Ingredient: diethylpropion hydrochloride
Equivalent Products: Maruate Spantab, North American Pharmacal; o.b.c.t., Pharmics, Inc.; Ro-Diet, Robinson Laboratory, Inc.; Tepanil Ten-Tab, Riker Laboratories, Inc.
Dosage Forms: Controlled-release tablet; 75 mg (white). Tablet: 25 mg (blue)
Use: Short-term treatment of obesity
Minor Side Effects: Diarrhea; dizziness; dry mouth; headache; insomnia; nausea; palpitations; restlessness; unpleasant taste in the mouth; vomiting
Major Side Effects: Chest pain; high blood pressure; overstimulation of nerves
Contraindications: This drug should not be taken by people who have heart disease (certain types), thyroid disease, or glaucoma. People who have demonstrated a potential for drug abuse, those who are allergic to the drug, those who are in an agitated state, and those who are taking or recently have taken a monoamine oxidase inhibitor (ask your pharmacist if you are unsure) should not use this drug. Consult your doctor immediately if this drug has been prescribed for you and you fit into any of these categories. • This drug is not recommended for use in children under age 12.
Warnings: This drug should be used cautiously by people who have high blood pressure, heart disease, diabetes, or epilepsy; or by those who are pregnant. Be sure your doctor knows if you have any of these conditions. • This drug interacts with acetazolamide, guanethidine, phenothiazines, sodium bicarbonate, and antidepressants; if you are currently taking any drugs of these types, consult your doctor about their use. If you are unsure

about the type or contents of your medications, ask your doctor or pharmacist. • While taking this drug, do not take any nonprescription item for cough, cold, or sinus problems without first checking with your doctor. • This drug may mask symptoms of extreme fatigue and decrease your ability to perform potentially dangerous or hazardous tasks, such as driving or operating machinery. • This drug has the potential for abuse and must be used with caution. Tolerance may develop quickly; do not increase the dose of this drug or take it more frequently than prescribed without first consulting your doctor. A serious overdose could result, especially with the sustained-action form of the drug.

Comments: To be effective, therapy with this drug must be accompanied by a low-calorie diet. • Weight loss is greatest during the first three weeks of drug therapy. • This drug's effects on appetite control wear off; do not take the drug for more than three weeks at a time. One way to get full benefit from this drug is to take it for three weeks, stop for three weeks, then resume taking the drug. Consult your doctor about this regimen. • To avoid sleeplessness, do not take the sustained-action form of this drug later than 3:00 P.M.

Tepanil Ten-Tab adrenergic (Riker Laboratories, Inc.), see Tenuate adrenergic.

OTC   terpin hydrate and codeine elixir expectorant cough remedy

Manufacturer: various manufacturers
Ingredients: terpin hydrate; codeine; alcohol
Dosage Form: Liquid (content per 5 ml, or one teaspoon): terpin hydrate, 85 mg; codeine, 10 mg; alcohol, 40%
Use: Temporary relief of cough due to colds or "flu"; also to convert a dry, nonproductive cough to a productive, phlegm-producing cough
Side Effects: Constipation; nausea; slight drying of respiratory passages; vomiting
Warnings: This product should be used with caution by persons who have asthma or other respiratory diseases. If you have such a condition, consult your doctor before taking this product. • Because this product contains codeine, it has the potential for abuse and must be used with caution. It usually should not be taken for more than seven to ten days. Tolerance may develop quickly, but do not increase the dose without consulting your doctor. • This product interacts with alcohol, guanethidine, monoamine oxidase inhibitors, sedative drugs, and tricyclic antidepressants. If you are currently taking any drugs of these types, check with your doctor before taking this product. If you are unsure of the type or contents of your medications, ask your doctor or pharmacist.
Comments: Do not use this product to treat chronic coughs, such as from smoking or asthma. • Do not use this product to treat productive (hacking) coughs that produce phlegm. • If you require an expectorant, you need more moisture in your environment. Drink eight to ten glasses of water daily. The use of a vaporizer or humidifier may also be beneficial. Consult your doctor. • Over-the-counter sale of this product may not be permitted in some states.

Rx   Terramycin antibiotic

Manufacturer: Pfizer Laboratories Division
Ingredient: oxytetracycline hydrochloride
Equivalent Products: Oxlopar, Parke-Davis; Oxybiotic, Star Pharmaceuticals, Inc.; Oxy-Tetrachel, Rachelle Laboratories, Inc.; oxytetracycline hydrochloride, various manufacturers; Tetramine, Tutag Pharmaceuticals, Inc.; Uri-Tet, American Urologicals, Inc.

588

Dosage Forms: Capsule: 125 mg; 250 mg (both are opaque yellow). Syrup (content per 5 ml): 125 mg. Tablet: 250 mg (film coated)

Use: Treatment of acne and wide variety of infections

Minor Side Effects: Diarrhea; increased sensitivity to light; loss of appetite; nausea; vomiting

Major Side Effects: Anemia; "black tongue;" mouth irritation; rash; rectal and vaginal itching; sore throat; superinfection

Contraindications: This drug should not be taken by people who are allergic to any tetracycline drug. Consult your doctor immediately if this drug has been prescribed for you and you have such an allergy.

Warnings: This drug may cause permanent discoloration of the teeth if used during tooth development; therefore, it should be used cautiously by pregnant or nursing women and infants and children under nine years of age. This drug should be used cautiously by people who have liver or kidney disease. Be sure your doctor knows if you have any of these conditions. • This drug interacts with antacids, barbiturates, carbamazepine, diuretics, iron-containing products, penicillin, and phenytoin; if you are currently taking any drugs of these types, consult your doctor about their use. If you are unsure of the type or contents of your medications, ask your doctor or pharmacist. • Milk and other dairy products interfere with the body's absorption of this drug, so separate taking this drug and any dairy product by at least one hour. Do not take this drug at the same time as any iron preparation; their use should be separated by at least one hour. •This drug may cause you to be especially sensitive to the sun, so avoid exposure to sunlight as much as possible. • This drug may affect syphilis tests; if you are being treated for this disease, make sure that your doctor knows you are taking this drug. • If you are taking an anticoagulant in addition to this drug, remind your doctor.

Comments: Take this drug on an empty stomach (one hour before or two hours after a meal). • When used to treat strep throat, this drug should be taken for at least ten full days, even if symptoms disappear within that time.

Tetra-Bid antibiotic (Rucker Pharmacal Co., Inc.), see tetracycline hydrochloride antibiotic.

Tetra-C antibiotic (Century Pharmaceuticals, Inc.), see tetracycline hydrochloride antibiotic.

Tetracap antibiotic (Circle Pharmaceuticals, Inc.), see tetracycline hydrochloride antibiotic.

Tetrachel antibiotic (Rachelle Laboratories, Inc.), see tetracycline hydrochloride antibiotic.

Tetra-Co and Tetra-Co B.I.D. antibiotics (Coastal Pharmaceutical Co., Inc.), see tetracycline hydrochloride antibiotic.

℞   **tetracycline hydrochloride antibiotic**

Manufacturer: various manufacturers

Ingredient: tetracycline hydrochloride

Equivalent Products: Achromycin V, Lederle Laboratories; Amtet, Amid Laboratories, Inc.; Bio-Tetra, General Pharmaceutical Prods., Inc.; Bristacycline, Bristol Laboratories; Centet, The Central Pharmacal Co.; Cyclopar, Parke-Davis; Deltamycin, Trimen Laboratories, Inc.; Desamycin, Pharmics, Inc.; Duratet, Meyer Laboratories, Inc.; G-Mycin, Coast Laboratories, Inc.; Maytrex, Mayrand Incorporated; M-Tetra 250, Misemer Pharmaceuticals, Inc.; Nor-Tet, North American Pharmacal, Inc.; Paltet, Palmedico, Inc.; Panmycin, The Upjohn Company; Partrex, Parmed Pharmaceuticals, Inc.; Piracaps,

Tutag Pharmaceuticals, Inc.; Retet, Reid-Provident Laboratories, Inc.; Robitet '250,' A. H. Robins Company; SK-Tetracycline, Smith Kline & French Laboratories; Sumycin, E. R. Squibb & Sons, Inc.; T-250, Paul B. Elder Company; Teline, Winston Pharmaceuticals, Inc.; Tet-250 and Tet-500, W. E. Hauck, Inc.; Tetra-Bid, Rucker Pharmacal Co., Inc.; Tetra-C, Century Pharmaceuticals, Inc.; Tetracap, Circle Pharmaceuticals, Inc.; Tetrachel, Rachelle Laboratories, Inc.; Tetra-Co and Tetra-Co B.I.D., Coastal Pharmaceutical Co., Inc.; Tetracyn, Pfipharmecs Division; Tetralan-250 and Tetralan-500, The Lannett Company, Inc.; Tetram, Dunhall Pharmaceuticals, Inc.; Tri-Tet, Tri-County Pharmaceuticals

Dosage Forms: Capsule; Liquid; Tablet (various strengths and colors)

Use: Treatment of acne and a wide variety of bacterial infections

Minor Side Effects: Diarrhea; increased sensitivity to light; loss of appetite; nausea; vomiting

Major Side Effects: Anemia; "black tongue;" mouth irritation; rash; rectal and vaginal itching; sore throat; superinfection

Contraindications: This drug should not be taken by people who are allergic to any tetracycline drug. Consult your doctor immediately if this drug has been prescribed for you and you have such an allergy.

Warnings: This drug may cause permanent discoloration of the teeth if used during tooth development; therefore, it should be used cautiously by pregnant or nursing women and infants and children under nine years of age. This drug should be used cautiously by people who have liver or kidney disease. Be sure your doctor knows if you have any of these conditions. • This drug interacts with antacids, barbiturates, carbamazepine, diuretics, iron-containing products, penicillin, and phenytoin; if you are currently taking any drugs of these types, consult your doctor about their use. If you are unsure of the type or contents of your medications, ask your doctor or pharmacist. • Milk and other dairy products interfere with the body's absorption of this drug, so separate taking this drug and any dairy product by at least one hour. Do not take this drug at the same time as any iron preparation; their use should be separated by at least one hour. • This drug may cause you to be especially sensitive to the sun, so avoid exposure to sunlight as much as possible. • This drug may affect syphilis tests; if you are being treated for this disease, make sure that your doctor knows you are taking this drug. • If you are taking an anticoagulant in addition to this drug, remind your doctor.

Comments: Take this drug on an empty stomach (one hour before or two hours after a meal). • When used to treat strep throat, this drug should be taken for at least ten full days, even if symptoms disappear within that time.

Tetracyn antibiotic (Pfipharmecs Division), see tetracycline hydrochloride antibiotic.

Tetralan-250 and Tetralan-500 antibiotics (The Lannett Company, Inc.), see tetracycline hydrochloride antibiotic.

Tetram antibiotic (Dunhall Pharmaceuticals, Inc.), see tetracycline hydrochloride antibiotic.

Tetramine antibiotic (Tutag Pharmaceuticals, Inc.), see Terramycin antibiotic.

Tet-250 and Tet-500 antibiotic (W. E. Hauck, Inc.), see tetracycline hydrochloride antibiotic.

Theocap bronchodilator (Meyer Laboratories, Inc.), see Elixophyllin bronchodilator.

Theo-Col expectorant and smooth muscle relaxant (Columbia Medical Co.), see Quibron expectorant and smooth muscle relaxant.

Theodrine antiasthmatic (Rugby Laboratories), see Tedral antiasthmatic.

Theo-Drox adrenergic, sedative, and smooth muscle relaxant (Columbia Medical Co.), see Marax adrenergic, sedative, and smooth muscle relaxant.

Theofensae antiasthmatic (Spencer-Mead, Inc.), see Tedral antiasthmatic.

Theophed antiasthmatic (Bowman Pharmaceuticals), see Tedral antiasthmatic.

Theophozine adrenergic, sedative, and smooth muscle relaxant (Spencer-Mead, Inc.), see Marax adrenergic, sedative, and smooth muscle relaxant.

Theoral antiasthmatic (Vangard Laboratories), see Tedral antiasthmatic.

Theozine adrenergic, sedative, and smooth muscle relaxant (Henry Schein, Inc.), see Marax adrenergic, sedative, and smooth muscle relaxant.

OTC   Thera-Combex H-P multivitamin

Manufacturer: Parke-Davis
Ingredients: ascorbic acid (vitamin C); thiamine mononitrate (vitamin B_1); riboflavin (vitamin B_2); pyridoxine hydrochloride (vitamin B_6); cyanocobalamin (vitamin B_{12}); nicotinamide (niacinamide); dl-panthenol
Dosage Form: Capsule: ascorbic acid, 500 mg; thiamine mononitrate, 25 mg; riboflavin, 15 mg; pyridoxine hydrochloride, 10 mg; cyanocobalamin, 5 mcg; nicotinamide, 100 mg; dl-panthenol, 20 mg
Use: Dietary supplement
Warnings: This product contains vitamin B_6 in an amount great enough that it may interact with levodopa (L-dopa). If you are currently taking L-dopa, check with your doctor before taking this product.
Comments: This product may interfere with the results of urine tests.

OTC   Theragran-M nutritional supplement

Manufacturer: E. R. Squibb & Sons, Inc.
Ingredients: copper; zinc; manganese; iodine; vitamin A; vitamin D; vitamin E; ascorbic acid (vitamin C); thiamine (vitamin B_1); riboflavin (vitamin B_2); niacinamide; pyridoxine hydrochloride (vitamin B_6); cyanocobalamin (vitamin B_{12}); calcium pantothenate; iron; magnesium
Dosage Form: Tablet: copper, 2 mg; zinc, 1.5 mg; manganese, 1 mg; iodine, 0.15 mg; vitamin A,10,000 IU; vitamin D, 400 IU; vitamin E, 15 IU; ascorbic acid, 200 mg; thiamine, 10 mg; riboflavin, 10 mg; niacinamide, 100 mg; pyridoxine hydrochloride, 5 mg; cyanocobalamin, 5 mcg; calcium pantothenate, 20 mg; iron, 12 mg; magnesium, 65 mg
Use: Dietary supplement
Side Effects: Constipation; diarrhea; nausea; stomach pain
Contraindications: This product should not be used by persons who have active peptic ulcer or ulcerative colitis.

Warnings: The minerals in this product interact with oral tetracycline antibiotics and reduce the absorption of the antibiotics. If you are currently taking tetracycline, consult your doctor or pharmacist before taking this product. If you are unsure of the type or contents of your medications, ask your doctor or pharmacist. • Alcoholics and persons who have chronic liver or pancreatic disease should use this product with special caution; such persons may have enhanced iron absorption and are therefore more likely than others to experience iron toxicity. • Accidental iron poisoning is common in children; be sure to keep this product safely out of their reach. • This product contains vitamin B₆ in an amount great enough that it may interact with levodopa (L-dopa). If you are currently taking L-dopa, check with your doctor before taking this product. • This product contains ingredients that accumulate and are stored in the body. The recommended dose should not be exceeded for long periods (several weeks to months) except by doctor's orders.

Comments: Because of its iron content, this product may cause constipation, diarrhea, nausea, or stomach pain. These symptoms usually disappear or become less severe after two to three days. Taking your dose with food or milk may help minimize these side effects. If they persist, ask your pharmacist to recommend another product. • Black, tarry stools are a normal consequence of iron therapy. If your stools are not black and tarry, this product may not be working for you. Ask your pharmacist to recommend another product. • If large doses are taken, this product may interfere with the results of urine tests. Inform your doctor and pharmacist you are taking this product.

OTC Theragran nutritional supplement

Manufacturer: E. R. Squibb & Sons, Inc.

Ingredients: vitamin A; vitamin D; vitamin E; ascorbic acid (vitamin C); thiamine (vitamin B₁); riboflavin (vitamin B₂); niacinamide; pyridoxine hydrochloride (vitamin B₆); cyanocobalamin (vitamin B₁₂); calcium pantothenate

Dosage Form: Tablet: vitamin A, 10,000 IU; vitamin D, 400 IU; vitamin E, 15 IU; ascorbic acid, 200 mg; thiamine, 10 mg; riboflavin, 10 mg; niacinamide, 100 mg; pyridoxine hydrochloride, 5 mg; cyanocobalamin, 5 mcg; calcium pantothenate, 20 mg

Use: Dietary supplement

Warnings: This product contains vitamin B₆ in an amount great enough that it may interact with levodopa (L-dopa). If you are currently taking L-dopa, check with your doctor before taking this product. • This product contains ingredients that accumulate and are stored in the body. The recommended dose should not be exceeded for long periods (several weeks to months) except by doctor's orders.

Comments: If large doses are taken, this product may interfere with the results of urine tests. Inform your doctor and pharmacist you are taking this product.

Thermoloid thyroid hormone (Mills Pharmaceuticals, Inc.), see thyroid hormone.

Thia-Serpa-Line diuretic and antihypertensive (Robinson Laboratory, Inc.), see Ser-Ap-Es diuretic and antihypertensive.

Thia-Serp diuretic and antihypertensive (Robinson Laboratories, Inc.), see Hydropres diuretic and antihypertensive.

Thiaserp diuretic and antihypertensive (Spencer-Mead, Inc.), see Diupres diuretic and antihypertensive.

Thoradol phenothiazine (H. R. Cenci Laboratories), see Thorazine phenothiazine.

℞   **Thorazine phenothiazine**

Manufacturer: Smith Kline & French Laboratories
Ingredient: chlorpromazine hydrochloride
Equivalent Products: Chloramead, Spencer-Mead, Inc.; chlorpromazine hydrochloride, various manufacturers; Chlor-PZ, USV (P.R.) Development Corporation; Promapar, Parke-Davis; Thoradol, H.R. Cenci Laboratories
Dosage Forms: Concentrate (content per 1 ml): 30 mg; 100 mg. Suppository, 25 mg; 100 mg. Syrup (content per 5 ml): 10 mg. Tablet: 10 mg; 25 mg; 50 mg; 200 mg (all brown). Time-release capsule: 30 mg; 75 mg; 150 mg; 200 mg; 300 mg (all brown/clear with brown and white beads)
Use: Management of certain psychotic disorders; treatment of intractable hiccups; nausea; vomiting
Minor Side Effects: Blurred vision; change in urine color; constipation; diarrhea; drooling; drowsiness; dry mouth; jitteriness; menstrual irregularities; nasal congestion; nausea; rash; reduced sweating; restlessness; uncoordinated movements; vomiting
Contraindications: This drug should not be given to people who are comatose. This drug should not be taken by people who have blood diseases or by those who are in a drug-induced depression. • People who have previously had an allergic reaction to any phenothiazine should not take this drug. Consult your doctor immediately if you have such a condition and this drug has been prescribed for you.
Warnings: This drug should be used cautiously by pregnant or nursing women. • This drug may cause motor restlessness, uncoordinated movements, or muscle spasms. Contact your doctor immediately if you notice any such symptoms. • This drug may cause drowsiness; avoid tasks that require alertness. To prevent oversedation, avoid the use of alcohol or other drugs that have sedative properties. • This drug interacts with antacids, anticholinergics, central nervous system depressants, and guanethidine; if you are currently taking any drugs of these types, consult your doctor about their use. If you are unsure of the type or contents of your medications, ask your doctor or pharmacist. • This drug has persistent action; never take it more frequently than your doctor prescribes. A serious overdose may result. • While taking this drug, do not take any nonprescription item for cough, cold, or sinus problems without first checking with your doctor. • The antivomiting activity of this drug may mask symptoms of severe disease or toxicity due to overdose of other drugs.
Comments: The effects of this drug may not be apparent for at least two weeks. • Chew gum or suck on ice chips or a piece of hard candy to reduce mouth dryness. • Because this drug reduces sweating, avoid excessive exercise or work in hot weather. • To avoid dizziness or light-headedness when you stand, contract and relax the muscles of your legs for a few moments before rising. Do this by pushing one foot against the floor while raising the other foot slightly, alternating feet so that you are "pumping" your legs in a pedaling motion. • The liquid concentrate form of this drug should be added to 60 ml (two fluid ounces) or more of water, milk, juice, coffee, tea, or a carbonated beverage, or to pulpy foods immediately prior to administration.

T.H.P. antiparkinson drug (Spencer-Mead, Inc.), see Artane antiparkinson drug.

OTC   **Throat Discs throat lozenges**

Manufacturer: Marion Laboratories, Inc.

Ingredients: capsicum; peppermint; anise; cubeb; glycyrrhiza extract (licorice); linseed
Dosage Form: Lozenge (amounts of ingredients not specified)
Use: Temporary relief of minor throat irritations
Contraindications: Unless directed otherwise by your doctor, do not give this product to children under three years of age.
Warnings: A sore throat in a child under age six should never be treated without medical supervision. Consult your doctor. • If your sore throat is severe; is accompanied by headache, high fever, nausea, or vomiting; or lasts for more than two days, consult your doctor promptly.
Comments: The value of this product lies in its throat-soothing quality.

Thyrar thyroid hormone (Armour Pharmaceuticals Company), see thyroid hormone.

Thyrocrine thyroid hormone (Lemmon Company), see thyroid hormone.

℞   **thyroid hormone**

Manufacturer: various manufacturers
Ingredient: thyroid
Equivalent Products: Thermoloid, Mills Pharmaceuticals, Inc.; Thyrar, Armour Pharmaceuticals Company; Thyrocrine, Lemmon Company; Thyro-Teric, Mallard Incorporated
Dosage Form: Chewable tablet; Enteric-coated tablet; Sustained-release capsule; Tablet (various dosages and various colors)
Use: Thyroid replacement therapy
Minor Side Effects: None when drug is used as directed.
Major Side Effects: Chest pain; diarrhea; headache; heat intolerance; insomnia; nervousness; palpitations; sweating; weight loss
Contraindications: This drug should not be used to treat obesity.
Warnings: This drug should be used cautiously by people who have heart disease, high blood pressure, or diabetes. Be sure your doctor knows if you have any of these conditions. • This drug interacts with cholestyramine, digitalis, oral anticoagulants, oral antidiabetics, and phenytoin; if you are currently taking any drugs of these types, consult your doctor about their use. If you are unsure of the type or contents of your medications, ask your doctor or pharmacist. • While taking this drug, do not take any nonprescription item for cough, cold, or sinus problems without first checking with your doctor. • If you are taking digitalis in addition to this drug, watch carefully for symptoms of increased toxicity (e.g., nausea, blurred vision, palpitations) and notify your doctor immediately if they occur.
Comments: Be sure to follow your doctor's dosage instructions exactly. Most side effects from this drug can be controlled by dosage adjustment; consult your doctor if you experience side effects. • Although many thyroid products are on the market, they are not all bioequivalent; that is, they may not all be absorbed into the bloodstream at the same rate or have the same overall pharmacologic activity. Don't change brands of this drug without consulting your doctor or pharmacist to make sure you are receiving an identically functioning product.

Thyro-Teric thyroid hormone (Mallard Incorporated), see thyroid hormone.

R_X   **Tigan antinauseant**

Manufacturer: Beecham Laboratories
Ingredients: trimethobenzamide hydrochloride; benzocaine (suppository form only)
Dosage Forms: Capsule: trimethobenzamide hydrochloride, 100 mg (blue/white); 250 mg (blue). Pediatric suppository: trimethobenzamide hydrochloride, 100 mg; benzocaine, 2%. Suppository: trimethobenzamide hydrochloride, 200 mg; benzocaine, 2%.
Use: Control of nausea and vomiting
Minor Side Effects: Blurred vision; depression; diarrhea; drowsiness; headache; tremor
Contraindications: This drug should not be taken by people who are allergic to it. Consult your doctor immediately if this drug has been prescribed for you and you have such an allergy. • The suppository form of this drug should not be given to premature or newborn infants.
Warnings: This drug should be used with extreme caution in children for the treatment of vomiting. This drug is not recommended for treatment of uncomplicated vomiting in children and its use should be limited to prolonged vomiting of known cause. • Since this drug may cause drowsiness, patients should not operate motor vehicles or dangerous machinery until their individual responses to the drug have been determined. • This drug should be used cautiously by pregnant women and nursing mothers. • This drug should be used with caution in patients with acute febrile illness, encephalitis, gastroenteritis, dehydration, and electrolyte imbalance (especially in children and the elderly or debilitated), or various central nervous system reactions. Be sure your doctor knows if you have any of these conditions. • This drug may render diagnosis more difficult in such conditions as appendicitis and obscure signs of toxicity due to overdose of other drugs. • This drug should be discontinued at the first sign of sensitivity to it.
Comments: Since this drug may cause drowsiness, prevent oversedation by avoiding the use of alcohol or other sedative drugs.

R_X   **Timoptic ophthalmic solution**

Manufacturer: Merck Sharp & Dohme
Ingredient: timolol maleate
Dosage Form: Drop (content per ml): timolol, 0.25% (2.5 mg) and 0.5% (5 mg); monobasic and dibasic sodium phosphate; sodium hydroxide; benzalkonium chloride, 0.1%
Use: Treatment of some types of chronic glaucoma
Minor Side Effect: Mild eye irritation
Major Side Effects: Major side effects are rare when this product is used correctly. However, rare occurrences of bronchospasm, generalized rash, and slight reduction of the resting heart rate have been observed in some users of this drug.
Contraindications: This drug should not be used by people who are allergic to it. Consult your doctor immediately if this drug has been prescribed for you and you have such an allergy.
Warnings: This drug should be used with caution by people with bronchial asthma, heart disease, or narrow-angle glaucoma. Be sure your doctor knows if you have any of these conditions. • This drug is not recommended for use by children. • This drug should be used cautiously by pregnant women. If you are pregnant, be sure your doctor knows about your condition before you take this drug. • People taking beta blockers should use this drug with caution. If you are presently taking any drugs of this type, consult your doctor about their use. If you are unsure of the type or contents of your medications, ask your doctor or pharmacist.

Comments: This product is also available in a white plastic ophthalmic dispenser with a controlled drop tip, called an Ocumeter. Your pharmacist can give you details. • Be careful about the contamination of drops used for the eyes. Wash your hands before administering eyedrops. Do not touch the dropper to the eye. Do not wash or wipe the dropper before replacing it in the bottle. Close the bottle tightly to keep out moisture. • This product may sting at first, but this is normal and usually goes away after continued use. Like other eyedrops, this product may cause some clouding or blurring of vision. This symptom will go away quickly.

OTC Tinactin athlete's foot remedy

Manufacturer: Schering Corporation
Ingredients: tolnaftate; polyethylene glycol-400; propylene glycol; carboxypolymethylene; monoamylamine; titanium dioxide; butylated hydroxytoluene; corn starch; talc; polyethylenepolypropylene glycol monobutyl ether; denatured alcohol; isobutane (propellant) (Ingredients vary with dosage forms; see below.)
Dosage Forms: Cream: tolnaftate, 1%; polyethylene glycol-400; propylene glycol; carboxypolymethylene; monoamylamine; titanium dioxide; butylated hydroxytoluene. Solution: tolnaftate, 1%; butylated hydroxytoluene; polyethylene glycol-400. Powder: tolnaftate, 1%; corn starch; talc. Powder aerosol: tolnaftate, 1%; butylated hydroxytoluene; talc; polyethylenepolypropylene glycol monobutyl ether; denatured alcohol, 14%; isobutane (propellant)
Use: Treatment of athlete's foot and jock itch (all dosage forms); treatment of ringworm of the body exclusive of the nails and scalp (cream and solution only)
Side Effects: Allergy; local irritation
Warnings: Do not apply this product to mucous membranes. • If your condition worsens, or if irritation occurs, stop using this product and consult your pharmacist. • When using the aerosol form of this product, be careful not to inhale any of the powder.
Comments: Some lesions take months to heal, so it is important not to stop treatment too soon. • If foot lesions are consistently a problem, check the fit of your shoes. • Wash your hands thoroughly after applying this product. • The cream and solution forms of this product are preferable to the powders for effectiveness; the best action of the powders may be in drying the infected area. • When using the solution form of this product, avoid contaminating the contents of the bottle by squeezing some of the liquid into a separate container for each use. • The powder aerosol may be more expensive than the other forms of this product; check prices before paying for convenience you do not need.

℞ Tofranil antidepressant

Manufacturer: Geigy Pharmaceuticals
Ingredient: imipramine hydrochloride
Equivalent Products: Antipress, Lemmon Company; Imavate, A. H. Robins Company; imipramine hydrochloride, various manufacturers; Janimine, Abbott Laboratories; Norfranil, North American Pharmacal, Inc.; Presamine, USV (P.R.) Development Corp.; SK-Pramine, Smith Kline & French Laboratories; W.D.D., Tutag Pharmaceuticals, Inc.
Dosage Form: Tablet: 10 mg; 25 mg; 50 mg (all coral)
Use: Control of bed-wetting; relief of depression
Minor Side Effects: Diarrhea; difficult urination; dizziness; drowsiness; fatigue; hair loss; headache; increased sensitivity to light; loss of appetite;

nausea; numbness in fingers or toes; palpitations; rash; reduced sweating; uncoordinated movements; vomiting; weakness

Major Side Effects: Enlarged or painful breasts (in both sexes); imbalance; heart attack; high or low blood pressure; impotence; jaundice; mouth sores; nervousness; ringing in the ears; sleep disorders; sore throat; stroke; tremors; weight loss or gain (in children)

Contraindications: This drug should not be taken by people who are allergic to it, or by anyone who has recently had a heart attack. The drug should not be taken by people who are using monoamine oxidase inhibitors (ask your pharmacist if you are unsure). Consult your doctor immediately if this drug has been prescribed for you and you have any of these conditions.

Warnings: This drug should be used cautiously by the elderly and by people who have glaucoma, heart disease, epilepsy, thyroid disease, liver or kidney disease, or who have ever had urinary retention problems. Pregnant or nursing women, people who receive electroshock therapy, or those who use drugs that lower blood pressure should also use this drug cautiously. Be sure your doctor knows if you have any of these conditions. • This drug must be used cautiously in children; its safety has not been established for children under six years of age, or for long-term use by children over six years of age. • Notify your doctor if you experience abrupt changes in mood. • If you are going to have any type of surgery, be sure your doctor knows that you are taking this drug; the drug should be discontinued before surgery. (Consult your doctor before stopping the drug.) • This drug interacts with alcohol, amphetamine, barbiturates, central nervous system depressants, clonidine, epinephrine, guanethidine, methylphenidate hydrochloride, monoamine oxidase inhibitors, oral anticoagulants, and phenylephrine; if you are currently taking any drugs of these types, consult your doctor about their use. If you are unsure of the type or contents of your medications, ask your doctor or pharmacist. • While taking this drug, do not take any nonprescription item for cough, cold, or sinus problems without first checking with your doctor. • This drug may cause drowsiness; avoid tasks that require alertness. To prevent oversedation, avoid the use of alcohol or other drugs that have sedative properties. • Because this drug reduces sweating, avoid excessive work or exercise in hot weather. • This drug may cause you to be especially sensitive to the sun, so avoid exposure to sunlight as much as possible.

Comments: The effects of therapy with this drug may not be apparent for at least two weeks. • Chew gum or suck on ice chips or a piece of hard candy to reduce mouth dryness. • Many people receive as much benefit from taking a single dose of this drug at bedtime as from taking multiple doses throughout the day. Talk to your doctor about this dosage plan. • Tofranil antidepressant is also available in capsules that contain larger doses of the drug than the tablets. The capsule form, called Tofranil-PM, should not be used in children because the greater potency increases the risk of overdose.

℞   **Tolectin anti-inflammatory**

Manufacturer: McNeil Laboratories
Ingredient: tolmetin sodium
Dosage Forms: Capsule: 400 mg (orange). Tablet: 200 mg (white)
Use: Relief of pain and swelling due to arthritis
Minor Side Effects: Bloating; cramps; diarrhea; drowsiness; flatulence; headache; heartburn; nausea; ringing in the ears; vomiting
Major Side Effects: Blood in stools; depression; fluid retention; hearing loss; jaundice; palpitations; tremors; visual disturbances; weight gain
Contraindications: This drug should not be taken by people who are allergic to it or to aspirin. Consult your doctor immediately if this drug has

been prescribed for you and you have either allergy.

Warnings: This drug should be used with extreme caution in patients with upper gastrointestinal tract disease, peptic ulcer, heart disease, kidney disease, or bleeding diseases. Be sure your doctor knows if you have any of these conditions. • Persons taking this drug should have eye examinations shortly after beginning therapy and at periodic intervals thereafter. • This drug should be used cautiously in pregnant women and in nursing mothers. Persons using this drug should have periodic urine tests performed. • This drug interacts with anticoagulants, aspirin, oral antidiabetics, phenytoin, or sulfonamides. If you are currently taking any drugs of these types, consult your doctor about their use. If you are unsure of the type or contents of your medications, ask your doctor or pharmacist.

Comments: In numerous tests, this drug has been shown to be as effective as aspirin in the treatment of arthritis, but aspirin is still the drug of choice for the disease. Because of the high cost of this drug consult your doctor about prescribing proper doses of aspirin instead. • If you are allergic to aspirin, you may not be able to use this drug. • Do not take aspirin or alcohol while taking this drug without first consulting your doctor. • This drug may cause drowsiness; avoid tasks that require alertness, such as driving and operating machinery. • You should note improvement of your condition soon after you start using this drug; however, full benefit may not be obtained for as long as a month. It is important not to stop taking this drug even though symptoms have diminished or disappeared. • This drug is not a substitute for rest, physical therapy, or other measures recommended by your doctor to treat your condition. • If this drug upsets your stomach, take it with food or an antacid.

℞   **Tolinase oral antidiabetic**

Manufacturer: The Upjohn Company
Ingredient: tolazamide
Dosage Form: Tablet: 100 mg; 250 mg; 500 mg (all white)
Use: Treatment of diabetes mellitus
Minor Side Effects: Diarrhea; dizziness; fatigue; headache; loss of appetite; nausea; rash; vomiting; weakness
Major Side Effects: Jaundice; low blood sugar; sore throat
Contraindications: This drug should not be taken by diabetic patients who have infections, severe trauma, or who are undergoing surgery, who have ketosis, acidosis, or coma, or a history of repeated bouts of ketoacidosis or coma. This drug is not indicated for persons with juvenile or "brittle" diabetes. This drug is not to be taken by people with liver disease, kidney disease, endocrine disease, or uremia. Be sure your doctor knows if you have any of these conditions. • This drug should not be taken by pregnant women, and probably not by women of childbearing age. Be sure your doctor knows if you are pregnant or might become so.

Warnings: Careful control over the administration of this drug must be maintained, as is the case for the administration of insulin. Persons receiving this drug must be given full and complete instructions about the nature of their disease, what they must do to prevent and detect complications, and how to control their condition. Persons taking this drug cannot neglect their dietary restrictions, develop a careless attitude, or disregard instructions about body weight, exercise, personal hygiene, and avoidance of infection. Persons taking this drug must know how to recognize and counteract hypoglycemia, as well as how and when to test for glycosuria and ketonuria. • During the trial period with this drug, when insulin is being withdrawn, care should be taken to avoid ketosis, acidosis, and coma. Careful observation of persons taking this drug is required. • This drug should be given with caution when thiazide-type diuretics are also being given, since such combinations can aggravate diabetes mellitus. • Close observation and careful adjustment of dosage is required in persons who are debilitated or malnourished; severe hypoglycemic reactions may occur. • This drug should be used cautiously in persons with liver disease, kidney disease, malnutrition, debility, advanced age, alcoholism, and adrenal and pituitary gland problems. Be sure your doctor knows if you have any of these conditions. • This drug interacts with alcohol, anabolic steroids, anticoagulants, aspirin, chloramphenicol, guanethidine, monoamine oxidase inhibitors, phenylbutazone, probenecid, propranolol, steroids, sulfonamides, tetracycline, thiazide diuretics, or thyroid hormone. If you are currently taking any drugs of these types, consult your doctor about their use. If you are unsure of the type or contents of your medications, ask your doctor or pharmacist.

Comments: Studies have shown that a good diet and exercise program may be just as effective as oral antidiabetic drugs. However, these drugs allow diabetics a bit more leeway in their lifestyle. Nonetheless, persons taking this drug should carefully watch their diet and exercise program. • Oral antidiabetic drugs are not effective in treating diabetes in children under age 12. • Take the dose of this drug at the same time each day. Ask your doctor how to recognize the first signs of low blood sugar and how and when to test for glucose and ketones in the urine. • During the first six weeks of therapy with this drug, visit your doctor at least once a week. • A patient taking this drug will have to be switched to insulin therapy if complications (e.g., ketoacidosis, severe trauma, severe infection, diarrhea, nausea, or vomiting) or the need for major surgery develop. • Do not take alcohol while taking this drug. Avoid any other drugs unless your doctor tells you to take them. Especially be careful of nonprescription cold remedies. • You may sunburn easily while taking this product. Avoid exposure to the sun as much as possible.

OTC   Topex acne preparation

Manufacturer: Vicks Toiletry Products Division
Ingredient: benzoyl peroxide
Dosage Form: Lotion: benzoyl peroxide, 10%
Use: Treatment of acne
Side Effects: Allergy; local irritation
Warnings: Do not get product in or near the eyes. • Persons having known sensitivity to benzoyl peroxide should not use this product.
Comments: If the condition worsens, stop using this product and call your pharmacist. • Wash the area gently with warm water and pat dry before applying this lotion. • Avoid exposure to heat lamps, sunlamps, or direct sunlight when using this product. • This product may be especially active on fair-skinned people. • This product may damage certain fabrics including rayon.

Topsyn steroid hormone (Syntex Laboratories, Inc.), see Lidex steroid hormone.

Totacillin antibiotic (Beecham Laboratories), see ampicillin antibiotic.

Tranmep sedative and hypnotic (Reid-Provident Laboratories, Inc.), see meprobamate sedative and hypnotic.

Tranqui-Tabs sedative and hypnotic (General Pharmaceutical Prods., Inc.), see meprobamate sedative and hypnotic.

℞   Tranxene sedative and hypnotic

Manufacturer: Abbott Laboratories

Ingredient: clorazepate dipotassium
Dosage Forms: Capsule: 3.75 mg (gray/white); 7.5 mg (gray/maroon); 15 mg (gray). Sustained-action tablet: 11.25 mg (blue); 22.5 mg (tan)
Use: Relief of anxiety, nervousness, tension; withdrawal from alcohol addiction
Minor Side Effects: Confusion; constipation; depression; difficult urination; dizziness; drowsiness; dry mouth; fatigue; headache; nausea; rash; slurred speech; uncoordinated movements
Major Side Effects: Blurred vision; decreased sexual drive; double vision; jaundice; low blood pressure; stimulation; tremors
Contraindications: This drug should not be taken by people who are allergic to it or who have acute narrow-angle glaucoma. Consult your doctor immediately if this drug has been prescribed for you and you have such an allergy or condition.
Warnings: This drug is not recommended for persons with depressive neuroses or psychotic reactions. • This drug may cause drowsiness; avoid tasks that require alertness, such as driving a car or operating machinery. • This drug should not be taken with alcohol or other central nervous system depressants. Taken alone, this drug is safe; when it is combined with alcohol or other sedative drugs, serious adverse reactions may develop. If you are currently taking any drugs of this type, consult your doctor about their use. If you are unsure about the type or contents of your medications, ask your doctor or pharmacist. • This drug is not recommended for use in patients less than 18 years of age. • This drug should be taken cautiously by persons considered to have psychological tendencies for drug dependence. Withdrawal symptoms have been reported in patients following abrupt discontinuance of the drug after long-term use of high dosages. Do not stop taking this drug without informing your doctor. • This drug should be used with caution in pregnant women and nursing mothers. • In those persons in which a high degree of depression accompanies the anxiety, suicidal tendencies may be present. The least amount of the drug that is feasible should be available to the patient. • This drug should be used with caution in elderly and debilitated persons, and in persons with impaired liver or kidney function. Patients using this drug for prolonged periods should have blood counts and liver function tests periodically. • This drug has the potential for abuse and must be used with caution. Tolerance may develop quickly; do not increase the dose without first consulting your doctor. • Never take the sustained-action tablets more frequently than your doctor prescribes. A serious overdose may result.
Comments: This drug currently is used by many people to relieve nervousness. It is effective for this purpose, but it is important to try to remove the cause of the anxiety as well. Phenobarbital is also effective for this, and it is less expensive. Consult your doctor. • This drug may cause dryness of the mouth. To reduce this feeling, chew gum or suck on ice chips or a piece of hard candy. • Do not stop taking this drug suddenly.

Trates Granucaps antianginal (Tutag Pharmaceuticals, Inc.), see Nitro-Bid Plateau Caps antianginal.

Tremin antiparkinson drug (Schering Corporation), see Artane antiparkinson drug.

Triafed adrenergic and antihistamine (Henry Schein, Inc.), see Actifed adrenergic and antihistamine.

OTC   Triaminic Expectorant cough remedy

Manufacturer: Dorsey Laboratories
Ingredients: phenylpropanolamine hydrochloride; guaifenesin; alcohol

Dosage Form: Liquid (content per 5 ml, or one teaspoon): phenylpropanolamine hydrochloride, 12.5 mg; guaifenesin, 100 mg; alcohol, 5%

Use: Temporary relief of cough and nasal congestion due to colds or "flu"; also to convert a dry, nonproductive cough to a productive, phlegm-producing cough

Side Effects: Mild stimulation; occasional nausea, vomiting

Warnings: This product should be used with special caution by children under two years of age, and by persons who have diabetes, heart disease, high blood pressure, or thyroid disease. If you have any of these conditions, consult your doctor before taking this product. • This product interacts with guanethidine and monoamine oxidase inhibitors. If you are currently taking any drugs of these types, check with your doctor before taking this product. If you are unsure of the type or contents of your medications, ask your doctor or pharmacist.

Comments: Do not use this product to treat chronic coughs, such as those from smoking or asthma. • Do not use this product to treat productive (hacking) coughs that produce phlegm. • If you require an expectorant, you need more moisture in your environment. Drink eight to ten glasses of water daily. The use of a vaporizer or humidifier may also be beneficial. Consult your doctor.

OTC   Triaminic Expectorant with Codeine cough remedy

Manufacturer: Dorsey Laboratories

Ingredients: codeine phosphate; guaifenesin; phenylpropanolamine hydrochloride; pheniramine maleate; pyrilamine maleate; alcohol

Dosage Form: Liquid (content per 5 ml, or one teaspoon): codeine phosphate, 10 mg; guaifenesin, 100 mg; phenylpropanolamine hydrochloride, 12.5 mg; pheniramine maleate, 6.25 mg; pyrilamine maleate, 6.25 mg; alcohol, 5%

Use: Temporary relief of cough, nasal congestion, and other symptoms of colds or "flu"; also to convert a dry, nonproductive cough to a productive, phlegm-producing cough

Side Effects: Anxiety; blurred vision; chest pain; confusion; constipation; diarrhea; difficult and painful urination; dizziness; drowsiness; dry mouth; headache; heartburn; increased blood pressure; insomnia; loss of appetite; low blood pressure; nasal congestion; nausea; nervousness; palpitations; rash; reduced sweating; severe abdominal pain; sore throat; sweating; tension; tremor; vomiting

Contraindications: This product should not be used by persons who have severe heart disease or severe high blood pressure. This product should not be given to newborn or premature infants.

Warnings: This product should be used with special caution by the elderly or debilitated, and by persons who have asthma or respiratory disease, diabetes, enlarged prostate, glaucoma (certain types), heart disease, high blood pressure, kidney disease, obstructed bladder, obstructed intestine, peptic ulcer, or thyroid disease. If you have any of these conditions, consult your doctor before taking this product. • This product may cause drowsiness. Do not take it if you must drive, operate heavy machinery, or perform other tasks requiring mental alertness. To prevent oversedation, avoid the use of alcohol or other drugs that have sedative properties. • This product interacts with alcohol, guanethidine, monoamine oxidase inhibitors, sedative drugs, and tricyclic antidepressants. If you are currently taking any drugs of these types, check with your doctor before taking this product. If you are unsure of the type or contents of your medications, ask your doctor or pharmacist. • Because this product reduces sweating, avoid excessive work or exercise in hot weather. • Because this product contains codeine, it has the potential for abuse and must be used with caution. It usually should not be taken for more than seven to ten days. Tolerance may develop quickly, but do not increase the dose without consulting your doctor.

Comments: Many other conditions (some serious) mimic the common cold. If symptoms persist beyond one week or if they occur regularly without regard to season, consult your doctor. • Do not use this product to treat chronic coughs, such as from smoking or asthma. • Do not use this product to treat productive (hacking) coughs that produce phlegm. • If you require an expectorant, you need more moisture in your environment. Drink eight to ten glasses of water daily. The use of a vaporizer or humidifier may also be beneficial. Consult your doctor. • Chew gum or suck on ice chips or a piece of hard candy to reduce mouth dryness. • Over-the-counter sale of this product may not be permitted in some states.

OTC   Triaminicin cold and allergy remedy

Manufacturer: Dorsey Laboratories

Ingredients: phenylpropanolamine hydrochloride; chlorpheniramine maleate; aspirin; caffeine

Dosage Form: Tablet: phenylpropanolamine hydrochloride, 25 mg; chlorpheniramine maleate, 2 mg; aspirin 450 mg (7 grains); caffeine, 30 mg

Use: Temporary relief of nasal congestion, fever, aches, pains, and general discomfort due to colds or upper respiratory allergies

Side Effects: Anxiety; blurred vision; chest pain; confusion; constipation; difficult and painful urination; dizziness; drowsiness; headache; increased blood pressure; insomnia; loss of appetite; nausea; nervousness; palpitations; rash; reduced sweating; ringing in the ears; slight blood loss; tension; tremor; vomiting

Contraindications: This product should not be used by persons who have aspirin sensitivity, asthma, blood-clotting disease, gout, severe heart disease, severe high blood pressure, significant drug or food allergies, or vitamin-K deficiency. • This product should not be given to newborn or premature infants.

Warnings: This product should be used with special caution by the elderly or debilitated, and by persons who have diabetes, enlarged prostate, glaucoma (certain types), heart disease, high blood pressure, kidney disease, obstructed bladder, obstructed intestine, peptic ulcer, or thyroid disease. If you have any of these conditions, consult your doctor before taking this product. • This product may cause drowsiness. Do not take it if you must drive, operate heavy machinery, or perform other tasks requiring mental alertness. To prevent oversedation, avoid the use of alcohol or other drugs that have sedative properties. • This product interacts with alcohol, ammonium chloride, guanethidine, methotrexate, monoamine oxidase inhibitors, oral anticoagulants, oral antidiabetics, probenecid, sedative drugs, steroids, sulfinpyrazone, tricyclic antidepressants, and vitamin C. If you are currently taking any drugs of these types, check with your doctor before taking this product. If you are unsure of the type or contents of your medications, ask your doctor or pharmacist. • Because this product reduces sweating, avoid excessive work or exercise in hot weather.

Comments: Many other conditions (some serious) mimic the common cold. If symptoms persist beyond one week or if they occur regularly without regard to season, consult your doctor. • The effectiveness of this product may diminish after being taken regularly for seven to ten days; consult your pharmacist about substituting another product containing a different antihistamine if this product begins to lose its effectivenss for you. • Chew gum or suck on ice chips or a piece of hard candy to reduce mouth dryness.

OTC   Triaminicin nasal decongestant

Manufacturer: Dorsey Laboratories

Ingredients: phenylpropanolamine hydrochloride; phenylephrine hydrochloride; pheniramine maleate; pyrilamine maleate; benzalkonium chloride

Dosage Form: Nasal spray: phenylpropanolamine hydrochloride, 0.75%; phenylephrine hydrochloride, 0.25%; pheniramine maleate, 0.125%; pyrilamine maleate, 0.125%; benzalkonium chloride, 1:10,000

Use: Temporary relief of nasal congestion due to colds, sinusitis, hay fever, or other upper respiratory allergies

Side Effects: Burning, dryness of nasal mucosa, increased nasal congestion or discharge, sneezing, and/or stinging; blurred vision; dizziness; drowsiness; headache; insomnia; nervousness; palpitations; slight increase in blood pressure; stimulation

Contraindications: This product should not be used by persons who have glaucoma (certain types).

Warnings: This product should be used with special caution by persons who have diabetes, advanced hardening of the arteries, heart disease, high blood pressure, or thyroid disease. If you have any of these conditions, consult your doctor before taking this product. • This product interacts with guanethidine, monoamine oxidase inhibitors, thyroid preparations, and tricyclic antidepressants. If you are currently taking any drugs of these types, check with your doctor before taking this product. If you are unsure of the type or contents of your medications, ask your doctor or pharmacist. • To avoid side effects such as burning, sneezing, or stinging, and a "rebound" increase in nasal congestion and discharge, do not exceed the recommended dosage and do not use this product for more than three or four continuous days. • This product should not be used by more than one person; sharing the dispenser may spread infection.

OTC   Triaminicol cough remedy

Manufacturer: Dorsey Laboratories

Ingredients: phenylpropanolamine hydrochloride; pheniramine maleate; pyrilamine maleate; dextromethorphan hydrobromide; ammonium chloride

Dosage Form: Liquid (content per 5 ml, or one teaspoon): phenylpropanolamine hydrochloride, 12.5 mg; pheniramine maleate, 6.25 mg; pyrilamine maleate, 6.25 mg; dextromethorphan hydrobromide, 15 mg; ammonium chloride, 90 mg

Use: Temporary relief of cough, nasal congestion, and other symptoms of colds or "flu"

Side Effects: Anxiety; blurred vision; chest pain; confusion; constipation; difficult and painful urination; dizziness; drowsiness; headache; increased blood pressure; insomnia; loss of appetite; mild stimulation; nausea; nervousness; palpitations; rash; reduced sweating; tension; tremor; vomiting

Contraindications: This product should not be used by persons who have severe heart disease or severe high blood pressure. • This product should not be given to newborn or premature infants.

Warnings: This product should be used with special caution by the elderly or debilitated, and by persons who have asthma, diabetes, enlarged prostate, glaucoma (certain types), heart disease, high blood pressure, kidney disease, obstructed bladder, obstructed intestine, peptic ulcer, or thyroid disease. If you have any of these conditions, consult your doctor before taking this product. • This product may cause drowsiness. Do not take it if you must drive, operate heavy machinery, or perform other tasks requiring mental alertness. To prevent oversedation, avoid the use of alcohol or other drugs that have sedative properties. • This product interacts with alcohol, guanethidine, monoamine oxidase inhibitors, sedative drugs, and tricyclic antidepressants.

If you are currently taking any drugs of these types, check with your doctor before taking this product. If you are unsure of the type or contents of your medications, ask your doctor or pharmacist. • Because this product reduces sweating, avoid excessive work or exercise in hot weather.

Comments: Many other conditions (some serious) mimic the common cold. If symptoms persist beyond one week or if they occur regularly without regard to season, consult your doctor. Do not use this product to treat chronic coughs, such as those from smoking or asthma. • Do not use this product to treat productive (hacking) coughs that produce phlegm. • Chew gum or suck on ice chips or a piece of hard candy to reduce mouth dryness.

Rx   **Triavil phenothiazine and antidepressant**

Manufacturer: Merck Sharp & Dohme

Ingredients: amitriptyline hydrochloride; perphenazine

Equivalent Products: Etrafon, Schering Corporation; Perphenyline, Henry Schein, Inc.; Triptazine, Spencer-Mead, Inc.

Dosage Forms: Tablet 2-10: amitriptyline hydrochloride, 10 mg; perphenazine, 2 mg (blue). Tablet 2-25: amitriptyline hydrochloride, 25 mg; perphenazine, 2 mg (orange). Tablet 4-10: amitriptyline hydrochloride, 10 mg; perphenazine, 4 mg (salmon). Tablet 4-25: amitriptyline hydrochloride, 25 mg; perphenazine, 4 mg (yellow). Tablet 4-50: amitriptyline hydrochloride, 50 mg; perphenazine, 4 mg (orange)

Use: Relief of anxiety or depression

Minor Side Effects: Aching or numbness of arms and legs; blurred vision; change in urine color; constipation; difficult urination; dizziness; drowsiness; diarrhea; dry mouth; fatigue; headache; increased salivation; loss of appetite; loss of hair; jitteriness; menstrual irregularities; nasal congestion; nausea; palpitations; rash; reduced sweating; restlessness; vomiting; weakness

Major Side Effects: Enlarged or painful breasts (in both sexes); fluid retention; heart attack; high or low blood pressure; imbalance; impotence; insomnia; involuntary movements of the face, mouth, jaw, and tongue; jaundice; mouth sores; muscle stiffness; nervousness; ringing in the ears; sore throat; stroke; tremors; weight gain or loss

Contraindications: This drug should not be taken by persons with drug-induced depression, heart disease, or blood disease. This drug should not be taken by people who are allergic to either of its components. Consult your doctor immediately if this drug has been prescribed for you and you have any of these conditions or such an allergy.

Warnings: This drug should be used with caution in persons with thyroid disease, certain types of glaucoma, impaired liver function, certain types of heart disease, epilepsy, difficult urination, asthma, and other respiratory disorders. Be sure your doctor knows if you have any of these conditions. • This drug may cause drowsiness; avoid tasks requiring alertness, such as driving a motor vehicle or operating machinery. • This drug should also be used with caution in pregnant women and is not recommended for use in children. • Use of this drug may cause mood changes (including possible suicide attempts), paralyzed ileum, cross allergy, and rise in body temperature. • This drug should be used with caution in persons undergoing elective surgery and electroshock therapy. • This drug has been shown to result in both elevation and lowering of blood sugar levels. This drug should not be administered in large amounts. • The antiemetic effect of this drug may obscure signs of toxicity due to overdosage of other drugs, or render more difficult diagnosis of disorders such as brain tumors or intestinal obstruction. • This drug should not be taken with alcohol, amphetamine, barbiturates, epinephrine, guanethidine, monoamine oxidase inhibitors, oral anticoagulants, phenylephrine, ant-acids, anticholinergics, central nervous system depressants, or clonidine. If you are currently taking any drugs of these types, consult your doctor about their use. If you are unsure of the type or contents of your medications, ask your doctor or pharmacist. • Deaths by deliberate or accidental overdose have been reported with the use of this drug.

Comments: The effects of this drug may not be apparent for at least two weeks. • While taking this drug, avoid using alcohol, and do not start or stop taking any other drug, including nonprescription items, without consulting your doctor. • This drug may cause dryness of the mouth. To reduce this feel-ing, chew gum or suck on ice chips or a piece of hard candy. • This drug reduces sweating; avoid excessive work or exercise in hot weather. • To avoid dizziness or light-headedness when you stand, contract and relax the muscles of your legs for a few moments before rising. Do this by pushing one foot against the floor while raising the other foot slightly, alternating feet so that you are "pumping" your legs in a pedaling motion. • Three products equivalent to this drug are available and they differ in cost from this product. Have your doctor prescribe a generic preparation, and ask your pharmacist to fill your prescription with the least expensive brand.

Tri-Ergone vasodilator (Columbia Medical Co.), see Hydergine vasodilator.

Trigot vasodilator (E. R. Squibb & Sons, Inc.), see Hydergine vasodilator.

Trihexane antiparkinson drug (Rugby Laboratories), see Artane an-tiparkinson drug.

Trihexidyl antiparkinson drug (Henry Schein, Inc.), see Artane an-tiparkinson drug.

Tri-Hydroserpine diuretic and antihypertensive (Rugby Laboratories), see Ser-Ap-Es diuretic and antihypertensive.

Trimox antibiotic (E. R. Squibb & Sons, Inc.), see amoxicillin antibiotic.

OTC   Trind cough remedy

Manufacturer: Mead Johnson Nutritional Division

Ingredients: guaifenesin; phenylephrine hydrochloride; acetaminophen; alcohol

Dosage Form: Liquid (content per 5 ml, or one teaspoon): guaifenesin, 50 mg; phenylephrine hydrochloride, 2.5 mg; acetaminophen, 120 mg; alcohol, 15%

Use: Temporary relief of cough, nasal congestion, fever, aches, and pains due to colds or "flu"; also to convert a dry, nonproductive cough to a produc-tive, phlegm-producing cough

Side Effects: Drowsiness; mild stimulation; nausea; vomiting

Warnings: This product should be used with special caution by children under three years of age, and by persons who have diabetes, heart disease, high blood pressure, or thyroid disease. If you have any of these conditions, consult your doctor before taking this product. • This product interacts with guanethidine and monoamine oxidase inhibitors. If you are currently taking any drugs of these types, check with your doctor before taking this product. If you are unsure of the type or contents of your medications, ask your doctor or pharmacist. • When taken in overdose, acetaminophen is more toxic than aspirin. Follow dosage instructions carefully.

Comments: Do not use this product to treat chronic coughs, such as those from smoking or asthma. • Do not use this product to treat productive (hacking) coughs that produce phlegm. • If you require an expectorant, you need more moisture in your environment. Drink eight to ten glasses of water daily. The use of a vaporizer of humidifier may also be beneficial. Consult your doctor.

OTC **Trind-DM cough remedy**

Manufacturer: Mead Johnson Nutritional Division

Ingredients: phenylephrine hydrochloride; dextromethorphan hydrobromide; guaifenesin; acetaminophen; alcohol

Dosage Form: Liquid (content per 5 ml, or one teaspoon): phenylephrine hydrochloride, 2.5 mg; dextromethorphan hydrobromide, 7.5 mg; guaifenesin, 50 mg; acetaminophen, 120 mg; alcohol, 15%

Use: Temporary relief of cough, nasal congestion, fever, aches, and pains due to colds or "flu"; also to convert a dry, nonproductive cough to a productive, phlegm-producing cough

Side Effects: Drowsiness; mild stimulation; nausea; vomiting

Warnings: This product should be used with special caution by children under three years of age, and by persons who have diabetes, heart disease, high blood pressure, or thyroid disease. If you have any of these conditions, consult your doctor before taking this product. • This product interacts with guanethidine and monoamine oxidase inhibitors. If you are currently taking any drugs of these types, check with your doctor before taking this product. If you are unsure of the type or contents of your medications, ask your doctor or pharmacist. When taken in overdose, acetaminophen is more toxic than aspirin. Follow dosage instructions carefully.

Comments: Do not use this product to treat chronic coughs, such as from smoking or asthma. • Do not use this product to treat productive (hacking) coughs that produce phlegm. • If you require an expectorant, you need more moisture in your environment. Drink eight to ten glasses of water daily. The use of a vaporizer or humidifier may also be beneficial. Consult your doctor.

Tri-Pavasule smooth muscle relaxant (Tri-State Pharmaceutical Co., Inc.), see Pavabid Plateau Caps smooth muscle relaxant.

Triphed adrenergic and antihistamine (Lemmon Pharmacal Co.), see Actifed adrenergic and antihistamine.

Tri-Phen-Chlor adrenergic and antihistamine (Rugby Laboratories), see Naldecon adrenergic and antihistamine.

Triphenyl Plus adrenergic and antihistamine (Spencer-Mead, Inc.), see Naldecon adrenergic and antihistamine.

Triple Sulfa vaginal cream (E. Fougera and Co.), see Sultrin vaginal anti-infective.

Triptazine phenothiazine and antidepressant (Spencer-Mead, Inc.), see Triavil phenothiazine and antidepressant.

Tri-Tet antibiotic (Tri-County Pharmaceuticals), see tetracycline hydrochloride antibiotic.

Tri-Vi-Flor vitamin and fluoride supplement (Mead Johnson Nutritional Division), see Poly-Vi-Flor vitamin and fluoride supplement.

Tri-Zide diuretic and antihypertensive (Tri-County Pharmaceuticals), see hydrochlorothiazide diuretic and antihypertensive.

T-250 antibiotic (Paul B. Elder Company), see tetracycline hydrochloride antibiotic.

OTC   Tucks hemorrhoidal preparation

Manufacturer: Parke-Davis
Ingredients: Medicated pad: benzalkonium chloride USP; glycerin USP; hamamelis water; methylparaben. Cream; Ointment: hamamelis water; lanolin; petrolatum
Dosage Forms: Medicated pad: benzalkonium chloride USP, 0.003%; glycerin USP, 10%; hamamelis water, 50%; methylparaben, 0.1%. Cream; Ointment: hamamelis water, 50%; lanolin; petrolatum
Use: Relief of discomfort of hemorrhoids, anorectal wounds, episiotomies, and other superficial irritations
Warnings: Sensitization (continued itching and redness) may occur with long-term and repeated use.
Comments: Hemorrhoidal (pile) preparations relieve itching, reduce pain and inflammation, and check bleeding, but do not heal, dry up, or give lasting relief from the hemorrhoids. • Certain ingredients in this product may cause an allergic reaction; do not use for longer than seven days at a time unless your doctor has advised you otherwise. • Never self-medicate for hemorrhoids if pain is continuous or throbbing, if bleeding or itching is excessive, or if you feel a large pressure within the rectum.

Tudecon T. D. adrenergic and antihistamine (Tutag Pharmaceuticals, Inc.), see Naldecon adrenergic and antihistamine.

Tumol-750 muscle relaxant (Tutag Pharmaceuticals, Inc.), see Robaxin muscle relaxant.

OTC   Tums antacid

Manufacturer: Norcliff Thayer Inc.
Ingredients: calcium carbonate; peppermint oil
Dosage Form: Tablet: calcium carbonate, 500 mg; peppermint oil
Use: For relief from acid indigestion, heartburn, sour stomach, and/or hyperacidity
Side Effects: Constipation
Contraindications: Persons with kidney disease or hypercalcemia, and those drinking large quantities of milk should not use this product.
Comments: Self-treatment of severe or repeated attacks of heartburn, indigestion, or upset stomach is not recommended. If you do self-treat, limit therapy to two weeks, then call your doctor if symptoms persist. Never self-medicate with this product if your symptoms occur regularly (two to three times or more a month); if they are particularly worse than normal; if you feel "tightness" in your chest, have chest pains, or are sweating; or if you are short of breath. Consult your doctor. • This product is safe and effective when used on an occasional basis only. Repeated administrations for longer than one to two weeks may cause "rebound acidity," resulting in increased gastric acid production. If this happens, your symptoms get worse. • This product works best when taken one hour after meals or at bedtime, unless otherwise directed by your doctor or pharmacist. • Do not take this product within two hours of a dose of a tetracycline antibiotic. Also, if you are taking iron, a vitamin-mineral product, chlorpromazine, phenytoin, digoxin, quinidine, or warfarin, remind your doctor or pharmacist that you are taking this product.

R̷ **Tussionex cough suppressant**

Manufacturer: Pennwalt Pharmaceutical Division

Ingredients: hydrocodone and phenyltoloxamine in a resin complex

Dosage Forms: Capsule (green/white); Liquid (content per 5 ml, or one teaspoon); Tablet (light brown): hydrocodone, 5 mg; phenyltoloxamine, 10 mg

Use: Cough suppressant

Minor Side Effects: Blurred vision; confusion; constipation; diarrhea; difficult urination; dizziness; drowsiness; dry mouth; headache; insomnia; nasal congestion; nausea; nervousness; palpitations; rash; reduced sweating; restlessness; vomiting

Major Side Effects: Low blood pressure; severe abdominal pain; sore throat

Warnings: This drug should be used carefully with young children. Estimation of dosage relative to the age and weight of the child is of great importance.

Comments: The liquid form of this drug must be shaken well before measuring each dose. • This drug is intended to be taken at 12-hour intervals. Never take more than one dose every 12 hours unless specifically directed to do so by your doctor. • Since this drug may cause drowsiness, avoid the use of sedative drugs or alcohol while taking it to prevent oversedation. Also, do not drive or operate machinery. • While taking this drug, do not take any nonprescription item for cough, cold, or sinus problems without first checking with your doctor. • This drug may cause dryness of the mouth. To reduce this feeling, chew gum or suck on ice chips or a piece of hard candy. • This drug reduces sweating; avoid excessive work or exercise in hot weather. • Products containing narcotics (e.g., hydrocodone) are usually not used for more than seven to ten days. This drug has the potential for abuse and must be used with caution. Tolerance may develop quickly; do not increase the dose of this drug without first consulting your doctor. An overdose usually sedates an adult but may cause excitation leading to convulsions and death in a child.

R̷ **Tuss-Ornade cough and cold remedy**

Manufacturer: Smith Kline & French Laboratories

Ingredients: caramiphen edisylate; chlorpheniramine maleate; isopropamide iodide; phenylpropanolamine hydrochloride; alcohol (liquid form only)

Dosage Forms: Liquid (content per 5 ml, or one teaspoon): caramiphen edisylate, 5 mg; chlorpheniramine maleate, 2 mg; isopropanamide iodide, equivalent to 0.75 mg isopropamide; phenylpropanolamine hydrochloride, 15 mg; alcohol, 7.5%. Sustained-release capsule: caramiphen edisylate, 20 mg; chlorpheniramine maleate, 8 mg; isopropamide iodide, equivalent to 2.5 mg isopropamide; phenylpropanolamine hydrochloride, 50 mg (white/clear with multicolored pellets)

Use: Relief of symptoms of allergy, sinusitis or the common cold.

Minor Side Effects: Blurred vision; confusion; constipation; diarrhea; difficult urination; dizziness; drowsiness; dry mouth; headache; heartburn; insomnia; loss of appetite; nasal congestion; nausea; palpitations; rash; reduced sweating; restlessness; vomiting; weakness

Major Side Effects: Chest pain; high blood pressure; low blood pressure; severe abdominal pain; sore throat

Contraindications: This drug should not be taken by people who are allergic to any of its components. Consult your doctor immediately if this drug has been prescribed for you and you have such an allergy. • The liquid form of this drug should not be used in children under 15 pounds or in children less than 6 months old. • The capsule form of this drug should not be used in children under 12 years of age. • This drug should not be taken concurrently with monoamine oxidase inhibitors. If you are currently taking any drugs of this type, consult your doctor about their use. If you are unsure of the type or contents of your medications, ask your doctor or pharmacist. • This drug should not be taken by persons with severe high blood pressure, bronchial asthma, coronary artery disease, peptic ulcer, or obstructed bladder or intestine. Be sure your doctor knows if you have any of these conditions.

Warnings: This drug should be used with caution in people with heart disease, glaucoma, enlarged prostate, or thyroid disease. Be sure your doctor knows if you have any of these conditions. • This drug may cause drowsiness; avoid tasks requiring alertness, such as driving a motor vehicle or operating machinery. To prevent oversedation, avoid the use of other sedative drugs or alcohol. • This drug should be used cautiously in pregnant women and nursing mothers. • This drug interacts with alcohol, guanethidine, monoamine oxidase inhibitors, and other sedative drugs. If you are currently taking any drugs of these types, consult your doctor about their use. If you are unsure of the type or contents of your medications, ask your doctor or pharmacist.

Comments: This drug has sustained action; never take it more frequently than your doctor prescribes. A serious overdose may result. • While taking this drug, do not take any nonprescription item for cough, cold, or sinus problems without first checking with your doctor. • This drug may cause dryness of the mouth. To reduce this feeling, chew gum or suck on ice chips or a piece of hard candy. • This drug reduces sweating; avoid excessive work or exercise in hot weather. • Be sure to tell your doctor that you are taking this drug if you are scheduled for a thyroid function test. The drug may affect the results of the test.

Tuzon analgesic (Tutag Pharmaceuticals, Inc.), see Parafon Forte analgesic.

OTC   2/G cough remedy

Manufacturer: Dow Pharmaceuticals
Ingredients: guaifenesin; alcohol; corn derivatives
Dosage Form: Liquid (content per 5 ml, or one teaspoon): guaifenesin, 100 mg; alcohol, 3.5%; corn derivatives
Use: Temporary relief of cough due to colds or "flu"; also to convert a dry, nonproductive cough to a productive, phlegm-producing cough
Side Effects: Occasional nausea, vomiting
Contraindications: Do not give this product to children under two years of age unless directed to do so by your doctor.
Comments: Do not use this product to treat chronic coughs, such as from smoking or asthma. • Do not use this product to treat productive (hacking) coughs that produce phlegm. • If you require an expectorant, you need more moisture in your environment. Drink eight to ten glasses of water daily. The use of a vaporizer or humidifier may also be beneficial. Consult your doctor.

OTC   2/G-DM cough remedy

Manufacturer: Dow Pharmaceuticals
Ingredients: dextromethorphan hydrobromide; guaifenesin; alcohol; corn derivatives; invert sugar; sorbitol
Dosage Form: Liquid (content per 5 ml, or one teaspoon): dextromethorphan hydrobromide, 15 mg; guaifenesin, 100 mg; alcohol, 5%; corn derivatives; invert sugar, 27.8%; sorbitol, 10.3%
Use: Temporary relief of cough due to colds or "flu"; also to convert a dry, nonproductive cough to a productive, phlegm-producing cough
Side Effects: Drowsiness; nausea; vomiting

Warnings: This product interacts with monoamine oxidase inhibitors; if you are currently taking any drugs of this type, check with your doctor before taking this product. If you are unsure of the type or contents of your medications, ask your doctor or pharmacist.

Comments: Do not use this product to treat chronic coughs, such as from smoking or asthma. • Do not use this product to treat productive (hacking) coughs that produce phlegm. • If you require an expectorant, you need more moisture in your environment. Drink eight to ten glasses of water daily. The use of a vaporizer or humidifier may also be beneficial. Consult your doctor.

Tylaprin analgesic (H. R. Cenci Laboratories, Inc.), see Tylenol with Codeine analgesic.

OTC   Tylenol analgesic

Manufacturer: McNeil Consumer Products Company
Ingredient: acetaminophen
Dosage Forms: Chewable tablet: acetaminophen, 80 mg. Drop (content per 0.6 ml, or one dropperful): acetaminophen, 60 mg. Elixir (content per 5 ml, or one teaspoon): acetaminophen, 120 mg. Tablet: acetaminophen, 325 mg
Use: Relief of pain of headache, toothache, sprains, muscular aches, nerve inflammation, menstruation; relief of discomforts and fever following immunizations or of colds or "flu"; temporary relief of minor aches and pains of arthritis and rheumatism
Side Effects: When taken in overdose: blood disorders, rash
Warnings: When taken in overdose, this product is more toxic than aspirin. The dosage instructions listed on the package should be followed carefully; toxicity may occur in adults or children with repeated doses.
Comments: The chewable tablets, drops, and elixir forms of this product are intended for use by children. • The drops and elixir forms are 7 percent alcohol.

OTC   Tylenol Extra Strength analgesic

Manufacturer: McNeil Consumer Products Company
Ingredient: acetaminophen
Dosage Forms: Capsule; tablet: acetaminophen, 500 mg. Liquid (content per 15 ml, or one tablespoon): acetaminophen, 500 mg
Use: Relief of pain of headache, toothache, sprains, muscular aches, nerve inflammation, menstruation; relief of discomforts and fever of colds or "flu"; temporary relief of minor aches and pains of arthritis and rheumatism
Side Effects: When taken in overdose: blood disorders, rash
Warnings: When taken in overdose, this product is more toxic than aspirin. The dosage instructions listed on the package should be followed carefully.
Comments: The liquid form of this product is 8½ percent alcohol.

Rx   Tylenol with Codeine analgesic

Manufacturer: McNeil Laboratories
Ingredients: acetaminophen; codeine phosphate
Equivalent Products: Capital with Codeine, Carnrick Laboratories, Inc.; Coastaldyne, Coastal Pharmaceuticals Co., Inc.; Empracet with Codeine, Burroughs Wellcome Co.; Pavadon, Coastal Pharmaceutical Co., Inc.; SK-APAP with Codeine, Smith Kline & French Laboratories; Tylaprin, H. R. Cenci Laboratories, Inc.
Dosage Forms: Liquid (content per 5 ml): acetaminophen, 120 mg; codeine, 12 mg. Tablet (#1, #2, #3, #4): acetaminophen, 300 mg; codeine (see "Comments") (all white)

Use: Symptomatic relief of mild to severe pain, depending on strength

Minor Side Effects: Constipation; drowsiness; dry mouth; flushing; light-headedness; nausea; palpitations; rash; sweating; urine retention; vomiting

Major Side Effects: Breathing difficulties; jaundice; low blood sugar; rapid heartbeat; tremors

Contraindications: This drug should not be taken by people who are allergic to either of its components. Consult your doctor immediately if this drug has been prescribed for you and you have such an allergy.

Warnings: This drug should be used cautiously by the elderly and by people who have asthma or other respiratory problems, epilepsy, head injury, liver or kidney disease, thyroid disease, acute abdominal conditions, prostate disease; and by pregnant women. Be sure your doctor knows if you have any of these conditions. • This drug may cause drowsiness; avoid tasks that require alertness. To prevent oversedation, avoid the use of alcohol or other drugs that have sedative properties. • Because this product contains codeine, it has the potential for abuse and must be used with caution. It usually should not be taken for more than ten days. Tolerance may develop quickly, but do not increase the dose without consulting your doctor.

Comments: The name of this drug is followed by a number that refers to the amount of codeine present (e.g., Tylenol with Codeine #1). Hence, #1 contains 1/8 grain (gr) codeine; #2 has 1/4 gr; #3 has 1/2 gr; and #4 contains 1 gr codeine. • Phenaphen with Codeine analgesic (A. H. Robins Company) differs from the products listed above only in the amount of acetaminophen it contains.

Ultimox antibiotic (Parke-Davis), see amoxicillin antibiotic.

OTC   Unicap M multivitamin and mineral supplement

Manufacturer: The Upjohn Company

Ingredients: vitamin A; vitamin D; vitamin E; vitamin C; folic acid; thiamine; riboflavin; niacin; vitamin B_6; vitamin B_{12}; pantothenic acid; iodine; iron; copper; zinc; manganese; potassium

Dosage Form: Tablet: vitamin A, 5000 IU; vitamin D, 400 IU; vitamin E, 15 IU; vitamin C, 60 mg; folic acid, 0.4 mg; thiamine, 1.5 mg; riboflavin, 1.7 mg; niacin, 20 mg; vitamin B_6, 2 mg; vitamin B_{12}, 6 mcg; pantothenic acid, 10 mg; iodine, 150 mcg; iron, 18 mg; copper, 2 mg; zinc, 15 mg; manganese, 1 mg; potassium, 5 mg

Use: Dietary supplement

Side Effects: Constipation; diarrhea; nausea; stomach pain

Contraindications: This product should not be used by persons who have active peptic ulcer or ulcerative colitis.

Warnings: The minerals in this product interact with oral tetracycline antibiotics and reduce the absorption of the antibiotics. If you are currently taking tetracycline, consult your doctor or pharmacist before taking this product. If you are unsure of the type or contents of your medications, ask your doctor or pharmacist. • Alcoholics and persons who have chronic liver or pancreatic disease should use this product with special caution; such persons may have enhanced iron absorption and are therefore more likely than others to experience iron toxicity. • Accidental iron poisoning is common in children; be sure to keep this product safely out of their reach. • This product contains ingredients that accumulate and are stored in the body. The recommended dose should not be exceeded for long periods (several weeks to months) except by doctor's orders.

Comments: Because of its iron content, this product may cause constipation, diarrhea, nausea, or stomach pain. These symptoms usually disappear or become less severe after two to three days. Taking your dose with food or milk may help minimize these side effects. If they persist, ask your pharmacist to recommend another product. • Black, tarry stools are a normal consequence of iron therapy. If your stools are not black and tarry, this product may not be working for you. Ask your pharmacist to recommend another product. • If large doses are taken, this product may interfere with the results of urine tests. Inform your doctor and pharmacist you are taking this product.

OTC Unicap multivitamin

Manufacturer: The Upjohn Company

Ingredients: vitamin A; vitamin D; vitamin E; vitamin C; folic acid; thiamine; riboflavin; niacin; vitamin B_6; vitamin B_{12}

Dosage Forms: Capsule; Chewable tablet; Tablet: vitamin A, 5000 IU; vitamin D, 400 IU; vitamin E, 15 IU; vitamin C, 60 mg; folic acid, 0.4 mg; thiamine, 1.5 mg; riboflavin, 1.7 mg; niacin, 20 mg; vitamin B_6, 2 mg; vitamin B_{12}, 6 mcg

Use: Dietary supplement

Warnings: This product contains ingredients that accumulate and are stored in the body. The recommended dose should not be exceeded for long periods (several weeks to months) except by doctor's orders.

Comments: If large doses are taken, this product may interfere with the results of urine tests. Inform your doctor and pharmacist you are taking this product. • Chewable tablets should never be referred to as "candy" or as "candy-flavored" vitamins. Your child may take you literally and swallow toxic amounts.

OTC Unicap T multivitamin and mineral supplement

Manufacturer: The Upjohn Company

Ingredients: vitamin A; vitamin D; vitamin E; vitamin C; folic acid; thiamine; riboflavin; niacin; vitamin B_6; vitamin B_{12}; pantothenic acid; iodine; iron; copper; zinc; manganese; potassium

Dosage Form: Tablet: vitamin A, 5000 IU; vitamin D, 400 IU; vitamin E, 15 IU; vitamin C, 300 mg; folic acid, 0.4 mg; thiamine, 10 mg; riboflavin, 10 mg; niacin, 100 mg; vitamin B_6, 6 mg; vitamin B_{12}, 18 mcg; pantothenic acid, 10 mg; iodine, 150 mcg; iron, 18 mg; copper, 2 mg; zinc, 15 mg; manganese, 1 mg; potassium, 5 mg

Use: Dietary supplement

Side Effects: Constipation; diarrhea; nausea; stomach pain

Contraindications: This product should not be used by persons who have active peptic ulcer or ulcerative colitis.

Warnings: The minerals in this product interact with oral tetracycline antibiotics and reduce the absorption of the antibiotics. If you are currently taking tetracycline, consult your doctor or pharmacist before taking this product. If you are unsure of the type or contents of your medications, ask your doctor or pharmacist. • Alcoholics and persons who have chronic liver or pancreatic disease should use this product with special caution; such persons may have enhanced iron absorption and are therefore more likely than others to experience iron toxicity. • Accidental iron poisoning is common in children; be sure to keep this product safely out of their reach. • This product contains vitamin B_6 in an amount great enough that it may interact with levodopa (L-dopa). If you are currently taking L-dopa, check with your doctor before taking this product. • This product contains ingredients that accumulate and are stored in the body. The recommended dose should not be exceeded for long periods (several weeks to months) except by doctor's orders.

Comments: Because of its iron content, this product may cause constipation, diarrhea, nausea, or stomach pain. These symptoms usually disappear or become less severe after two to three days. Taking your dose with food or milk may help minimize these side effects. If they persist, ask your pharmacist to recommend another product. • Black, tarry stools are a normal consequence of iron therapy. If your stools are not black and tarry, this product may not be working for you. Ask your pharmacist to recommend another product. • If two or more tablets are taken daily, this product may interfere with the results of urine tests. Inform your doctor and pharmacist you are taking this product.

Unipres diuretic and antihypertensive (Reid-Provident Laboratories, Inc.), see Ser-Ap-ES diuretic and antihypertensive.

OTC   Unisom Nightime sleep aid

Manufacturer: Leeming Division
Ingredients: doxylamine succinate
Dosage Form: Tablet: doxylamine succinate, 25 mg
Use: Gentle relaxant to help induce sleep
Side Effects: Blurred vision; confusion; constipation; diarrhea, difficult urination; dizziness; drowsiness; dry mouth; headache; insomnia; low blood pressure; nasal congestion; nausea; nervousness; palpitations; rash; rash from exposure to sunlight; reduced sweating; restlessness; severe abdominal cramping; sore throat; vomiting
Contraindications: Persons with asthma, certain types of glaucoma, certain types of peptic ulcer, enlarged prostate, obstructed bladder, obstructed intestine, and pregnant and nursing women should not take this medication.
Warnings: If you are currently taking another medication or wish to take any nonprescription drug for cough, cold, or sinus problems do not take this product without first checking with your doctor.
Comments: This product interacts with alcohol; avoid the use of alcohol or other central nervous system sedatives while taking this product. • This product may cause dryness of the mouth. To reduce this feeling, chew gum or suck on ice chips or a piece of hard candy. • The elderly are more likely to suffer side effects when taking this product than other people. Children taking this product may become restless and excited. • There is probably no reason to purchase this item. Try to find and correct the cause of your insomnia. A warm glass of milk and a soak in a hot tub may do as much good as this product. • Do not take this product for longer than two weeks without consulting your doctor.

Uri-Tet antibiotic (American Urologicals, Inc.), see Terramycin antibiotic.

Urodine analgesic (Robinson Laboratory, Inc.), see Pyridium analgesic.

Uticillin VK antibiotic (The Upjohn Company), see penicillin potassium phenoxymethyl antibiotic.

Valdrene antihistamine (The Vale Chemical Co., Inc.), see Benadryl antihistamine.

Rx   Valisone steroid hormone

Manufacturer: Schering Corporation
Ingredient: betamethasone valerate
Dosage Forms: Aerosol spray: 0.15%. Cream: 0.01%, 0.1%. Lotion: 0.1%. Ointment: 0.1%

Use: Relief of skin inflammation associated with conditions such as dermatitis, eczema, or poison ivy

Minor Side Effects: Burning sensation; dryness; irritation of the affected area; itching; rash

Major Side Effects: Secondary infection

Contraindications: This drug should not be used by people who are allergic to it. Consult your doctor immediately if this drug has been prescribed for you and you have such an allergy.

Warnings: If irritation develops when using this drug, immediately discontinue its use and notify your doctor. • This drug should be used with caution during pregnancy. • These products are not for use in the eyes or other mucous membranes. • Systemic absorption of this drug will be increased if extensive areas of the body are treated, particularly if occlusive bandages are used. Therefore, suitable precautions should be taken under this circumstance and under long-term use, particularly in children and infants.

Comments: When the spray is used about the face, cover the eyes and do not inhale the spray; inhalation of spray can prove fatal. • The spray produces a cooling response which may be uncomfortable for some people. • The spray form is packed under pressure. Do not puncture the container or store near heat or open flame. • When using the spray form, avoid freezing of the tissue by not spraying for more than three seconds, and by spraying at a distance of not less than six inches. • If the affected area is extremely dry or is scaling, the skin may be moistened before applying the medication by soaking in water or by applying water with a clean cloth. The ointment form is probably better for dry skin. • Do not use this product with an occlusive wrap unless your doctor directs you to do so. If it is necessary for you to use this drug under a wrap, follow your doctor's instructions exactly; do not leave the wrap in place longer than specified.

℞ Valium sedative and hypnotic

Manufacturer: Roche Products Inc.

Ingredient: diazepam

Dosage Form: Tablet: 2 mg (white); 5 mg (yellow); 10 mg (blue)

Use: Relief of anxiety, nervousness, tension; relief of muscle spasms; withdrawal from alcohol addiction

Minor Side Effects: Confusion; constipation; depression; difficult urination; dizziness; drowsiness; dry mouth; fatigue; headache; nausea; rash; slurred speech; uncoordinated movements

Major Side Effects: Blurred vision; decreased sexual drive; double vision; jaundice; low blood pressure; stimulation; tremors

Contraindications: This drug should not be given to children under six months of age. This drug should not be taken by persons with certain types of glaucoma. This drug should not be taken by people who are allergic to it. Consult your doctor immediately if this drug has been prescribed for you and you have glaucoma or such an allergy.

Warnings: This drug is not of value in the treatment of persons with psychoses. • This drug may cause drowsiness; avoid tasks requiring alertness, such as driving a motor vehicle or operating machinery. • Use of this drug may worsen seizures in persons with grand mal epilepsy. Abrupt withdrawal of this drug may also temporarily increase the frequency and/or the severity of seizures. • This drug should not be taken simultaneously with alcohol, or other central nervous system depressants. Taken alone, this drug is safe; when it is combined with alcohol or other sedative drugs, serious adverse reactions may develop. • Use of this drug may cause physical and psychological dependence, similar to that which is noted with alcohol and barbiturates. Do not stop taking this drug without informing your doctor. If you have been taking the drug regularly, and wish to discontinue the drug's use, you must decrease the dose gradually, following your doctor's instructions. This drug has the potential for abuse and must be used with caution. Tolerance may develop quickly; do not increase the dose without first consulting your doctor. • This drug should be used with caution in pregnant women, especially during the first trimester, and in the elderly and debilitated patients. • Persons taking this drug should have periodic blood counts and liver function tests. • This drug should be used cautiously in persons with impaired liver or kidney function. Be sure your doctor knows if you have either of these conditions.

Comments: This drug currently is used by many people to relieve nervousness. It is effective for this purpose, but it is important to try to remove the cause of the anxiety as well. Phenobarbital is also effective for this purpose, and it is less expensive. Consult your doctor. • This drug may cause dryness of the mouth. To reduce this feeling, chew gum or suck on ice chips or a piece of hard candy.

R̥   **Vanceril anti-asthmatic**

Manufacturer: Schering Corporation
Ingredient: beclomethasone dipropionate
Dosage Form: Pressurized inhaler for oral use (content per one actuation from mouthpiece): 42 mcg
Use: Treatment of chronic asthma
Minor Side Effects: Dry mouth; bronchospasm; hoarseness; rash
Major Side Effects: Suppression of function of hypothalamus, pituitary, and adrenal glands on overdose
Contraindications: This drug should not be used in the primary treatment of static asthmaticus or other acute episodes of asthma where intensive measures are required. • This drug should not be used for treating asthma that is controlled by other drugs. It should also not be used by people who must take oral steroid drugs frequently. • This drug should not be used by people who are allergic to it. Consult your doctor immediately if this drug has been prescribed for you and you have such an allergy or fit into any of these categories.
Warnings: This drug should be used with caution in patients withdrawing from oral steroids. This drug should be used with caution if long-term need for the drug is indicated. Pregnant women, nursing mothers, and women of child-bearing age should use this drug with caution. Consult your doctor immediately if this drug has been prescribed for you and you fit into any of these categories. • This drug is not to be regarded as a bronchodilator and is not indicated for rapid relief of bronchospasm. • This drug should be used cautiously in children under the age of six. • The dosage of this drug should be monitored very carefully. • The use of this drug may have to be discontinued if localized infections occur.
Comments: The contents of one canister of this drug should provide at least 200 oral inhalations. • This drug is sealed in the canister under pressure. Do not puncture the canister. Do not store the canister near heat or an open flame. • Rinsing the mouth after inhalation of this drug is advised.

Van-Mox antibiotic (Vangard Laboratories), see amoxicillin antibiotic.

OTC   **Vanoxide acne preparation**

Manufacturer: Dermik Laboratories, Inc.
Ingredients: benzoyl peroxide; chlorhydroxyquinoline
Dosage Form: Lotion: benzoyl peroxide, 5%; chlorhydroxyquinoline, 0.25%

Use: Treatment of acne
Side Effects: Allergy; local irritation
Contraindications: Persons having known hypersensitivity to benzoyl peroxide or chlorhydroxyquinoline should not use this product.
Warnings: Do not get product in or near the eyes. • Harsh, abrasive cleaners should not be used simultaneously with lotion.
Comments: If condition worsens, stop using this product and call your pharmacist. • This acne preparation may be especially active on fair-skinned people. • Wash area gently with warm water and pat dry before applying this product. • Avoid exposure to heat lamps, sunlamps, or direct sunlight when using these acne preparations. • This product may damage certain fabrics including rayon. • There may be a slight, transitory stinging or burning sensation on initial application of product. • Reduce the amount and frequency of use if excessive redness or peeling occurs.

OTC   Vanquish analgesic

Manufacturer: Glenbrook Laboratories
Ingredients: aspirin; acetaminophen; caffeine; dried aluminum hydroxide gel; magnesium hydroxide
Dosage Form: Caplet: aspirin, 227 mg (3½ grains); acetaminophen, 194 mg; caffeine, 33 mg; dried aluminum hydroxide gel, 25 mg; magnesium hydroxide, 50 mg
Use: Relief of pain of headache, toothache, sprains, muscular aches, nerve inflammation, menstruation; relief of discomforts and fever of colds or "flu"; temporary relief of minor aches and pains of arthritis and rheumatism
Side Effects: Dizziness; mental confusion; nausea and vomiting; ringing in the ears; slight blood loss; sweating
Contraindications: This product may cause an increased bleeding tendency and should not be taken by persons with a history of bleeding, peptic ulcer, or stomach bleeding.
Warnings: Persons with kidney disease, asthma, hay fever, or other allergies should be extremely careful about using this product. The product may interfere with the treatment of gout. If you have any of these conditions, consult your doctor or pharmacist before using this medication. • Do not use this product if you are currently taking alcohol, methotrexate, oral anticoagulants, oral antidiabetics, probenecid, steroids, and/or sulfinpyrazone; if you are unsure of the type or contents of your medications, ask your doctor or pharmacist. • When taken in overdose, this product is more toxic than plain aspirin. The dosage instructions should be followed carefully.
Comments: Magnesium interacts with tetracycline antibiotics. There may not be enough magnesium in this product to cause any problem, but if you are taking a tetracycline antibiotic in addition to this product, separate the dosages by at least two hours. • Pain-relief tablets, such as this product, that contain salts of magnesium or aluminum are known as buffered tablets. Such products dissolve faster than unbuffered products, but there is no evidence that they relieve pain faster or better than those products that do not contain buffers. Buffered tablets may be less likely to cause gastric upset in some people. • There is no evidence that combinations of ingredients are more effective than similar doses of a single-ingredient product. The caffeine in this product may have a slight stimulant effect but has no pain-relieving value.

Vasal Granucaps smooth muscle relaxant (Tutag Pharmaceuticals, Inc.), see Pavabid Plateau Caps smooth muscle relaxant.

616

OTC   **Vaseline Hemorr-Aid hemorrhoid remedy**

Manufacturer: Cheesebrough-Pond's Inc.
Ingredients: Specially formulated highly refined white petrolatum
Dosage Form: Ointment
Use: Relief of pain, burning, and itching of hemorrhoids
Warnings: Sensitization (continued itching and redness) may occur with long-term and repeated use.
Comments: Hemorrhoidal (pile) preparations relieve itching, reduce pain and inflammation, and check bleeding, but do not heal, dry up, or give lasting relief from the hemorrhoids. • Never self-medicate for hemorrhoids if pain is continuous or throbbing, if bleeding or itching is excessive, or if you feel a large pressure within the rectum. • It is doubtful that this product is worth the money since is it basically similar to the lower-priced Vaseline petroleum jelly.

Vaseline petrolatum gauze (Chesebrough-Pond's Inc.), see Vaseline petroleum jelly.

OTC   **Vaseline petroleum jelly**

Manufacturer: Chesebrough-Pond's Inc.
Ingredient: petroleum jelly
Dosage Form: Gel
Use: To soothe minor skin irritations such as burns, scrapes, or chapped skin; to help prevent diaper rash
Comments: This product is not intended for use on puncture wounds, serious burns, or cuts. • A related product made by Chesebrough-Pond's Inc. is Vaseline petrolatum gauze, an absorbent gauze saturated with white petrolatum. It is applied directly to the skin as a protective dressing.

Vasocap-150 smooth muscle relaxant (Keene Pharmaceuticals, Inc.), see Pavabid Plateau Caps smooth muscle relaxant.

℞   **Vasodilan vasodilator**

Manufacturer: Mead Johnson Pharmaceutical Division
Ingredient: isoxsuprine hydrochloride
Equivalent Products: isoxsuprine hydrochloride, various manufacturers; Vasoprine, Spencer-Mead, Inc.
Dosage Form: Tablet: 10 mg; 20 mg (both white)
Use: To increase blood supply to the extremities; to relieve symptoms associated with cerebrovascular insufficiency
Minor Side Effects: Dizziness; nausea; vomiting
Major Side Effects: Palpitations; severe rash
Comments: This drug is effective in increasing the flow of blood to the brain and other areas of the body, but the benefits of this action have not been established. Discuss the relative merits of the drug with your doctor.

Vasoglyn Unicelles antianginal (Reid-Provident Laboratories, Inc.), see Nitro-Bid Plateau Caps antianginal.

Vasoprine vasodilator (Spencer-Mead, Inc.), see Vasodilan vasodilator.

Vasospan smooth muscle relaxant (Ulmer Pharmacal Co.), see Pavabid Plateau Caps smooth muscle relaxant.

Vasotrate antianginal (Reid-Provident Laboratories, Inc.), see Isordil antianginal.

V-Cillin K antibiotic (Eli Lilly and Company), see penicillin potassium phenoxymethyl antibiotic.

Vectrin antibiotic (Parke-Davis), see Minocin antibiotic.

Veetids '250' antibiotic (E. R. Squibb & Sons, Inc.), see penicillin potassium phenoxymethyl antibiotic.

OTC — Vergo wart remover

Manufacturer: Daywell Laboratories Corporation
Ingredients: ascorbic acid; calcium pantothenate; starch
Dosage Form: Ointment (quantities of ingredients not specified)
Use: Removal of common warts
Side Effects: Local irritation
Contraindications: Do not use this product if you have diabetes or poor circulation unless directed to do so by your doctor.
Warnings: Use externally only. • Do not apply wart remover to mucous membranes. Avoid contact with skin around the wart.
Comments: Do not use this product for more than one week. If the condition worsens, stop using wart remover and call your pharmacist. • After applying product, wash your hands thoroughly.

Rx — Vibramycin antibiotic

Manufacturer: Pfizer Laboratories Division
Ingredient: doxycycline
Equivalent Products: Doxy-II, USV (P.R.) Development Corp.; Doxychel, Rachelle Laboratories, Inc.
Dosage Forms: Capsule: 50 mg (blue/white); 100 mg (blue). Suspension (content per 5 ml): 25 mg. Syrup (content per 5 ml): 50 mg
Use: Treatment of a wide variety of bacterial infections
Minor Side Effects: Diarrhea; increased sensitivity to light; loss of appetite; nausea; vomiting
Major Side Effects: Anemia; "black tongue," mouth irritation; rash; sore throat; rectal and vaginal itching; superinfection
Contraindications: This drug should not be taken by people who are allergic to any tetracycline drug. Consult your doctor immediately if this drug has been prescribed for you and you have such an allergy.
Warnings: This drug may cause permanent discoloration of the teeth if used during tooth development; therefore, it should be used cautiously by pregnant or nursing women and infants and children under nine years of age. • This drug interacts with antacids, barbiturates, carbamazepine, diuretics, iron-containing products, penicillin, and phenytoin; if you are currently taking any drugs of these types, consult your doctor about their use. If you are unsure of the type or contents of your medications, ask your doctor or pharmacist. Do not take this drug at the same time as any iron preparation or antacid; their use should be separated by at least two hours. • This drug may cause you to be especially sensitive to the sun, so avoid exposure to sunlight as much as possible. • This drug may affect syphilis tests; if you are being treated for this disease, make sure that your doctor knows you are taking this drug. • If you are taking an anticoagulant in addition to this drug, remind your doctor. • Do not increase the dose of this drug unless instructed to do so by your doctor.

Comments: Try to take this drug on an empty stomach (one hour before or two hours after a meal). If the drug upsets your stomach, you may take your dose with food. • When used to treat strep throat, this drug should be taken for at least ten full days, even if symptoms disappear within that time.

OTC   Vicks cough remedy

Manufacturer: Vicks Health Care Division
Ingredients: dextromethorphan hydrobromide; guaifenesin; sodium citrate; alcohol
Dosage Form: Liquid (content per 15 ml, or one tablespoon): dextromethorphan hydrobromide, 10.5 mg; guaifenesin, 75 mg; sodium citrate, 600 mg; alcohol, 5%
Use: Temporary relief of cough due to colds or "flu"; also to convert a dry, nonproductive cough to a productive, phlegm-producing cough
Side Effects: Drowsiness; nausea; vomiting
Contraindications: Do not give this product to children under two years of age unless directed otherwise by your doctor.
Warnings: This product interacts with monoamine oxidase inhibitors; if you are currently taking any drugs of this type, check with your doctor before taking this product. If you are unsure of the type or contents of your medications, ask your doctor or pharmacist.
Comments: Do not use this product to treat chronic coughs, such as those from smoking or asthma. • Do not use this product to treat productive (hacking) coughs that produce phlegm. • If you require an expectorant, you need more moisture in your environment. Drink eight to ten glasses of water daily. The use of a vaporizer or humidifier may also be beneficial. Consult your doctor.

OTC   Vicks Inhaler nasal decongestant

Manufacturer: Vicks Health Care Division
Ingredients: levodesoxyephedrine; menthol; camphor; methyl salicylate; bornyl acetate
Dosage Form: Inhaler: levodesoxyephedrine, 50 mg; menthol, camphor, methyl salicylate, bornyl acetate, 150 mg total
Use: Temporary relief of nasal congestion due to colds, sinusitis, hay fever, or other upper respiratory allergies
Side Effects: Blurred vision; burning, dryness of nasal mucosa, increased nasal congestion or discharge, sneezing, and/or stinging; dizziness; drowsiness; headache; insomnia; nervousness; palpitations; slight increase in blood pressure; stimulation
Contraindications: This product should not be used by persons who have glaucoma (certain types).
Warnings: This product should be used with special caution by persons who have diabetes, advanced hardening of the arteries, heart disease, high blood pressure, or thyroid disease. If you have any of these conditions, consult your doctor before taking this product. • This product interacts with monoamine oxidase inhibitors, thyroid preparations, and tricyclic antidepressants. If you are currently taking any drugs of these types, check with your doctor before taking this product. If you are unsure of the type or contents of your medications, ask your doctor or pharmacist. • To avoid side effects such as burning, sneezing, or stinging, and a "rebound" increase in nasal congestion and discharge, do not exceed the recommended dosage and do not use this product for more than three or four continuous days. • This product should not be used by more than one person; sharing the dispenser may spread infection.

OTC　　　　**Vicks Vaporub external analgesic**

Manufacturer: Vicks Health Care Division
Ingredients: camphor; cedar leaf oil; eucalyptus oil; menthol; myristica oil; thymol; turpentine spirits
Dosage Form: Ointment: camphor, cedar leaf oil, eucalyptus oil, menthol, myristica oil, thymol, turpentine spirits, 14% in petrolatum base
Use: Temporary relief of pain in muscles and muscular tightness
Side Effects: Allergic reactions (rash, itching, soreness); local irritation; local numbness
Warnings: Use this product externally only. • Do not use on broken or irritated skin or on large areas of the body; avoid contact with eyes.
Comments: To relieve muscle tightness apply a hot, moist towel to affected area. Remove the towel and massage well with this ointment. • This product is traditionally rubbed on children's chests for colds. There is little objective evidence, however, to support this use.

℞　Vioform-Hydrocortisone steroid hormone and anti-infective

Manufacturer: CIBA Pharmaceutical Company
Ingredients: hydrocortisone; iodochlorhydroxyquin
Equivalent Products: Cortin, C & M Pharmacal, Inc.; Domeform-HC, Dome Division; Formtone-HC, Dermik Laboratories, Inc.; HCV, Saron Pharmacal Corp.; Heb-Cort, Barnes-Hind Pharmaceuticals, Inc.; Hexaderm I.Q., Amfre-Grant, Inc.; Hydroquin, Robinson Laboratory, Inc.; Hysone, Mallard Incorporated; Iodocort, Ulmer Pharmacal Company; Mity-Quin, Reid-Provident Laboratories, Inc.; Racet, Lemmon Company; Vioquin-HC, Scott-Alison Pharmaceuticals, Inc.; Viotag, Tutag Pharmaceuticals, Inc.
Dosage Forms: Cream; Ointment: hydrocortisone, 1%, 0.5%; iodochlorhydroxyquin, 3%
Use: Symptomatic relief of skin inflammation associated with such conditions as dermatitis, eczema
Minor Side Effects: Burning sensation; irritation of affected area; itching (all rare)
Major Side Effects: Secondary infection
Contraindications: This drug should not be used by people who are allergic to any of its components or to related compounds. The drug should not be used by people who have eye damage, tuberculosis of the skin, or viral skin disease. Consult your doctor immediately if this drug has been prescribed for you and you have any of these conditions.
Warnings: This drug should be used cautiously in or around the eyes. • Notify your doctor if irritation develops. • If it is necessary for you to use this drug under a wrap, follow your doctor's instructions exactly; do not leave the wrap in place longer than specified. Do not use a wrap unless directed to do so by your doctor. • This product may affect the results of thyroid function tests; if you are scheduled to have such a test, be sure your doctor knows that you are using this drug.
Comments: Apply this product as thinly as possible to the skin. • The cream form of this drug is better than the ointment for use on the scalp or other hairy areas of the body. • The ointment form of the drug is preferable for people with dry skin. • If the affected area is extremely dry or is scaling, the skin may be moistened before applying the medication by soaking in water or by applying water with a clean cloth.

Vioquin-HC steroid hormone and anti-infective (Scott-Alison Pharmaceuticals, Inc.), see Vioform-Hydrocortisone steroid hormone and anti-infective.

Vio-Serpine antihypertensive (Rowell Laboratories, Inc.), see reserpine antihypertensive.

Viotag steroid hormone and anti-infective (Tutag Pharmaceuticals, Inc.), see Vioform-Hydrocortisone steroid hormone and anti-infective.

OTC   Viro-Med cold remedy

Manufacturer: Whitehall Laboratories
Ingredients: acetaminophen; pseudoephedrine hydrochloride; dextromethorphan hydrobromide; sodium citrate; alcohol
Dosage Form: Liquid (content per fluid ounce, or two tablespoons): acetaminophen, 648 mg; pseudoephedrine hydrochloride, 30 mg; dextromethorphan hydrobromide, 20 mg; sodium citrate, 500 mg; alcohol, 16.63%
Use: Temporary relief of nasal congestion, fever, coughing, aches, pains, and general discomfort due to colds or "flu"
Side Effects: Mild to moderate stimulation; nausea; vomiting
Warnings: This product should be used with special caution by persons who have diabetes, heart disease, high blood pressure, or thyroid disease. If you have any of these conditions, consult your doctor before taking this product. • This product interacts with alcohol, guanethidine, monoamine oxidase inhibitors, sedative drugs, and tricyclic antidepressants. If you are currently taking any drugs of these types, check with your doctor before taking this product. If you are unsure of the type or contents of your medications, ask your doctor or pharmacist. • When taken in overdose, acetaminophen is more toxic than aspirin. Follow dosage instructions carefully.
Comments: Many other conditions (some serious) mimic the common cold. If symptoms persist beyond one week or if they occur regularly without regard to season, consult your doctor. • The effectiveness of this product may diminish after being taken regularly for seven to ten days; consult your pharmacist about substituting another medication if this product begins to lose its effectiveness for you.

OTC   Viro-Med cold remedy (tablet)

Manufacturer: Whitehall Laboratories
Ingredients: aspirin; chlorpheniramine maleate; pseudoephedrine hydrochloride; dextromethorphan hydrobromide; guaifenesin
Dosage Form: Tablet: aspirin, 324 mg (5 grains); chlorpheniramine maleate, 1 mg; pseudoephedrine hydrochloride, 15 mg; dextromethorphan hydrobromide, 7.5 mg; guaifenesin, 50 mg
Use: Temporary relief of nasal congestion, fever, coughing, aches, pains, and general discomfort due to colds or "flu'
Side Effects: Anxiety; blurred vision; chest pain; confusion; constipation; difficult and painful urination; dizziness; drowsiness; headache; increased blood pressure; insomnia; loss of appetite; nausea; nervousness; palpitations; rash; reduced sweating; ringing in the ears; slight blood loss; tension; tremor; vomiting
Contraindications: This product should not be used by persons who have allergies, aspirin sensitivity, asthma, blood-clotting disease, gout, severe heart disease, severe high blood pressure, or vitamin-K deficiency. • This product should not be given to newborn or premature infants.
Warnings: This product should be used with special caution by the elderly or debilitated, and by persons who have diabetes, enlarged prostate, glaucoma (certain types), heart disease, high blood pressure, kidney disease, obstructed bladder, obstructed intestine, peptic ulcer, or thyroid disease. If you have any of these conditions, consult your doctor before taking this prod-

uct. • This product may cause drowsiness. Do not take it if you must drive, operate heavy machinery, or perform other tasks requiring mental alertness. To prevent oversedation, avoid the use of alcohol or other drugs that have sedative properties. • This product interacts with alcohol, ammonium chloride, guanethidine, methotrexate, monoamine oxidase inhibitors, oral anticoagulants, oral antidiabetics, probenecid, sedative drugs, steroids, sulfinpyrazone, tricyclic antidepressants, and vitamin C. If you are currently taking any drugs of these types, check with your doctor before taking this product. If you are unsure of the type or contents of your medications, ask your doctor or pharmacist. • Because this product reduces sweating, avoid excessive work or exercise in hot weather.

Comments: Many other conditions (some serious) mimic the common cold. If symptoms persist beyond one week or if they occur regularly without regard to season, consult your doctor. • The effectiveness of this product may diminish after being taken regularly for seven to ten days; consult your pharmacist about substituting another product containing a different antihistamine if this product begins to lose its effectiveness for you. • Chew gum or suck on ice chips or a piece of hard candy to reduce mouth dryness.

OTC   Visine decongestant eyedrops

Manufacturer: Leeming Division
Ingredients: benzalkonium chloride; boric acid; disodium ethylene diamine tetraacetate; sodium borate; sodium chloride; tetrahydrozoline hydrochloride
Dosage Form: Drop: benzalkonium chloride, 0.01%; disodium ethylene diamine tetraacetate, 0.1%; tetrahydrozoline hydrochloride, 0.05% (quantities of other ingredients not specified)
Use: Relief of minor eye irritation
Side Effects: Allergic reactions (rash, itching, soreness); local irritation; momentary blurred vision
Contraindications: Do not use this product if you have glaucoma.
Warnings: Do not use this product for more than two consecutive days without checking with your doctor.
Comments: Use this product only for minor eye irritations. • A child who accidentally swallows this product is likely to become overstimulated. Call your doctor at once. • Do not touch the dropper or bottle top to the eye or other tissue because contamination of the solution will result. • This product contains boric acid which many medical authorities believe should not be used because it is toxic. Follow the directions on package. • The use of more than one eye product at a time may cause severe irritation to the eye. Consult your pharmacist before doing so.

Vistaril sedative (Pfizer Laboratories Division), see Atarax sedative.

OTC   vitamin A (retinol)

Manufacturer: various manufacturers
Ingredient: vitamin A
Dosage Forms: Capsule; Tablet: vitamin A is available in various strengths per dose; common strengths are 5000, 10,000, 25,000, and 50,000 IU (international units)
Use: Dietary supplement
Warnings: Large doses of vitamin A can cause loss of appetite and hair; intense headaches; dry, flaky skin; blurred vision; inflamed optic nerve and eye damage; brain or liver damage; and lymph node and spleen enlargement. There is no reason to take vitamin A supplements unless you have a true vitamin-A deficiency, which only your doctor can diagnose. • Always keep

vitamin A supplements out of the reach of children.

Comments: Vitamin A is readily available in liver; yellow-orange fruits and vegetables, dark green leafy vegetables, whole milk, vitamin A-fortified skim milk, butter, and margarine. Many ready-to-eat breakfast cereals are also fortified with vitamin A. • In spite of claims, there is no proof that taking vitamin A supplements will prevent or cure dry or wrinkled skin, respiratory diseases, visual defects, or eye diseases. Oral supplementation is not effective as a treatment for acne, but a topical form of vitamin A, retinoic acid, has been used effectively against acne.

OTC   vitamin B₁ (thiamine)

Manufacturer: various manufacturers
Ingredient: vitamin B₁
Dosage Forms: Liquid; Tablet: vitamin B₁ is available in various strengths per dose; common strengths are 5, 10, 25, 50, 100, 250, and 500 mg
Use: Dietary supplement
Comments: Vitamin B₁ is present in tiny amounts in most foods. Enriched and whole-grain cereal products, and meat, especially pork, are good sources of the vitamin. An ordinary mixed diet is sufficient to prevent severe deficiency of vitamin B₁, and severe deficiency of this vitamin rarely occurs in the Western world nowadays. A subclinical deficiency—occurring when the amount of vitamin B₁ in the diet is barely adequate—could occur, however, with a less-than-well-balanced diet. A subclinical deficiency does not produce symptoms, but can be confirmed by blood or urine tests. • There is some evidence that if you require vitamin B₁ supplementation you will also need supplements of other B vitamins. Therefore, there is probably no reason to take plain vitamin B₁ supplements unless your doctor specifically prescribes it for vitamin B₁ deficiency (beriberi)—a disease that only he or she can diagnose. • In spite of claims, there is no proof that taking supplements of vitamin B₁ will give you increased energy, stimulate your appetite, or reduce fatigue, nor will it be effective in the prevention or treatment of dermatitis, multiple sclerosis, neuritis, or mental disorders.

OTC   vitamin B₂ (riboflavin)

Manufacturer: various manufacturers
Ingredient: vitamin B₂
Dosage Form: Tablet: vitamin B₂ is available in various strengths, commonly 5, 10, 25, 50, and 100 mg
Use: Dietary supplement
Comments: Vitamin B₂ is readily available in milk and dairy products, meats, green leafy vegetables, and in enriched bread and cereal products. Most Americans get sufficient vitamin B₂ in their diets to prevent deficiency without the use of supplementation via tablets. A medical examination is required to determine the existence of a B vitamin deficiency, and there is some evidence that if you require vitamin B₂ supplementation you will also need supplements of the other B vitamins. Therefore, there is probably no reason to take plain vitamin B₂ supplements unless your doctor specifically prescribes it for a deficiency state that only he or she can diagnose. • In spite of claims, there is no proof that taking large amounts of B vitamins will prevent or cure various diseases such as glaucoma, cataracts, night blindness, diabetes, peptic ulcer, or vaginitis, nor will it relieve stress. • If you take large doses of vitamin B₂, your urine may become bright yellow in color.

OTC   vitamin B₆ (pyridoxine)

Manufacturer: various manufacturers

Ingredient: vitamin B₆

Dosage Forms: Tablet; Timed-release capsule: vitamin B₆ is available in various strengths per dose; common strengths are 5, 10, 25, 50, 100, 200, and 500 mg

Use: Dietary supplement

Warnings: Large doses (200 to 300 mg) of vitamin B₆ taken daily for over a month have produced a temporary dependency, and unpleasant reactions have occurred when dosage was stopped. • Large doses of vitamin B₆ interfere with the drug levodopa (L-dopa), used in the treatment of Parkinson's disease. If you are taking L-dopa, avoid taking vitamin B₆ supplements and do not eat excessive quantities of foods that are rich in the vitamin.

Comments: Vitamin B₆ is found in all foods; bananas, lima beans, meats, potatoes, and whole-grain cereals are especially rich sources. Most Americans get sufficient vitamin B₆ in their diets to prevent deficiency without the use of supplementation via tablets or capsules. A medical examination is required to determine the existence of a B vitamin deficiency, and there is some evidence that if you require vitamin B₆ supplementation you will also need supplements of the other B vitamins. Therefore, there is probably no reason to take plain vitamin B₆ supplements unless your doctor specifically prescribes it for a deficiency state that only he or she can diagnose, or for use in conjunction with the prescription drug isoniazid. (Vitamin B₆ is frequently prescribed with isoniazid to reduce side effects from the latter drug.) • In spite of claims, there is no proof that taking supplements of vitamin B₆ will reduce the morning sickness of pregnancy, nor will it be effective in the prevention or treatment of kidney stones, migraine headaches, or hemorrhoids.

OTC   **vitamin B₁₂ (cyanocobalamin)**

Manufacturer: various manufacturers

Ingredient: vitamin B₁₂

Dosage Forms: Capsule; Tablet: vitamin B₁₂ is available in various strengths per dose; common strengths are 10, 25, 50, 100, and 250 mcg (micrograms)

Use: Dietary supplement

Comments: Dietary deficiencies of vitamin B₁₂ are practically never seen; the body requires only minute amounts daily, and the liver stores small amounts of the vitamin as well. Vitamin B₁₂ is found only in animal foods—meats (especially liver), seafood, egg yolk, and cheese, for example—so strict vegetarians (those who eat no eggs or cheese, and do not drink milk) should supplement their diets with B₁₂. • It is important to note that pernicious anemia, resulting from vitamin B₁₂ deficiency, is not caused by a lack of the vitamin in the diet. People with pernicious anemia suffer from a disease that makes them incapable of absorbing vitamin B₁₂, even though it is present in their diets. Oral supplements of the vitamin will not cure them, because they cannot absorb the supplements, unless another medication is taken at the same time. To effectively treat pernicious anemia, vitamin B₁₂ must be injected. Therefore, there is no reason to take oral vitamin B₁₂ supplements unless you are a strict vegetarian. • In spite of claims, there is no proof that taking supplements of vitamin B₁₂ will give you increased energy or ensure mental health.

OTC   **vitamin C (ascorbic acid)**

Manufacturer: various manufacturers

Ingredient: vitamin C

Dosage Forms: Capsule; Chewable tablet; Drop; Liquid; Tablet; Wafer:

vitamin C is available in various strengths per dose; common strengths are 25, 50, 100, 250, and 500 mg

Use: Dietary supplement

Warnings: The use of megadoses (4 grams or more daily) of vitamin C has been associated with the formation of kidney stones in some people. If you have a predisposition to kidney stones, do not take massive doses of vitamin C. • A few people have complained of abdominal discomfort, cramps, and diarrhea after taking large doses of this vitamin. However, the effects apparently occur in only a small percentage of the people who take megadoses of vitamin C. • If you take massive doses of this vitamin for an extended period of time, you may become conditioned to the increased intake and develop symptoms of vitamin C deficiency (scurvy) if you discontinue or reduce the dosage. • Large doses of vitamin C may counteract the effect of oral anticoagulant drugs and may interfere with urine and blood tests, causing errors in the diagnosis of disease. If you are taking vitamin C, be sure to inform your doctor and pharmacist of the fact. • Vitamin C may interfere with the common over-the-counter urinalysis tests for determining blood glucose levels. If you use these urine-testing products, consult your doctor or pharmacist about your concurrent use of vitamin C.

Comments: Vitamin C is readily available in fruits (especially citrus fruits) and vegetables. Most Americans get sufficient vitamin C in their diets to prevent deficiency without the use of OTC supplements. • Take your dose of vitamin C with at least a full glass of water, and drink eight to ten glasses of water daily. • In spite of claims, there is no proof that taking supplemental vitamin C will prevent colds or reduce their seriousness. Vitamin C is not effective in the treatment of hardening of the arteries, allergies, mental illness, corneal ulcers, blood clots, or pressure sores. • Although the concentration of vitamin C in the blood of smokers is lower than that of nonsmokers, it is still within normal range, and smokers who eat an adequate diet do not need vitamin C supplements.

OTC   vitamin D (calciferol)

Manufacturer: various manufacturers

Ingredient: vitamin D

Dosage Forms: Capsule; Drop; Tablet: vitamin D is available in various strengths per dose; common strengths are 400, 8000, 25,000, and 50,000 IU (international units)

Use: Dietary supplement

Warnings: Excess amounts of vitamin D cause absorption of abnormally large amounts of calcium, which become deposited in body tissues. Irreversible damage to the kidney or lungs may result, or irregular heartbeats and abnormal nervous activity may occur, leading to cardiac arrhythmias and to convulsions and death. Never take a vitamin supplement containing more than 400 IU of vitamin D per dose. • Always keep vitamin D supplements out of the reach of children.

Comments: Although fish liver oils and some fish are the only naturally occurring foods containing significant amounts of vitamin D, many ready-to-eat breakfast cereals and all the milk sold commercially in this country are fortified with vitamin D. Furthermore, humans manufacture their own vitamin D when exposed to direct sunlight or ultraviolet light from a sunlamp. Because of the hazards of vitamin D overdose, there is no reason to take vitamin D supplements unless you have a true vitamin D deficiency, which only your doctor can diagnose. Children and young adults under the age of 22, and pregnant and nursing women should drink three to four glasses of fortified milk daily to meet their requirements for vitamin D; people over the age of 22 (whose bone development is complete) are able to meet their daily requirements by exposure to sunlight. If you are seldom exposed to sunshine by reason of occupation, living habits, or mode of dress, you should probably drink fortified milk regularly to ensure an adequate intake. • In spite of claims, there is no proof that taking supplemental vitamin D will prevent or cure arthritis or nervousness.

OTC   vitamin E (tocopherol)

Manufacturer: various manufacturers
Ingredient: vitamin E
Dosage Forms: Capsule; Chewable tablet; Drop; Liquid: vitamin E is available in various strengths per dose; common strengths are 30, 50, 100, 200, 400, 600, 800, and 1000 IU (international units)
Use: Dietary supplement
Warnings: Some people taking more than 400 IU of vitamin E daily for long periods have suffered nausea, intestinal distress, fatigue, and other flu-like symptoms.
Comments: There is no evidence of even marginal vitamin E deficiency in the American people. Vitamin E is readily available in vegetable and seed oils, and to a lesser extent, in meats, cereal and dairy products, and vegetables. Supplemental vitamin E is advised only when a doctor determines that there is evidence of a deficiency or risk of deficiency in a newborn baby (a circumstance that occasionally occurs, but is easily diagnosed), or in a patient suffering from diseases that inhibit absorption of the vitamin. • In spite of the abundance of claims made for it, there is no proof that vitamin E is effective in the prevention, treatment, or cure of conditions including acne, aging, bee stings, liver spots on the hands, bursitis, diaper rash, frostbite, heart attacks, labor pains, miscarriage, muscular dystrophy, poor posture, sexual impotence, sterility, infertility, sunburn, or scarring. If you accept the unfounded claims for vitamin E and use the vitamin to treat a physical condition yourself, the delay in getting proper medical treatment might have serious consequences.

Wampocap vitamin supplement (Wallace Laboratories), see nicotinic acid vitamin supplement.

OTC   Wart-Off wart remover

Manufacturer: Pfipharmecs Division
Ingredients: salicylic acid in flexible collodion
Dosage Form: Liquid: salicylic acid, 17% in flexible collodion
Use: Removal of warts
Side Effects: Allergy; local irritation
Contraindications: This product should not be used by diabetics or persons with impaired circulation. • This product should not be used on moles, birthmarks, or unusual warts with hair growing from them.
Warnings: Do not use this product near the eyes or on mucous membranes. • This product is flammable; do not use around an open flame. • If the condition worsens, or if pain develops, stop using this product and consult your doctor or pharmacist.
Comments: This product is extremely corrosive. Follow directions carefully and exactly. Protect surrounding skin with petroleum jelly before use. • This product creates a film over the area as it is applied. Do not be alarmed and do not remove the film. • Do not use this product for more than one week. • A small brush is provided with this product to aid in brushing away loose tissue.

W.D.D. antidepressant (Tutag Pharmaceuticals, Inc.), see Tofranil antidepressant.

626

Wehvert antinauseant (W. E. Hauck, Inc.), see Antivert antinauseant.

WescoHEX detergent cleanser (West Chemical Products, Inc.), see pHisoHex detergent cleanser.

Wintrocin antibiotic (Winston Pharmaceuticals, Inc.), see erythromycin antibiotic.

Wyamycin antibiotic (Wyeth Laboratories), see erythromycin antibiotic.

OTC   Wyanoid hemorrhoidal preparation

Manufacturer: Wyeth Laboratories
Ingredients: Suppository: belladonna extract; bismuth oxyiodide; bismuth subcarbonate; boric acid; cocoa butter; ephedrine sulfate; Peruvian balsam; zinc oxide. Ointment: benzocaine; boric acid; castor oil; ephedrine sulfate; Peruvian balsam; petrolatum; zinc oxide
Dosage Form: Suppository: belladonna extract, 15 mg; bismuth oxyiodide, 30 mg; bismuth subcarbonate, 146 mg; boric acid, 543 mg; cocoa butter; ephedrine sulfate, 3 mg; Peruvian balsam, 30 mg; zinc oxide, 176 mg. Ointment: benzocaine, 2%; boric acid, 18%; castor oil; ephedrine sulfate, 0.1%; Peruvian balsam, 1%; petrolatum; zinc oxide, 5%
Use: Relief of pain, burning, and itching of hemorrhoids
Warnings: Sensitization (continued itching and redness) may occur with long-term and repeated use.
Comments: Hemorrhoidal (pile) preparations relieve itching, reduce pain and inflammation, and check bleeding, but do not heal, dry up, or give lasting relief from the hemorrhoids. • Certain ingredients in this product may cause an allergic reaction; do not use for longer than seven days at a time unless your doctor has advised you otherwise. • The suppository is not recommended for external hemorrhoids or bleeding internal hemorrhoids. Use the ointment form. Use caution when inserting applicator. • Never self-medicate for hemorrhoids if pain is continuous or throbbing, if bleeding or itching is excessive, or if you feel pressure within the rectum. Consult your doctor. • This product contains boric acid which many medical authorities believe should not be used because it is toxic. Follow directions on package.

Wymox antibiotic (Wyeth Laboratories), see amoxicillin antibiotic.

X-Aqua diuretic and antihypertensive (General Pharmaceutical Prods., Inc.), see hydrochlorothiazide diuretic and antihypertensive.

OTC   yellow mercuric oxide ophthalmic ointment

Manufacturer: various manufacturers
Ingredient: mercuric oxide
Dosage Form: Ointment: mercuric oxide, 5%; 10%
Use: Relief of mild inflammations of the eyes
Side Effects: Minor burning, itching, stinging of the eye; redness and watering of the eye
Warnings: This product should not be used for more than a day or two. Consult your doctor if the condition persists.
Comments: To administer an eye ointment, pull the lower eyelid down to form a pouch. Then, squeeze a one-quarter to one-half inch line of ointment into the pouch, and close your eye. Roll your eye a few times to spread the ointment.

Zetran sedative and hypnotic (W. E. Hauck, Inc.), see Librium sedative and hypnotic.

Zide diuretic and antihypertensive (Tutag Pharmaceuticals, Inc.), see hydrochlorothiazide diuretic and antihypertensive.

OTC   **zinc oxide ointment**

Manufacturer: various manufacturers
Ingredient: zinc oxide
Dosage Form: Ointment
Use: Treatment of diaper rash; minor burns; sunburn; other minor skin conditions
Comments: This product is excellent for treating diaper rash.

OTC   **Ziradryl poison ivy remedy**

Manufacturer: Parke-Davis
Ingredients: alcohol; camphor; diphenhydramine hydrochloride; zinc oxide
Dosage Form: Lotion: alcohol, 2%; camphor, 0.1%; diphenhydramine hydrochloride, 2%; zinc oxide, 2%
Use: Relief of itching due to poison ivy and poison oak
Side Effects: Allergic reactions (rash, itching, soreness); local irritation
Warnings: Do not apply this product to extensive or raw, oozing areas or for a prolonged time except as directed by a physician.
Comments: To prevent irritation and secondary infection, avoid scratching.
• Before applying medication, soak the area in warm water or apply towels soaked in water for five to ten minutes. Dry the area gently by patting with a soft towel, then apply medication.

℞   **Zyloprim uricosuric**

Manufacturer: Burroughs Wellcome Co.
Ingredient: allopurinol
Dosage Form: Tablet: 100 mg (white); 300 mg (peach)
Use: Treatment of gout
Minor Side Effects: Diarrhea; nausea; vomiting
Major Side Effects: Fatigue; paleness; rash; sore throat; visual disturbances
Contraindications: This drug should not be used by children, with the exception of those children with hyperuricemia secondary to cancer. • This drug should not be used by nursing mothers. • This drug should not be used in persons who have had a severe reaction to it. Consult your doctor immediately if this drug has been prescribed for you and you have had such a reaction.
Warnings: This drug should be discontinued at the first sign of skin rash or any sign of adverse reaction. Notify your doctor immediately if reactions occur. • This drug should be used with caution in persons with blood disease, liver disease, or kidney disease. Be sure your doctor knows if you have such conditions. • This drug should be used by pregnant women and women of child-bearing age only if potential benefits to the patient are weighed against the possible risk to the fetus. • Some investigators have reported an increase in acute gout attacks during the early stages of use of this drug. • Drowsiness may occur as a result of using this drug; avoid tasks that require alertness. • A fluid intake sufficient to yield a daily urinary output of at least 2 liters is desirable when taking this drug. • Periodic determination of liver and kidney function and complete blood counts should be performed during therapy with this drug, especially during the first few months of therapy. • Iron salts should not be given simultaneously with this drug. • This drug should not be given in conjunction with azathioprine, cyclophosphamide, mercaptopurine, or oral anticoagulants. If you are currently taking any drugs of these types, consult your doctor about their use. If you are unsure about

the type or contents of your medications, ask your doctor or pharmacist. •
This drug should be used with caution in patients receiving other uricosuric
agents.

Comments: It is common for persons beginning to take this drug to also
take colchicine for the first three months. Colchicine helps minimize painful
attacks of gout. • If one tablet of this drug is prescribed three times a day, ask
your doctor if a single dose (either three 100-mg tablets or one 300-mg tablet)
can be taken as a convenience. • The effects of this drug therapy may not be
apparent for at least two weeks. • Drink at least eight glasses of water each
day to help minimize the formation of kidney stones. • While you are on this
drug, do not drink alcohol without first checking with your doctor.

Part IV
Health Care
Accessories

Health Care Accessories

Fever Thermometers

A clinical or fever thermometer measures the temperature of the inside of the body. Most are made of glass and contain a column of mercury to register temperature. The thermometer is usually placed in either the mouth or the rectum, although the armpit, navel, and the vagina are also used occasionally.

Three types of thermometers are generally available: the oral thermometer, with a long, thin-walled bulb; the rectal thermometer with a pear-shaped, blunt bulb designed to avoid tearing or irritating the rectal wall; and the security or stubby thermometer, with a short stubby bulb. The stubby model can be used in either the mouth or rectum. It is preferred for use with children because it is harder to break. However, it does not register as quickly as the other types and should be left in place a few minutes longer.

Use and Maintenance

To take a temperature orally, the patient should sit or lie down, and the thermometer should be placed in the mouth, with the bulb under the tongue. The lips, but not the teeth should be closed around the stem. An oral thermometer should be left in place for two to four minutes; a stubby, for four or five. Oral temperatures should not be taken for 30 minutes after eating or drinking either hot or cold foods or beverages.

Before taking a temperature rectally, you should lubricate the thermometer with a small amount of K-Y lubricating jelly, mineral oil, or petroleum jelly. Then insert it carefully, far enough so that the 98.6 mark is within the rectum. About half the thermometer should be outside the body. The thermometer should be left in place for two to four minutes (longer if using a stubby). Generally considered the most accurate reading of body temperature, the rectal temperature usually registers about a degree higher than the oral.

If a thermometer breaks while being inserted into the rectum, do not try to remove it, but go to the nearest emergency room at once. If a thermometer breaks in the mouth, remove as much of the glass and mercury as possible, and then contact your doctor. In such situations the broken glass is more dangerous than the mercury.

The best way to read a thermometer is to stand with your back to a light and hold the end opposite the bulb between two fingers. Rotate the thermometer until you see the column of mercury. Follow the mercury with your eyes. Each small line usually indicates two-tenths of a degree.

After reading the temperature, shake down the thermometer. Hold the stem end firmly between the fingers of one hand and snap your wrist as

---

Note: If you are unable to find one of the items described in this chapter, or if you wish to consult the manufacturer, talk to your pharmacist, who may be able to special order the item or give you the manufacturer's address.

though you were snapping water off your fingers.

After each use, the thermometer should be cleaned with soap and water, rinsed, and then disinfected. To disinfect a thermometer, soak it in 70-percent alcohol for at least 15 minutes. Rinse it in cold water, and then wipe dry. Do not store the thermometer in the disinfectant.

Buying a Thermometer

Thermometers are tested for accuracy before being placed on sale—check that the thermometer you purchase comes with a certificate that describes how accurate it is.

Before buying a thermometer, test it (if possible) by holding the bulb between your fingers to make sure that the mercury column moves. After it has moved, test how difficult it is to shake down the thermometer.

If you have trouble reading thermometers, look for one with a colored background for the mercury, one that uses some liquid other than mercury, or one with a red strip along the side (the most easily read). Another feature to look for is a case with an inner spring or clamp to secure the thermometer and protect it from possible breakage.

Avoid thermometers being sold at "bargain" prices. Sometimes thermometers are made as promotional items for a special sale, and such thermometers may be less carefully made and tested than other thermometers.

You may want to consider purchasing one of the electronic thermometers now available. They give a quick and accurate reading, but they are rather expensive. Plastic strip thermometers, another recent introduction, are designed to be placed on the patient's forehead. They indicate temperature by changing color. The accuracy of these thermometers has not been proven, and they cannot be recommended for other than occasional use.

Recommendations

Choose a thermometer according to the criteria already described. The following companies are among the largest manufacturers of thermometers: Becton, Dickinson Consumer Products; Biomedical Division; and Chesebrough-Pond's Inc. Remember that a bargain-priced thermometer may be less accurate and less carefully tested than higher-priced models.

Recommended Unique Thermometers

The Asepto Tab Top thermometer (Becton, Dickinson Consumer Products) features a hand grip that makes it easier to hold while reading the temperature and shaking down the thermometer. The feature is available in both oral and rectal models.

The Unitemp thermometer (Biomedical Division) is a thin, flexible flat plastic strip with yellow dots that change to red to indicate a temperature. It is used orally and provides a reading after one minute. These thermometers are accurate to within two-tenths of a degree. They are sold in packs of 25 (cost about $2.00). Each disposable thermometer is individually wrapped and sterilized—no need to clean and disinfect a thermometer each time you take someone's temperature.

The Basal Temperature thermometer (Becton, Dickinson Consumer Products) is used to help determine the time of ovulation during the menstrual cycle, either to help a woman become pregnant or help her avoid pregnancy. This method of controlling conception is based on the slight rise in body temperature at ovulation. An ordinary fever thermometer is not sensitive enough to record this change; thus, the Basal thermometer has only a short range of temperatures (95° to 100°) and is graduated in one-tenth rather than two-tenth degree increments. It can be used orally or rectally, and it comes with a helpful chart to be used to keep track of the temperature cycle. Consult a gynecologist for further information on this method of birth control.

Blood Pressure Kits and Pulsemeters

Blood Pressure Kits

Blood pressure measurement kits are a fairly new arrival on the home health care product market, and their availability is largely due to increased awareness of the dangers of hypertension. But keeping track of one's blood pressure is not just for hypertensives. Blood pressure is an important indicator of your health, and should be checked regularly and recorded in your personal health history. This is especially important, of course, if you have hypertension, heart problems, or a family history of these ailments.

Home blood pressure kits generally consist of a sphygmomanometer, which measures the pressure of the blood in the arteries, and a stethoscope, which is used to listen to the pulse in the arm. The electronic models do not require the use of a stethoscope.

The heart of all the kits is the sphygmomanometer, generally a cloth-covered cuff encasing an inflatable bag. There is a rubber bulb to inflate the bag, a valve for deflating it, and a gauge for reading the pressure.

Use

Complete instructions for taking your blood pressure should be included with all the kits. General instructions adaptable to most models are included in the chapter on health records.

Learning to use your kit properly takes practice. Typically you must squeeze the rubber bulb, turn the pressure release valve, and hold the stethoscope to your arm, all with one hand, since the arm wearing the cuff must be held still and relaxed. In addition, you need to hear well enough to recognize the pulse sounds indicating when to read the pressure off the gauge.

This may prove difficult at first, but keep trying. You may find it helpful to ask your doctor for a demonstration or to practice with a friend or family member.

Choosing a Blood Pressure Kit

The three main types of blood pressure kits are: the mercury type, with a thermometer-like gauge filled with mercury; the aneroid type, with a dial-like gauge on which a needle indicates the pressure; and the electronic type, which uses a microphone built into the cuff instead of a stethoscope to pick up the pulse. Some electronic models display the pressure on an aneroid type dial gauge, while others have a digital display.

The mercury type kits have one major advantage—superior accuracy. They are more accurate when new and more likely to remain accurate over the long run. There is, however, a major disadvantage to the mercury type kits, especially for home use. Mercury and its vapors are toxic, and this presents a hazard if the gauge is broken. As a result, an aneroid type kit would be a safer choice for a family with young children. The mercury type kits are slightly more difficult to read than other types, and they are frequently more expensive than the aneroid type.

If you buy an aneroid type kit, it is wise to have the gauge checked for accuracy by your doctor. And have it rechecked every six months, since rough handling can easily knock the gauge out of accurate calibration. It is notable that on some models, such as model 705204 (from Taylor Instrument of Ohio) and the Marshall Electronics Inc. Home Blood Pressure Kit 105, you can see when the gauge is out of calibration. The indicator needle does not fall exactly on zero when the cuff is deflated. However, other kits have gauges with a hidden pin preventing the needle from going below zero. So it points to zero even when the gauge is inaccurate. Try to avoid models with this feature.

The accuracy of the electronic kits varies greatly. It all depends on how well the microphone built into the cuff picks up pulse sounds. This in turn depends on the character of the sounds—a factor that differs from one person to the next. As a result, electronic kits are highly accurate for some people, inaccurate for others. In addition, the built-in microphones are often so sensitive they pick up background noises, resulting in inaccurate readings.

If you buy an electronic type blood pressure kit, get a promise of return privileges from the seller. Then have your doctor check it for accuracy. If it works properly, fine. If not, return it and consider buying one of the manual kits.

The great advantage of the electronic kits is their convenience. Simply strap on the cuff, pump it up, and release the pressure. You take a reading off the gauge when a light blinks or a tone sounds. The digital models make it even easier. Both systolic and diastolic pressure, as well as pulse rate, are displayed on the readout until the device is turned off.

The price for this convenience is high, from approximately $60 for the simplest electronic kits to $200 for those with digital readout. By contrast, prices for the manual kits range from about $20 to $40. Except for people with impaired hearing, vision, or coordination, electronic kits are probably not worth the extra expense.

The convenience of using mercury and aneroid type kits varies from model to model, depending on the design. One feature that adds greatly to ease of operation, especially when you are taking your blood pressure by yourself, is a D-ring on the cuff. (This is sometimes called a slide bar.) The D-ring is an elongated metal ring that makes it much easier to put the cuff on your arm. You slide one end of the cuff through the D-ring, which is attached to the other end, then pull the cuff tight around your arm.

Some kits have an automatic deflating valve. This is slightly more convenient than having to release the pressure by turning a control knob. On some models, the automatic valve is activated by a push button. One problem with an automatic deflation valve is that it may release the pressure too fast, making it difficult for you to get an accurate reading.

On other kits the stethoscope is permanently attached beneath the bottom edge of the cuff. This may be less awkward, but it may also put the stethoscope in the wrong position on your arm. If you buy a kit with a permanently attached stethoscope, ask your doctor to check its position.

An extra convenience feature offered on some of the electronic devices is a low battery indicator. Most of the other electronic kits simply stop working when the power falls from nine to five volts. If you notice that your kit is giving erratic readings, you should buy a new battery.

Manufacturers of blood pressure kits include Bristoline Inc.; Clayton Division, Marshall Electronics Inc.; and Taylor Instrument of Ohio, a division of Sybron Corporation.

Pulsemeters

Blood pressure kits are not the only item on the health care market that enables you to monitor the function of your circulatory system. There are also electronic pulsemeters, devices that measure your pulse rate, the number of heartbeats per minute. These have come onto the market in the wake of the booming interest in physical fitness, since a person's pulse rate while exercising and at rest are two indicators of fitness.

The Instapulse by Sharper Image is a rod-shaped unit that is held in the user's hands. Built-in sensors carry electronic impulses from the fingertips to a digital readout where the pulse rate is displayed.

The Roadrunner Electronic Pulse Meter by Nissei is a box-shaped device with a hole in the side where the user inserts a finger. A sensor reads the pulse and displays the rate on a meter.

Considering the price of these devices (as much as $150) and that they reveal nothing about the strength and character of your pulse, pulsemeters are probably an unjustified expense for most people. In addition, almost everyone can do manually what these devices do electronically. Simply count your pulse for 15 seconds and multiply by four to get your pulse rate.

Sickroom Utensils

Dosage Teaspoons and Cups

Studies have shown that the usual household teaspoon may hold from three to nine milliliters of liquid. With such an inaccurate tool, measuring a proper dose of medication is difficult. Dosage teaspoons and cups are calibrated to allow for careful measurement of liquid medications. A medicinal teaspoon holds exactly five milliliters, and by using such a device you are always sure to receive the correct amount of medication. An additional advantage is that children seem less likely to resist taking medication when it is administered in a special spoon or cup.

Many variations of the medicine spoon or cup are available. One model is a calibrated medicine dropper that can be used to inject medicine into the back of a child's mouth. For general use, we recommend a spoon with a hollow calibrated handle and tiny feet that allow the spoon to be set down without spilling its contents.

Some people find it difficult to swallow pills, capsules, and tablets. For these people, a medicine cup with a shelf on which to place the medication may be helpful. When using this device, the glass is partially filled with water or other liquid, and the medication is placed on the shelf. When the patient drinks the liquid, the pill is swallowed almost automatically.

Manufacturers of these products include Apex Medical Supply, Inc.; Precision Plastics; and Samuel's Products Incorporated.

Invalid Cushions

Several styles of cushions are available for use by patients who are bedridden or for whom sitting is painful, for example, those who have hemorrhoids or who have had recent surgery on the rectal area. The most common type of invalid cushion is a circular or oval shape with an opening in the center. Generally these cushions are either a foam or an inflatable rubber ring.

If an inflatable cushion is used, it should be filled until it is comfortably soft, not firm and hard. Sitting on a rubber ring cushion may become uncomfortable after some time because air trapped within the center hole area becomes heated. To solve this problem, horseshoe-shaped inflatable cushions are available. They are likely to be more comfortable; however, they are also more expensive.

Small inflatable ring cushions, usually eight by ten inches, are also available. They are designed to fit under the elbows or heels of bedridden patients, places where bedsores are likely to develop. Your pharmacist may have to special order these for you if you want them.

All these cushions, whether foam or rubber, must be periodically washed with a mild soap solution and allowed to dry completely. They should be stored in a dry, dark place. Make sure that they do not come into contact with oil or oily materials. Such substances may cause deterioration of the cushions.

For most people, the foam cushion is more comfortable than the inflatable rubber design. Because the foam is more porous than the rubber, the air in the center hole is less likely to become unbearably hot. However, after prolonged use, the foam cushion is likely to deteriorate somewhat.

Buying Invalid Cushions

No matter which type cushion is chosen, the size desired should be determined carefully. The patient's weight should be borne along the edge of the central hole. A center hole that is too large will squeeze the pelvic bones together, while a center hole that is too small will force the pelvic bones apart. The proper dimension can be determined by measuring the distance between the bones of the buttocks. The bones of most adults are four to six inches apart, and for most people, either the 14- or 16-inch cushion is the right size.

Incidentally, some authorities believe that invalid cushions should only be used temporarily because after long use they may cause a change in the relative positions of the pelvic bones.

Before purchasing such cushions, inspect them carefully. Inflate a rubber cushion to check for leaks, and examine foam cushions carefully for cracks or tears. Double check to make sure that you are purchasing the correct size. Manufacturers of invalid cushions include Davol Inc.; Faultless Rubber Company (Division of Abbott Laboratories); and 3M.

Sheepskin Pads

Sheepskin or sheepskin-like pads are used commonly by bedridden patients to protect certain parts of the body from constant pressure and resultant bedsores. The body parts most commonly affected include the heels, buttocks, and elbows.

The fleece side of a natural sheepskin pad is trimmed to a thickness of about one inch. The reverse side is tanned. An entire pad usually measures about 36 by 42 inches, although smaller pieces may be purchased to protect smaller body areas.

If you decide to purchase a sheepskin pad, consult your pharmacist about how it is to be cleaned. Most can be laundered as long as they are dried flat. Do not put sheepskin pads in the dryer. If you want to test the pad's washability, wash a small section of a corner in warm water with mild soap. Allow to dry, and compare the washed portion with the rest of the pad.

Synthetic sheepskin-like or fleecy pads are far less expensive than natural sheepskin, and they are easier to clean. A natural pad is likely to be more durable, but, for short-term use, synthetic sheepskin is an acceptable purchase.

When these pads are used, they should be placed directly under the patient. Neither sheets nor clothing should come between the patient's skin and the pad. We recommend the use of these pads for bedridden patients. However, because they are of no special benefit unless they contact the skin directly, we do not recommend them for people confined to wheelchairs.

Disposable Underpads

Disposable underpads are used to prevent the soiling of bed linens by incontinent patients. They are also useful when placed beneath a bedpan to protect against accidental spills. They are usually made from an absorbent filler placed between a soft facing and a waterproof backing. The standard underpad measures 17½ by 24 inches, but both larger and smaller sizes are available.

The best underpads have a soft, nonrolling, fabric-like facing, a cellulose filler, and a polyethylene or polypropylene backing. Underpads of poorer quality usually have a paper facing, a pulp filler, and a moisture-repellent paper backing. Johnson & Johnson and Parke-Davis manufacture disposable underpads.

Rubber Sheeting

Rubber sheeting is placed under invalids or infants to protect mattresses. Rubber sheeting is available in sizes ranging from 36 to 54 inches in width, and up to several yards in length.

When using rubber sheeting under a patient, never allow the patient's bare skin to come into contact with the rubber. Always place a bedsheet, a piece of cloth, or item of clothing between the rubber and the skin. Otherwise, the skin may become severely irritated due to friction as well as to an accumulation of moisture on the rubber. For invalids who are confined to bed, it is preferable to use a disposable underpad. Disposable underpads are absorbent and less likely to cause irritation or bedsores than rubber sheeting.

Do not fold rubber sheeting; it may become crimped and permanently creased. Rather, when storing the rubber sheeting, roll it into a cylinder. Following use, wash the sheeting in warm water and a mild soap solution and allow it to dry completely. Never use oils or oily products on it, as these may cause deterioration of the rubber. Always keep the sheeting out of sunlight and away from heat. Jung Products, Inc. manufactures rubber sheeting.

Bedpans, Urinals, and Vomit Basins

Bedpans

Bedpans are shallow containers that can be slid under patients confined to bed to allow them to have bowel movements and to urinate. Bedpans are more difficult to use and far less convenient than bedside commodes, and any patient capable of using a commode instead should be encouraged to do so.

Bedpans are made of plastic, enamelware, or stainless steel. Stainless steel is the most durable, but plastic is less expensive, does not require warming before use, and is recommended for most home use. An unwarmed bedpan can be a sudden shock to an invalid, so enamelware and stainless steel bedpans should be warmed before use. This can be done by running the pan under warm water, putting a heating pad or hot water bottle on it, or putting it under the blankets with the patient. Also make sure the seat of the bedpan is dry before bringing it to the patient; a light dusting of talcum powder may be helpful.

All bedpans are shaped in basically the same way, although child-sized and fracture bedpans are also available. A fracture bedpan is smaller and more slanted than a regular bedpan. Fracture bedpans are supposedly easier to use, especially with children and overweight or immobilized people. However, they are also more shallow than other bedpans and are therefore easier to spill.

Before a bedpan is used, a disposable underpad or several layers of newspaper should be spread under the patient when possible in case of accidental spillage. After emptying, the bedpan should be cleaned with soap and water.

Urinals

Urinals are special containers in which bedridden patients can urinate. Both male and female urinals are available, but female urinals are seldom used because most women seem to prefer to use bedpans. Urinals are made of the same materials used for bedpans and should be cared for in the same way. Plastic is preferred, again because it does not need to be warmed before use. In certain diseases it is important to keep track of the amount of urine eliminated, and for this reason, calibrated urinals are available.

Vomit Basins

A vomit basin is a kidney-shaped pan used to collect vomit or sputum. It is also called a kidney basin. Vomit basins are made of stainless steel, enamelware, and plastic and require thorough washing after each use.

Manufacturers of bedpans, urinals, and vomit basins include Davol Inc.; Jones-Zylon, Inc.; Jung Products, Inc.; and The Vollrath Company.

Surgical, Cold Weather, and Filter Masks

Surgical Masks

Surgical masks are worn to help prevent the spread of infection. Your doctor may advise you to wear a surgical mask when attending to a sick child or if you are sick and must care for someone extremely susceptible to illness, such as an infant.

Surgical masks may be made from a single layer of a finely woven cloth, from several layers of finely woven gauze, or from a nonwoven synthetic fiber. Masks are maximally useful for only 30 minutes or so. After one to two hours they become wet and are not effective. If you must use a surgical mask, we recommend one, such as the Aseptex surgical mask made by 3M, that is made of a nonwoven synthetic fiber with an elastic headband and an adjustable metal nosepiece.

Cold Weather Masks

Cold weather masks are worn by people with serious heart or lung diseases. Such conditions may be made worse by the inhalation of large quantities of cold air. Normally, the nose and throat warm inhaled air before it reaches sensitive lung tissue. In extremely cold weather, especially if a person is exercising vigorously, the quantity of cold air inhaled may be more than the system can manage, and when the cold air reaches the lungs, the lung tissue contracts. Such contraction is not serious in a healthy individual, but it may be fatal in someone whose respiratory capacity is already impaired. Cold weather masks are worn to warm the air before it enters the nose.

Usually a cold weather mask consists of a synthetic foam material shaped to fit around the nose and mouth. An elastic band is used to hold it in place. When choosing a mask, look for one made of a lint-free material and about ⅛ inch thick. It should not restrict the flow of air when held to the face. It should be comfortable and resistant to damage by moisture. A mask that is washable and reusable is the most economical. The Micropore cold weather mask made by 3M is made of hypoallergenic foam and is recommended.

Filter Masks

Filter masks are worn by people with serious lung diseases during times of severe air pollution. They may also be beneficial to those whose work exposes them to a variety of airborne dust and irritants, particularly if the irritants are known to cause serious disease (for example, coal dust, beryllium, and asbestos). Filter masks are designed to screen out potentially harmful particles that might otherwise reach the lungs. Either a surgical mask or a cold weather mask will serve to filter out such particles but there are also special masks designed for this purpose. Some are designed with disposable filters and durable rubber headpieces. Others are entirely disposable. We recommend the disposable Mircopore pollen and dust mask, made by 3M.

Rubber Gloves

In the sickroom, rubber gloves are used to guard against infection and to protect the hands. If you need gloves for the insertion of rectal suppositories or thermometers, you can purchase surgical gloves similar to those used in the operating room or disposable gloves made of a vinyl film. Surgical gloves are very thin to allow great freedom and sensitivity. They are not sterile when purchased. Sizes range from 6½ to 10. When purchasing surgical gloves, grasp the open end of the glove and apply pressure to check for air holes. After use, the gloves should be washed with soap and water and hung up to dry. After the outside has dried, turn the glove inside out to allow the inside to dry as well.

Disposable gloves can also be used as an occlusive wrap over a medicated ointment on your hands. Do not wear rubber or vinyl gloves over medication unless directed to do so by your doctor, however.

If your doctor specifies that you need sterile gloves, you can purchase disposable sterilized gloves. Becton, Dickinson Consumer Products; Davol, Inc.; and Faultless Rubber Company (a division of Abbott Laboratories) all manufacture rubber gloves.

Fingercots

A fingercot is a thin sheath placed over a finger. Fingercots are usually made from the kind of rubber used to make surgical gloves. They are used for purposes such as suppository insertion, both to protect the rectal wall (if, for example, fingernails are long) and for sanitary reasons. Some people also use fingercots for sorting papers, because they permit a better grip. Fingercots should not be used to cover bandages or wounds; they prevent airflow and allow water leakage.

Fingercots are generally available in small, medium, large, and thumb sizes. Davol Inc. is one manufacturer.

Humidifiers and Vaporizers

Doctors and pharmacists agree that one of the best measures of protection against, as well as treatment for, respiratory illness is to add moisture to the air you breathe. When the air is dry—as it is especially indoors during the fall and winter months—the mucous membranes lining the nose, throat, and lungs become dry. This mucous lining helps the body rid itself of inhaled bacteria, viruses, and dust particles that cause colds and other respiratory diseases. This lining also contains enzymes and antibodies that help decrease the chance of an invasion of germs into the body. But if the mucous lining becomes dried and thus thickened, some of the body's resistance against infections and irritation is lost. With this decreased resistance, a person is likely to get more frequent and severe coughs, colds, and various other respiratory problems.

Humidifiers and vaporizers are two devices sold for adding moisture to the air. Humidifiers blow minute droplets of water into the air. Vaporizers heat water to boiling and produce moisture as steam. Although some manufacturers now offer "cool mist vaporizers" and vaporizer-humidifiers, vaporizers and humidifiers are not the same. However, therapeutically, either type of device is beneficial. The important factor is the water content of the air, not the method by which the water was put there.

Choosing Between the Two

There are several differences between a humidifier and a vaporizer. Humidifiers usually cost more than vaporizers to purchase, but they are less expensive to operate. The cool mist produced by a humidifier may deposit a light coating of minerals on furniture and on walls, particularly if hard water is being used. Humidifiers take slightly longer to produce complete humidification of a room. But because humidifiers are usually run continuously, this should not be an important consideration.

Vaporizers generate heat and, therefore, take more energy to operate than humidifiers take. The vaporizer may be a potential hazard; the reservoir of hot water could be spilled and the steam could burn anyone who should accidentally get too close. A vaporizer should be set on the floor. If it is placed on furniture, a cloth or a pad of newspaper should be placed underneath to protect the furniture from droplets of water that may condense on the unit and fall onto the furniture.

Vaporizers are usually less expensive than humidifiers, and when they are used properly, they are relatively safe. Many people use vaporizers in sickrooms. Vaporizers have a reservoir in which volatile medications can be placed. The steam will distribute the medication throughout the room. However, these medications have no therapeutic benefit and their cost is unwarranted. Vaporizers usually shut off automatically when they run out of water, while humidifiers do not.

Use and Maintenance

Occasionally, a vaporizer will spit large droplets of water instead of delivering a fine steam. If this happens, replace part of the tap water with distilled water. For example, use three parts tap water to one part distilled water. Adjust the proportions until a steady flow of steam is obtained.

If a vaporizer doesn't give off steam, you may need to add minerals to the water. Add table salt to the water, pinch by pinch, until the steam flows.

After each use, completely rinse the water reservoir of a humidifier or of a vaporizer to help eliminate mineral deposits. If you see a whitish film collecting on the reservoir wall, add a small amount of vinegar to the container and let it soak for a couple of hours, then rinse well. Do not run the unit with vinegar in the water.

A problem that has been noted with the use of humidifiers is the buildup of fungi within the units. Once these plant organisms are in the unit, they can become airborne when propelled from the unit during its use. The airborne fungi can be potentially dangerous, since they can cause asthma attacks, stuffy nose, and various other reactions to airborne organisms. Because of the potential problem related to fungi, it is important that humidifiers be cleaned out weekly, and that fresh water be used after each day's operation. In addition, there are antifungal tablets that can be purchased over-the-counter. These tablets are simply dropped into the water of the units each day.

Finally, be sure to follow carefully the directions that are supplied with your unit. The continuous use of humidifiers and vaporizers poses no health problems so long as the units are properly maintained. Both humidifiers and vaporizers require regular maintenance to make sure that they will continue to perform properly.

Recommendations

When purchasing either a humidifier or a vaporizer, make sure that it is guaranteed against defects. A humidifier should have a water reservoir that holds at least two gallons; a vaporizer's reservoir should hold at least one gallon. These quantities of water are required to make sure that the unit will run all night. Also, make sure the vaporizer has a device that automatically shuts off the unit when the water has been used up.

Among the most well known manufacturers of humidifiers and vaporizers are the following companies: the DeVilbiss Company, Health Care Division; Gerber Products Company, Hankscraft Division; Rexall Drug Co.; and Walton Laboratories.

Hot and Cold Application Devices

Heating Pads

In most homes electric heating pads are now preferred over hot water bottles because they can be adjusted and are more convenient. Heating pads are constructed of a wire heating element wound over an insulating core and covered with more insulation. This element is then sewn in a criss-cross fashion to a flat object such as a piece of burlap. Thermostats and a cordset are added, and the unit is covered with layers of soft cotton and then sealed in a rubberized cover. Finally, a soft material covering is slipped over the rubber.

Buying a Heating Pad

Before purchasing a heating pad, consumers should determine whether they want a heating pad that is moisture resistant or wet proof, and a three-speed or a three-positive (variable) model.

The rubberized cover of a moisture-resistant heating pad is not completely sealed. The heating pad that is labeled wet proof is completely sealed and has been subjected to immersion tests. It may be used with moist heat, as when a wet towel is placed beneath the pad. Some wet proof heating pads are sold with a sponge insert for moist heat. The user soaks the sponge, wrings it out, and then inserts it beneath the cloth cover of the heating pad.

With a three-speed heating pad, the user can choose how quickly the pad will heat. At all three speeds—low, medium, and high—the pad will eventually arrive at a final temperature of about 165° to 180° F. The difference is that at a low speed the pad will take longer to heat.

With a three-positive (variable) pad, the user can choose how hot he or she wants the pad to be. Set at low, the pad will generally heat to 115° to 130°

F; at medium, 140° to 158° F; and at high, 167° to 180° F. Generally, maximum temperature is reached on each switch setting within 15 to 20 minutes. We recommend the selection of the three-positive or variable model rather than a three-speed heating pad.

Push-button switches seem to be more convenient than other designs. We also recommend a model with a light on the heat selector, a convenient feature for use in dimly lighted areas or for persons with limited vision. The pad size should be about 12 by 15 inches. Make sure that the pad has a consumer-based seal of approval and the UL listing mark on the box. Guarantees may range from one to five years. Make sure that the guarantee does not require that you send a large amount of money with the pad in case you need to have it repaired. A five dollar repair charge on a seven dollar heating pad doesn't make sense.

Look for a model with an outer cloth cover that can be removed for cleaning. Generally those heating pads that are manufactured for sale in massive promotions are three-speed models with a very limited guarantee. They usually are not wet proof. You should avoid these heating pads.

Use

When using a heating pad, never use a pin or other metallic item to fasten the pad in place. Never fold or crush the pad, and never fall asleep while using the pad, since burns on the skin may result. People with diabetes or insensitivity to heat should not use heating pads. They may get burned before they realize the pad is overheating. Heating pads should not be used on infants or on people who are sleeping or unconscious; they may not react in time if the pad overheats. Always make sure the pad is unplugged when not in use.

Follow the directions that come with the pad; do not use a heating pad for moist heat applications unless it is labeled wet proof. Do not use a pad without its removable cover.

Special Shapes and Designs

In addition to the standard rectangular designs, heating pads are now available in a number of different shapes to warm particular parts of the body. All of the following devices have rather specialized uses. For most people, their expense is probably not justified. However, people with certain problems (arthritis, chronic sinus infections, or frequent athletic injuries) may find such products both useful and extremely satisfying.

Wrap-around heating bands with ties or other closures are available from several manufacturers (Ricar Industries, Gillette, Northern Electric). These are useful for fastening around a sore shoulder or thigh, and they can also be used around the waist for low back pain. Some come with moist heat inserts.

Other specially shaped heating pads include face masks for sinus relief, mitts and booties for arthritic hands and cold feet, collars for the neck, and angle heat pads for use on joints such as the elbow, knee, and shoulder.

The Foot Warmer (Northern Electric) is a two-footed boot that comes with a thermostatically controlled warming pad to be placed beneath the feet.

The Thermophore heat pack (Battle Creek Equipment) draws moisture from the air to produce continuous intense moist heat. The unit has a heavy canvas-lined pad, and a thick flannel cover, and it comes in three sizes. While using the pad, the user must keep the switch depressed; when pressure is released the unit shuts off. This safety feature assures that burns will not occur should the user fall asleep. The unit is expensive, and unless it is going to be used frequently over a long period of time, its purchase is not recommended.

The Deluxe Heat Wrap/Cold Pack (Gillette) and the Moist Heat Band with Cold Pack (Northern Electric) are wrap-around heating pads with both sponge inserts for moist heat and flexible gel inserts for use as cold packs. The cold insert must be placed in the freezer before use, although the substance does not freeze but remains flexible so that it can be wrapped and fastened around a sprained or bruised limb. Both have three heat settings and a night light. They have shoulder straps, Velcro fasteners, and belt loops so that the unit can be wrapped and fastened to apply heat or cold where it is needed.

The Muscle Relaxer (Conair) is a similar product, but rather than a simple cold pack, it offers a cold/hot pack. Similar to the gel inserts offered by Gillette and Northern Electric, the cold/hot pack can also be immersed in hot water and inserted into the velour cover for non-electric wrap-around heat.

Water Bottles

Traditionally, water bottles have been used to apply heat to relieve muscle and joint soreness. Most water bottles are rectangular rubber bags formed by fusing two sheets of rubber together around the edge. The seam is usually reinforced with glue or an extra strip of rubber sheeting. The neck of a water bottle has a threaded closing so that a water-tight, hard rubber stopper can be inserted.

Use

Heat should not be applied to a freshly swollen sprained ankle, to an infected tooth, to a pus-laden infection, or to the abdomen if signs of appendicitis are evident. However, heat is comforting for several other conditions—sore muscles, backache, and sinus conditions, for example.

The water used in a water bottle should be uncomfortably hot, but not unbearably so. For adults, a temperature of 120° to 130° F is best, while 110° to 120° F is ideal for children. Most home hot water tanks heat water to 140° F or slightly higher. Therefore, the water bottle should not be filled directly from the hot water tap. Rather, fill a basin or pitcher with hot water and allow it to cool. Check the temperature with a thermometer or place your hand in it. If it feels uncomfortably hot but not unbearably hot to your hand, the temperature is correct.

Fill the bottle to about one-half to three-fourths of its capacity, to warm the rubber. Squeeze the bottle to see if it leaks. Empty and refill the bottle—again to about one-half to three quarters of its capacity. Lay the bottle on its side with the neck held up and gently press along the flat side to expel any air. Stopper the bottle and again test for leaks.

Never fill a water bottle until it bulges out. Overfilling causes stretching and deterioration of the rubber. If the bottle is too full, it cannot conform to the body's shape.

Most people wrap the bottle in a towel or place it in a cover before putting it on the skin. The bottle should be refilled about every two hours, and after use it should be hung upside down by its tab until it is dry. After it is dry, it should be filled with air, closed tightly, and kept in a cool place out of the sunlight.

Buying a Water Bottle

The durability of a water bottle depends upon the quality of the rubber used in its construction and the thickness of the bottle wall. Cheaper models may be made of reclaimed rubber or rubber with a mineral filler, resulting in loss of durability and elasticity. A poor quality bottle is also likely to have a short guarantee, as little as one year perhaps. Better models are likely to be guaranteed for up to five years. Consumers should remember that differences among water bottles at the same price range are usually insignificant, but differences between the cheapest water bottle from one manufacturer and the same manufacturer's more expensive line are likely to be significant.

Because the standard hot water bottle varies little from brand to brand, we suggest you consider the length of the guarantee as a gauge of quality. And because the range of prices is not wide (approximately four to seven dollars), we suggest you consider water bottles at the upper end of the price range.

Manufacturers of water bottles include Davol Inc., Faultless Rubber Company (Division of Abbott Laboratories), and Textile Rubber Company.

Ice Bags

Ice bag applications can be useful for conditions such as sprained ankles. Cold application immediately after an injury helps minimize bruising, and cold applied to the bridge of the nose may help stop a nosebleed.

Two styles of ice bags are generally available. One style is made much the same way that water bottles are made. In fact combination water bottle-ice bag products are available. This style ice bag may be made in particular shapes to fit specific parts of the body—for example, the throat or spine.

The most common and popular style of ice bag is the English type, formed by fusing a layer of rubber between two layers of thick cloth. Pieces of this material are cut to size and then drawn together, forming an opening in the center. A gasketed plastic screw-on cap is fitted into the opening for a water-tight seal. English style ice bags can be telescoped into a long flat shape or pushed into a round flat shape, depending on where they will be placed. The size of an English type ice bag is determined by its diameter when the bag is flattened out. A wide range of sizes is available.

Use

Before being put in an ice bag, the ice should be broken into small pieces, about the size of a walnut, and then rinsed with water in order to melt the sharp edges that could otherwise damage the bag. The bag should be filled from one-half to two-thirds full; the air should be pressed out, and the stopper then put on. The bag should then be squeezed to test it for leaks. The ice will have to be replaced approximately every two hours. The bag should be washed after use, dried, and stored in a cool, dark place.

Buying an Ice Bag

To determine whether the ice bag is of good quality, check its finishing details—does the cap screw on tightly? Do the seams appear to be straight and neatly finished? Does the bag feel thick and not flimsy? Check for weak spots around the center opening, the weakest part in many ice bags. A high quality ice bag will have a complete money-back guarantee.

Manufacturers of ice bags include Davol Inc., Faultless Rubber Company (Division of Abbott Laboratories), and Textile Rubber Company.

Gel Hot and Cold Packs

A relatively recent introduction, these hot and cold packs consist of sturdy plastic bags containing a gel. 3M's product, Cold Hot Pack, can be used for applications of both heat and cold. For cold application, the 4½ inch by 10½ inch bag is put in the freezer. For maximum cold, it should be left in the freezer for two hours. The gel does not freeze but remains flexible so that it can be folded and will conform to body contours. To use the pack for heat application, it should be immersed in water that has been brought to a boil. If the bag has been stored in the freezer, it should be left in the water for ten minutes for maximum heat. If the bag is at room temperature, it should be left in the water for no more than seven minutes.

Col Pac (Chattanooga Pharmacol Company) is a similar product, but it can be used only for cold application. These cold packs are available in sizes suited for use on the throat, hand and wrist, foot and ankle, and eye.

Iceband (Norcliff-Thayer Inc.) is a gel cold pack approximately 3 inches by 12 inches with ties on the end so that it can be fastened around the head, neck, or other body parts.

These products are, in some ways, more convenient than the conventional water bottle and ice bag. They are not as messy, will not drip, and do not require that you break up ice cubes or fill a water bottle. While they are generally sturdy, they may break or develop leaks if handled very roughly. And they do require some forethought in use. If you are willing to store one in the freezer for immediate use as a cold pack, or if you can anticipate when you will need a cold pack, they are very satisfactory.

Disposable Hot and Cold Packs

Instant hot and cold packs are disposable, one-time-use plastic pouches filled with chemicals. When the pouch is squeezed or shaken, the chemicals inside mix, and within a very short time (seconds to minutes) the pouches become hot or cold enough to use wherever you may want to apply heat or cold.

Instant hot and cold packs are convenient for emergency use, for traveling, at athletic events, and on camping trips—wherever it would be difficult to obtain hot water or ice. However, over a period of time the instant packs are more expensive than the more conventional products used for hot or cold applications, and if you need a hot or cold pack frequently, it will be more economical to purchase a water bottle, heating pad, or ice bag than to stock up on these instant pouches.

Kwik Kold (Kwik Kold, Inc.) and Cutter Instant Ice Cold Compress (Cutter Laboratories, Inc.) are two instant cold packs. Kwik Heat (Kwik Kold, Inc.) is an instant hot pack.

Surgical Dressings and Related Supplies

Adhesive Bandages

An adhesive bandage is basically a small sterile dressing attached to a piece of adhesive tape. Adhesive bandages are available under a variety of different trade names. Although it is frequently used to refer to any adhesive bandage, the word "Band-Aid" is a trade name referring specifically to the adhesive bandage made by Johnson & Johnson.

The dressing on an adhesive bandage may be made of gauze or of nonadhering plastic. Some brands of adhesive bandages have dressings impregnated with an antiseptic medication. The benefits to be gained from using such a bandage are questionable.

The tape portion of an adhesive bandage may be made of plastic or cloth. Plastic tape is generally preferred; it is thinner, it sticks better, and it is less conspicuous.

A relatively recent introduction is the liquid or spray-on bandage. This is usually a collodion or plastic film that is said to keep the wound clean and sealed. It is generally believed that these products retard healing somewhat, and they are not recommended.

Use

Adhesive bandages are frequently used when they are not actually needed. They do provide some protection against bumping a tender or sore spot, and applied to a fresh wound, they keep blood from dripping onto clothing or other items. A crying child who has a minor cut or abrasion can often be quieted by the application of a bandage and a show of concern. However, once the child has stopped crying and the wound has stopped bleeding, there is usually little need to continue to wear such a bandage on a minor wound. Adhesive bandages do allow dirt to get to the wound, and if the wound needs to be kept closed, a "butterfly" (a small strip of adhesive tape with wing-shaped ends) may be more effective. A deep wound, of course, demands a doctor's attention and possibly some sutures.

Buying Adhesive Bandages

We recommend that you buy nationally-advertised brands of adhesive bandages, for example, Band-Aid brand. Although generic adhesive bandages are available and may be less expensive, they may also be less adherent. Most people prefer adhesive bandages made with plastic tape. A box of bandages of assorted sizes is usually a better buy than a box with single-size strips. A bandage that is too small serves no real purpose, and one that is too large is likely to come off or be cumbersome. Whichever brand of bandages you buy, make sure that they are waterproof.

In addition to Johnson & Johnson, Bauer & Black (part of The Kendall Company) and 3M manufacture adhesive bandages.

Dressings

Dressings are generally divided into two types. Primary dressings are those placed directly on the wound; they must be sterile and absorbent. Secondary dressings are used to hold the primary dressing in place. They also cushion the wound somewhat and provide extra protection from dirt. Rolled gauze can be used as a primary or secondary dressing.

Primary dressings are usually made of gauze. Rolled gauze may be made into a dressing and applied to a wound, but ready-made gauze pads precut into convenient sizes (such as two-inch or four-inch squares) are probably more convenient for most people. "Sponge" dressings incorporate absorbent cotton between layers of gauze. They are more absorbent than other dressings and are used for seeping wounds or wounds that require additional cushioning.

Many of the variations among dressings are made in an attempt to solve the problem of removing the dressing. With most dressings, as the wound heals, the scab dries within the threads of the gauze. When the bandage is removed, part of the scab is often torn off with it, causing pain and possibly damaging the wound. One type of "nonadhering" dressing is made from gauze impregnated with a lubricating dressing such as petrolatum jelly. The nonadhering dressing that we recommend is gauze covered with a nonwoven plastic facing that is pierced with holes for ventilation, for example, Telfa Sterile Pads from Bauer & Black (part of The Kendall Company). Johnson & Johnson and Chesebrough-Pond's Inc. also manufacture dressings.

Gauze and Gauze Bandages

Cotton gauze is an open-weave cloth sometimes used for dressing wounds. Gauze is classified by how closely the mesh is woven; type I is the most closely woven, type VIII is the most loosely woven. The looser the weave, the softer the gauze, and the closer the weave, the stronger and more protective the gauze.

Gauze bandage stocked in pharmacies is usually type I gauze. Rolls of gauze bandage are available in widths from one to four inches and in lengths up to ten yards. As sold, gauze bandage is sterile. As soon as the package is open, the bandage loses its sterility.

Gauze bandage is generally used to hold primary dressings in place; it may also be used to provide some pressure and support on the wound area and to absorb blood from wounds.

Special Types of Gauze Bandage

It is difficult for an inexperienced person to bandage a wound neatly with the traditional gauze bandage, and consumers can now purchase special types of gauze bandage that make this task easier. We recommend any of the following products as alternatives to the more conventional gauze bandage for general household use. They form neat, comfortable dressings that don't slip. In fact, they can be used in place of adhesive bandages for most applications.

Surgitube, made by the Carlton Corporation, is a tubular seamless bandage. To hold on a dressing with this product, simply open the tube, slip it over the injury, and cut it off at the appropriate length. It is self-adhering; a slight twist will secure it. Surgitube bandage is available in five sizes: one for small fingers and toes; one for large fingers and toes; one for hands, feet, knees, and elbows; one for wrist and foot injuries; and one for head and leg injuries. It is available in either white or flesh tone cotton. It comes packed in an applicator with instructions for use.

Kling elastic gauze bandage from Johnson & Johnson is an example of a "clinging" gauze bandage, that is, one made to conform readily to the body's contours. This self-adhering bandage is made from a loosely woven mesh and has crimped edges. A slight twist causes the bandage to stick to itself to decrease slippage. Its loose mesh permits great absorbency. This conforming gauze bandage is available in sizes ranging from one to four inches in width and in rolls of five yards.

Gauztex from General Bandages, Inc. is a self-adhering gauze bandage that has been treated with rubber latex. It sticks only to itself, not to skin or hair. It is dry to the touch. It is available in widths of one or two inches.

Adhesive Tape

Adhesive tape is a strip of fabric, plastic film, or other material with one sticky surface. Adhesive tape is used to hold primary dressings in place and to immobilize an injured limb or joint. Broken ribs may be stabilized by strapping the chest, that is, wrapping the chest with adhesive tape. Many athletes tape certain joints to provide extra support. Adhesive tape cut into butterfly strips (strips with wing-like ends) can be used to suture wounds.

Standard tape products come on metal roll dispensers with snap-on metal lids. Tape is available in widths from one-half inch to four inches, and one to ten yards may be wound on one spool. Plastic tape often comes in a special easy-to-use dispenser. Some hypoallergenic tapes are commonly sold without any dispenser at all.

Use

Adhesive tape should be applied to clean, dry skin. If the skin feels moist, or if the user sweats a great deal, dab a little rubbing alcohol on the area and allow it to dry before applying the tape. If tape is to be applied repeatedly to a particular location, the skin in that area should be shaved to make it easier and less painful to remove the tape. A solvent such as mineral oil can be used to ease the removal of adhesive tape. Apply the mineral oil to the tape and allow it to soak through. After a few minutes the tape will be easy to pull away.

Hypoallergenic Tapes

From one to five percent of the people who use adhesive tape have allergic type reactions to it. The longer the tape is left on, the more likely it is that the user will have some reaction. If you have a reaction to adhesive tape, we suggest that you try one of the hypoallergenic or hyposensitive tapes. These tapes have a special nonirritating adhesive spread on a nonwoven paper-like backing. Because the backing allows air to get to the skin, these tapes are less likely to cause reactions. They are somewhat less adhesive than other tapes, but when applied properly (carefully smoothed down and pressed against the skin), they are satisfactorily adhesive.

When you are ready to remove this tape, a gentle tug pulls it free with little effort and only a minimum of discomfort.

Hypoallergenic tape is available in widths of one-half to three inches for hospital and home use. If you wish to purchase the three-inch tape, your pharmacist will probably have to order it. It should be noted that some people react even to hypoallergenic types of tape.

Choosing Tape

Tapes of different materials have different uses. Cloth tape is usually chosen for strapping or taping joints, limbs, or other parts of the body because it provides the most support. Plastic film tape is generally more adhesive than the "paper" tapes, and so it is used to hold dressings on wounds that are likely to get wet or anywhere that great adhesiveness is necessary. "Paper" tapes are least likely to cause irritation, although they are somewhat less adhesive than other types.

You can rely on adhesive tape from nationally advertised manufacturers such as Johnson & Johnson, The Kendall Company, and 3M. Generic tapes may be less expensive, but they may also be less adhesive.

Gauze Eye Pads

Eye pads are oval-shaped gauze pads covered with cotton. They are usually about two by three inches. They are used to protect an injured eye from dust and infection and to help it heal. They are sterile and are held in place with a piece of clear plastic tape. Johnson & Johnson manufactures eye pads.

Finger Stalls

Finger stalls, also called finger splints, finger guards, or finger cots, are devices meant to be slipped over injured fingers to protect them from bumps and to keep them immobile until the wound heals. Finger stalls are usually made of aluminum or plastic. Some are lined with foam rubber. A finger stall usually has a cap-like top that fits over the fingertip and four legs to keep the finger from bending.

Use

If your finger is accidentally jammed against something, even if it is not broken, a finger stall can be used to protect it while it is healing. If your finger has a cut that would open were the finger bent, a finger stall will keep it from bending.

To use a finger stall for an injury like a cut, you should bandage the wound, slip the finger stall over the finger, and apply adhesive tape to hold the finger stall on the finger. Finger stalls come in three different sizes, and the legs can be cut to fit the length of different fingers exactly. A finger stall can also be cut to fit on an injured toe.

Buying Finger Stalls

There is little difference between metal and plastic finger stalls, although the plastic ones may be slightly less expensive. Be sure to buy the proper size to fit your finger.

Emergency First Aid Kits

Every family should have emergency first aid supplies, and keeping such supplies separate from those in the home medicine cabinet is a good idea. Ideally, emergency supplies should be kept in a portable case in a place that is easily accessible, yet out of the reach of children.

Rather than assembling your own supplies, you may prefer to purchase a prepackaged emergency first aid kit. Such kits can be a good starting point from which a family can tailor a collection of supplies suited for the needs of their particular household. It is unlikely that a prepackaged kit will include all the items you want, and most will include some things that may never be used. However, they are convenient, and buying a kit will probably cost you less than it would to assemble all the supplies yourself.

Buying or Assembling a Kit

A good kit will include a selection of sterile gauze dressings and adhesive bandages in assorted sizes, adhesive tape, a roll of gauze bandage, an analgesic, scissors, and a first aid guide. Useful additions could include a medicated first aid dressing, an antiseptic, a tweezers, a collection of safety pins, and a flashlight. Depending on your needs, you may also want an insect sting kit (if anyone in the family is hypersensitive to insect stings and bites), a snake bite kit, and ipecac syrup and activated charcoal for poisoning.

Johnson & Johnson manufactures a number of first aid kits from which you can choose. Add to the basic supplies according to your particular needs.

Foot Care Products

Your feet take an incredible amount of wear and tear each day. Every time you take a step, your foot bears the full weight of your body. And if your shoes are not properly fitted, friction and pressure compound the normal strain.

The foot comfort products on the market fall into three general categories: supports to reinforce the bones, muscles and ligaments of the foot; cushions to lessen pressure caused by walking or other activity; and pads to protect the foot from friction. In addition, there are products to aid in the removal of corns and calluses and others to massage and relax aching feet.

All of these products offer some relief from foot discomfort. Considering that they are relatively inexpensive, and that a visit to a podiatrist or an orthopedic doctor, plus x-rays, may cost over $100, it makes sense to try these supports, cushions and pads. However, you should seek medical attention if redness and pain persist for 10 to 14 days.

It is possible your problem is nothing worse than poorly fitting shoes. On the other hand, some foot problems, such as severe bunions, require surgery for lasting relief.

Supports

Products aimed at supporting the foot range from arch supports to braces for straightening the toes.

Arch supports work by lifting the muscles and ligaments of the foot and creating a slight arch. This increases the foot's mechanical efficiency, which in turn reduces fatigue in both the leg and foot.

The Flexo Foam Arch by Dr. Scholl's is a useful product for active people with slighty weak arches. Because it is made of leather and foam rubber, the Flexo arch provides both support and cushioning. A better product for less active people with weaker arches is the Foot-Eazer by Dr. Scholl's. Although more expensive than the Flexo arch ($15 to $20 as opposed to about $5), it is made of leather and metal and provides greater support.

Another product to support the arch is the Dr. Scholl's Arch Binders, an elastic bandage worn around the foot. These are less effective than in-shoe arch supports; the bandage would have to be custom-fitted to work effectively.

Devices that straighten the toes prevent them from rubbing against each other and against the inside of the shoe. One such product is Dr. Scholl's Toe Flex, a rubber wedge placed between overlapping toes. This may relieve the pain of a corn between the toes, or it may only shift the problem to another toe where friction will form another corn. If this happens, you can often get relief simply by lubricating the toes with petroleum jelly.

The Toe Flex is also useful for straightening the large toe bent inward by a mild bunion. However, while straightening will reduce friction on other toes, only surgical correction will provide complete relief if the deformity is severe.

Cushions

Products aimed at cushioning the foot range from the familiar foam insoles to small cushions for specific areas of the foot, such as the ball or the heel.

The insoles are useful in relieving discomfort from mild calluses on the foot bottom. They also add an extra measure of comfort to any pair of shoes.

Insoles are generally sold by shoe size and come in a variety of materials, from foam rubber, to special insulation for warmth, to foam impregnated with charcoal to absorb odors.

Probably the most familiar insole is the Dr. Scholl's Air-Pillo Insole, which sells for about a dollar a pair. The insulated types, such as Dr. Scholl's Thermocushion, and the deodorant types, such as Johnson's Odor-Eaters (Combe Incorporated), cost about twice as much, but it is doubtful that either product will totally solve the problems of cold feet or foot odor.

Cushioning products for specific foot areas include heel pads, bunion pads, toe caps, and metatarsal (ball of foot) cushions. While none of them can totally relieve excess pressure, one that is particularly effective in relieving

650

heel pain is the Dr. Scholl's Foam-Eaze Cupped Heel Rest. Some podiatrists actually prescribe this product.

Friction Reducers

The foot care products aimed at reducing friction include adhesive-backed material that can be cut to size and pressed onto the foot wherever painful rubbing occurs, as well as precut pads for covering calluses and corns.

One of the most well-known friction reducing products is Dr. Scholl's Moleskin, an adhesive-backed felt. Other similar products are made of more durable cloths or rubber foam. These are more expensive than Moleskin, but are worthwhile if your problem is caused by a combination of pressure and friction.

The precut pads come in various sizes and shapes; the main difference among them is that some are cut out in the center, like rings. This shape is best for deep, painful corns and calluses, while the patches are more suited to shallower, less painful irritations.

Corn and Callus Removers

Many precut corn and callus pads come with discs impregnated with salicylic acid. Placed over the callus or corn, the disc is designed to remove it through the action of the acid. Zino Corn Pads and Zino Callus Pads by Dr. Scholl's come with these removal discs. A similar product is the Dr. Scholl's Fixo Corn Plaster, a salicylic acid-impregnated tape that can be cut to size and applied to the foot.

Acid-type products should be strictly avoided by anyone with diabetes or poor circulation. The acid action on their sensitive tissues could produce a sore that would not easily heal. These people should also avoid OTC liquid corn and callus removers. Corn- and callus-removing products may also cause problems for people with especially sensitive skin.

This is not to say that people in normal health should avoid these products. They can be useful, especially in removing hard, deep calluses and corns. However, you should apply them carefully to avoid irritating the tissue around the dead skin being removed. Another caution is not to use them for corns between the toes. The natural moisture there increases the penetration of the acid, which can cause painful irritation.

It is possible to have an allergic reaction to the ingredients in corn and callus removers. If you develop a rash, redness, or swelling, stop using the product and see your doctor immediately.

Other products for removing calluses and hard corns are pumice stones and abrasive sticks, such as Dr. Scholl's Corn and Callus File and Dr. Scholl's Hard Skin Remover. These are particularly useful in removing shallow, spread-out calluses. As with the acid-based products, it is important to use abrasives carefully to avoid damaging live tissue. In addition, the foot must be dry when using an abrasive stick or file.

One method for removing calluses that does not require any additional purchase is simply to rub the callus firmly with a towel when the foot is still moist after a bath or shower. This will remove some of the dead skin. When repeated several times, the process may remove the entire callus.

Sports Foot Care

Along with the recent increase in the popularity of exercise has come a great increase in the number of foot problems. Several new foot care products have been introduced for use by joggers, walkers, and other fitness seekers.

Some of these products, such as Dr. Scholl's Sports Cushions, are simply more durable versions of conventional foot care accessories. The Sports Cushion is an insole guaranteed to last the life of your athletic shoe. It also costs more than twice as much as a standard foam insole.

On the other hand, a few sports-oriented foot products are new designs, and some podiatrists recommend them. The Dr. Scholl's Runner's Wedge is an arch support that causes the foot to roll in such a way that the arch is raised, taking stress off foot and leg muscles. At about $10, the Wedge is a good buy for the serious jogger or walker with foot or knee pains, especially before going to the much greater expense of having a podiatrist make a custom-fitted orthotic support.

Vibrators and Baths

Besides foot care products designed to relieve specific foot problems, you can get overall relief by using foot vibrators and massage baths. These products relax the muscles and relieve the burning sensation of tired feet. Whether they actually stimulate blood circulation, as some manufacturers claim, is doubtful.

Two popular foot vibrators are the Dr. Scholl's Dual-Head Electric Foot Massager, and the Dr. Scholl's Deluxe Electric Foot Massager With Heat. With both the user sits on a chair, sets the vibrator on the floor and places his or her feet on vibrating pads. The Deluxe model has foot-shaped vibrating pads with built-in heating elements. The heat adds to the soothing effect, but it also increases the price by about $10.

There are two main types of foot massage baths: whirlpools, with jets that circulate the water; and vibrators, with electric motors that vibrate the water in the tub. Some people find the whirlpool effect more soothing, but these types generally cost from $10 to $20 more than the vibrators.

Most baths are designed to be used while the user is sitting in a chair. Some, though, are strong enough for a person to stand in the tub.

Since foot massage baths are electric devices, users should guard against shock hazards. Look for the Underwriters Laboratories (UL) label when buying a bath. Then follow the manufacturers instructions carefully. Do not overfill the tub, nor immerse the bath in water. Nor should you use the bath when any part of your body is in contact with plumbing, a radiator, or any other electrically grounded object.

A feature that makes some whirlpool baths slightly more desirable than others is a movable nozzle, which allows you to change the direction of the water jet. Models with this feature include the Han-D-Jet (Dazey Products Co.), the Sears Compact Whirlpool Bath, and the Pollenex Deluxe Portable Whirlpool Bath.

Two especially durable foot baths are the Pollenex Deluxe Portable Whirlpool Bath, and the Pollenex Hydro Action Foot Bath. Both are built so that the user can stand in the tub. In the former, the entire bottom of the tub is in contact with the floor. The bottom of the latter is well supported by five rubber feet.

Another bath with several attractive features is the Foot Fixer by Clairol. It is a vibrator type bath that heats and thermostatically controls the temperature of the water. In addition, it can be used without water, and the vibrating surface has mounds that will massage the arches of your feet.

Dental Equipment

Toothbrushes

Proper use of a good toothbrush is an important part of preventing the loss of teeth, either from decay or from gum (periodontal) disease. By brushing carefully and regularly, along with careful and regular flossing, bacterial plaque can effectively be removed from the teeth and gum line. Plaque is the sticky, colorless material containing harmful bacteria that is constantly forming on the teeth and at the gum line. Plaque combines with sugars in the mouth, creating acids that inflame the gums and eat away at tooth enamel.

Toothbrush bristles are made either of a synthetic material, such as nylon, or from a natural fiber. The bristles come in various degrees of hardness, ranging from very hard to very soft. Some toothbrushes come with a floss holder or a rubber dental stimulator on the end of the handle.

For most people, the best toothbrush to use is one with soft, rounded-end, nylon bristles that are firmly anchored into the plastic. The brushing surface, or head, of the toothbrush should be as flat as possible, and small enough to reach every tooth in the mouth. This type of toothbrush will help prevent scratching of the teeth and gums, and the bristles can be maneuvered into most nooks and crannies around the teeth. By getting into these hard-to-reach places, you will scrub most of the plaque in your mouth many times every time you brush your teeth.

The handle design of a toothbrush also affects its utility. Though there are some angled-handled toothbrushes on the market today, there is no clear evidence that they are superior to the more traditional straight-handled models. It seems that any angle chosen will always be ineffective in reaching some surface in the mouth. Furthermore, the angled models are generally more expensive than the straight-handled models. Regardless of its shape, the handle should be wide and flat to allow for a good grip and for ease of manipulation.

A toothbrush should be replaced as soon as the bristles become bent, frayed, broken, or worn down. Any one of these conditions can make the bristles ineffective in removing plaque. A toothbrush usually lasts most people about three to four months before the bristles become worn. Some dentists recommend that a person have two toothbrushes, alternating between them so that a dry toothbrush is always available.

There are many companies that manufacture toothbrushes. Among those companies producing quality toothbrushes are the following: Squibb Corporation, Oral B Company, John O. Butler Co., Block Drug Co., Inc., and Johnson & Johnson. When considering the purchase of a toothbrush, ask your dentist or pharmacist for a recommendation.

Electric Toothbrushes

Though most people can brush their teeth effectively using a hand-operated toothbrush, there are some people who might benefit from using an electrically-powered model. For example, some handicapped persons may be unable to make all the hand and arm motions necessary to manipulate the hand toothbrush. And because of their novelty, electric toothbrushes may be especially motivating for some children, though the novelty may soon wear off.

Some electrically-powered toothbrushes work off wall current, while others are battery-operated. We prefer the battery-operated models for safety reasons. But regardless of which type is used, it should carry the UL label, which means that it has been tested and approved for use by Underwriters Laboratories Incorporated.

The most important factor regarding electric toothbrushes is that they should have a dual action motion. That is, the brush should be capable of going up and down and back and forth. The brush chosen for use in an electric toothbrush handle should have many soft bristles with rounded tips, just as the standard brush should have.

Although several companies manufacture electrically-powered toothbrushes, only three models are rated acceptable by the American Dental Association. The three are as follows: Broxident Automatic Toothbrush, Squibb Corporation; General Electric Automatic Toothbrush Arcuate, Dual, Corded, General Electric Co.; and J.C. Penney Automatic Toothbrush, Dual, J.C. Penney Co., Inc.

Dental Floss

Dental floss helps clean unwanted food particles and plaque from between the teeth and around the gum line. (Plaque is a sticky, colorless material that contains harmful bacteria. Plaque is constantly forming on the teeth and gums.) By removing unwanted food particles and plaque, you are helping to prevent tooth decay (dental caries) and gum (periodontal) disease.

Use

To learn to floss correctly and safely, you should be taught by a dentist, a dental hygienist, or some other trained health professional whose specialty is related to the teeth and gums. Children need to be given special assistance, since incorrect flossing techniques can lead not only to cavities but also to gum damage.

One method of flossing is as follows: Break off between 18 and 24 inches of floss. Wrap the ends of the floss around your middle fingers, allowing more floss on one finger than the other. As you floss, roll the used or frayed portion of the floss onto the finger with the least floss. Use your thumbs and forefingers to guide the floss between your teeth. Always maintain about one inch of floss between your fingers while flossing. Without allowing any slack on the floss between your fingers, use a gentle sawing motion to insert the floss between two teeth. Don't "snap" the floss between your teeth—you can damage your gum. When the floss reaches your gum line and you can feel some resistance, curve the floss into a "C shape" against one tooth and gently slide the floss into the space between the gum and the tooth. Continue to hold the floss tightly against the tooth. Then move the floss away from the gum, scraping the side of the tooth in the process. Scrape the floss down on the upper teeth and up on the lower teeth. Do not use a "back-and-forth" motion when scraping the teeth, since gum damage can result.

Floss Holder

A dental-floss holder may make the use of floss easier for some people, particularly those people who have some manual dexterity problems. Also, a person with a very small mouth or a person who tends to gag easily may find the floss holder a desirable tool to use.

The floss holder is a device with a plastic handle, with a fork on one end. A piece of floss is fastened to each prong of the fork. The holder is then used to pass the floss between the teeth. Some holders have a container for the floss in the handle. Angled floss holders fit in the mouth better. The floss holder should be made of a durable plastic.

In general, the floss holder does not do as good a flossing job as does a person manipulating the floss by hand. The main reason for this is that the floss in the holder tends to bow, resulting in possibly uneven pressure against the side of a tooth. Such uneven pressure can prevent the floss from scraping the tooth effectively.

Buying Dental Floss

Dental floss comes in various weights, or gauges. The difference in the weight is related to the thickness of the fiber or fibers used in manufacturing. In addition, the floss is available either coated with wax or waxless. The unwaxed form is very fibrous, thereby better able to cut through and remove plaque than the waxed form. The waxed form of floss is really nothing more than a simple thread encased in wax. Some of that wax can get caught between the teeth when flossing, resulting in gum irritation and/or tooth discomfort. Therefore, we recommend the use of unwaxed dental floss, and the thinner the floss the better.

Dental floss is manufactured by various companies. Among the most popular are Johnson & Johnson and John O. Butler Co.

There is another product on the market that is also used to remove plaque. That product is called dental tape. Though used in a fashion similar to that of dental floss, dental tape does not seem to work as efficiently as dental floss. It is easier to manipulate the floss than it is to manipulate the tape, mainly because the tape is wide. The tape comes only in a waxed form, which means that some of the wax can get caught between the teeth during cleaning. Because the tape is not as fibrous as the floss, the tape cannot cut through and remove plaque as easily as the floss. Therefore, we recommend that unwaxed dental floss be used instead of dental tape, whenever possible.

Dental Mirrors

A dental mirror can help you locate areas in the mouth that have not been brushed or flossed well. This tool can also help you look for any sores or irritations on the gums, the palate, the tongue, or the cheeks. We think this tool is a handy and useful accessory in promoting good oral health.

Dental mirrors come in two types: one with a metal handle and holder, and the other with a plastic handle and holder. In either case, the mirrored end of the device is slanted to give a better viewing angle of all corners of the mouth, including the back side of the teeth and gums.

We recommend the purchase of a plastic model. A plastic dental mirror will be less expensive than the metal mirror. However, metal dental mirrors often have a metal screw that secures the mirror, an advantage because it makes the mirror replaceable.

Dental mirrors have a tendency to fog up at the time of use. A defogging solution can be purchased; however, there is a simple defogging procedure. Place the mirror against the moist inside of the cheek for a second or two, before use. The moisture will prevent the fogging of the glass.

Purchasing a Dental Mirror

When purchasing any type of dental mirror, be sure that the mirrored portion is distortion free. Look for what are called front-surface mirrors, mirrors constructed with a special backing for the glass. Flat-surface mirrors are often distorted, and should be avoided. Also, the dental mirror that you select should not have any chips in the glass, nor should the mirror be loose in its mounting.

There are also some dental mirrors on the market today that have a light source as part of their construction. If you always make sure that you are looking into your mouth in a well-lighted room, you will find that the extra expense for the lighted models is unwarranted. The John O. Butler Co. is one manufacturer of dental mirrors.

Disclosing Agents

Disclosing agents are made from a vegetable dye that stains, or "discloses," the plaque that remains on the teeth and at the gum line. They are a very important part of good oral hygiene, and we recommend their use, especially for persons with a history of poor brushing and flossing techniques.

Disclosing agents basically come in two forms: tablets and solutions. Although both forms serve the same function, the tablets are less expensive and not quite as messy as the solution. However, the solutions may prove to be easier to use with young children, since they are already in uniform consistency.

To use disclosing agents, all you need to do is to chew a tablet or swish a solution around in your mouth. Spit out or swallow any excess; the vegetable dye is harmless. Then examine your teeth, particularly at the gum line. Be sure to examine your teeth in good light. The use of a dental mirror at this time may be very helpful in locating the plaque. The color that you see on your teeth and at the gum line, usually bright red, indicates the location of plaque that must be removed by brushing and by flossing. (There are some solutions that are painted on with a cotton swab. These solutions, though messy and expensive, indicate new plaque in red and old, built-up plaque in blue.) Don't be concerned if your tongue and gums remain a little stained after the plaque has been removed. The color will soon fade as the dye continues to mix with the saliva in your mouth.

Until you become a proficient flosser and brusher of your teeth, you should use a disclosing agent every time you floss and brush. Then, when you have mastered the flossing and brushing techniques, you will need to use a disclosing agent only periodically to spot check for missed plaque.

Dental Stimulators

Dental stimulators are tapered pieces of wood or rubber that are used to massage the gum tissue between the teeth. The rubber tip found on the end of some toothbrushes is one kind of dental stimulator, and these tips are usually helpful in massaging the gums. Although toothbrush stimulators are less expensive, they are not as easy to manipulate as the stimulator sold on a special angled handle. These tools are usually made of metal and have replaceable tips.

Dental stimulators should not be used unless specifically prescribed by a dentist. Dentists usually recommend the use of a dental stimulator following certain kinds of dental surgery or in persons with periodontal disease. The benefit of a stimulator in those situations is that it toughens the tissue around the tooth as the stimulator is pushed between the teeth. Also, the dental stimulator seems to hasten the maturation of gum tissue right after surgery for periodontal disease. Periodontists will often recommend that a dental stimulator be used for at least two to three months after surgery. Johnson & Johnson is one manufacturer of dental stimulators.

Oral Irrigating Devices

Oral irrigating devices use a pulsating spray of water to remove food particles from between the teeth. Such devices will also massage the gums and stimulate blood circulation. The most popular device of this kind on the market today is the Teledyne Water Pik.

Oral irrigating devices should be used only by persons who are incapable of mastering correct toothbrushing and flossing techniques. Though some dentists recommend this kind of device for patients wearing braces or having bridgework (caps and crowns), oral irrigating devices have not been proved to be effective in removing bacterial plaque from the teeth and gums. Plaque has been found to be the major cause of dental caries and gum (periodontal) disease. In addition, the pressure of the pulsating water against the gums can cause them to separate from the teeth, which can result in plaque being pushed deep into the space between the teeth and the gums. Another problem is that if the water-pressure regulator on these devices is turned to maximum strength, the force of the water may loosen some bridgework or cause some marginal fillings to fall out.

Because the sensation of pulsating water makes the mouth feel as though it is being cleaned effectively, many people tend to rely on an oral irrigating device to clean their teeth and gums. Unfortunately, most of the plaque between the teeth and at the gum line is not being removed; only regular, proper brushing and flossing can accomplish this. Therefore, we do not generally recommend the use of oral irrigating devices except in conjunction with thorough brushing and flossing.

Denture Aids

Dentures require care unlike that prescribed for normal teeth. Two important aids are the denture brush and the denture cup.

The denture brush, which some dentists will supply to their patients, should have a wide, flat handle. We prefer one that is about one inch wide and about one-fourth inch thick. The bristles should be stiff. Longer bristles at one end of the brush head will allow the brush to get into the inside surfaces of the denture. Examples of quality denture brushes are those made by the John O. Butler Co. and the Block Drug Co.

Most any container large enough to hold your dentures will serve as a denture cup. However, the container should have a cover and should be unbreakable. The outside surface should not be slippery; the cup should be easy to hold. Some dentists supply denture cups to their patients.

It is very important that dentures be cleaned over a sink filled with water. Should the denture slip from your hand while you are brushing it, the water will help cushion the fall to help prevent breakage. Also, dentures should be placed only in water that is of room temperature. Hot water can cause dentures to warp. Dentures that have been left out of the mouth for an extended period without being placed in water, can dry out, resulting in warping.

Contraceptive Aids

Diaphragms

A diaphragm is a round latex dome rimmed with a metal spring or band. Prior to intercourse, it is smeared with a spermicidal agent and inserted through the vagina to fit over the cervix. Although it also serves as a physical barrier to the sperm, its primary contraceptive value is that it holds the spermicidal

657

agent against the cervix. To be effective, a diaphragm must be used with a contraceptive cream, jelly, or foam.

When used carefully, a diaphragm is nearly as effective as oral contraceptives (98 percent). However, less careful use may result in an effectiveness rate as low as 80 percent. It has virtually no major side effects, although some couples find that either the latex or the spermicide may cause irritation.

Obtaining a Diaphragm

Diaphragms are fitted by doctors or other health professionals (nursemidwife, nurse-practitioner). The doctor may supply the diaphragm, or you may have to take a prescription to the pharmacy to purchase the diaphragm. You should not leave the doctor's office without being instructed in inserting and removing the diaphragm. While in the office you should practice inserting and removing it, and the doctor should check to make sure that you have inserted it properly. Diaphragms can be inserted with the fingers or with a special applicator.

The fit of the diaphragm is an important factor in its effectiveness and the woman's comfort. A week or two after having the diaphragm fitted, you should go back and have the fit checked. Thereafter, you should have it checked whenever you have your periodic gynecological examination. A woman will not be able to feel a properly fitted diaphragm. A diaphragm that is too large may be painful; one that is too small may move excessively during intercourse, thus lessening its effectiveness. A woman may need to have the diaphragm refitted after gaining or losing ten pounds, delivering a child, and having surgery or a miscarriage. Diaphragms should routinely be replaced about every two years.

Use

Before using the diaphragm, fill it with water or hold it in front of a light to check for leaks. The diaphragm can be inserted approximately two hours before intercourse, and it must be left in place for six to eight hours after intercourse. Do not leave the diaphragm in place for more than 24 hours.

Before inserting the diaphragm, apply about a tablespoon of the spermicidal agent inside the dome of the diaphragm, i.e., the part that rests against the cervix. Also, spread the spermicide around the rim of the diaphragm with your fingers. It is believed that one reason for failure with the diaphragm is the use of an insufficient amount of the spermicide.

If you wait more than two hours after insertion to have intercourse, you must reapply the spermicide, although it's not necessary to remove the diaphragm to do so. Simply insert an applicator-full of the spermicidal agent. If you have intercourse more than once, you must reapply the spermicide every time.

After use, both the diaphragm and the applicator must be thoroughly cleaned with mild soap, rinsed well, and then thoroughly dried. The diaphragm may be dusted with cornstarch (to help keep it dry) and should be stored in its special case.

Buying a Diaphragm

There are three basic types of diaphragms; they differ in the type of spring they have. The differences between them are most apparent when they are bent prior to insertion. The arcing spring is the most commonly used. It is believed to be easier to insert by hand and to provide a better and tighter fit. The coil spring may be more comfortable for some women. The flat spring type may be prescribed for women with poor muscle tone in the wall of the bladder or rectum. Your doctor will determine which type you should get.

When you get the diaphragm you should also get an applicator (if you use one to insert the diaphragm) and spermicide. Usually, a special storage case is also provided.

There are few differences among brands of diaphragms. Ask your pharmacist to double-check that your diaphragm is being sold within the time period specified by the manufacturer. If fitted properly and used conscientiously, a diaphragm provides a high degree of protection against pregnancy. Ortho Pharmaceutical Corporation is a prominent manufacturer of diaphragms.

Condoms

A condom, or prophylactic, is a thin sheath worn over the penis during sexual intercourse. Condoms are worn as a birth control device or to prevent the transmission of venereal disease between sexual partners. Condoms are, currently, the only method of temporary contraception that is used by the male. Used properly, condoms provide a high degree of protection (up to 97 percent). Some couples use condoms with a spermicidal agent (cream, jelly, or foam) either in the woman's vagina or as a lubricant applied to the condom. With an effectiveness rate over 99 percent, such combined use offers extremely reliable birth control protection.

Condoms are available in a single size: one and one-half to two inches in diameter by about seven inches in length. They may be used more than once, but must be carefully cleaned, dried, and rerolled after use. Most men simply discard them after use.

Condoms may be made of latex or of animal membrane. Condoms made of animal membrane are more expensive than those made of latex, however many men believe them to be more sensitive. Condoms may be purchased lubricated or dry. Lubricated condoms are said to be less likely to tear and to minimize irritation. The closed-end may have a nipple-like receptacle for the sperm or it may be plain-ended. Choices among these alternatives are based mainly on personal considerations. Latex condoms are tested for holes, strength, and aging, and they must meet United States standards for size, thickness, and weight.

Use

Condoms prevent pregnancy by containing the ejaculate. To be effective, the condom must be applied before intercourse, not before ejaculation. Having intercourse before putting the condom on risks pregnancy because the lubricating fluid secreted at the tip of the penis may contain sperm.

If you use a plain-ended condom, be sure to leave a little space for the semen at the tip. This lessens the possibility of tearing or rupture. As the man withdraws, he should hold onto the rim of the condom to prevent leakage or slipping. Before discarding the condom, look to see if it is leaking anywhere. If so, consider using a spermicidal cream, jelly, or foam immediately. You may apply a lubricant to the condom after it has been put on. Use a spermicidal agent or a water soluble lubricant such as K-Y jelly. Do not use petroleum products such as Vaseline petroleum jelly on latex condoms. Such products may cause the latex to deteriorate.

If irritation develops while using condoms, try changing to a different type—from latex to animal membrane, or from dry to lubricated. Additional lubrication may also help.

Store condoms in a cool, dry place away from heat and sunlight. Even body heat may cause a condom to deteriorate. Don't carry condoms in a pocket or wallet for very long. Sometimes condoms don't work because they are defective; they may have a small puncture or they may break during use. Sometimes the condom slips off during intercourse or as the man withdraws. However, the most common cause of failure is not using the condom—it may not be applied at all or it may be applied too late.

Buying Condoms

Condoms should be purchased at a reliable drugstore, at family planning agencies, or through a reliable mail order house. Condoms purchased from a vending machine may be defective or old.

Never purchase condoms advertised as having special "sensory" devices attached. Typically, these condoms have projections of hard rubber along the shaft or tip. Although they are claimed to increase the sexual pleasure of the female partner, these projections usually cause a great deal of irritation.

Purchase condoms with the receptacle end. Many authorities believe that they are less likely to break during use. We also recommend that a contraceptive cream, jelly, or foam product be used along with a condom; their combined effectiveness approaches that of the oral contraceptive tablets.

Condoms are sold in packages of three or twelve. Generally, you can save money by buying the larger packages, assuming that you will use them within two years, the approximate shelf life of condoms. Condoms are available in many different styles and colors, but high quality condoms vary little in safety or effectiveness. Two prominent manufacturers of condoms are Schmid Products, Inc. and Youngs Drug Products Corp.

Elastic Goods

Elastic Bandages

Elastic bandages are worn as part of the treatment for injuries such as sprains. Athletes may wear them to provide extra support to certain joints. And they may be worn to treat varicose veins. Elastic bandages are beneficial in that they somewhat limit movement of an injured joint, provide additional support, and help to reduce swelling.

Elastic bandages may be made of fabric with a rubber or spandex thread sewn in, or they may be made of a specially knit cotton fiber. The cotton bandages are likely to be more durable, but they do not provide as much support as those made with rubber. Because rubber bandages are somewhat occlusive, they cause the area on which they are worn to become warm. This warmth is an advantage in the treatment of injuries such as a sprained muscle. Bandages that contain spandex instead of rubber are usually lighter in weight and are stronger. We feel the spandex bandages are the most comfortable and the most useful.

Elastic bandages are usually about five yards long when stretched. They come in widths ranging from two to six inches. The narrow widths (two or two and one-half inches) are used for wrists and feet; the middle widths (three to four inches) are used for ankles, elbows, or knees; the widest (four to six inches) are for the shoulders, ribs, and other large areas.

Use

Normally a pamphlet is included with the elastic bandage showing how it should be wrapped on a particular part of the body. We urge you to follow that pattern. Be careful not to apply too much or too little pressure. Too much pressure can lead to a loss of blood supply, and too little doesn't provide any support. A bandage that is wrapped too tightly may cause swelling, numbness, or throbbing.

Between uses, elastic bandages should be washed in warm, soapy water and rinsed well. They should be thoroughly dry before they are stored.

Elastic bandages are usually fastened in place with one or two metal clips near the end of the bandage. If you lose these clips, they can be replaced in most drug stores. We recommend the purchase of an elastic bandage that comes with metal clips attached (such as the Tensor Elastic Bandage from the Kendall Company) or one that sticks to itself (such as the Coban Elastic Bandage from 3M).

Elastic Hosiery

People who have "tired" feet and legs are often advised to wear elastic hosiery for the relief it provides. Elastic hosiery is part of the prescribed treatment for varicose veins, and pregnant women often wear it to keep from developing varicosities. Elastic hosiery is used for these purposes because it provides support and pressure to the veins in the legs. It is through these veins that blood must travel upward back to the heart. If the veins have lost their elasticity, the upward trip is more difficult than normal and the blood tends to pool in the legs, possibly leading to swollen feet and ankles and the tired feeling. Elastic hosiery, by supporting the veins, makes the trip easier.

Elastic hosiery basically can be divided into two types: two-way stretch, which provides both circular and longitudinal stretch; or one-way stretch, which provides only circular stretch.

Two-way stretch hosiery is suitable for relieving tired feet and legs, but it has no other therapeutic benefits. One-way stretch hosiery is heavier and provides greater support; it is the only style that should be chosen by people with varicose veins or other medical reasons to wear support hose.

Use

People who wear elastic hosiery for medical reasons should put the stockings on before they get out of bed in the morning; that way, blood never gets the chance to pool in the legs. If the stocking is difficult to put on, normal nylon hose can be worn under the support hosiery. Wearing the hose in this way may also extend the life of the support stockings; it keeps the sensitive elastic away from sweat and body oils.

All stockings should be washed regularly in warm soap and water and rinsed thoroughly. After washing, they should not be reworn for a day or two to allow them time to recover their elasticity. To prevent deterioration of the elastic, ointments, oils, and similar items should not come in contact with the hosiery.

Buying Elastic Hosiery

Two-way stretch hosiery is available in sheer-weight or heavier styles. They are easier to fit and put on than the one-way stretch stocking, however all elastic hosiery must be correctly fit to provide support without cutting off the blood supply. Consult your doctor if you feel you need support stockings, and make sure that you purchase the appropriate style—one-way or two-way stretch—for your use. Consult your pharmacist about your choice and about how to fit the stockings properly.

Elastic hosiery is available as panty-hose, regular stockings, and knee-length stockings. Some elastic hosiery is toe-less and heel-less, a style preferred by women who wear dress hosiery over the support stockings. However, the open toe and heel styles may be uncomfortable for women who have severe swelling of the feet.

Elastic ankles, kneecap, and elbow supports are modifications of elastic hosiery used to provide support to a particular part of the body. Athletes find them useful, and they may be more convenient than elastic bandages for frequent or long-term support of a particular joint.

Manufacturers of elastic hosiery include Becton, Dickinson Consumer Products; Harcourt Co.; Johnson & Johnson; Jung Products, Inc.; and The Kendall Company.

Suspensory

A suspensory is a pouch worn to support the scrotum. It consists of a cloth pouch attached to a waistband. Some styles have leg straps. In the center of the pouch is a hole through which the penis is inserted. A suspensory should be worn only at a doctor's direction. It is not meant to be a substitute for an athletic supporter or to protect the scrotum during strenuous activity.

The size of suspensory you need will be determined by your doctor. It should be large enough to hold the entire scrotum, but if it is too large it will cause intense discomfort. A wide variety of suspensories are available, and before buying one you should ask your pharmacist for a recommendation based on your build and weight as well as your doctor's instructions.

After use, a suspensory must be washed with warm, soapy water, rinsed thoroughly, and dried completely.

Ambulation Aids

Canes

A cane is a hand-held staff used as an aid in walking. Canes do help a patient balance, but they tend to be wobbly and unstable, and they do not actually provide much support. No cane should bear more than about 20 percent of the body weight.

Canes can generally be classified as one of three types. The standard single support model is the most common. The blind person's cane is 42 inches long, has a white top, a red bottom, and a metal tip. The third type has a straight stem with three or four short legs; it offers the best support and balance.

Use and Maintenance

Cane length should be such that with the rubber tip in place the elbow is bent about 20 to 30 degrees. The tip should touch the floor at about six inches to the side of the foot. Aluminum canes are frequently adjustable. Wooden canes can be shortened by sawing off the end.

Learning to walk with a cane is a little difficult but it is important that you are able to use the cane properly. A cane is most often carried beside the sound leg. The cane is advanced first, then the weak leg is advanced followed by the good leg. For climbing or descending steps, hang the cane in a belt or a pocket. Hold onto the rail. When going down stairs, the disabled leg goes first.

While still new, a wooden cane should be given several coats of a good wax to preserve its appearance and make it easier to clean. Wax should be reapplied at least once every six months.

Recommendations

Remember that a three- or four-legged cane provides the greatest support and stability. If you are buying a standard single support cane, remember that a good hardwood cane is the most durable. Aluminum canes are lighter, but not as strong. Avoid the canes with fancy handles if you are buying one for support. The carved handles are likely to break off. Make sure that you have tips for your cane; they prevent slippage. Prominent manufacturers of canes include Jung Products, Inc.; Professional Convalescent Products Co., and Tri-Med Surgical Company, Inc.

Crutches

Crutches are supports, typically fitted under the armpit, used to help the disabled walk. When using crutches, the patient puts weight on the arms and wrists rather than on an injured leg. Crutches are usually recommended for short term use following an accident or trauma to one or both legs. Occasionally they are also used by people who are permanently disabled.

Crutches are available in several styles and many sizes. They are generally made of wood or aluminum, and may be adjustable or nonadjustable. The standard nonadjustable double upright underarm crutches are made in lengths of 26 to 60 inches. Aluminum models are adjustable, lighter, stronger, and more expensive. For adults, the nonadjustable crutch is satisfactory and less expensive than adjustable models. For growing children who will be using crutches for a long time, the adjustable model may be preferred.

Forearm crutches are supports topped by cuffs or bands that encircle the patient's forearms. They are often used by people who must use crutches for an extended period. They are more expensive and are harder to use initially. Once the technique of using them is learned, however, they are easier to maneuver. Forearm crutches can support up to 40 to 50 percent of the total body weight.

Use and Maintenance

Properly sized or adjusted crutches are important to the patient's comfort. The top of an underarm crutch should come to about two inches below the armpit. The hand piece should be placed so that the arm bends at the elbow only about 20 to 30 degrees. This measurement should be taken while the patient is standing erect with legs slightly apart. If the patient is bedridden, measure from the armpit to the heel and add four inches.

Forearm crutches should be adjusted so that the forearm cuff comes to about one inch below the elbow, and the handgrip is placed at the distance from the floor to the patient's clenched fist.

Crutches should come equipped with rubber tips to prevent slipping and armpads on the top of the crutch. The crutch should be adjusted or measured while these tips and pads are on. Crutch armpads are made of foam rubber and they make the device more comfortable. Hand pads for the crosspieces of the crutches also make using crutches more comfortable.

There are several different ways of walking with crutches. Which way is used depends on the condition of both legs. Before you leave the pharmacy with crutches, you should practice whichever technique you have been instructed to use. You should also know how to go up and down stairs with the crutches, how to sit, and how to rise from a sitting position. Remember also, that when you are using crutches, your weight is borne on the hands and wrists, and not on the armpits.

Wooden crutches should be given several coats of a good wax while they are still new. The wax will preserve the appearance and make cleaning easier. The wax application should be repeated at least every six months.

Recommendations

Crutches may be rented or purchased. If they are to be used for a month or longer, it may be more economical to purchase them. For short term use, renting is generally less expensive. Also, make sure that the crutch-renting service provides armpads and rubber tips as part of the crutch rather than requiring that you purchase these separately. Among the most common manufacturers of crutches are Jung Products, Inc. and Tri-Med Surgical Company, Inc.

Walkers

Walkers are metal frameworks used by handicapped or crippled people to aid them in walking. The usual walker allows its user to rest his or her body weight on the handgrips rather than on possibly unsteady legs, thus affording greater stability. Walkers are frequently used when someone "graduates" from a wheelchair, but is still not able to walk unassisted. They might also be used by people with diseases, such as arthritis, that make walking difficult or painful.

Use

To use a walker, the person grasps it with both handgrips, moves the walker ten or twelve inches forward, and then steps into it, one leg after the other. Then, the walker is again advanced forward. An individual with one disabled leg should place the disabled leg inside the walker first and then the other leg. Walkers are almost completely useless on steps; and if someone must walk up or down steps, crutches would be preferable.

Recommendations

Walkers can be purchased or rented. Generally, they are required for many months, and if this is the case, purchasing a walker rather than renting one, will be more attractive. Walkers are available as adjustable or nonadjustable models. Most are made of aluminum, stainless steel, or chrome-plated steel. Some have attachable seats, some have underarm support rests, and others even have wheels. Some units are foldable, a useful feature for storage or for those who drive.

Manufacturers of walkers include Jung Products, Inc.

Syringes and Tubing

Bulb Syringes

Bulb syringes are hollow, usually pear-shaped containers connected to a hollow tip or pipe or tubing. The size and composition of the bulb and pipe or tubing vary according to the intended use, but all designs work basically the same way. Squeezing creates pressure inside the bulb. The pressure can be used to force fluid out of the bulb and into a body cavity, or it can be used to suction fluid out of a body cavity (nasal aspirators and breast pumps work this way).

Common types of bulb syringes include the ear syringe, the feminine bulb syringe, the rectal syringe, the breast pump, and the nasal aspirator.

Ear syringe. Ear syringes are used to irrigate the ear. They are filled with hydrogen peroxide or water to soften and rinse impacted wax out of the ear. Ear syringes range in capacity from one to three ounces and are usually molded in a single piece. Because they have a flexible tip, ear syringes can be used to irrigate other body cavities as well.

When using an ear syringe, you should warm the fluid to body temperature, but not hotter. When irrigating the ear of an adult, the lobe should be pulled up and backward to straighten the canal. An infant's earlobe, however, should be drawn downward and back. Squeeze on the bulb gently and steadily to avoid damaging the eardrum. Do not insert the tip deeply into the ear.

Feminine bulb syringes. Feminine bulb syringes are used for vaginal douching. Although they do not hold as much fluid, they are smaller and easier to transport than fountain syringes and combination syringe-water bottles—the other devices used for douching. To douche with a bulb syringe, you simply fill the syringe with your douching solution, sit on the toilet or in the bath, insert the tip into the vagina, and squeeze gently to release the fluid into the vagina.

Consult your gynecologist if you feel you need to douche. Douching on a routine basis for purposes of hygiene is no longer generally recommended.

Rectal syringe. Rectal syringes are used to give enemas. They are used in much the same way as a fountain syringe is used, although the pressure comes from squeezing the bulb rather than suspending the bag. Consult your doctor or pharmacist if you think you need an enema. Constipation can usually be better treated with a change in diet than with an enema.

Breast pump. Breast pumps are syringes used to remove milk from the breasts. The bulb of a breast pump is connected to a horn-shaped shield made of glass or plastic. Attached to the bottom of the shield is a receptacle for the milk pumped from the breast. In use, the bulb is depressed and the horn is placed over the breast. The bulb is released, and the milk is suctioned from the breast. This procedure may be done to collect milk for a baby who cannot nurse, to encourage the flow of milk, or to empty the breast completely. Many authorities believe that manual expression is a better way to empty the breasts and therefore that a breast pump should not be used without a doctor's advice.

Nasal aspirator. The infant nasal aspirator is a bulb syringe used by adults to remove mucus from a baby's nose. The syringe is first compressed and the tip is placed gently in the nose while the bulb is released. This creates a gentle suction that removes mucus from the nose.

Use

All bulb syringes should be washed and allowed to dry thoroughly after use. Whenever the tip of any syringe is inserted into any body cavity, care should be taken not to insert it too deeply. Pressure on the bulb should always be gentle; too much force may cause damage.

Buying Bulb Syringes

Judge the quality of the bulb syringes you buy in the same way you would judge the quality of other rubber goods—look for a smooth finish and a tight fit between tip and bulb. Make sure the syringe is not cracked. Abbott Laboratories and Davol Inc. manufacture a variety of bulb syringes.

Fountain Syringes and Combination Syringe-Water Bottles

Fountain syringes and combination syringe-water bottles are usually rectangular rubber bags formed by fusing two sheets of rubber together around the edge. After the seam is assured it is usually covered and reinforced with glue or an extra strip of rubber sheeting.

A fountain syringe has a large opening at the top and a short piece of hollow pipe extending out of the base. Flexible tubing attaches to this pipe.

The neck of a combination syringe-water bottle has a threaded closing. A combination syringe-water bottle usually comes with two stoppers: one, a water-tight plug to use when you want to apply heat with a water bottle; the other, a plug with a short piece of hollow pipe in the center. A length of flexible tubing is attached to this hollow pipe when the device is used as a syringe.

Combination syringe-water bottles and fountain syringes are usually marketed with a length of appropriate tubing, a shut-off valve for the tubing, and at least one vaginal tip and one rectal tip. Three tips are furnished with the better models—a vaginal tip, an adult rectal tip, and an infant rectal tip. These may be made of hard rubber, plastic, or nylon.

Use

These products are used for douching or for the administration of enemas. The combination product may also be used, as is a regular water bottle, for the application of heat. We suggest that you consult your doctor if you feel you need to douche or have an enema. Most medical authorities now believe that douching is not necessary for normal personal hygiene and that changes in one's diet or lifestyle are preferable to enemas for treating constipation.

After either use, the tip should be washed with soap and water; soaked in an antiseptic solution (such as diluted Lysol disinfectant solution) for 15 minutes, then rinsed with rubbing alcohol, and allowed to dry before storage. The syringe and tubing should be rinsed with water and hung up to drain and dry. The shut-off valve should always be removed from the tubing to prevent kinking.

Choosing a Fountain Syringe or Combination Product

Consider carefully how you plan to use the product you're buying. Don't buy a combination syringe-water bottle unless you use both a water bottle and a syringe. The combination product is more expensive than either a water bottle or a syringe purchased alone.

Differences between syringes made by different manufacturers for the same price range are usually insignificant. But differences between cheaper and more expensive models may affect the durability of the product and your satisfaction with it.

The single factor that most affects the performance of a particular syringe or syringe-water bottle is the quality of the rubber used. Cheaper models may use reclaimed rubber or rubber with mineral filler, making the bag less durable and less elastic. Unfortunately, it's difficult for most consumers to determine the quality of rubber. However, other indicative features can be noted.

Examine the tubing. It should be at least five feet long, and it should be rubber, not plastic. Plastic is more likely to pinch and crimp than rubber. Avoid syringes with a simple spring or snap to close off the flow of fluid through the tubing. Models with a threaded or lever closure device are easier to operate. Tips that screw onto the tubing are less likely to leak than those that slip into the tubing. Finally, read the guarantee. Better models have a longer guarantee (up to five years) while poorer quality products may be guaranteed for only one year.

Davol Inc. and Faultless Rubber Company (Division of Abbott Laboratories) manufacture fountain syringes and combination syringe-water bottles.

Tubing

Tubing may be made of either rubber or plastic. Rubber is preferred because it is less likely to tear or become crimped. Tubing may be purchased for use with fountain syringes as well as for general household purposes such as siphoning liquids from one container into another container. Tubing is sized by its internal diameter. Be sure you buy the right size to prevent leakage. Tubing may be purchased in precut lengths of five or six feet, or your pharmacist can cut it to your specifications. Tubing is manufactured by Bel-Art Products and Davol Inc.

Emergency Medical Identification

People with certain diseases or allergies should carry identification describing their condition in case of emergencies. Such information can be life-saving in situations—an auto accident perhaps—in which a person may lose consciousness. Various tags and bracelets are available at pharmacies for just this purpose. Usually the information is engraved on one side of a small metal tag with a medical symbol on the other side. The tag may be sold on a bracelet, or it may be designed to be worn on a necklace, bracelet, or watch.

Examples of information generally available on such tags include that the wearer is diabetic, has an allergy to penicillin or other drugs, has epileptic seizures, is a heart patient, or wears contact lenses. Special messages can be ordered through the pharmacist. Manufacturers of such tags include the National Identification Co., Inc.

Hypodermic Syringes and Needles

A hypodermic syringe is a syringe used with a hollow needle to inject liquids into the body beneath the surface of the skin. A syringe basically consists of a barrel that holds the liquid and a plunger that pushes the liquid out.

You may buy either reusable or disposable syringe sets. Reusable units may be made so that the barrel and plunger are interchangeable or not interchangeable. The latter type of syringe set will have a serial number printed on both the barrel and plunger. If one part breaks, the entire unit must be replaced.

Disposable syringes may be made of glass or plastic and often have a rubber gasket on the plunger tip. With disposable syringes there is no need to sterilize the unit after use. They are more convenient and less likely to cause infection than reusable units, and we recommend their purchase.

Luer-Lok reusable syringes have a metal device on the tip that in theory serves as a lock for the needle. These devices make the syringe somewhat more cumbersome to use and add to the cost of the device. Correctly placed needles will not slip off a syringe.

Syringes come in sizes from 1 to 100 cc. Specialized syringes, such as those used by diabetics, come in smaller sizes. Reusable syringes are graduated with marks either etched in or scratched in. Disposables may be marked with paint instead of etching. All syringes are tested before they are sold, and the graduations must be accurate within 5 percent.

Three special types of syringes include the vaccine syringe, the tuberculin syringe, and the insulin syringe. The standard vaccine syringe is intended to hold about 1 cc and is graduated in 1/20 of a cc intervals. It can be used with medications other than vaccines. Tuberculin syringes come in various sizes and allow the measurement of amounts as small as 1/100 of a cc. Insulin syringes are usually graduated in units of insulin rather than in cc intervals. Insulin syringes are currently calibrated for 40 units, 80 units, and 100 units. At some point in the future, the 40 unit and 80 unit syringes will be discontinued in an attempt to standardize insulin preparation and reduce the dangers to patients using multiple concentrations of insulin and syringes. Meanwhile, always make sure to use the insulin syringe that is correct for the strength of insulin you use. To help you, insulin syringes are often color-coded to match the colors on insulin labels. Forty unit insulin labels and syringes are red; 80 unit insulin labels and syringes are green; and 100 unit insulin labels and syringes are orange.

Hypodermic needles are designated by two numbers—gauge and shaft length. Gauge refers to the width of the needle and may range from 27 to 13. The larger the number, the smaller the diameter, and vice versa. The size needle to choose depends on the type of medication and where it is being injected. If the medication is thick, a heavy needle will have to be used. If the medication is watery, a thinner needle is preferred because it makes the injection more comfortable.

Most needles used for home injections do not need to be longer than about ⅜ or ½ inch because most home injections are made by placing the medication directly under the skin. If the medication is to be injected into the muscle or into a vein, a longer needle will be required.

Use

You should be fully instructed in the proper use of a hypodermic syringe and needle before you buy one. The instruction should include an actual injection performed by whoever will be doing the injections at home—whether that is the patient or someone else. Be careful to remove all air from the syringe before the injection. Any air left in the syringe takes up space that should be filled with medication. If this air is not removed, a dosage error may result. Tip the needle upward so that any air bubbles rise to the top of the syringe, then press the plunger in until a drop of liquid comes out of the needle.

Reusable equipment should be carefully sterilized after each use. If a glass plunger ever gets stuck within the barrel, place the entire unit in a pan of boiling water and allow it to boil gently for a few minutes. The two parts should then easily pull apart. But be careful to pick up the unit carefully; it will be hot. When discarding syringes and needles, always make sure you destroy the needle first by bending it.

Buying Syringes and Needles

When buying syringes and needles, always buy the brand that you have been using. With a brand different than your usual, you may inject slightly more or less medication. If you think you want to change brands, talk to your doctor first.

When purchasing a reusable syringe, examine it to make sure there are no cracks or chips in the glass. Make sure that the serial numbers on the barrel and plunger match. If you purchase reusable needles, be sure to get needle wires to clean out the inside of the needle. Disposable needles may cost a little more, but they are sterile and they tend to be sharper and better lubricated than reusable needles, making them more comfortable to use.

When you go into a pharmacy, you will have to ask your pharmacist for the syringes and needles. These supplies must be kept in a locked case or behind the prescription counter. You may also have to sign your name in a registry book to show that you purchased the item.

In some states, the pharmacist cannot sell this equipment without a written prescription. In other states, only state residents may purchase such equipment. If you are traveling, therefore, it's a good idea to take a supply of syringes and needles sufficient to last until you return home. And for diabetics, it's always a good idea to have an extra syringe if reusable equipment is being used. If disposable equipment is used, the diabetic will find it economical and convenient to keep a few extra units on hand.

Recommendation

For most people, the ideal combination of syringe and needle is the disposable product that has the needle sealed into the end of the barrel of the syringe (for example, the Plastipak syringe/needle combinations available from Becton, Dickinson Consumer Products). Such products give consistent results, and a diabetic can save money on insulin by using them because less of the drug is lost in the hub of the needle. We recommend these all-in-one units because they are both convenient and safe.

Urine-Testing Products

Urine contains the products of metabolism of the body's cells and is a most extensively studied body fluid. It is a valuable means for diagnosing several disease processes. In addition, many drugs can be detected in the urine, and testing for them is one way to assure patient compliance as well as to identify possible overdose or drug abuse problems.

Use

OTC urine-testing products are easy to use and are inexpensive. And you can get in minutes the same information that may not come from a laboratory for several days, but you must learn how to use them properly.

First, completely wash, rinse, and dry the urine collection container. Or, use a disposable paper cup. Unless otherwise directed, collect the urine immediately before testing. Sometimes, a urine sample must be taken in the early morning or at some other specific time but usually testing immediately follows collection. If the urine sample must be kept for more than a few minutes, put it in the refrigerator and indicate the time the sample was taken on a piece of tape placed on the container. Then, before you do the actual test, allow the urine to reach room temperature for a few minutes. The following are among the most commonly used urine tests.

Testing for glucose. One of the most common urine tests is a test for sugar, or glucose. It can be used to detect the presence of diabetes, or it can be used by diabetics to determine if they have been using too little insulin.

These tests may be of two types: dip-and-read tests or tablet tests. A dip-and-read product is dipped into a urine sample, kept there for a specific length of time, withdrawn, and read by comparing its color against a color chart.

The tablet test products include test tubes and tablets. A tablet is added to the urine sample in the test tube. As soon as the testing period is up, the color of the sample in the test tube is "read" by comparing it to a color chart.

Dip-and-read tests rely on enzyme action and are susceptible to damage from exposure to heat or humidity. These products must be stored in a cool, dry place (not in the refrigerator). Tablet tests also should be stored in a cool, dry place. Cotton should not be placed in the bottle. The tablets are toxic if swallowed; keep them out of the reach of children. Dip-and-read products that have turned brown or tablets that develop black spots should be discarded.

Testing for ketones. Dip-and-read products and tablets also test for ketones, chemicals that are released into the urine when the body is burning fat. The presence of ketones in the urine may be due to diabetes, but only a doctor can tell for sure. See a doctor whenever a ketone test is positive.

Testing for protein. Protein is normally present in the blood but not in the urine. The presence of protein in the urine indicates kidney disease. Tests for protein are of the dip-and-read type. Because residue on the inside of the urine collection container may influence test results, the container should be washed with a strong soap—not a detergent—rinsed well, and allowed to dry completely. If a urine sample has been refrigerated, allow it to warm before testing. Discard the sample if it appears cloudy after it has warmed. To detect cloudiness, hold the container against a black background and shine a light on it.

Pregnancy tests. To conduct a pregnancy test, the test material is added to a urine sample in a special glass tube. The tube is allowed to stand undisturbed for two hours. A brown ring in the bottom of the tube indicates pregnancy. If these tests are performed nine days or more after the first missed menstrual period and the results are positive (i.e., pregnancy is indicated), they are 97 percent accurate. If, however, the results are negative there is a 25 percent chance that the woman is pregnant (i.e., the result is false negative). The chance of having false negative results is greater the earlier the test is done. Therefore, negative results indicate the need for a second test.

A woman considering the use of one of these tests may want to consult her gynecologist or obstetrician. Most doctors will want to confirm the test's results if they are positive—meaning that the woman will probably end up paying for two tests no matter what the result.

Tests for pH determination. The pH value reflects the acidity or alkalinity of a substance. Determination of the pH of urine is an important diagnostic test for diseases of the kidneys or lungs. Normal urine has a pH range of 4.8 to 8.5. In case of severe ketosis (acidosis) the pH value may drop to below 4.8. In periods of urinary infection, the pH may rise to 9 or more.

Determination of urinary pH is also used in managing certain diseases. For example, if you are using certain drugs to treat a urinary tract infection your urine should be kept acidic to maximize the therapeutic benefits of these drugs. Urine should also be kept acidic when treating certain urinary tract stones (kidney stones) because the stones are more soluble in an acid urine.

Overdoses of certain drugs can be treated by maintaining a certain pH value. For example, if you were to take too much of an acidic drug such as aspirin or a barbiturate such as phenobarbital, the drugs would be excreted from the body in greater amounts if a basic urine were maintained. Amphetamine (a basic drug), on the other hand, would be excreted in greater amounts if the urine were acidic.

When used alone, urinary pH measurement has little value—urine pH normally fluctuates throughout the day. However, combined with the results of other tests or with the presence of specific symptoms, the pH figure serves as an invaluable aid to confirm or deny the presence of a specific disease. For example, in a patient with marked clinical symptoms of acidosis (diabetes), but with a urinary pH of 6.7, diagnosis of acidosis or diabetes is probably not valid. However, if with symptoms of acidosis the patient has a urinary pH of about 5 (acid), diabetes is indicated. Thus, it is important not to look at urinary pH without considering other factors as well.

A number of methods are available for determining urine pH. An electronic pH meter covers the entire pH range (1 to 14) but is expensive, cumbersome, not easily portable, and unrealistic for home use. Litmus paper determines whether the urine is acid, but it does not provide specific values. Nitrazine indicator paper has a limited pH range and must be compared with a color chart when it is used with urine. The most convenient method for measuring urinary pH is the dip-and-read pH indicator sticks (available from your pharmacist) that measure a pH ranging from 5 to 9.

Whenever you use a dip-and-read stick for determining pH, the last drop of urine remaining on the strip should be removed by touching the strip to the side of the container before reading to prevent the "run-over" of chemicals from one area of the strip to another.

It is important that you collect urine samples in clean containers and measure for pH immediately upon voiding. If your urine stands for 30 to 60 minutes or longer, certain bacteria present in the urine may cause the urine to change pH. Thus, your reading would be false. Note also, that if you are using a urinary pH test to monitor a disease, you should do the test at a specific time each day and try to avoid drinking a large quantity of water before the test.

Tests for blood, hemoglobin, or myoglobin. The presence of blood, hemoglobin, or myoglobin in the urine may result from a number of diseases. Blood in the urine may be visible to the naked eye, or it may cause the urine to look smoky or dark. Sometimes, blood is detectable only when a chemical is added.

The term "hematuria" refers to the presence of whole blood cells in the urine, resulting specifically from some kidney disease. Hemoglobinuria results when blood cells are destroyed and hemoglobin is added to the urine. Infections and certain allergic conditions are the usual causes of hemoglobinuria. Myoglobinuria refers to the presence of myoglobin in the urine. Myoglobin is a constituent of muscle and whenever a muscle is damaged, myoglobin is released into the blood and enters the urine. Thus, the presence of myoglobin reflects some muscular disease such as muscular dystrophy. Myoglobin is also frequently present in the urine of persons involved in contact sports, following heart attacks, as well as during kidney disease.

The most convenient way to measure blood, hemoglobin, or myoglobin in the urine is to use a dip-and-read product. Immerse the stick in urine and 30 seconds later, compare the color to a color chart.

Tests for bilirubin. The presence of bilirubin, a bile pigment, in the urine is one indicator of several types of liver disease. Ictotest tablets (Ames Company) are a convenient testing procedure. This test involves using a special asbestos cellulose mat and a tablet. Urine is added to the asbestos cellulose mat and the tablet is placed thereon. If a purple color appears after a small quantity of water is added to the tablet, bilirubin is present.

Combination products. Combination products are useful for many diagnostic situations. If you are involved in monitoring a specific disease, a single test product will be more economical. If you need to keep track of several conditions, then a combination product will be easier to use and cheaper in the long run.

Buying Urine-Testing Products

There are dozens of different kinds of urine testing products. Your doctor or pharmacist will advise you on which is appropriate for your needs.

Index

672

Adsorbocarpine ophthalmic solution, 298
adverse reaction, 17–25
See also drug eruptions
aerosol sprays, application of, 42–3
Afrin nasal decongestant, 299
in treatment of: allergy, 108; common cold, 93; earache, 95; middle ear infection, 99; nasal congestion, 100; nosebleeds, 101; sinus infection, 103; sore throat, 105
Aftate athlete's foot remedy, 299
in treatment of ringworm infections, 78
Agoral laxative, 300
Air-Pillo Insole foot cushion, 650
alcoholic hepatitis, 145
See also alcoholism; cirrhosis
alcoholism, 201–3
See also alcoholic hepatitis; cirrhosis
Aldactazide diuretic and antihypertensive, 300
and breast enlargement, 275, 286
Aldactone diuretic and antihypertensive, 301
and breast enlargement, 275, 286
interaction with potassium, 24
Aldomet antihypertensive, 302
effect on gastrointestinal system, 18
See also methyldopa
Aldoril diuretic and antihypertensive, 303
aldosterone, and adrenal diseases, 275–76
aldosteronism, primary, 275–76
Alka-Seltzer analgesic and antacid, 304
Alka-Seltzer antacid, 304–5
sodium bicarbonate in, 173
Alka-Seltzer Plus cold remedy, 305
Alka-2 antacid, 306
calcium carbonate in, 174
Allbee multivitamin, 306
Allerest decongestant eyedrops, 306–7
Allerest hay fever and allergy remedy, 307
Allerest nasal decongestant, 307
Allerfrin adrenergic and antihistamine, 308
allergen, 107
allergy, 107–8
allergy and congestion remedy
℞ drugs profiled: Disophrol Chronotab, 394; Drixoral, 405–6; Duo-Hist, 406; Histodrix T.D., 441
allergy remedy
OTC drugs profiled: Allerest, 307; A.R.M., 320; Dimetane, 391; Teldrin, 586–87
Allernade antihistamine, anticholinergic, and adrenergic, 308
Allerphed adrenergic and antihistamine, 308
Allerphed C expectorant, 308

allopurinol (Zyloprim), 628–29
in treatment of: gout, 232; kidney stones, 185
Almocarpine ophthalmic solution, 308
aloe, in laxatives, 150
Alophen laxative, 308–9
alumina gel, in diarrhea remedies, 151–52
aluminum
acetate, 96
chloride, in treatment of hyperhidrosis, 67
salts, in OTC antacids, 173–74
amantidine
in treatment of: influenza, 117; Parkinson's disease, 219
ambenonium, in treatment of myasthenia gravis, 218
Ambenyl expectorant, 309–10
ambulation aids, 662–64
Amcill antibiotic, 310
amebiasis. *See* amebic dysentery
amebic dysentery, 145–46
amenorrhea, 197
Amen progesterone hormone, 310
Americaine hemorrhoidal preparation, 310
Americaine local anesthetic, 310
in treatment of burns and sunburn, 241; chicken pox, 250
Ameri-EZP antibacterial and analgesic, 310
Aminodur Dura-Tabs bronchodilator, 310
aminophylline bronchodilator, 310–11
in treatment of asthma, 109–10
Amitril antidepressant, 311
amitriptyline hydrochloride antidepressant (Elavil), 409–10
Ammens Medicated Powder rash remedy, 311
ammonium chloride, in treatment of emphysema, 116
amoxicillin antibiotic, 311–12
Amoxil antibiotic, 312
amphetamine
and drug dependence, 207
definition, 12
interaction with other drugs, 24–25
in treatment of: hiccups, 164; hyperkinesis, 214
Amphojel antacid, 312–13
amphotericin B
in treatment of: candidiasis, 249; histoplasmosis, 253
ampicillin antibiotic, 313
in treatment of: appendicitis, 147; erysipelas, 252; gonorrhea, 262; meningitis, 216; salpingitis, 200; typhoid fever, 267; whooping cough, 123
Ampico antibiotic, 313
Amplin antibiotic, 313

bedpan, 637–38
bedsore, 56–67
bed-wetting, 182
Benadryl antihistamine, 335
    in treatment of Parkinson's disease,
    219
Benadryl Cream local anesthetic, 336
Bendectin antinauseant, 336
    in treatment of: morning sickness,
    169; nausea and vomiting, 170
Benemid uricosuric, 336–37
    interaction with other drugs, 24
Ben-Gay external analgesic, 337
    in treatment of backache, 231
Bentyl antispasmodic, 337–38
    in treatment of: colic, 148; peptic
    ulcer, 174
Bentyl antispasmodic with
    phenobarbital, 338
Benylin DM cough remedy, 338
Benzedrex nasal decongestant, 338–39
benzocaine
    in eardrops, 94–95
    in OTC drugs: diet aids, 271;
    hemorrhoidal preparations, 160–61;
    local anesthetics, 241; poison ivy
    remedies, 74; throat lozenges, 104;
    toothache remedies, 176
Benzodent toothache and sore gums
    remedy, 339
    in treatment of toothache, 177
benzoyl peroxide, in OTC acne
    preparations, 56
beriberi, 269–70
beta blocker
    definition, 14
    R̲ drugs profiled: Inderal, 446–47;
    Lopressor, 466
Betapen-VK antibiotic, 339
Bexophene analgesic, 339
B.F.I. Powder external anti-infective,
    339–40
    in treatment of canker sores and
    fever blisters, 59
bilirubin, 166
    urine-testing kits for, 671
Bio-Tetra antibiotic, 340
Biphetamine anorectic, 340
    in treatment of obesity, 271–72
birth control pills. See contraceptives,
    oral
birth defects, 21–23
bisacodyl, in laxatives, 150
bismuth subgallate, in diarrhea
    remedies, 151–52
bites
    animal, 240
    insect, 60–61, 69–70
black eye, 83–84
black lung disease. See occupational
    lung disease
bladder
    cancer, 287

infection, inflammation, 186–88
bleeding
    eye, 86
    postmenopausal vaginal, 199–200
    unusual internal, 142–43
    See also hemorrhage; stools, black
blepharitis, 84
Blistex Ointment canker sore and
    fever blister remedy, 340–41
Blis-To-Sol athlete's foot remedy, 341
blood clots, 129–30
    and angina pectoris, 127
    and heart attack, 133
    See also heart attack; stroke,
    thrombophlebitis of the deep veins
blood pressure kits, 633–34
    and high blood pressure, 138
    use, 46
    See also high blood pressure
Blupav smooth muscle relaxant, 341
boils, 57–58
bones, disorders affecting, 227–39
Bonine antinauseant, 341–42
    in treatment of: motion sickness,
    169; nausea and vomiting, 171
Borofax rash remedy, 342
botulism, 155–56
brain
    cancer, 289
    encephalitis, 208
    See also nervous system
Brasivol acne preparation, 342
Breacol cough remedy, 342–43
breast
    abnormal enlargement, 275, 286
    cancer, 286–87
    self-examination, 49–50, 286
Brethine bronchodilator, 343
Bricanyl bronchodilator, 343
Bristacycline antibiotic, 343
Bristamycin antibiotic, 343
Brocon antihistamine, 343
Bromatapp antihistamine, 343
Bromepaph antihistamine, 344
Bromophen antihistamine, 344
Bromo-Seltzer analgesic, 344
bronchiectasis, 110–11
bronchitis, 111–12
    See also cough; emphysema;
    pneumonia
bronchodilator
    definition, 14
    R̲ drugs profiled: Aminodur Dura-
    Tabs, 310; aminophylline, 310–11;
    Brethine, 343; Bricanyl, 343;
    Bronkodyl, 345; Choledyl, 357;
    Elixophyllin, 410; Lanophyllin, 459;
    Somophyllin, 575; Somophyllin-T,
    575; Theocap, 590; theophylline,
    410
bronchopneumonia. See pneumonia
Bronitin asthma remedy, 344
Bronkaid asthma remedy, 345

Bronkaid mist asthma remedy, 345
   in treatment of asthma, 110
Bronkodyl bronchodilator, 345
Broxident Automatic Toothbrush, 654
bruises, 240
Buerger's disease, 130-31
buffered analgesics, 54
Bufferin analgesic, 345-46
bulk-forming laxatives, 149-51
bunion, 58
burn, 241-42
burn remedy
   OTC drugs profiled: Americaine, 310;
      Foille, 427
burn remedy and antiseptic
   OTC drugs profiled: Medi-Quik, 472;
      Noxzema, 503; Solarcaine, 573
bursitis. See arthritis
busulfan, taken during pregnancy, 22
Butazolidin Alka anti-inflammatory, 346
Butazolidin anti-inflammatory, 346-47
   and gastritis, 157
   and gastroenteritis, 158
   interaction with other drugs, 24
Butisol Sodium hypnotic, 347

Cafergot migraine remedy, 347-48,
   in treatment of headache, 214
Cafergot P-B migraine remedy, 348
Cafermine migraine remedy, 348
Cafertrate migraine remedy, 348
caffeine
   and anxiety, 204
   in OTC analgesics, 53
   in prevention of migraine headache,
      211
Caladryl poison ivy remedy, 348
calamine lotion, 348
   in treatment of: chicken pox, 250;
      measles, 257; poison ivy/poison
      oak, 74-75; scabies, 79; shingles,
      81
calciferol, in treatment of tetany, 225
   See also vitamin D
Calcimar, in treatment of Paget's
   disease, 236
calcium carbonate, in OTC antacid,
   173-74
callus, 62
   See also foot care product
Campho-Phenique athlete's foot
   remedy and antiseptic, 349
camphor spirits, in treatment of canker
   sores and fever blisters, 59
cancer, 284-92
   and drug use, 23
Candex antifungal agent, 349
candidiasis, 249
cane, 662-63
canker sore and fever blister remedy
   OTC drugs profiled: Blistex
      Ointment, 340-41; Gly-Oxide,
      437-38

canker sore, 58-59
Capade antihistamine, anticholinergic,
   and adrenergic, 349
Capital with Codeine analgesic, 349
capsule, administration of, 40
carbamazepine, in treatment of tic
   douloureux, 226
carbamide peroxide
   in product for: canker sores and
      fever blisters, 59; impacted earwax,
      96-97
carbohydrate, as nutrient, 268
carbuncle, 57-58
carcinogen, 285
cardiovascular system, 124-143
Carter's Little Pills laxative, 349
casanthranol, in laxative, 150
cascara sagrada laxative, 349-50
   in treatment of constipation, 150
castor oil laxative, 350
   in treatment of: constipation, 150;
      hives, 67; ingrown toenails, 69
Catapres antihypertensive, 350-51
cataract, 84
cathartic, 14
   See also laxative
CAT scanner, in diagnosis of cancer,
   288
cavity, tooth. See tooth decay
Centet antibiotic, 351
central nervous system depressant, 14
   See also hypnotic; sedative; sedative
      and hypnotic
Cēpacol throat lozenge, 351
   in treatment of sore throat, 104
Cēpacol Troches anesthetic throat
   lozenge, 351-52
cerebrovascular accident. See stroke
cerebrovascular disease. See stroke
Cerespan smooth muscle relaxant, 352
cerumen, 96
cervical cancer, 289
cervicitis, 190
Cerylin expectorant and smooth muscle
   relaxant, 352
Cetaphil Lotion skin cleanser, 352
   in treatment of eczema, 64-65
chafing, 59-60
chemotherapy, in treatment of cancer,
   286-92
Cheracol cough remedy, 352-53
   in treatment of: bronchitis, 111-12;
      common cold, 93; coughing,
      113-14; influenza, 117; occupational
      lung disease, 119; pneumonia, 121;
      whooping cough, 123
Cheracol D cough remedy, 353
   in treatment of: bronchitis, 111-12;
      common cold, 93; coughing,
      113-14; influenza, 117; occupational
      lung disease, 119; pneumonia, 121;
      sore throat, 105; whooping cough,
      123

chicken pox, 250
chigger bites, 60-61
Chloramead phenothiazine, 353
chloramphenicol
    in treatment of: Rocky Mountain
        spotted fever, 259; tularemia, 266;
        typhoid fever, 267; typhus, 267
Chloraseptic throat lozenges, 353
    in treatment of: common cold, 93;
        sore throat, 105
Chlordiazachel sedative and hypnotic,
    353
Chlorofon-F analgesic, 353
Chlorserpine diuretic and
    antihypertensive, 353
chlorothiazide diuretic and
    antihypertensive. See Diuril diuretic
    and antihypertensive
chlorpheniramine maleate
    in products used to treat: allergy,
        108; itching, 71
chlorpromazine hydrochloride
    and breast enlargement, 286
    in treatment of hiccups, 164
    See also Thorazine phenothiazine
chlorpropamide. See Diabinese oral
    antidiabetic drug
Chlor-Trimeton decongestant cold and
    allergy remedy, 354
    in treatment of: conjunctivitis, 85;
        hay fever, 96; hives, 67
Chlor-Trimeton Expectorant cough
    remedy, 354-55
Chlor-Trimeton Expectorant with
    Codeine cough remedy, 355-56
Chlorzide diuretic and antihypertensive,
    356
Chlorzone Forte analgesic, 356
chlorzoxazone w/APAP. See Parafon
    Forte analgesic
Chocks multivitamin, 356
Chocks Plus Iron multivitamin, 356-57
cholecystitis. See gallstones
Choledyl bronchodilator, 357
cholelithiasis. See gallstones
cholera, 251
cholestyramine, in treatment of drug-
    induced liver disease, 168
chorea minor. See St. Vitus' dance
chronic simple glaucoma, 88
Cin-Quin antiarrhythmic, 357
Circanol vasodilator, 357
cirrhosis, 147-48
    and liver cancer, 287
    See also alcoholic hepatitis;
        alcoholism
Clearasil Antibacterial Acne Lotion, 358
Clearasil Medicated Cleanser acne
    preparation, 358
Cleocin antibiotic, effect on
    gastrointestinal system, 18
climacteric. See menopause
clindamycin, in treatment of acne, 56

Clinoril anti-inflammatory, 358-59
clofibrate, in prevention of
    atherosclerosis, 129
Clomid synthetic estrogen, in treatment
    of infertility, 195
Clostridium, botulinum, 155
clotrimazole
    in treatment of: candidiasis, 249;
        ringworm infections, 72
clove oil, in treatment of toothache,
    176
cluster headache, 211-12
coal tar
    in OTC products used to treat:
        eczema, 65; psoriasis, 76
Coastaldyne analgesic, 359
Coban Elastic Bandage, 661
cocaine. See drug dependence
coccidioidomycosis, 251-52
Cocillin V-K antibiotic, 359
codeine
    and drug dependence, 206
    in cough suppressant, 111, 113, 117,
        119, 121
    in treatment of: diarrhea, 152;
        pneumonia, 121
Cogentin antiparkinson drug, 359
coitus, painful, 199
    See also cervicitis; endometriosis
Colace laxative, 359
    in treatment of constipation, 151;
        heart attack, 134
ColBENEMID uricosuric, 359
colchicine gout remedy, 359-60
    in treatment of gout, 232
cold, 91-94
cold and allergy remedy
    OTC, discussion, 92
    OTC drugs profiled: Bayer
        Decongestant, 333-34; Chlor-
        Trimeton decongestant, 354;
        Congespirin children's, 364-65;
        Contac, 365-66; Contac Jr.
        children's, 366; Coricidin, 367;
        Coricidin 'D' decongestant, 368;
        Coricidin Demilets children's, 369;
        Covangesic, 376-77; Dristan, 402-3;
        Dristan timed-release, 404-5;
        Novahistine, 500; Ornade 2 for
        Children, 512; Sinarest, 564-65;
        Sine-Off, 566-67; Sinutab, 569-70;
        Sinutab-II, 570-71; Triaminicin, 602
Col-Decon adrenergic and
    antihistamine, 360
Cold Hot Pack, 644-45
cold pack
    disposable, 645
    gel, 644-45
cold remedy
    OTC drugs profiled: Alka-Seltzer Plus,
        305; Bayer children's, 333; Comtrex,
        363-64; Coryban-D decongestant,
        372-73; CoTylenol children's,

373-74; CoTylenol, 374-75; CoTylenol (liquid), 375; 4-Way, 429; Neo-Synephrine Compound decongestant, 493-94; Ornex, 513; Sudafed, 578; Sudafed Plus, 578-79; Viro-Med (liquid), 621; Viro-Med (tablet), 621-22

colic, 148

colloidal oatmeal bath. See Aveeno Colloidal Oatmeal bath product

Collyrium Drops eyewash, 360
   in treatment of conjunctivitis, 85
   in treatment of sty, 90

colon
   cancer, 290-91
   irritable, 166

Colonil anticholinergic and antispasmodic, 360

colostomy
   in treatment of cancer, 291;
   ulcerative colitis, 180

Col Pac, 645

Colsalide (colchicine) gout remedy, 360

Combid Spansule anticholinergic and phenothiazine, 360-61

common cold, 91-94

Compazine phenothiazine, 361-62
   in treatment of: cancer, 292-92;
   nausea and vomiting, 170;
   pneumonia, 120-21

Compound W wart remover, 362-63
   in treatment of warts, 82

Compoz Tablets sleeping aid, 363

Com-Pro-Span anticholinergic and phenothiazine, 363

Comtrex cold remedy, 363-64

Conceptrol contraceptive cream, 364

concussion, 242

condom, 192, 659-60

Congens No. 1 estrogen hormone, 364

Congespirin children's cold and allergy remedy, 364-65

congestion, rebound, due to nasal spray or drops, 93, 100

congestive heart failure, 131-32

conjugated estrogens. See Premarin estrogen hormone

conjunctivitis, 85

Conn's syndrome, 275-76

constipation, 148-51

Contac cold and allergy remedy, 365-66
   Contac Jr. children's cold and allergy remedy, 366

contact dermatitis, 61

contraception, 190-93

contraceptive
   condom, 659-60
   definition, 14
   diaphragm, 657-59
   OTC drugs profiled: Conceptrol, 364; Dalkon Kit, 378; Delfen, 382; Emko, 411; Encare Oval, 412-13; Intercept Contraceptive Inserts, 449; Ortho-

Creme, 513-14; Ortho-Gynol, 514; Semicid, 560
   See also contraception

contraceptive, oral, 191, 509-10
   in treatment of: endometriosis, 195; menstrual disorders, 197-98; salpingitis, 200

Coprobate sedative and hypnotic, 366

Cordran steroid hormone, 366-67

Coricidin cold and allergy remedy, 367

Coricidin cough remedy, 367-68

Coricidin 'D' decongestant cold and allergy remedy, 368

Coricidin Demilets children's cold and allergy remedy, 369

Coricidin nasal decongestant, 369-70

corn and callus remedy
   OTC drugs profiled: Dr. Scholl's Corn/Callus Salve, 397; Dr. Scholl's "2" Drop Corn-Callus Remover, 398; Freezone Corn and Callus Remover, 429-30
   See also foot care products

corneal ulcer, 85-86

corns, 62
   See also foot care products

coronary thrombosis. See heart attack

Corphed adrenergic and antihistamine, 370

Correctol laxative, 370

Cortaid topical steroid product, 370-71
   in treatment of poison ivy/poison oak 75

Cortan steroid hormone, 371

corticosteroids. See steroid hormone

Cortin steroid hormone and anti-infective, 371

cortisol. See hydrocortisone

Cortisporin ophthalmic suspension, 371

Cortisporin otic solution/suspension, 371-72

Coryban-D cough remedy, 372

Coryban-D decongestant cold remedy, 372-73

Co-Salt salt substitute, 373
   in treatment of: edema, 132; menstrual disorders, 198

CoTylenol children's cold remedy, 373-74

CoTylenol cold remedy, 374-75

CoTylenol liquid cold formula, 375

cough, 112-14
   See also cold

cough and cold remedy
   ℞ drug profiled: Tuss-Ornade, 608-9

cough remedy, 113
   OTC drugs profiled: Benylin DM, 338; Breacol, 342-43; Cheracol, 352-53; Cheracol D, 353; Chlor-Trimeton Expectorant, 354-55; Chlor-Trimeton Expectorant with Codeine, 355-56; Coricidin, 367-68; Coryban-D, 372; Dimacol, 390-91;

Demi-Regroton diuretic and antihypertensive, 383
dental equipment, 653-57
dependence
on alcohol, 201-3
on drugs, 206-8
depression, 204-5
dermatitis
atopic, 64
contact, 61
medicamentosa, 63-64
Dermolate anal-itch ointment, 383-84
in treatment of hemorrhoids, 161
Dermolate topical steroid, 384
DES. See diethylstilbestrol
Desamycin antibiotic, 384
Desenex athlete's foot remedy, 384
in treatment of ringworm infections, 78
desert fever (coccidioidomycosis), 251-52
Desitin Ointment rash remedy, 385
Desitin rash remedy, 385
detergent cleanser
℞ drugs profiled: pHisoHex, 530-31; Soy-Dome Cleanser, 575; WescoHEX, 627
deviated septum, 103
De Witt's Pills analgesic, 385
Dexedrine (dextroamphetamine sulfate)
anorectic, 271, 385
in treatment of narcolepsy, 218
taken during pregnancy, 22
dextromethorphan, in cough suppressants, 105, 111, 113, 117, 119, 121, 123
diabetes insipidus, 276-77
diabetes mellitus, 277-80
See also antidiabetic; antidiabetic, oral
Diabinese oral antidiabetic drug, 385-86
in treatment of diabetes mellitus, 279-80
taken during pregnancy, 22
Diacin vitamin supplement, 386
Dialex antianginal, 386
Dialose laxative, 386-87
Dialose Plus laxative, 387
Diamox diuretic, 387-88
interaction with other drugs, 24
in treatment of glaucoma, 88
Diaparene Baby Powder rash remedy, 388
Diaparene Peri-Anal Cream rash remedy, 388
diaper rash, 63
diaphragms, 192, 657-59
See also contraception; contraceptive
Diaqua diuretic and antihypertensive, 388
diarrhea, 151-52
diarrhea remedy, 151-52

OTC drugs profiled: Donnagel, 398; Donnagel-PG, 398-99; Kaopectate, 454-55; Kaopectate Concentrate, 454-55; Lactinex, 459; Parepectolin, 517-18; Pepto-Bismol, 522
See also anticholinergic and antispasmodic; antidiarrheal
diarrhea, travelers', 179
diastolic pressure, 137
Diazachel sedative and hypnotic, 388
Di-Azo analgesic, 388
diazoxide, in treatment of hypoglycemia, 280
Dibent antispasmodic, 389
dibucaine
in OTC drugs: hemorrhoidal preparations, 160-61; poison ivy remedies, 74
dicyclomine hydrochloride antispasmodic. See Bentyl antispasmodic
dienestrol, taken during pregnancy, 22
diet
for weight loss, 271-72
guidelines for nutritious, 269
diethylstilbestrol
and cancer, 23, 289
taken during pregnancy, 22
Di-Gel antacid and antiflatulent, 389
simethicone content of, 174
digitalis
and heartbeat irregularities, 135-36
definition, 14
effect on vision, 18
in treatment of: congestive heart failure, 132; heart attack, 134; obesity, 271
digoxin. See Lanoxin
dihydrotachysterol, in treatment of tetany, 225
See also calciferol; vitamin D
Dilantin anticonvulsant, 389-90
interaction with other drugs, 24
Dilantin with Phenobarbital anticonvulsant, 390
Dilart smooth muscle relaxant, 390
dilation and curettage
in treatment of: cervicitis, 190; postmenopausal vaginal bleeding, 200
Dimacol cough remedy, 390-91
dimenhydrinate, in OTC antinauseants, 169
Dimetane allergy remedy, 391
Dimetane DC expectorant, 391-92
Dimetane expectorant, 392-93
Dimetapp antihistamine, 393-94
dioctyl calcium sulfosuccinate. See docusate
dioctyl sodium sulfosuccinate. See docusate
Diothane hemorrhoidal preparation, 394
Dipav smooth muscle relaxant, 394

Duchenne type of muscular dystrophy, 233
Dulcolax laxative, 406
  in treatment of constipation, 150–51
Duo-Hist allergy and congestion remedy, 406
Duratet antibiotic, 406
Duration nasal decongestant, 406–7
dusty lung diseases. *See* occupational lung diseases
Dyazide diuretic and antihypertensive, 407–8
Dymelor antidiabetic drug, in treatment of diabetes mellitus, 279
dysentery, 145–46
dysmenorrhea, 197–98
dyspareuni. *See* coitus, painful
dyspepsia, 164–66

ear. *See* ear, nose, and throat
earache, 94–95
Eardro otic solution, 408
eardrops
  administration, 40–41
  in treatment of swimmer's ear, 106
  OTC drugs profiled: Auro, 327; Debrox, 381
eardrum, perforated, 98, 101–2
ear infection, middle, 98–99
ear, nose, and throat disorders of, 91–106
ear, swimmer's, 106
earwax, impacted, 96–97
ecchymosis, 142
Ecotrin analgesic, 408–9
  in treatment of: arthritis, 228; pain and fever, 54
eczema, 64–65
edema, 132
edrophonium, in treatment of myasthenia gravis, 218
E.E.S. antibiotic, 409
Elavil antidepressant, 409–10
Eldatapp antihistamine, 410
Eldefed adrenergic and antihistamine, 410
Elder 65 Compound analgesic, 410
Eldezine antinauseant, 410
electroshock therapy, in treatment of depression, 205
Elixophyllin bronchodilator, 410
embolism, pulmonary. *See* blood clots; thrombophlebitis of the deep veins
embolus. *See* blood clots; heart attack; thrombophlebitis of the deep veins
emetic, 14
Emetrol antinauseant, 410–11
  in treatment of nausea and vomiting, 171
Emko contraceptive, 411
emphysema, 115–16
  See also bronchitis; cough; occupational lung diseases

Empirin Compound analgesic, 411–12
Empirin Compound with Codeine analgesic, 412
Empracet with Codeine analgesic, 412
E-Mycin antibiotic, 412
Encare Oval contraceptive, 412–13
encephalitis, 208
Endep antidepressant, 413
endocarditis, 132
endometriosis, 194–95
Enduron diuretic and antihypertensive, 413–14
Enoxa anticholinergic and antispasmodic, 414
enteric-coated analgesics, 54
enteric fever. *See* typhoid fever
enteritis, regional, 164–65
enuresis, 182
Enzactin athlete's foot remedy, 414
Epi-Clear acne preparation, 414
Epi-Clear Scrub Cleanser acne preparation, 414
Epi-Clear Soap for Oily Skin acne preparation, 414–15
epigastric pain, 153
epileptic seizures, 209–10
epinephrine
  in products used to treat:
    asthma, 109–10; glaucoma, 88
  in treatment of shock, 247
epsom salts, in treatment of constipation, 151
Equagesic analgesic, 415
Equanil sedative and hypnotic, 415
  and drug dependence, 206
Ergocaf migraine remedy, 415
ergot alkaloids, taken during pregnancy, 22
ergotamine tartrate, in prevention of migraine headache, 211
Erypar antibiotic, 415
erysipelas, 252
Erythrocin antibiotic, 415
erythromycin antibiotic, 415–16
  in treatment of: acne, 56; boils and carbuncles, 58; impetigo, 68; syphilis, 263; whooping cough, 123
Esidrix diuretic and antihypertensive, 416
Eskabarb sedative and hypnotic, 416
Eskatrol adrenergic and phenothiazine, 416–17
esophagitis, 154
Estroate estrogen hormone, 417
Estrocon estrogen hormone, 417
estrogen hormone
  action, 275
  and cancer, 289
  and osteoporosis, 235
  and postmenopausal vaginal bleeding, 199
  in oral contraceptives, 191
  ℞ drugs profiled: Congens No. 1, 364;

conjugated estrogens, 536-37; Estroate, 417; Estrocon, 417; Kestrin, 456; Menogen, 474; Menotab, 474; Ovest, 514; Premarin, 536-37; Sodestrin, 573

E.T.H. Compound adrenergic, sedative, and smooth muscle relaxant, 417

ethionamide, taken during pregnancy, 22

Ethril antibiotic, 417

Etrafon phenothiazine and antidepressant, 417

Excedrin analgesic, 418

Excedrin P.M. analgesic, 418-19

Ex-Lax laxative, 419

expectorant
  definition, 14-15
  Rx drugs profiled: Actifed-C, 297-98; Allerphed C, 308; Ambenyl, 309-10; Dimetane, 392-93; Dimetane DC, 391-92; Dri-Phed-C, 402; HRC-Proclan with Codeine, 441; HRC-Proclan VC with Codeine, 441; J-Gan-VC, 454, K-Phen with Codeine, 458; Mallergan, 470; Mallergan VC with Codeine, 470; Mallergan with Codeine, 470; Midatane, 478; Midatane DC, 478; Normatane, 499; Normatane DC, 499; Pentazine, 522; Pentazine with Codeine, 522; Phenergan, 526; Phenergan VC, 526-27; Phenergan VC with Codeine, 527-28; Phenergan with Codeine, 528; Proclan, 540; Proclan VC, 540; Promethazine Hydrochloride, 541; Promethazine Hydrochloride VC with Codeine, 541; Promethazine Hydrochloride with Codeine, 541; Promex, 541; Promex with Codeine, 541; Prothazine, 542; Prothazine with Codeine, 542; Puretane DC, 543; Puretane, 543; Sherafed-C, 563; Spentane, 576; Spentane DC, 576
  See also cough remedy

expectorant and smooth muscle relaxant
  Rx drugs profiled: Cerylin, 352; Glyceryl-T, 437; Lanophyllin-GG, 459; Quibron, 544; Slo-Phillin, 572; Theo-Col, 591

expiration date, 37-38

Exsel seborrheic shampoo, 419

external analgesics. See analgesic

eye disorders, 83-90

eyedrops
  administration, 40
  OTC drugs profiled: Isopto-Frin, 452; Murine, 484; Visine decongestant, 622
  See also ophthalmic solution

eye pad, gauze, 648

eyewash, OTC, Collyrium Drops, 360

fainting, 210

family planning, natural, 192-93
  See also Basal Temperature thermometer; contraception; contraceptive

Fastin anorectic, 419-20

fats, as nutrients, 268

Feen-A-Mint laxative, 420

female
  reproductive tract, disorders of, 189-200
  sex hormone. See estrogen; progesterone; steroid hormone

Femiron iron supplement, 420-21

Femiron multivitamin and iron supplement, 421

Fenbutal analgesic and sedative, 421

fenoprofen calcium, in treatment of arthritis, 228
  See also Nalfon anti-inflammatory

Fenylhist antihistamine, 422

Feosol iron supplement, 422

Fergon iron supplement, 422-23

Fer-In-Sol iron supplement, 423

Fernisone steroid hormone, 423

ferrous gluconate, in treatment of iron-deficiency anemia, 126-27
  See also Fergon iron supplement

fever
  as a symptom, 53-54
  blisters, 58-59

filiform warts. See warts

fingercots, 639

finger stalls, 648

Fiorinal analgesic and sedative, 423-24

Fiorinal with Codeine analgesic and sedative, 424

first aid
  for miscellaneous injuries, 240-47
  kits, emergency, 649

5-FU, in treatment of cancer, 285, 286, 291

Fixo Corn Plaster, 651

Fizrin Powder analgesic and antacid, 424-25
  ingredients of, 173

Flagyl anti-infective, 425-26
  in treatment of amebic dysentery, 146

flatulence, 154-55

Fleet Enema laxative, 426

Fletcher's Castoria laxative, 426

Flexeril analgesic and muscle relaxant, 426-27

Flexo Foam Arch, 650

floss, dental, 654-55
  holder, 654-55

Fluonid steroid hormone, 427

fluoride, in prevention of tooth decay, 178

"flu." See influenza

F.M.-200 sedative and hypnotic, 427

688

grisOwen antifungal, 438
guaifenesin, in OTC cough remedies, 113, 117, 121, 123
Gull's disease. *See* myxedema
gum disorders
  gingivitis, 158–59
  periodontal disease, 175–76
  trench mouth, 179–80
gynecomastia. *See* breast, abnormal enlargement
Gyne-Lotrimin antifungal, 438

Habdryl antihistamine, 438
hair loss, 65
  See also ringworm infections
Haldol antipsychotic agent, 438–39
Haley's M-O laxative, 439
haloprogin, in products used to treat ringworm infections, 77
Han-D-Jet whirlpool foot bath, 652
hangover, alcoholic, treatment of, 203
Hansen's disease. *See* leprosy
hay fever, 95–96
  See also allergy; asthma; eczema
hay fever and allergy remedy, OTC, Allerest, 307
Hazel-Balm hemorrhoidal preparation, 439–40
HVC steroid hormone and anti-infective, 440
headaches, 210–14
Head & Shoulders Cream dandruff treatment, 440
Head & Shoulders Shampoo dandruff treatment, 440
health care accessories, 631–72
health records, 44–50
heart attack, 133–35
heartbeat irregularities, 135–36
heartburn, 159–60
  and esophagitis, 154
heart drug
  Rx drugs profiled: digoxin, 460; Lanoxin, 460
heart failure. *See* congestive heart failure
heat collapse. *See* heatstroke
heat exhaustion, 245
heating pads, 641–43
heat prostration, 65–66
heat rash, 65–66
heatstroke, 244–45
Heb-Cort steroid hormone and anti-infective, 440
Heet external analgesic, 440
Hematest Tablets, 136
Hemoccult Slides, 136
hemoglobin, urine-testing kit for, 671
hemolytic anemia, 126–27
hemorrhage, 136–37
hemorrhoidal preparation
  OTC drugs profiled: Americaine, 310; Anusol, 316–17; Diothane, 394;

Gentz Wipes, 434; Hazel-Balm, 439–40; Lanacane, 459; Nupercainal (ointment and suppository), 505; Preparation H, 537; Tucks, 607; Vaseline Hemorr-Aid, 616–17; Wyanoid, 627
hemorrhoids, 160–61
Henotal sedative and hypnotic, 440
heparin
  in treatment of: blood clots, 130; heart attack, 134; stroke, 141
hepatitis, 161–62
  alcoholic, 145
  and cirrhosis, 147
hepatitis, toxic. *See* liver disease, drug-induced
herpes simplex virus
  fever blisters, 59
  genital infection, 261
herpes zoster. *See* shingles
Hexaderm I.Q. steroid hormone and anti-infective, 440
Hexyphen antiparkinson drug, 441
hiatus hernia, 162–63
hiccups, 163–64
high blood pressure, 137–38
hirsutism, 66
  and anorexia nervosa, 203
Hiserpia antihypertensive, 441
histamine
  role in: allergy, 107–8; the common cold, 92
Histatapp antihistamine, 441
Histodrix T.D. allergy and congestion remedy, 441
histoplasmosis, 253
hives, 66–67
  See also allergy; contact dermatitis; drug eruptions; itching
HMG, 196
Hodgkin's disease, 288
Hold cough suppressant lozenges, 441
Hold liquid cough suppressant and decongestant, 441
homatropine methylbromide for diarrhea, 152
hookworm, 253–54
hordeolum. *See* sty
hormonal disorders, 274–83
hormone
  definition, 15
  in oral contraceptives, 191
  in treatment of endometriosis, 195
  taken during pregnancy, 22
hosiery, elastic, 661
hot packs
  disposable, 645
  gel, 644
housemaid's knee. *See* arthritis
HRC-Proclan VC with Codeine expectorant, 441
HRC-Proclan with Codeine expectorant, 441

human menopausal gonadotropin, 196
humidifiers, 639-41
Huntington's chorea, 222
Hydergine vasodilator, 442
  in treatment of stroke, 141
hydralazine hydrochloride
    antihypertensive
  and systemic lupus erythematosus,
    238
  in treatment of high blood pressure,
    137-38
  See also Apresoline antihypertensive
Hydro-Chlor diuretic and
    antihypertensive, 442
hydrochlorothiazide diuretic and
    antihypertensive, 442-43
hydrocortisone
  action, 275
  seborrheic dermatitis, 80
  in treatment of: hemolytic anemia,
    126-27; hemorrhoids, 161;
    seborrheic dermatitis, 80; ulcerative
    colitis, 180
HydroDIURIL diuretic and
    antihypertensive, 443
  in treatment of edema, 132
hydrogen peroxide, 443
Hydromal diuretic and antihypertensive,
    443
Hydrophed adrenergic, sedative, and
    smooth muscle relaxant, 444
Hydropres diuretic and
    antihypertensive, 444-45
Hydroquin steroid hormone and
    anti-infective, 445
Hydroserp diuretic and
    antihypertensive, 445
Hydroserpine diuretic and
    antihypertensive, 445
Hydrotensin diuretic and
    antihypertensive, 445
hydroxychloroquine, 238
hydroxyzine hydrochloride sedative.
  See Atarax sedative
Hydro-Z-50 diuretic and
    antihypertensive, 445
Hygroton diuretic and antihypertensive,
    445-46
hyoscine hydrobromide, in diarrhea
    remedies, 152
hyoscyamine sulfate, in diarrhea
    remedies, 152
hyperactivity. See hyperkinesis
hyperemia, 129
hyperhidrosis, 67
hyperkinesis, 214-15
hypermenorrhea, 198
hypersensitivity to sunlight, 72-73
  See also allergy
hypertension. See high blood pressure
hyperthyroidism. See thyroid diseases
hypnotic
  definition, 15

R drugs profiled: Butisol Sodium,
    347; Dalmane, 378-79; Nembutal
    Sodium, 491-92; pentobarbital,
    491-92; Seconal Sodium, 559
  See also sedative; sedative and
    hypnotic
hypodermic syringes and needles,
    667-68
hypoglycemia, 280-81
  See also adrenal diseases; diabetes
    mellitus
hypoglycemic agents, oral. See
    antidiabetic drugs, oral
hyposensitization, for hay fever, 96
hypothyroidism. See thyroid diseases
Hysone steroid hormone and
    anti-infective, 446
hysterectomy, 289
Hytakerol (dihydrotachysterol), in
    treatment of tetany, 225

ibuprofen, in treatment of arthritis, 228
  See also Motrin anti-inflammatory
ice bags, 644
Iceband gel cold band, 645
ICN 65 Compound analgesic, 446
Ictotest urine-testing tablets, 671
identification, emergency medical, 667
idoxuridine, in treatment of keratitis, 89
ileitis, 164-65
Ilosone antibiotic, 446
Ilotycin antibiotic, 446
Imavate antidepressant, 446
imipramine hydrochloride
    antidepressant, in treatment of bed-
    wetting, 182
  See also Tofranil antidepressant
impacted earwax, 96-97
  See also earache; ear infection,
    middle; earwax, impacted
impetigo, 67-68
impotence, 215
Inderal beta blocker, 446-47
  and heartbeat irregularities, 135-36
  effect on respiratory system, 19
  interaction with other drugs, 24
indigestion, 164-66
Indocin anti-inflammatory, 447-48
  effect on vision, 18
indomethacin, in treatment of arthritis,
    228
  See also Indocin anti-inflammatory
infantile paralysis. See polio
infectious diseases, 248-67
infertility, 195-96
influenza, 116-17
Infra-Rub external analgesic, 448
ingrown toenails, 68-69
  OTC drug profiled, Outgro, 514
INH. See isoniazid
injuries, 240-47
insect sting and bite remedy, OTC, 70
insomnia, 215-216

Instapulse, 635
insulin antidiabetic, 448-49
    action, 275
    and diabetes mellitus, 277-80
    and hypoglycemia, 280
interactions, drug, 23-25
Intercept Contraceptive Inserts, 449
interferon, 53
intestinal flu, see influenza
intrauterine devices, 191
    See also contraception;
    invalid cushions, 635-36
iodides, taken during pregnancy, 22
iodine, in treatment of thyroid diseases, 283
iodine tincture, 449
    in treatment of Rocky Mountain
    Spotted fever, 259
iodochlorhydroxyquin, in products used
    to treat eczema, 65
    See also Vioform-hydrocortisone
    steroid hormone and anti-infective
Iodocort steroid hormone and anti-infective, 449
Ionamin anorectic, 271, 449
Ionax Foam acne preparation, 449-50
Ionax Scrub acne preparation, 450
Iosel 250 seborrheic shampoo, 450
I-PAC analgesic and sedative, 450
ipecac syrup, 450
    in treatment of iron toxicity, 270;
    poisoning, 34-35
iritis, 88-89
    See also eye
iron
    deficiency, 125-26
    interaction with tetracycline, 23
    symptoms of overdose, 33
    toxicity, 270
iron-deficiency anemia. See anemia
iron supplement, OTC
    drug names: Femiron, 420-21;
    Feosol, 422; Fergon, 422-23; Fer-In-
    Sol, 423
irrigating devices, oral, 657
irritable bowel syndrome, 166
irritable colon, 166
Isollyl analgesic and sedative, 450
isoniazid, 451
    interaction with other drugs, 24-25
    in treatment of: salpingitis, 200;
    tuberculosis, 122
isoproterenol, in treatment of asthma, 109
Isopto Carpine ophthalmic solution, 451-52
Isopto-Frin eyedrops, 452
Isopto Plain artificial tears, 452
    in treatment of foreign body in eye, 87
Isordil (isosorbide) antianginal, 452-53
isosorbide, in treatment of angina
    pectoris, 128

Isotrate Timecelles antianginal, 453
isoxsuprine hydrochloride vasodilator.
    See Vasodilan vasodilator
itch, the. See scabies
itching, 70-71
IUDs, 191
Ivy Dry Cream poison ivy remedy, 453

Janimine antidepressant, 453
jaundice, 166-67
    symptoms of hepatitis, 162
J.C. Penney Automatic Toothbrush, 654
Jen-Diril diuretic and antihypertensive, 453
J-Gan-VC expectorant, 454
Jock itch, 77-78
Johnson & Johnson Medicated Powder
    rash remedy, 454
Johnson's Baby Cream rash remedy, 454
Johnson's Baby Powder rash remedy, 454
    in treatment of: chafing, 60; contact
    dermatitis, 61; diaper rash, 63; heat
    rash, 66
Johnson's Odor-Eaters insoles, 650
joints, disorders affecting, 227-39

Kaochlor-Eff potassium chloride
    replacement, 454
Kaochlor potassium chloride
    replacement, 454
kaolin, in diarrhea remedies, 151-52
Kaon-Cl potassium chloride
    replacement, 454
Kaopectate Concentrate diarrhea
    remedy, 454-55
Kaopectate diarrhea remedy, 454-55
    interaction with other drugs, 23-24
    in treatment of diarrhea, 152
Kavrin smooth muscle relaxant, 455
Kay Ciel potassium chloride
    replacement, 455
KEFF potassium chloride replacement, 455
Keflex antibiotic, 455
Kemadrin antiparkinson drug, 455
Kenacort steroid hormone, 455
Kenalog steroid hormone, 456
keratitis, 89
keratolytic
    definition, 15
    in OTC products for treatment of:
    corns and calluses, 62; psoriasis,
    76; ringworm infections, 77
kernicterus, 167
Kestrin estrogen hormone, 456
ketones, urine-testing kit for, 670
ketosis, and glomerulonephritis, 184
kidney failure, acute, 181-82
kidney stones, 184-85
kissing disease. See mononucleosis,
    infectious

691

Kling gauze bandage, 647
KLOR-CON potassium chloride
    replacement, 456
Kloride potassium chloride
    replacement, 456
K-Lor potassium chloride replacement,
    456
KLOR potassium chloride replacement,
    456
Klorvess potassium chloride
    replacement, 456
K-Lyte/Cl potassium chloride
    replacement, 457
K-Lyte DS potassium replacement, 457
K-Lyte potassium replacement, 457
knee, trick, 239
Kolantyl antacid, 457-58
Komed acne preparation, 458
Korostatin antifungal agent, 458
K-Pava smooth muscle relaxant, 458
K-Pen antibiotic, 458
K-Phen with Codeine expectorant, 458
K-10 potassium chloride replacement,
    458
Kwell pediculocide and scabicide,
    458-59
  in treatment of lice-infestation, 72;
    scabies, 79
Kwik Heat disposable hot pack, 645
Kwik Kold disposable cold pack, 645

Lactinex diarrhea remedy, 459
  and canker sores, 59
laetrile, 291
Lanacane hemorrhoidal preparation,
    459
Laniazid antitubercular, 459
Lanophyllin bronchodilator, 459
Lanophyllin-GG expectorant and
    smooth muscle relaxant, 459
Lanorinal analgesic and sedative, 460
Lanoxin heart drug, 460
  in treatment of congestive heart
    failure, 132
Lapav Graduals smooth muscle
    relaxant, 460
Larotid antibiotic, 460
laryngitis, 97
  See also sore throat
Lasix diuretic and antihypertensive,
    460-61
  in treatment of edema, 132
laxative
  and abdominal pain, 146
  definition, 15
  OTC drugs profiled: Agoral, 300;
    Alophen, 308-9; Carter's Little Pills,
    349; cascara sagrada, 349-50;
    castor oil, 350; Colace, 359;
    Correctol, 370; Dialose, 386-87;
    Dialose Plus, 387; Dorbane, 400;
    Dorbantyl, 400-1; Dorbantyl Forte,
    400-1; Doxidan, 401; Dulcolax, 406;

Ex-Lax, 419; Feen-A-Mint, 420; Fleet
    Enema, 426; Fletcher's Castoria,
    426; glycerin suppositories, 437;
    Haley's M-O, 439; magnesium
    citrate solution, 469-70; Metamucil,
    475-76; Modane, 482; Modane Bulk,
    481-82; Modane Mild, 482; Nature's
    Remedy, 491; Neoloid, 492; Nujol,
    504-5; Peri-Colace, 524; Regutol,
    548; Senokot, 560; Serutan, 563;
    Surfak, 580-81
  types of OTC, 149-51
laxative and antacid, OTC, Phillips'
    Milk of Magnesia, 529-30
L-dopa. See levodopa
Ledercillin VK antibiotic, 461
leprosy, 254-55
leukemia, 288
leukoplakia, 167
levodopa
  interaction with other drugs, 24
  in treatment of Parkinson's disease,
    219
Levoid thyroid hormone, 461
Levothroid thyroid hormone, 461
Lexor diuretic and antihypertensive, 461
Li-Ban Spray lice control spray, 461-62
  in treatment of: lice infestation, 72;
    scabies, 79
Librax sedative and anticholinergic, 462
  effect on vision, 18
Librium sedative and hypnotic, 462-63
  and drug dependence, 206
  in treatment of: heart attack, 134;
    hyperkinesis, 214-15
lice-control spray, OTC, Li-Ban Spray,
    461-62
lice infestation, 71-72
Lidex steroid hormone, 463-64
Lidinium sedative and anticholinergic,
    462
lidocaine, in treatment of heart attack,
    134
Lincocin, interaction with other drugs,
    24
lindane, 79
liquid medication, administration of,
    39-40
Liquifilm Tears ocular lubricant, 464
Liquimat acne preparation, 464
Liquiprin analgesic, 464
Listerine throat lozenges, 464-65
  in treatment of sore throat, 104
lithium carbonate
  in treatment of manic-depressive
    illness, 205
  taken during pregnancy, 22
liver
  cancer, 287
  drug-induced disease, 168
Lobac analgesic, 465
lobar pneumonia, 120-21
lobectomy, 286

Metho-500 muscle relaxant, 476
methotrexate antimetabolite, 476–77
 interaction with other drugs, 25
 in treatment of psoriasis, 76–77
 taken during pregnancy, 22
methyldopa
 and hemolytic anemia, 126
 in treatment of high blood pressure,
 137–38
 See also Aldomet
methylphenidate hydrochloride
 adrenergic
 in treatment of: hyperkinesis, 214;
 narcolepsy, 218
 See also Ritalin adrenergic
methylprednisolone steroid hormone.
 See Medrol steroid hormone
methyl salicylate, in OTC external
 analgesics, 230–31
methyltestosterone steroid hormone,
 477–78
 in treatment of: impotence, 215;
 menstrual disorders, 198
methysergide, in prevention of
 migraine headache, 211–12
Meticorten steroid hormone, 478
metronidazole, in treatment of
 trichomoniasis, 263
Mexate antimetabolite, 478
Mexsana Medicated Powder rash
 remedy, 478
miconazole
 in treatment of candidiasis, 259;
 ringworm infections, 77
Micropore cold weather mask, 639
Micropore pollen and dust mask, 639
Microsyn acne preparation, 478
Midatane DC expectorant, 478
Midatane expectorant, 478
Midatap antihistamine, 478
middle ear infection, 98–99
migraine headache, 211–12
migraine remedy, 212
 ℞ drugs profiled: Cafergot, 347–48;
 Cafergot P-B, 348; Cafermine, 348;
 Cafertrate, 348; Ergocaf, 415;
 Migrastat, 478
Migrastat migraine remedy, 478
miliaria. *See* heat rash
milk of magnesia, 478–79
 in treatment of bedsores, 57
Miltown (meprobamate) sedative and
 hypnotic, 479
 and drug dependence, 206
mineralocorticoid, 275
mineral oil, 479
 in treatment of: chigger bites, 60;
 constipation, 150–51; vitamin D
 toxicity, 273
minerals, as nutrients, 268
minimal brain dysfunction. *See*
 hyperkinesis
Minipress antihypertensive, 479–80

Minocin antibiotic, 480–81
Mi-Pilo ophthalmic solution, 481
Mistura ophthalmic solution, 481
Mitran sedative and hypnotic, 481
Mity-Quin steroid hormone and anti-
 infective, 481
Modane Bulk laxative, 481–82
 in treatment of constipation, 151
Modane laxative, 482
 in treatment of constipation, 150–51
Modane Mild laxative, 482
Moist Heat Band with Cold Pack
 heating pad, 642–43
moisturizer, OTC, Aveeno Lotion, 328
Moleskin adhesive-backed felt, 651
moniliasis, 249
Monistat 7 antifungal agent, 482
monoamine oxidase (MAO) inhibitor
 definition, 15
 interaction with other drugs, 24–25
mononeuritis. *See* neuritis
mononucleosis, infectious, 254
morning sickness, 168–69
morphine
 and drug dependence, 206
 in treatment of peritonitis, 176
motion sickness, 169
Motrin anti-inflammatory, 483
M-Tetra 250 antibiotic, 483
mucous colitis, 166
Multicebrin multivitamin, 483–84
multiple sclerosis, 216–17
multivitamin
 OTC drugs profiled: Allbee, 306;
 Chocks, 356; Chocks Plus Iron,
 356–57; Geritol Junior (liquid),
 434–35; Geritol Junior (tablet),
 435–36; Geritol (liquid), 436; Geritol
 (tablet), 436–37; Multicebrin,
 483–84; One-A-Day, 507; Poly-Vi-Sol,
 533; Stresscaps, 577; Stresstabs
 600, 577; Thera-Combex H-P, 591;
 Unicap, 612
multivitamin and iron
 OTC drugs profiled: Femiron, 421;
 One-A-Day Plus Iron, 507–8
multivitamin and mineral
 OTC drugs profiled: Myadec, 485;
 One-A-Day Plus Minerals, 508–9;
 Unicap M, 611–12; Unicap T, 612–13
mumps, 257
Murcil sedative and hypnotic, 484
Murine eyedrops, 484
Murine Plus decongestant eyedrops,
 484
muscle relaxant
 ℞ drugs profiled: Delaxin, 382;
 Forbaxin, 427; methocarbamol, 553;
 Metho-500, 476; Robaxin, 553;
 Spenaxin, 576; Tumol-750, 607
 See also smooth muscle relaxant
muscle relaxant and analgesic, ℞
 ℞ drugs profiled: Robaxisal, 553;

Soma Compound, 573-74; Soprodol Compound, 575
muscle relaxer, 643
muscles, disorders affecting, 227-39
muscle spasm headaches, 212
muscular dystrophy, 233
Myadec multivitamin and mineral supplement, 485
myasthenia gravis, 217-18
Mycelex antifungal agent, 485
Mycelex-G antifungal agent, 485
Mycitracin external anti-infective, 485-86
  in treatment of: boil and carbuncle, 60; chicken pox, 250; chigger bite, 60; cut, 242-43; impetigo, 68; scrape, 246
Mycolog steroid hormone and anti-infective, 486
Mycostatin antifungal agent, 486-87
myeloma, malignant, 285-86
Mylanta antacid and antiflatulent, 487
  ingredients of, 174
Mylanta-II antacid and antiflatulent, 487-88
Mylicon antiflatulent, 488
  in treatment of: flatulence, 154-55; heartburn, 160; hiatus hernia, 163; indigestion, 165; peptic ulcer, 175
Mylicon-80 antiflatulent, 488
Myobid smooth muscle relaxant, 488
myoglobin, urine-testing kit for, 671
myxedema, 282

Naldecon adrenergic and antihistamine, 488-89
Nalfon anti-inflammatory, 489-90
naloxone, in treatment of narcotic overdose, 207
Naprosyn anti-inflammatory, 490-91
  in treatment of arthritis, 229
Narcan antidote, in treatment of narcotic overdose, 207
narcolepsy, 218
narcotic
  and drug dependence, 206-7
  definition, 15
  symptoms of overdose, 33
narrow angle glaucoma, 88
nasal aspirator, 665
nasal congestion, 99-100
  See also allergy; cold; influenza
nasal decongestant
  OTC drugs profiled: Afrin, 299; Allerest, 307-8; Benzedrex nasal decongestant, 338-39; Coricidin, 369-70; Dristan Long-Lasting Nasal Mist, 403; Dristan (inhaler) 403-4; Dristan (spray), 404; Duration, 406-7; Neo-Synephrine Intranasal, 494; Neo-Synephrine II, 494; NTZ, 504; Privine, 538-39; Sine-Off Once-A-Day, 567; Sinex Long-Acting,

568-69; Sinex, 569; Sinutab Long-Lasting, 570; Vicks Inhaler, 619
Nature's Remedy laxative, 491
nausea, 169-71
  See also antinauseant; morning sickness; motion sickness
Nembutal Sodium hypnotic, 491-92
Neocurtasal salt substitute, 492
Neoloid laxative, 492
neomycin
  in diarrhea remedies, 152
  in OTC external anti-infectives, 79
Neo-Polycin Ointment external anti-infective, 492
  in treatment of: boil and carbuncle, 58; chicken pox, 250; chigger bite, 60; cut, 242-43; impetigo, 68; scrape, 246
Neosporin antibiotic ophthalmic solution, 492-93
Neosporin Ointment external anti-infective, 493
  in treatment of: boil and carbuncle, 55; chicken pox, 250; chigger bite, 60; cut, 242-43; impetigo, 68; scrape, 246
neostigmine, in treatment of myasthenia gravis, 218
Neo-Synephrine Compound decongestant cold remedy, 493-94
  interaction with other drugs, 25
Neo-Synephrine Intranasal nasal decongestant, 494
  interaction with other drugs, 25
  in treatment of: allergy, 108; common cold, 93; earache, 95; middle ear infection, 99; nasal congestion, 100; nosebleeds, 101; sinus infection, 103; sore throat, 105
Neo-Synephrine II nasal decongestant, 494
Neoxyn poison ivy remedy, 494-95
nephritis. See glomerulonephritis
Nervine Nightime Sleep-Aid, 495
nervous indigestion, 166
nervous system, disorders of, 201-26
  See also brain
Neuramate sedative and hypnotic, 495
neuritis, 218-19
niacin. See vitamin B₃
niacinamide. See nicotinamide
Niac vitamin supplement, 495
Nicalex vitamin supplement, 495
niclosamide, in treatment of tapeworm, 264
NICL vitamin supplement, 495
Nicobid vitamin supplement, 495
Nicocap vitamin supplement, 495
Nico-400 Plateau Caps vitamin supplement, 495
Niconyl antitubercular, 495
nico-Span vitamin supplement, 496

695

nicotinamide, in treatment of pellagra, 272
nicotine, effects of and withdrawal from, 224
nicotinic acid vitamin supplement, 496
in treatment of: atherosclerosis, 129; blood clots, 130; Buerger's disease, 130-31; pellagra, 272; Raynaud's disease, 139; stroke, 141
night blindness, 89
Nilstat antifungal agent, 496
Nitrine-TDC antianginal, 496
Nitro antianginal, 496
Nitro-Bid Plateau Caps antianginal, 496-97
Nitrobon-TR antianginal, 497
Nitrocap T.D. antianginal, 497
Nitrocels Diacels antianginal, 497
Nitrocot antianginal, 497
nitrofurantoin antibacterial. See Macrodantin antibacterial
nitroglycerin
in treatment of heart attack, 134
See also Nitro-Bid Plateau caps antianginal; Nitrostat antianginal
Nitrospan antianginal, 497
Nitrostat antianginal, 497-98
Nitrosule Pellsules antianginal, 498
Nitro T.D. antianginal, 498
Nitrotym antianginal, 498
nits. See lice infestation
nocardiosis, 117-18
nocturia. See urinary habits, change in
Norafed adrenergic and antihistamine, 498
Nordryl antihistamine, 498
Norfranil antidepressant, 498
Norgesic analgesic, 498-99
Normatane antihistamine, 499
Normatane DC expectorant, 499
Normatane expectorant, 499
Nor-Mil anticholinergic and antispasmodic, 499
Noroxine thyroid hormone, 499
Norpace antiarrhythmic, 499-500
Norpanth anticholinergic, 500
Nor-Pres antihypertensive, 500
Nor-Tet antibiotic, 500
nose, disorders of. See ear, nose, and throat
nosebleeds, 100
nose drops, administration of, 41
nose sprays, administration of, 41
Novahistine cold and allergy remedy, 500
Novahistine DH expectorant cough remedy, 501
Novahistine DMX cough remedy, 501-2
Novahistine Expectorant cough remedy, 502-3
Noxzema Medicated burn remedy and antiseptic, 503
NP-27 athlete's foot remedy, 503

NTZ nasal decongestant, 504
Nujol laxative, 504-5
Nupercainal hemorrhoidal preparation (ointment), 505
Nupercainal hemorrhoidal preparation (suppository), 505
Nupercainal local anesthetic, 505-6
nutritional disorders, 268-73
nutritional supplement
need for, 269
OTC drugs profiled: Theragran-M, 591-92; Theragran, 592
See also multivitamin; multivitamin and iron; multivitamin and mineral, vitamin supplement
nyctalopia, 89
Nydrazid antitubercular, 506
Nyquil cough remedy, 506
nystatin
in treatment of: candidiasis, 249; genital herpes, 261
Nytol Tablets sleeping aid, 506-7

o.b.c.t. adrenergic, 507
obesity, 270-72
obstruction, complication of peptic ulcer, 173
occupational lung diseases, 118-19
ocular lubricant, OTC, Liquifilm Tears, 464
Ocusol Drops eye decongestant, 507
ointment and cream, topical application, 42
ointment, eye administration, 40
ointment, vaginal administration, 41
oligomenorrhea, 197
Omnipen antibiotic, 507
One-A-Day multivitamin, 507
One-A-Day Plus Iron multivitamin and iron, 507-8
One-A-Day Plus Minerals multivitamin and mineral, 508-9
onychomycosis. See ringworm infections
open angle glaucoma, 88
ophthalmic herpes zoster. See shingles
ophthalmic ointment, R_x, Sodium Sulamyd, 573
ophthalmic solution
R_x drugs profiled: Adsorbocarpine, 298; Almocarpine, 308; Isopto Carpine, 451-52; Mi-Pilo, 481; Mistura, 481; Pilocar, 531; pilocarpine hydrochloride, 451; Pilomiotin, 531; P.V. Carpine Liquifilm, 543; Sodium Sulamyd, 573; Timoptic, 595-96
ophthalmic solution, antibiotic
R_x drug profiled, Neosporin, 492-93
ophthalmic suspension
R_x drug profiled, Cortisporin, 371
Orajel toothache and sore gums remedy, 509

oral contraceptives, 509-10
  See also contraception
Orapav Timecelles smooth muscle
  relaxant, 510
Orasone steroid hormone, 510
Oretic diuretic and antihypertensive,
  510
Oreton Methyl steroid hormone, 510
Orinase oral antidiabetic drug, 510-11
  in treatment of diabetes mellitus,
  279-80
Ornacol Capsules cough remedy, 511
Ornacol Liquid cough remedy, 511
Ornade Spansule antihistamine,
  anticholinergic, and adrenergic, 512
Ornade 2 for Children cold and allergy
  remedy, 512-13
Ornex cold remedy, 513
Ortho-Creme contraceptive, 513-14
Ortho-Gynol contraceptive jelly, 514
osteitis deformans, 235-36
osteoarthritis. *See* arthritis
osteomalacia, 236-37
osteomyelitis, 234
osteoporosis, 234-35
  and menopause, 196
otic solution
  R̶ drugs profiled: Auralgan, 327;
    Aurasol, 327; Eardro, 408; Oto, 514
otic suspension, R̶ drug profiled,
  Otobione, 514
otitis, external. *See* ear, swimmer's
otitis media. *See* ear infection, middle
Otobione otic suspension, 514
Oto otic solution, 514
Outgro ingrown toenail remedy, 514
  in treatment of ingrown toenails, 69
ovarian cancer, 290
overdosage, 32-36
Ovest estrogen hormone, 514
Oxalid anti-inflammatory, 514
Oxlopar antibiotic, 514
Oxybiotic antibiotic, 514
Oxy-5 acne preparation, 514-15
  in treatment of acne, 56
Oxy-10 acne preparation, 514-15
  in treatment of acne, 56
Oxy-Tetrachel antibiotic, 515
oxytocin, 274

PAC analgesic, 515
Paget's disease, 235-36
Pain-A-Lay toothache, sore throat, and
  sore gums remedy, 515
pain, as a symptom, 52-54
pain remedies. *See* analgesics
Paltet antibiotic, 515
Panasol steroid hormone, 515
Panazid antitubercular, 516
Pancreas cancer, 288
pancreatitis, 171-72
Pan-Kloride potassium chloride
  replacement, 516

Panmycin antibiotic, 516
Panwarfin anticoagulant, 516
Pap-Kaps-150 Meta-Kaps smooth
  muscle relaxant, 516
Pap smear, 289, 292
para-aminobenzoic acid, in sunscreens,
  73
Parachlor analgesic, 516
Paracort steroid hormone, 516
Parafon Forte analgesic, 516
Paragesic-65 analgesic, 516
parathyroid hormone, 274-75
paregoric antidiarrheal, 516-17
  ingredient in diarrhea remedies,
  151-52
Parepectolin diarrhea remedy, 517-18
  in treatment of diarrhea, 151-52
Parest sedative and hypnotic, 518
Pargesic Compound 65 analgesic, 518
Parkinson's disease, 219-20
  See also antiparkinson drug
Partrex antibiotic, 518
Pavabid Plateau Caps smooth muscle
  relaxant, 518
  in treatment of blood clots, 130;
  stroke, 141
Pavacap Unicelles smooth muscle
  relaxant, 519
Pavacels smooth muscle relaxant, 519
Pavacen Cenules smooth muscle
  relaxant, 519
Pavacot T.D. smooth muscle relaxant,
  519
Pavacron smooth muscle relaxant, 519
Pavadon analgesic, 519
Pavadur smooth muscle relaxant, 519
Pavadyl smooth muscle relaxant, 519
Pavakey smooth muscle relaxant, 519
Pava-Mead smooth muscle relaxant,
  519
Pava-Par smooth muscle relaxant, 519
Pava-R̶ smooth muscle relaxant, 519
Pavased smooth muscle relaxant, 519
Pavasule smooth muscle relaxant, 519
Pavatran smooth muscle relaxant, 519
Pava-2 smooth muscle relaxant, 519
Pavatym smooth muscle relaxant, 519
Pava-Wol smooth muscle relaxant, 519
Paverine Spancaps smooth muscle
  relaxant, 519
Paverolan smooth muscle relaxant, 519
PBR/12 sedative and hypnotic, 520
PCP. *See* drug dependence
pectin, in diarrhea remedies, 151-52
Pediamycin antibiotic, 520
Pediaquil cough remedy for children,
  520
pediculocide and scabicide
  definition, 15
  R̶ drugs profiled: Gamene, 431;
    Kwell, 458-59
pediculosis. *See* lice infestation
pellagra, 272

697

pelvic inflammatory disease. *See*
    salpingitis
Pen A antibiotic, 520
Penapar VK antibiotic, 520
Penbritin antibiotic, 520
penicillamine, taken during pregnancy,
    22
penicillin
    in treatment of: appendicitis, 147;
    boil and carbuncle, 58; ear
    infection, middle, 99; endocarditis,
    133; erysipelas, 252; gonorrhea,
    262; impetigo, 68; mastoiditis, 256;
    meningitis, 216; pneumonia,
    120–21; rheumatic fever, 140;
    scarlet fever, 260; sore throat,
    104–5; syphilis, 263; tetanus, 265;
    trench mouth, 179
    overdose of, 126
penicillin G antibiotic, 520–21
penicillin potassium phenoxymethyl
    antibiotic, 521
Pensyn antibiotic, 521
pentaerythritol tetranitrate, in
    treatment of angina pectoris, 128
Pentazine expectorant, 522
Pentazine with Codeine expectorant,
    522
pentazocine
    and drug dependence, 207
    in treatment of heart attack, 134
Pentids antibiotic, 522
pentobarbital hypnotic. *See* Nembutal
    Sodium hypnotic
Pen-Vee K antibiotic, 522
peptic ulcer, 172–75
Pepto-Bismol diarrhea remedy, 522
    in treatment of travelers' diarrhea,
    179
Percodan analgesic, 522–23
Percodan-Demi analgesic, 523
Percogesic analgesic, 523
perforated eardrum, 101–2
    See also ear infection, middle
perforation, complication of peptic
    ulcer, 173
Periactin antihistamine, 523–24
pericarditis, 138–39
Peri-Colace laxative, 524
    in treatment of constipation, 151
periodontal disease, 175–76
peritonitis, 176
Perphenyline phenothiazine and
    antidepressant, 525
Persantine antianginal, 525
Pertussin 8-Hour Cough Formula, 525
pertussis. *See* whooping cough
petechiae, 142
Pethadol analgesic, 525
petroleum jelly
    in treatment of corns and calluses,
    62; fever blisters, 59
    See also Vaseline petroleum jelly

Pfiklor potassium chloride replacement,
    525
Pfizer-E antibiotic, 525
Pfizerpen G antibiotic, 525
Pfizerpen VK antibiotic, 525
pH, urine-testing kit for, 670–71
Phedral antiasthmatic, 526
phenacetin, in OTC analgesics, 53
Phen-Amin antihistamine, 526
Phenaphen with Codeine analgesic, 526
Phenazodine analgesic, 526
phenazopyridine hydrochloride
    analgesic. *See* Pyridium analgesic
phencyclidine. *See* drug dependence
Phenergan expectorant, 526
Phenergan VC expectorant, 526–27
Phenergan VC with Codeine
    expectorant, 527–28
Phenergan with Codeine expectorant,
    527–28
phenmetrazine, taken during
    pregnancy, 22
phenobarbital sedative and hypnotic,
    529
    in treatment of: anxiety, 204; asthma,
    109; croup, 114; encephalitis, 208;
    hiccups, 164; pneumonia, 120–21;
    tetanus, 265
phenocaine hydrochloride, in OTC
    hemorrhoidal preparations, 160–61
phenol, in throat lozenges, 104
Pheno-Squar sedative and hypnotic, 529
phenothiazine
    definition, 15
    R drugs profiled: Chloramead, 353;
    chlorpromazine hydrochloride, 593;
    Compazine, 361–62; Mellaril,
    473–74; Promapar, 541; Stelazine,
    576–77; Thoradol, 593; Thorazine,
    593
    taken during pregnancy, 22
phenothiazine and antidepressant, R
    R drugs profiled: Etrafon, 417;
    Perphenyline, 525; Triavil, 604–5;
    Triptazine, 606
phentermine hydrochloride anorectic.
    See Fastin anorectic
phenylbutazone anti-inflammatory.
    See Butazolidin anti-inflammatory
phenylpropanolamine hydrochloride, in
    OTC diet aids, 271
phenytoin sodium anticonvulsant
    in treatment of: hypoglycemia, 280;
    tetanus, 265; tic douloureux, 226
    See also Dilantin anticonvulsant
Phillips' Milk of Magnesia laxative
    and antacid, 529–30
pHisoDan dandruff remedy, 530
pHisoHex detergent cleanser, 530–31
    in treatment of cradle cap, 63
photodermatitis, 72–73
    See also burns and sunburn; contact
    dermatitis; drug eruptions

phytonadione, taken during pregnancy, 22

PID. *See* salpingitis

piles. *See* hemorrhoids

Pilocar ophthalmic solution, 531

pilocarpine hydrochloride, in products used to treat glaucoma, 88
  See also Isopto Carpine ophthalmic solution

Pilomiotin ophthalmic solution, 531

pimples. *See* acne

pinkeye. *See* conjunctivitis

pinworms, 258
  and pruritus ani/pruritus vulvae, 75

piperazine, in treatment of roundworm, 259

Piracaps antibiotic, 531

plantar warts. *See* warts

plaque, atherosclerotic, 128

plaque, dental
  and gingivitis, 158
  and periodontal disease, 175
  and tooth decay, 178

Plastipak hypodermic syringe/needle combination, 669

pleurisy, 119–120
  See also bronchitis; pneumonia; rheumatic fever; tuberculosis

pneumoconiosis. *See* occupational lung diseases

pneumonectomy, 286

pneumonia, 120–21

podophyllin, in treatment of venereal warts, 263

poisoning, food. *See* food poisoning

poison ivy, 73–75
  See also contact dermatitis

poison ivy remedy, 74, 75
  OTC drugs profiled: Caladryl, 348; Ivy Dry Cream, 453; Neoxyn, 494–95; Rhulicream, 550; Rhulihist, 550–51; Ziradryl, 628

poison oak, 73–75
  See also contact dermatitis

poison sumac. *See* poison ivy

poison treatment, 32–36

Polaramine antihistamine, 531–32

polio, 220

poliomyelitis. *See* polio

Pollenex Deluxe Portable Whirlpool Bath, 652

Pollenex Hydro Action Foot Bath, 652

Polycillin antibiotic, 532

polymenorrhea, 198

Polymox antibiotic, 532

polymyxin, in OTC external anti-infectives, 79

polyneuritis. *See* neuritis

polyps
  cervical, 189–90
  nasal, due to sinus infection, 103

Polysporin Ointment external anti-infective, 532

in treatment of: boil and carbuncle, 58; chicken pox, 250; chigger bite, 60; cut, 242–43; impetigo, 68; scrape, 246

polyuria, 183

Poly-Vi-Flor vitamin and fluoride supplement, 532

Poly-Vi-Sol multivitamin, 533

Porox7 acne preparation, 533

Potasalan potassium chloride replacement, 533

potassium chloride replacement, 533–34
  R̥ drugs profiled: Kaochlor-Eff, 454; Kaochlor, 454; Kaon-Cl, 454; Kay Ciel, 455; KEFF, 455; K-Lor, 456; KLOR, 456; KLOR-CON, 456; Kloride, 456; Klorvess, 456; K-Lyte/Cl, 457; K-10, 458; Pan-Kloride, 516; Pfiklor, 525; Potasalan, 533; Slow-K, 572
  See also potassium replacement; salt substitute

potassium iodide, in treatment of emphysema, 116

potassium permanganate, in treatment of hyperhidrosis, 67

potassium replacement
  interaction with other drugs, 24
  R̥ drug profiled: K-Lyte DS, 457; K-Lyte, 457
  See also potassium chloride replacement; salt substitute

Povan anthelmintic, 534

powders, application of, 42

Poxy Compound 65 analgesic, 534

pramoxine hydrochloride
  in OTC preparation for the treatment of: hemorrhoids, 160–61; poison ivy, 74

Prednicen-M steroid hormone, 534

prednisone steroid hormone, 534
  in treatment of: cirrhosis, 148; contact dermatitis, 61; shingles, 81

pregnancy
  drug use, 21–23
  morning sickness, 168–69
  prevention of. *See* contraception, contraceptive
  urine test for, 670
  See also infertility

Preludin anorectic, 535–36

Premarin estrogen hormone, 536–37

premenstrual tension, 198

Preparation H hemorrhoidal preparation, 537

Presamine antidepressant, 537

prescription, 27–30

prickly heat. *See* heat rash

primaquine, in treatment of malaria, 255

Primatene M asthma remedy, 537–38

Primatene P asthma remedy, 538

Principen antibiotic, 538
Privine nasal decongestant, 538-39
Probalan uricosuric, 539
Pro-Banthine anticholinergic, 539-40
    effect on gastrointestinal system, 18
probenecid
    in treatment of: gonorrhea, 262; gout,
    232
    See also Benemid uricosuric
Probenimead uricosuric, 540
procainamide hydrochloride
    in treatment of heart attack, 134
    See also Pronestyl antiarrhythmic
Procamide antiarrhythmic, 540
Prochlor-Iso anticholinergic and
    phenothiazine, 540
Proclan expectorant, 540
Proclan VC expectorant, 540
Progesic Compound-65 analgesic, 540
Progesic-65 analgesic, 540
progesterone hormone, 275
    ℞ drugs profiled: Amen, 310; Provera,
    542
progestin
    in oral contraceptives, 191, 509-10
    taken during pregnancy, 22
Proglycerin, in treatment of
    hypoglycemia, 280
Prolamine appetite suppressant, 540
Proloid thyroid hormone, 541
Promapar phenothiazine, 541
Promethazine Hydrochloride
    expectorant, 541
Promethazine Hydrochloride VC with
    Codeine expectorant, 541
Promethazine Hydrochloride with
    Codeine expectorant, 541
Promex expectorant, 541
Promex with Codeine expectorant, 541
Pronestyl antiarrhythmic, 541-42
    and heartbeat irregularities, 136
Propadrine, interaction with other
    drugs, 25
propantheline bromide anticholinergic.
    See Pro-Banthine anticholinergic
prophylactics. See condoms
propoxyphene hydrochloride
    and drug dependence, 206-7
    See also Darvon analgesic
propranolol
    in treatment of: angina pectoris, 128;
    migraine headache, 212
propylthiouracil
    in treatment of thyroid diseases, 283
    taken during pregnancy, 22
prostatic cancer, 287
prostatitis, 185-86
protein
    as nutrient, 268
    urine-testing kit for, 670
Prothazine expectorant, 542
Prothazine with Codeine expectorant,
    542

protozoans, infection with, 249
Protran sedative and hypnotic, 542
Provera progesterone hormone, 542
Proxagesic analgesic, 543
Proxagesic Compound-65 analgesic,
    543
Proxene analgesic, 543
pruritus ani, 75-76
pruritus vulvae, 75-76
psoriasis, 76-77
puberty, precocious, 281
pulsemeters, 634-35
pulse rate, 47
puncture wounds, 245-46
    See also tetanus
Puretane DC expectorant, 543
Puretane expectorant, 543
purpura, 142
P.V. Carpine Liquifilm ophthalmic
    solution, 543
pyelonephritis, 186-88
pyorrhea, 175
pyrantel pamoate, in treatment of
    roundworm, 259
Pyridiate analgesic, 543
Pyridium analgesic, 543
pyridostigmine, in treatment of
    myasthenia gravis, 218
pyridoxine. See vitamin B₆
pyrosis. See heartburn
pyrvinium pamoate, in treatment of
    pinworms, 258

Quaalude sedative and hypnotic,
    543-44
    See also drug dependence
Quadra-Hist adrenergic and
    antihistamine, 544
Quibron expectorant and smooth
    muscle relaxant, 544
    in treatment of asthma, 110
Quinidex Extentabs antiarrhythmic, 545
quinidine sulfate antiarrhythmic, 545
    and heartbeat irregularities, 136
    in treatment of heart attack, 134
quinine sulfate, in treatment of malaria,
    255
Quinora antiarrhythmic, 545

rabbit fever. See tularemia
rabies, 221
Racet steroid hormone and anti-
    infective, 545
radiation therapy, in treatment of
    cancer, 286-92
rash
    contact dermatitis, 61
    diaper, 63
    eczema, 64
    heat, 65
    hives, 66
    poison ivy/poison oak, 73-75
    psoriasis, 76-77

ringworm infections, 77–78
shingles, 80–81
rash remedy
OTC drugs profiled: A and D
Ointment, 295; Ammens Medicated
Powder, 311: Aveeno Colloidal
Oatmeal bath product, 328; Baby
Magic Lotion, 330; Baby Magic Oil,
330; Baby Magic Powder, 330–31;
Borofax, 342; Desitin Ointment,
385; Desitin, 385; Diaparene Baby
Powder, 388; Diaparene Peri-Anal
Cream, 388; Johnson & Johnson
Medicated Powder, 454; Johnson's
Baby Cream, 454; Johnson's Baby
Powder, 454; Mexsana Medicated
Powder, 478
Raurine antihypertensive, 545
Rau-Sed antihypertensive, 545
Rauzide diuretic and antihypertensive,
545–46
Raynaud's disease, 139
rebound congestion, resulting from use
of nasal spray or drops, 93, 100
rectal cancer, 290
Regroton diuretic and antihypertensive,
547–48
Regutol laxative, 548
renal failure, acute. See kidney
failure, acute
Repen-VK antibiotic, 548
Reposans sedative and hypnotic, 548
Repro Compound 65 analgesic, 548
reserpine antihypertensive, 548–49
and cancer, 23, 286
in treatment of: high blood
pressure, 137–38; St. Vitus' dance,
222
taken during pregnancy, 22
Reserpoid antihypertensive, 549
respiration rate, 47
respiratory tract, disorders of, 107–23
Retet antibiotic, 549
Retin-A acne preparation, 549–50
in treatment of acne, 56
retinitis, 90
retinol. See vitamin A
Reye's syndrome, 221–22
Rezamid acne preparation, 550
rheumatic chorea. See St. Vitus' dance
rheumatic fever, 139–40
rheumatism. See arthritis
rheumatoid arthritis. See arthritis
Rhulicream poison ivy remedy, 550
Rhulihist poison ivy remedy, 550–51
rhythm method. See family planning,
natural
riboflavin. See vitamin B₂
rickets, 236–37
Rid antilouse preparation, 551
in treatment of: lice infestation, 72;
scabies, 79
ringing in the ears, 102

ringworm infections, 77–78
Riopan antacid, 551–52
Ritalin adrenergic, 552
Roadrunner Electronic Pulse Meter, 635
Robamox antibiotic, 552
Robaxin muscle relaxant, 553
Robaxisal muscle relaxant and
analgesic, 553
Robenecid uricosuric, 553
Robicillin VK antibiotic, 553
Robimycin antibiotic, 553
Robitet "250" antibiotic, 553
Robitussin cough remedies
in treatment of: bronchitis, 111–12;
common cold, 93; coughing,
113–14; influenza, 117; pneumonia,
121; whooping cough, 123
Robitussin-A-C cough remedy,
553–54
Robitussin-CF cough remedy, 554
Robitussin cough remedy, 554–55
Robitussin-DM Cough Calmers cough
remedy, 555
Robitussin-DM cough remedy,
555
Robitussin-PE cough remedy, 556
Ro-Chlorozide diuretic and
antihypertensive, 556
Rocinolone steroid hormone, 556
Rocky Mountain spotted fever,
258–59
Ro-Cloro-Serp-500 diuretic and
antihypertensive, 556
Ro-Diet adrenergic, 556
Rolaids antacid, 556–57
Rolazine antihypertensive, 557
Rolserp antihypertensive, 557
Romilar CF cough remedy, 557
Romycin antibiotic, 557
Roniacol vasodilator, 557
Ropanth anticholinergic, 557
Ropred steroid hormone, 557
Rosoxol antibacterial, 557
Ro-Thyroxine thyroid hormone, 557
roundworm, 259
Rozolamide diuretic, 557
RP-Mycin antibiotic, 557
rubber gloves, 639
rubber sheeting, 637
rubella, 259–60
rubeola, 256–57

Sabin vaccine, 220
St. Anthony's fire. See erysipelas
St. Vitus' dance, 222
salicylates, 15
salicylic acid
in products used for treatment of:
corns and calluses, 62; ringworm
infections, 77–78; warts, 82
ointment. See sulfur and salicylic
acid ointment
saline laxatives, 149–51

Sine-Off cold and allergy remedy, 566–67
Sine-Off Once-A-Day nasal decongestant, 567
Sinequan antidepressant, 567–68
Sinex Long-Acting nasal decongestant, 568–69
Sinex nasal decongestant, 569
sinus
　headache, 212–13
　infection, 102–3
sinusitis. See sinus infection
Sinutab cold and allergy remedy, 569–70
Sinutab Long-Lasting nasal decongestant, 570
Sinutab-II cold and allergy remedy, 570–71
SK-Ampicillin antibiotic, 571
SK-APAP with Codeine analgesic, 571
SK-Bamate sedative and hypnotic, 571
SK-Diphenhydramine antihistamine, 571
SK-Diphenoxylate anticholinergic and antispasmodic, 571
SK-Erythromycin antibiotic, 571
skin cancer, 285–86
skin cleanser
　OTC drugs profiled: Aveeno Bar, 328; Cetaphil Lotion, 352
　OTC, in treatment of eczema, 65
skin, disorders of, 55–82
SK-Lygen sedative and hypnotic, 571
SK-Niacin vitamin supplement, 571
SK-Penicillin G antibiotic, 571
SK-Penicillin VK antibiotic, 571
SK-Phenobarbital sedative and hypnotic, 571
SK-Pramine antidepressant, 571
SK-65 analgesic, 571
SK-65 Compound analgesic, 572
SK-Soxazole antibacterial, 572
SK-Tetracycline antibiotic, 572
SK-Triamcinolone steroid hormone, 572
Sleep-Eze sleeping aid, 572
sleeping aid
　OTC drugs profiled: Compoz Tablets, 363; Nervine Nightime, 495; Nytol Tablets, 506–7; Sleep-Eze, 572; Sominex, 574–75; Unisom Nightime, 613
　OTC, in treatment of insomnia, 216
sleeping sickness. See encephalitis
SLE. See lupus erythematosus, systemic
Slim-Line Candy appetite suppressant, 572
slipped disc. See backache; sciatica
Slo-Phyllin expectorant and smooth muscle relaxant, 572
Slow-K potassium chloride replacement, 572
smallpox, 263–64
smoking, 224–25
　and cancer 285

smooth muscle relaxant
　definition, 15
　R_x drugs profiled: Blupav, 341; Cerespan, 352; Delapav, 382; Dilant, 390; Dipav, 394; Kavrin, 455; K-Pava, 458; Lapav Graduals, 460; Myobid, 488; Pavabid Plateau Caps, 488; Orapav Timecelles, 510; Pap-Kaps-150 Meta-Kaps, 516; Pavabid Plateau Caps, 518; Pavacap Unicelles, 519; Pavacels, 519; Pavacen Cenules, 519; Pavacot T.D., 519; Pavacron, 519; Pavadur, 519; Pavadyl, 519; Pavakey, 519; Pava-Mead, 519; Pava-Par, 519; Pava-R_x, 519; Pavased, 519; Pavasule, 519; Pavatran, 519; Pava-2, 519; Pavatym, 519; Pava-Wol, 519; Paverine Spancaps, 519; Paverolan, 519; Sustaverine, 581; Tri-Pavasule, 606; Vasal Granucaps, 616; Vasocap-150, 617; Vasospan, 617
Sodestrin estrogen hormone, 573
sodium bicarbonate, in OTC antacids, 173
Sodium Sulamyd ophthalmic solution and ointment, 573
　in treatment of corneal ulcer, 86
Solarcaine burn remedy and antiseptic, 573
Solfoton sedative and hypnotic, 573
Soma Compound muscle relaxant and analgesic, 573–74
Sominex sleeping aid, 574–75
Somophyllin bronchodilator, 575
Somophyllin-T bronchodilator, 575
Sopor sedative and hypnotic, 575
Soprodol Compound muscle relaxant and analgesic, 575
Sopronol athlete's foot remedy, 575
Sorate antianginal, 575
Sorbide antianginal, 575
Sorbitrate antianginal, 575
sore throat, 104–5
Soy-Dome Cleanser detergent cleanser, 575
Spalix sedative and anticholinergic, 575
Spasmolin sedative and anticholinergic, 575
spastic colon. See irritable colon
Spastyl antispasmodic, 576
Spenaxin muscle relaxant, 576
Spengine vasodilator, 576
Spentane DC expectorant, 576
Spentane expectorant, 576
sphygmomanometer, 633–34
spironolactone
　and breast enlargement, 286
　and cancer, 286
　in treatment of adrenal diseases, 276
　See also aldosterone

703

sprained, ankle, 237
sprained, wrist, 237–38
Stelazine phenothiazine, 576–77
Sterapred steroid hormone, 577
sterilization, 193
    See also contraception
steroid hormone
    definition, 15
    OTC topical drug profiled: Dermolate, 384
    ℞ drugs profiled: Android, 315;
        Aristocort (topical), 318–19;
        Aristocort (oral), 319–20;
        Aristoderm, 320; Aristogel, 320;
        Aristo-Pak, 320; Cordran, 366–67;
        Cortan, 371; Deltasone, 382;
        Fernisone, 423; Fluonid, 427;
        Kenacort, 455; Kenalog, 456; Lidex,
        463–64; Medrol, 472–73; Metandren,
        476; methylprednisolone, 472–73;
        methyltestosterone, 477–78;
        Meticorten, 478; Orasone, 510;
        Oreton Methyl, 510; Panasol, 515;
        Paracort, 516; Prednicen-M, 534;
        prednisone, 534; Rocinolone, 556;
        Ropred, 557; SK-Triamcinolone,
        572; Sterapred, 577; Synalar, 581;
        Synemol, 582; Topsyn, 599;
        Valisone, 613–14
    topical application of, 42
steroid hormone and anti-infective
    ℞ drugs profiled: Cortin, 371;
        Domeform-HC, 398; Formtone-HC,
        427; HCV, 440; Heb-Cort, 440;
        Hexaderm I.Q., 440; Hydroquin, 445;
        Hysone, 446; Iodocort, 449; Mity-
        Quin, 481; Mycolog, 486; Racet,
        545; Vioform-Hydrocortisone, 620;
        Vioquin-HC, 620; Viotag, 621
steroid-hormone-containing anorectal
    product, ℞, Anusol-HC, 316–17
stethoscope, 633–34
stimulant
    dependence on, 207
    in products used to treat common
    cold, 92
stomach cancer, 287
stool, black, 147
stool softener laxative, 149–51
strep throat. See sore throat;
streptomycin
    in treatment of: salpingitis, 200;
    tuberculosis, 122; tularemia, 266
Stresscaps multivitamin, 577
Stresstabs 600 multivitamin, 577
Stri-Dex acne preparation, 577–78
stroke, 140–41
sty, 90
Sub-Quin antiarrhythmic, 578
Sucrets throat lozenges, 578
Sudafed cold remedy, 578
    interaction with other drugs, 25
    in treatment of: allergy, 108; common

cold, 93; earache, 95; hay fever, 96;
    nasal congestion, 100; sore throat,
    105
Sudafed Plus cold remedy, 578–79
Sudahist adrenergic and antihistamine,
    579
Suda-Prol adrenergic and antihistamine,
    579
Sul-Blue seborrheic shampoo, 579
Suldiazo antibacterial and analgesic,
    579
sulfacetamide, in products used to
    treat corneal ulcer, 86
sulfa drug
    definition, 15
Sulfalar antibacterial, 579
sulfamethazole, in treatment of
    urinary tract infections, 187
sulfasalazine, in treatment of
    ulcerative colitis, 180
sulfisoxazole antibacterial. See
    Gantrisin antibacterial
sulfonamide
    and neuritis, 218
    in treatment of: blepharitis, 84;
    conjunctivitis, 85; malaria, 255;
    ulcerative colitis, 180
    taken during pregnancy, 22
Sulforcin acne preparation, 579
    in treatment of acne, 56
sulfoxone, in treatment of leprosy, 255
sulfur, in products used to treat
    scabies, 79
sulfur and salicylic acid ointment
    in treatment of: ringworm infections,
    77–78; seborrheic dermatitis, 80
Sultrin vaginal anti-infective, 579–80
Sumox antibiotic, 580
Sumycin antibiotic, 580
sunburn, 241–42
sunstroke. See heatstroke
Supen antibiotic, 580
superinfection, 20–21
Super Odrinex appetite suppressant,
    580
    in treatment of obesity, 271–72
suppositories
    administration of: rectal, 41; vaginal,
    41–42
Surfak laxative, 580–81
    in treatment of constipation, 151
Surgitube gauze bandage, 647
suspensory, 662
Sustaverine smooth muscle relaxant,
    581
swimmer's ear, 105–6
Sydenham's chorea. See St. Vitus'
    dance
sympathomimetic amine
    definition, 15
    in products used to treat: nasal
    congestion, 100; sinus headaches,
    212–14

Synalar steroid hormone, 581
Synalgos analgesic, 581
Synalgos-DC analgesic, 581–82
Synemol steroid hormone, 582
Synthaloids throat lozenges, 582–83
Synthroid thyroid hormone, 583
syphilis, 262–63
syringes, 664–67
systemic lupus erythematosus, 238

tablet administration, 40
  sublingually, 40
  vaginally, 41–42
Tagafed adrenergic and antihistamine,
  583
Tagamet antisecretory, 583–84
  in treatment of: heartburn, 160;
  hiatus hernia, 163; indigestion, 165;
  peptic ulcer, 174–75
Talwin analgesic, 584
Tandearil anti-inflammatory, 584
tape, adhesive, 647–48
tapeworm, 264
tear gland swelling, 86
Tedral antiasthmatic (R̥), 584–85
  in treatment of asthma, 110
Tedral asthma remedy (OTC), 585–86
Tega-Span vitamin supplement, 586
Tegrin antipsoriasis remedy, 586
  in treatment of: eczema, 65;
  psoriasis, 77
Teldrin allergy remedy, 586–87
Teledyne Water Pik oral irrigating
  device, 657
Telfa sterile pads, 646
Teline antibiotic, 587
temperature, body
  basal, 192–93
  measurement of, 631–32
  See also fever
Tempra analgesic, 587
Tenax sedative and hypnotic, 587
tennis elbow, 238–39
  See also bursitis
Ten-Shun analgesic and sedative, 587
Tensor Elastic Bandage, 661
Tenuate adrenergic, 587–88
Tepanil Ten-Tab adrenergic 588
terpin hydrate and codeine elixir
  expectorant cough remedy, 588
Terramycin antibiotic, 588–89
testosterone
  in treatment of: osteoporosis, 235;
  Paget's disease, 236
  See also methyltestosterone; steroid
  hormone
tetanus, 264–65
tetany, 225
Tetra-Bid antibiotic, 589
tetracaine hydrochloride
  in OTC preparations for the
  treatment of: hemorrhoids, 160–61;
  poison ivy, 74

Tetra-C antibiotic, 589
Tetracap antibiotic, 589
Tetrachel antibiotic, 589
Tetra-Co antibiotic, 589
Tetra-Co B.I.D. antibiotic, 589
tetracycline hydrochloride antibiotic,
  589–90
  expiration date of, 37
  interaction with other drugs, 23–25
  in treatment of: acne, 56; boil and
  carbuncle, 58; cholera, 251;
  pneumonia, 120–21; prostatitis, 186;
  Rocky Mountain spotted fever, 259;
  syphilis, 263; trench mouth, 179;
  tularemia, 266; typhus, 267
  taken during pregnancy, 22
Tetracyn antibiotic, 590
Tetralan-250 antibiotic, 590
Tetralan-500 antibiotic, 590
Tetram antibiotic, 590
Tetramine antibiotic, 590
Tet-250 antibiotic, 590
Tet-500 antibiotic, 590
thalidomide, 21–22
Theocap bronchodilator, 590
Theo-Col expectorant and smooth
  muscle relaxant, 591
Theodrine antiasthmatic, 591
Theo-Drox adrenergic, sedative, and
  smooth muscle relaxant, 591
Theofensae antiasthmatic, 591
Theophed antiasthmatic, 591
Theophozine adrenergic, sedative, and
  smooth muscle relaxant, 591
theophylline bronchodilator
  in treatment of asthma, 109
  See also Elixophyllin bronchodilator
Theoral antiasthmatic, 591
Theozine adrenergic, sedative, and
  smooth muscle relaxant, 591
Thera-Combex H-P multivitamin, 591
Theragran-M nutritional supplement,
  591–92
Theragran nutritional supplement, 592
Thermocushion insole, 650
Thermoloid thyroid hormone, 592
thermometer
  basal temperature, 632–33
  fever, 631–33
Thermophore heat pack, 642
thiamine. See vitamin B₁
Thia-Serpa-Line diuretic and
  antihypertensive, 592
Thiaserp diuretic and antihypertensive,
  592
thiazide diuretic. See diuretic
  diuretic and antihypertensive;
  hydrochlorothiazide
thiotepa, in treatment of cancer, 286
Thoradol phenothiazine, 593
Thorazine phenothiazine, 593
  and breast enlargement, 286
T.H.P. antiparkinson drug, 593

Triptazine phenothiazine and
antidepressant, 606
Tri-Tet antibiotic, 606
Tri-Vi-Flor vitamin and fluoride
supplement, 606
Tri-Zide diuretic and antihypertensive,
607
T-250 antibiotic, 607
tubal ligation, 193
tuberculosis, 121–22
tubing, 667
Tucks hemorrhoidal preparation, 607
in treatment of pruritus ani/pruritus
vulvae, 75–76
Tudecon T.D. adrenergic and
antihistamine, 607
tularemia, 266
Tumol-750 muscle relaxant, 607
Tums antacid, 607
ingredients, 174
Tussionex cough suppressant, 608
Tuss-Ornade cough and cold remedy,
608–9
in treatment of common cold, 94
Tuzon analgesic, 609
2/G cough remedy, 609
2/G-DM cough remedy, 609–10
Tylaprin analgesic, 610
Tylenol analgesic, 610
Tylenol Extra Strength analgesic, 610
Tylenol with Codeine, 610
typhoid fever, 266–67
typhus, 267

ulcerative colitis, 180
Ultimox antibiotic, 611
undecylenic acid, in products used to
treat ringworm infections, 77–78
underpads, disposable, 637
Unicap M multivitamin and mineral
supplement, 611–12
Unicap multivitamin, 612
in treatment of night blindness, 89
Unicap T multivitamin and mineral
supplement, 612–13
Unipres diuretic and antihypertensive,
613
Unisom Nightime sleep aid, 613
Unitemp Thermometer, 632
urethritis, 186–88
uricosuric
definition, 16
R drugs profiled: Benemid, 336–37;
ColBENEMID, 359; Probalan, 539;
probenecid, 336; Probenimead, 540;
Robenecid, 553; Zyloprim, 628–29
urinals, 638
urinary habits, change in, 183
urine-testing products, 669–672
Uri-Tet antibiotic, 613
Urodine analgesic, 613
urticaria. See hives
uterine cancer, 289

Uticillin VK antibiotic, 613
vaccine
antirabies, 221
definition, 16
DPT, 123
rubella/rubeola, 260
Sabin, 220
Salk, 220
vaginal cream, R, Triple Sulfa, 606
Valdrene antihistamine, 613
Valisone steroid hormone, 613–14
Valium sedative and hypnotic, 614–15
in treatment of: anxiety, 204; heart
attack, 134; tetanus, 265
valley fever. See coccidioidomycosis
Vanceril anti-asthmatic, 615
Van-Mox antibiotic, 615
Vanoxide acne preparation, 615–16
in treatment of acne, 56
Vanquish analgesic, 616
vaporizers, 639–41
varicose veins, 143
Vasal Granucaps smooth muscle
relaxant, 616
vascular headache, 211–12
vasectomy, 193
Vaseline Hemorr-Aid hemorrhoid
remedy, 616–17
Vaseline petrolatum gauze, 617
Vaseline petroleum jelly, 617
in prevention of diaper rash, 63
in treatment of: corns and calluses,
62; itching, 70, 71
Vasocap-150 smooth muscle relaxant,
617
vasoconstrictor
definition, 16
in OTC hemorrhoidal preparation, 161
Vasodilan vasodilator, 617
vasodilator
definition, 16
R drugs profiled: Circanol, 357;
cyclandelate, 377–78; Cyclanfor,
377; Cyclospasmol, 377–78; Cydel,
378; Deapril-ST, 381; Gerigine, 434;
Hydergine, 442; isoxsuprine
hydrochloride, 617; Roniacol, 557;
Spengine, 576; Tri-Ergone, 605;
Trigot, 605; Vasodilan, 617;
Vasoprine, 617
Vasoglyn Unicelles antianginal, 617
vasopressin
and diabetes insipidus, 276
secretion and action, 274
Vasoprine vasodilator, 617
Vasospan smooth muscle relaxant, 617
Vasotrate antianginal, 618
V-Cillin K antibiotic, 618
Vectrin antibiotic, 618
Veetids '250' antibiotic, 618
venereal disease. See sexually
transmitted disease
Vergo wart remover, 618

vertigo, 250
  See also Ménière's syndrome
Vibramycin antibiotic, 618–19
Vicks cough remedy, 619
Vicks Inhaler nasal decongestant, 619
Vicks Vaporub external analgesic, 620
Vincent's infection. See trench mouth
Vioform-Hydrocortisone steroid
  hormone and anti-infective, 620
  in treatment of: bedsores, 57;
    eczema, 65; pruritus ani/pruritus
    vulvae, 75–76
Vioquin-HC steroid hormone and
  anti-infective, 620
Vio-Serpine antihypertensive, 621
Viotag steroid hormone and anti-
  infective, 621
Viro-Med cold remedy (liquid), 621
Viro-Med cold remedy (tablet), 621–22
Visine decongestant eyedrops, 622
  in treatment of hay fever, 96
Vistaril sedative, 622
vitamin
  as nutrient, 268
  definition, 16
vitamin and fluoride supplement
  Rx drugs profiled: Poly-Vi-Flor, 532;
    Tri-Vi-Flor, 606
vitamin A (retinol), 622–23
  in treatment of: eczema, 64–65; night
    blindness, 89
  taken during pregnancy, 22
  toxicity, 273
vitamin B₁ (thiamine), 623
  deficiency of (beriberi), 269–70
vitamin B₂ (riboflavin), 623
vitamin B₃ niacin, deficiency of
  (pellagra), 272
vitamin B₆ (pyridoxine), 623–24
  interaction with other drugs, 24
vitamin B₁₂ (cyanocobalamin), 624
  and pernicious anemia, 126
  in treatment of: shingles, 81; tic
    douloureux, 226
vitamin C (ascorbic acid), 624–25
  in treatment of common cold, 93;
    Paget's disease, 236
vitamin D (calciferol), 625
  and rickets, 236–37
  in treatment of: osteoporosis, 235;
    Paget's disease, 236
  taken during pregnancy, 22
  toxicity, 273
vitamin E (tocopherol), 626
vitamin supplement
  Rx drugs profiled: Diacin, 386; Niac,
    495; Nicalex, 495; NICL, 495;
    Nicobid, 495; Nicocap, 495;

Nico-400 Plateau Caps, 495; nico-
  Span, 496; nicotinic acid, 496; SK-
  Niacin, 571; Tega-Span, 586;
  Wampocap, 626
vomit basins, 638
vomiting, 169–71
  See also antinauseant; morning
    sickness; motion sickness

walkers, 664
Wampocap vitamin supplement, 626
warfarin, in treatment of stroke, 141
wart, 81–82
  venereal, 263
Wart-off wart remover, 626
wart remover, OTC, 82
  OTC drugs profiled: Compound W,
    362–63; Vergo, 618; Wart-Off, 626
water, as nutrient, 268
water bottles, 643–44
W.D.D. antidepressant, 626
Wehvert antinauseant, 627
WescoHEX detergent cleanser, 627
whooping cough, 122–23
wide angle glaucoma, 88
Wintrocin antibiotic, 627
withdrawal syndrome
  from addiction to: alcohol, 202–3;
    narcotics, 207; sedatives, 206;
    stimulants, 207
Wyamycin antibiotic, 627
Wyanoid hemorrhoidal preparation, 627
  in treatment of hemorrhoids, 161
Wymox antibiotic, 627

X-Aqua diuretic and antihypertensive,
  627

yellow mercuric oxide ophthalmic
  ointment, 627
  in treatment of sty, 90

Zetran sedative and hypnotic, 627
Zide diuretic and antihypertensive, 628
zinc oxide ointment, 628
  in prevention of diaper rash, 63
  in treatment of poison ivy/poison
    oak, 74–75
Zino Callus Pads, 651
Zino Corn Pads, 651
Ziradryl poison ivy remedy, 628
zirconia. See zirconium oxide
zirconium oxide, in OTC poison ivy
  remedies, 74
Zyloprim uricosuric, 628–29
  interaction with other drugs, 25
  in treatment of: cancer, 292; gout,
    232; kidney stones, 185